Escourolle and Poirier's Manual of Basic Neuropathology

Escourolle and Poirier's MANUAL OF BASIC NEUROPATHOLOGY

SEVENTH EDITION

EDITED BY

DOUGLAS C. ANTHONY, MD, PHD

PROFESSOR OF PATHOLOGY AND LABORATORY MEDICINE,
PROFESSOR OF NEUROLOGY, BROWN UNIVERSITY,
PROVIDENCE, RI, USA

UMBERTO De GIROLAMI, MD

PROFESSOR OF PATHOLOGY, HARVARD MEDICAL SCHOOL, BOSTON, MA, USA
SENIOR STAFF NEUROPATHOLOGIST, BRIGHAM AND WOMEN'S HOSPITAL, BOSTON, MA, USA

FRANCK BIELLE, MD, PHD

PROFESSOR OF PATHOLOGY AND NEUROPATHOLOGIST, RAYMOND ESCOUROLLE
DEPARTMENT OF NEUROPATHOLOGY, ACADEMIC AND MEDICAL DEPARTMENT OF
NEUROSCIENCE (DMU NEUROSCIENCES), APHP-SORBONNE UNIVERSITY, PARIS, FRANCE
PARIS BRAIN INSTITUTE, HÔPITAL DE LA PITIÉ-SALPÊTRIÈRE, PARIS, FRANCE

DANIELLE SEILHEAN, MD, PHD

PROFESSOR OF NEUROPATHOLOGY, NEUROPATHOLOGIST,
HEAD OF THE RAYMOND ESCOUROLLE DEPARTMENT OF
NEUROPATHOLOGY, AND DIRECTOR OF THE ACADEMIC
AND MEDICAL DEPARTMENT OF NEUROSCIENCE (DMU NEUROSCIENCES),
APHP-SORBONNE UNIVERSITY, PARIS, FRANCE
PARIS BRAIN INSTITUTE, HÔPITAL DE LA PITIÉ-SALPÊTRIÈRE, PARIS, FRANCE

OXFORD
UNIVERSITY PRESS

OXFORD
UNIVERSITY PRESS

Oxford University Press is a department of the University of Oxford. It furthers the University's objective of excellence in research, scholarship, and education by publishing worldwide. Oxford is a registered trade mark of Oxford University Press in the UK and certain other countries.

Published in the United States of America by Oxford University Press
198 Madison Avenue, New York, NY 10016, United States of America.

Fifth Edition published in 2014
Sixth Edition published in 2019
Seventh Edition published in 2025

CIP data is on file at the Library of Congress

ISBN 978–0–19–766130–7

DOI: 10.1093/med/9780197661307.001.0001

Printed by Marquis Book Printing, Canada

FSC www.fsc.org MIX Paper | Supporting responsible forestry FSC® C103567

Contents

Foreword

The first edition of *Escourolle and Poirier's Manual of Basic Neuropathology* came out in 1971, published in French. I recall sitting in Raymond Adams' living room and seeing the volume on his table along with other neuropathology articles in the original French and German that he was reading. The third edition of the *Manual*, published in 1990 in English, was accessible to a wider audience. Rather than the ponderous tomes on neuropathology that were available at the time, it brought a beautiful and accessible view to what had been a specialized corner of the neurosciences. Early in my training, I admired the stunning micrographs and gross pathology photographs that had been curated to epitomize the main disorders of the nervous system. Suddenly, the connection of neuropathology to clinical work came alive. I even tried to stuff a paperback version into the pocket of my white coat so I could read it for enjoyment over a coffee break. With the refinements of each succeeding edition, culminating now in the seventh, the editors and authors have kept alive the traditional virtues of clarity and simplicity, eschewing unnecessary digressions and getting to the heart of the matter in every chapter.

There is no escaping the changes that have occurred in the neurosciences, but Raymond Adams statement that neuropathology is the basic science of neurology is now reified. Who would have thought decades ago that the molecular biology of nervous system tumors would become anchored in the specialty of neuropathology? By moving fluidly back and forth between pathology and pathobiology, *Escourolle and Poirier* informs the inquisitive reader in multiple specialties. All those interested in the neurosciences, including neurologists, neurosurgeons, pathologists, and basic scientists, profit by the thoughtful interspersing of pathologic specimens, instructive diagrams, and concise descriptions of neuropathology and correlative clinical neurology. In fact, it is neuropathology that is leading other related specialties into the 21st century.

Chapters on traditional diseases such as stroke, trauma, and degenerative and demyelinating disorders are thorough, and the explanations and examples of neuropathologic changes are outstanding. I was impressed with the material under general malformations and perinatal diseases and hereditary metabolic diseases that are often orphaned but round out material for the well-educated neurologist and neuropathologist.

This book in essence allows the telling of the "whole story" of disorders of the nervous system rather than the discursive and algorithmic, factoid approach that has overtaking medicine. It allows an understanding of diseases from the "ground up" and provides a view of what can, and what cannot, happen in the nervous system. This is one of the most powerful lessons available to the practitioner in the neurosciences, from trainee to senior clinician. The book brings clarity and enjoyment and reminds us that we live in a rich world that has intellectual, visual, and practical meaning.

No better foundation can be obtained than in this new edition, and if I could only put the book into the hands of everyone interested in the neurosciences, I believe it would enliven their daily work and professional lives.

Allan H. Ropper, MD
Professor of Neurology
Harvard Medical School
Fellow, American Academy of Physicians
Fellow, Royal College of Physicians
Associate Editor, *New England Journal of Medicine*

Preface to the Seventh Edition

This seventh edition of the *Manual of Basic Neuropathology* attempts to maintain the initial intention of Professors Escourolle and Poirier to provide a concise description of the pathologic findings of diseases of the nervous system, limiting pathophysiological considerations to basic principles needed by resident trainees and other medical learners. Historical and neurologic data have been deliberately kept to a minimum. Detailed information with reference citations, not included here but required for the practice of neuropathology, can be obtained in the many comprehensive treatises available on the topic. We also have made the assumption that the reader is familiar with introductory neuroanatomy, neurohistology, and general principles of pathology and clinical neurology.

With these guidelines in mind, our aim has been to present descriptive aspects of neuropathology, including principally cellular and molecular pathology together with selected illustrations.

We think that the time is now right for a new edition, following the sixth edition in 2019. During the past several years, the expansion of specialty training in neurology, neurosurgery, and pathology has required less time devoted to neuropathology. Thus, the trainee in these disciplines is now very much in need of a concise introductory text, and this *Manual* is specifically oriented to this readership.

Despite the worldwide decline in the number of autopsies performed in current medical practice, the anatomic distribution and the neuropathologic basis of lesions continue to be a fundamental body of information for the interpretation of clinical and imaging data. To support this aim, we have made use of macroscopic illustrations and whole-brain sections from the collections in our archives.

The past few years has seen tremendous progress in molecular biology and gene sequencing technologies that have revolutionized the diagnosis of many neurologic diseases. Progress in immunohistochemistry methods for in situ identification of abnormal proteins or their abnormal distribution in the brain ("proteomics"), the identification of DNA mutations and translocations ("genomics"), and changes in messenger RNA and its distribution ("transcriptomics") have led to greater understanding of many neurologic diseases. Neuropathology stands at the vanguard of the development and implementation of these methodologies, and recent consensus classification schemes now include molecular detail in diagnostic classification. Whether discussing degenerative and metabolic disorders, developmental disorders, neuromuscular diseases, or the classification of tumors, diagnostic classifications now incorporate molecular information along with histopathologic data, to deliver "integrated" diagnoses. This integrated neuropathologic information is now required, not only for diagnosis but also in order to establish prognostic categories and to guide treatment.

In the introduction to the first edition, Professors Escourolle and Poirier offered an apology to the reader that is still valid half a century later. This concise work, designed to familiarize early learners and physicians-in-training about such a highly specialized discipline as neuropathology, faces two opposing risks: Overcompression of the full complexity risks creating unintelligible text for beginners; in the alternative, oversimplification risks creating misunderstandings of the full complexity of neurologic disease. We hope we have reached a balance that gives the reader a concise but accurate understanding of neuropathology.

The Editors

Acknowledgments

We first acknowledge those individuals who have contributed to prior editions of this work, and those who have collaborated in this edition, collating the experience and expertise of experts across four continents. We also extend our deepest gratitude to Craig Panner at Oxford University Press, critical in the creation of the seventh edition and prior editions. He guided us along the entire publication processes, from our first conceptualization to the final publication, reviewing early ideas, collecting reviewer comments, and producing a compact manual.

Finally, on the occasion of this 50th golden anniversary edition, we recognize those whose vision created the original *Manuel Élémentaire de Neuropathologie* in 1971 and its subsequent editions. The first two editions were conceived, written, and edited by Raymond Escourolle and Jacques Poirier. After the death of Raymond Escourolle in 1984, Francoise Gray joined Jacques Poirier for the third edition. The first three editions reached the English-speaking public thanks to the friendship and translating ability of Lucien Rubinstein. For the fourth edition, Umberto De Girolami joined as co-editor, and the scope of the monograph was expanded with the collaborative efforts of multiple expert authors throughout the world. With the retirement of Jacques Poirier, Charles Duyckaerts joined the editorial team for the fifth and sixth editions. With the retirement of Francoise Gray and the untimely death of Charles Duyckaerts, Douglas Anthony, Danielle Seilhean, and Franck Bielle have joined the editorial team for the seventh edition.

Here we share brief biographies of the prior editors:

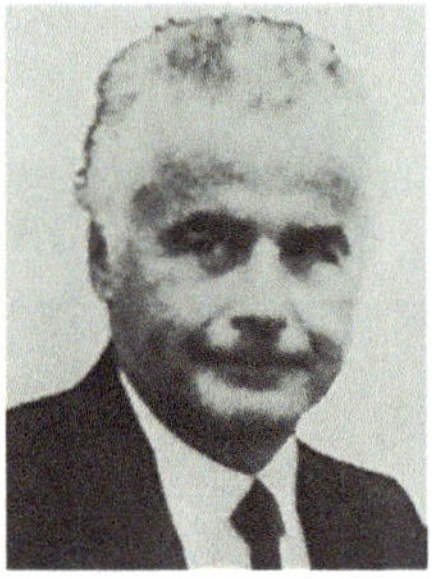 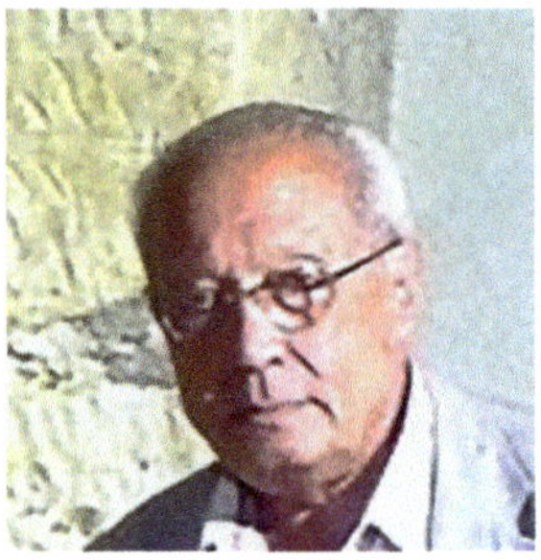

Raymond Escourolle (1924–1984) Professor Raymond Escourolle was born in the Auvergne region of France and graduated from the Medical School at the University of Paris. He had specialty training in neurology, psychiatry, and neuropathology at the Salpêtrière and the Sainte-Anne Hospitals in Paris. At that time, neuropathology was dependent on the neurology and neurosurgery departments: There were three separate laboratories at La Salpêtrière and another one in La Pitié, a hospital bordering La Salpêtrière. Pupil of neurologists Paul Castaigne and François Lhermitte and trained in neuropathology by Serge Brion, Escourolle assumed the Directorship of the new Neuropathology Laboratory of the Clinique des Maladies du Système Nerveux in La Salpêtrière in 1965, where he set up a separate Department of Neuropathology named after Charles Foix. His research interests covered the entire field of neuropathology, with 400 publications over the course of his career, and a special focus on cerebrovascular diseases. With Jacques Poirier, he first published the *Manuel Élémentaire de Neuropathologie* (first edition in 1971 and second edition in 1977). The third edition was translated into English by Lucien Rubinstein and had a wider readership with trainees in the neurological sciences throughout the world. One of his pupils and subsequent director of the newly named Laboratoire de Neuropathologie Raymond Escourolle at the Salpêtrière, Jean-Jacques Hauw, wrote a moving obituary of this remarkable man: *Acta Neuropathologica* (1984), 65, 89.

Jacques Poirier (1937–) Professor Jacques Poirier was born in Paris, France. He graduated from University of Paris Medical School in 1968. He was a resident in neurology and neuropathology at La Salpêtrière in Paris. He became Professor of Histology and Embryology at the University of Paris and Chair of the Department of Histology and Embryology at Henri Mondor (1970) and then Pitié-Salpêtrière (1995) hospitals in Paris. His practice covered the spectrum of neuropathology. His primary research interest focused on brain tumors and the history of medicine, both areas in which he attained expertise with international recognition. His charismatic personality attracted many neuropathologists, oncopathologists, and philosophers around him, most of whom subsequently became chairs in important Parisian centers. He published 350 articles and 47 books. As a leader of French histology, Poirier has published several widely acclaimed didactic books and drawings (the so-called histology sheets) that are still used by French medical students more than five decades after their first publication. When they met, Raymond Escourolle envisaged drafting a neuropathology handout for students. Poirier encouraged him to conceive and publish a more ambitious work combining the reliability of a handbook and clarity of an educational book to transmit in a synthetic way their complementary and in-depth knowledge of neuropathology. The high quality of organization, writing, and illustrations, bringing out the essential in all chapters, has undeniably contributed to the long-standing international success of the *Manuel Élémentaire de Neuropathologie* of Escourolle and Poirier. The first edition appeared in 1971, the second in 1977, and were translated in English by Lucien Rubinstein. From the third edition (1989), Poirier invited Françoise Gray to join him and share editorial responsibilities. The next three editions were written in English under the direction of Gray and Umberto De Girolami, and these editions retained the names of Escourolle and Poirier in the title of the *Manual.*

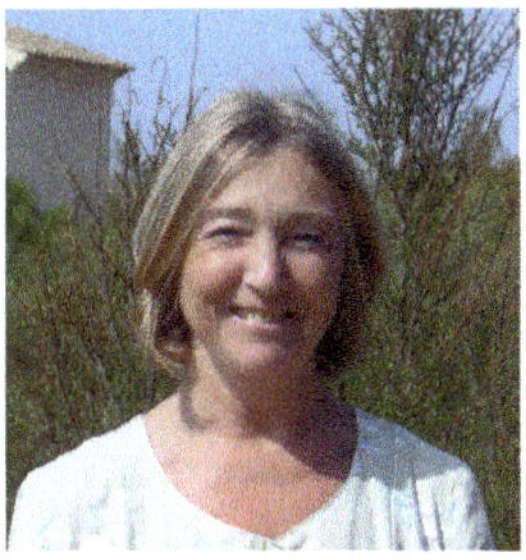

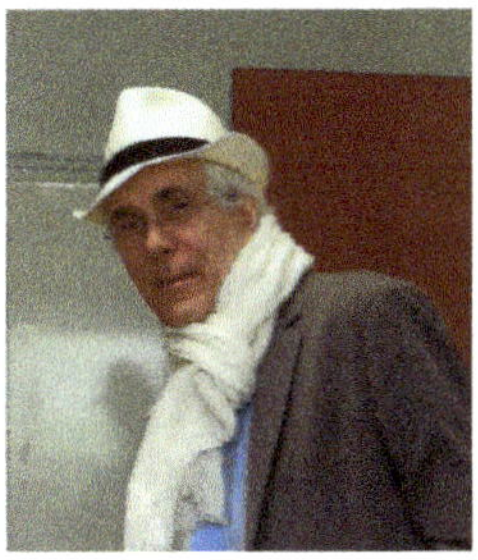

Françoise Gray (1944–) Professor Françoise Gray was born in Rouen Normandy, France. She graduated from the University of Paris Medical School in 1972. She trained in anatomic pathology, neurology, and neuropathology at La Salpêtrière in Paris and was certified in anatomic pathology and neurology. In 1983, she obtained a PhD in Human Biology from the University of Marseille, and she rose through the ranks to become Professor of Pathology at the University of Paris in 1991 and Chair of the Department of Pathology at the Lariboisière Hospital in Paris in 2005. In November 2014, she retired from professional activities. Her primary research interest was in the area of infectious disease, where she was recognized internationally as an expert, with more than 200 publications in the field and six books. She was on the editorial board of the principal journals of neuropathology and attained leadership roles in many scientific societies, including President of the International Society of Neuropathology. In 1989, she joined Jacques Poirier and Raymond Escourolle for the third edition of the *Manual of Neuropathology*. She was the lead editor of the fourth (2004), fifth (2014), and sixth editions (2019) of the *Manual*, which were subsequently published exclusively in English. Gray's contributions were to greatly expand the authorship of the chapters based on her many international contacts and to greatly expand the illustrations. She was instrumental in the worldwide dissemination and acclaim of the *Manual*.

Charles Duyckaerts (1951–2023) Charles Duyckaerts was born in 1951 in Liège, Belgium. He received his early education at the Jesuit college Saint-Servais. From this time, he kept a taste for ancient texts, but his erudition was above all nourished by a great curiosity for everything related to literature, music, and science. Attracted by engineering since childhood, he finally chose to study medicine in Paris from 1970 onwards. After obtaining his doctorate of medicine in 1983, he specialized in both pathological anatomy (1984) and clinical neurology (1985). In 1987, a doctorate in human biology marked the start of his academic career, first as associate professor, then as full professor from 1991, and finally as head of the Neuropathology Department at the Pitié-Salpêtrière Hospital from 2008 until his retirement in 2018. Recognized as an expert in the neuropathological approach to Alzheimer disease, Duyckaerts authored more than 500 publications. Over and above his internationally recognized talent as a researcher, he loved to spend hours explaining the state of research to the general public, to patients, and to students at all levels. He began contributing to the *Manual of Basic Neuropathology* as an author in the fourth edition (2004) and was one of the editors of the fifth (2014) and sixth (2019) editions, along with Françoise Gray and Umberto De Girolami. Illness prevented him from completing the seventh edition. During his outstanding career as a neuropathologist, Duyckaerts acquired an international reputation as a leading expert on neurodegenerative diseases. Since his departure, he remains a source of inspiration and courage for those who had the chance to know him.

Contributors

Homa Adle-Biassette, MD, PhD
Professor of Pathology, Faculté de Médecine Paris, Paris Cité, Paris, France
Pathologist, Neuropathologist, Department of Pathology, Hôpital Lariboisère, Paris, France

Pierre Amarenco, MD
Professor of Neurology, University of Paris-Cité, Bichat Hospital, Paris, France

Anthony A. Amato, MD
Professor of Neurology, Harvard Medical School, Boston, MA, USA
BWH Distinguished Chair in Neurology, Chief of the Neuromuscular Division, Department of Neurology, Brigham and Women's Hospital, Boston, MA, USA

Douglas C. Anthony, MD, PhD
Professor of Pathology and Laboratory Medicine, Professor of Neurology, Brown University, Providence, RI, USA

Franck Bielle, MD, PhD
Professor of Pathology and Neuropathologist, Raymond Escourolle Department of Neuropathology, Academic and Medical Department of Neuroscience (DMU Neurosciences), APHP-Sorbonne University, Paris, France
Paris Brain Institute, Hôpital de la Pitié-Salpêtrière, Paris, France

Susana Boluda, MD, PhD
Neuropathologist, Raymond Escourolle Department of Neuropathology, Academic and Medical Department of Neuroscience (DMU Neurosciences), APHP-Sorbonne University, Paris, France
Paris Brain Institute, Hôpital de la Pitié-Salpêtrière, Paris, France

Leila Chimelli, MD, PhD
Professor of Pathology, Federal University of Rio de Janeiro, Rio de Janeiro, Brazil
Neuropathologist, Laboratory of Neuropathology, State Institute of Brain, Rio de Janeiro, Brazil

Fabrice Chrétien, MD, PhD
Professor of Histology and Neuropathology, Université Paris Cité, Paris, France
GHU Paris Psychiatrie Neuroscience, Sainte Anne Hospital, Paris, France

Basil T. Darras, MD
Professor of Neurology, Joseph J. Volpe Distinguished Chair in Neurology, Harvard Medical School, Boston, MA, USA
Associate Neurologist-in-Chief, Director, Neuromuscular Program, Boston Children's Hospital, Boston, MA, USA

Umberto De Girolami, MD
Professor of Pathology, Harvard Medical School, Boston, MA, USA
Senior Staff Neuropathologist, Brigham and Women's Hospital, Boston, MA, USA

Teresinha Evangelista, MD
Sorbonne University—Pitié Salpêtrière Hospital—Assistance, Public Hôpitaux de Paris, Paris, France
Functional Unit of Neuromuscular Pathology, Neuropathology Department, Unité de Morphologie Neuromusculaire, Institut de Myologie, Paris, France

Mel Feany, MD, PhD
Professor of Pathology, Harvard Medical School, Boston, MA, USA
Neuropathologist, Brigham and Women's Hospital, Boston, MA, USA

Markus Glatzel, MD
Professor of Neuropathology, Director of the Institute of Neuropathology, Chairman of the Center of Diagnostics, University Medical Center Hamburg-Eppendorf, Hamburg, Germany

Hans H. Goebel, MD
Professor of Neuropathology, Johannes Gutenberg University, Mainz, Germany
Consultant Neuropathologist, Institute of Neuropathology, Charité, Berlin, Germany

Jeffrey A. Golden, MD
Professor of Pathology and Laboratory Medicine, and Biomedical Sciences, and Executive Vice Dean, Research and Education, Cedars-Sinai Medical Center, Los Angeles, CA, USA

Stéphane Haik, MD, PhD
Research Director, Paris Brain Institute, Sorbonne University, Paris, France
Inserm, CNRS, APHP, Paris, France
Coordinator of the French National Center of Reference for Prions, Hôpital de la Pitié-Salpêtrière, Paris, France

Brian Harding, MD, DPhil, BMBCh, FRCPath
Professor (Emeritus) of Pathology and Laboratory Medicine, University of Pennsylvania, Philadelphia, PA, USA
Neuropathologist, Children's Hospital of Philadelphia, Philadelphia, PA, USA

Jean-Jacques Hauw, MD
Professor of Neuropathology (ret.), Sorbonne University, Paris, France
Neuropathologist (ret.), APHP-Sorbonne University, Hôpital de la Pitié-Salpêtrière, Paris, France
Académie National de Médecine, Paris, France

Gabor G. Kovacs, MD, PhD, FRCPC
Professor of Neuropathology and Neurology, University of Toronto, Toronto, Ontario, Canada
Consultant Neuropathologist, Laboratory Medicine Program, University Health Network. Toronto, Ontario, Canada

Hans Lassman, MD, PhD
Professor, Medical University of Vienna, Vienna, Austria
Center for Brain Research, Vienna, Austria

Keith L. Ligon, MD, PhD
Associate Professor of Pathology, Harvard Medical School, Boston, MA, USA
Chief of Neuropathology, Brigham and Women's Hospital, Boston, MA, USA
Director, Center for Patient-Derived Models, Dana Farber Cancer Institute. Boston, MA, USA

David Meredith, MD, PhD
Assistant Professor of Pathology, Harvard Medical School, Boston, MA, USA
Neuropathologist, Brigham and Women's Hospital, Boston, MA, USA

Yann Nadjar, MD, PhD
Department of Neurology, Neuro-Metabolism Unit, Referral Center for Metabolic and Lysosomal Neurology Disorders, Hôpital Pitié-Salpêtrière, Paris, France

Luciano Neder, MD
Professor of Pathology and Forensic Medicine, Riberão Preto Medical School, University of São Paolo, São Paolo, Brazil

Vânia Nosé, MD, PhD
Professor of Pathology, Harvard Medical School, Boston, MA, USA
Director of Surgical Pathology, and Associate Chief for Anatomic and Molecular Pathology, Massachusetts General Hospital, Boston, MA, USA

Isabelle Plu, MD
Associate Professor of Forensic Medicine and Neuropathologist, Sorbonne University, Paris, France
Raymond Escourolle Department of Neuropathology, Academic and Medical Department of Neuroscience (DMU Neurosciences), APHP-Sorbonne University, Paris, France
Paris Brain Institute (ICM), Hôpital de la Pitié-Salpêtrière, Paris, France

Michael Punsoni, MD
Associate Professor of Pathology and Laboratory Medicine, Brown University, Providence, RI, USA
Neuropathologist, Director of Autopsy Services, and Director of Ophthalmic Pathology, Brown University Health, Providence, RI, USA

R. Ross Reichard, MD
Associate Professor of Pathology, Mayo Clinic Alix School of Medicine, Department of Laboratory Medicine and Pathology, Mayo Clinic, Rochester, MN, USA

Yuichi Riku, MD, PhD
Associate Professor of Neuropathlogy, Institute for Medical Science of Aging, Aichi Medical University, Aichi, Japan
Department of Neurology, Graduate School of Nagoya University, Aichi, Japan

Sandro Santagata, MD, PhD
Associate Professor of Pathology and Associate Professor of Systems Biology, Harvard Medical School, Boston, MA, USA
Neuropathologist, Brigham and Women's Hospital, Boston, MA, USA

Danielle Seilhean, MD, PhD
Professor of Neuropathology, Neuropathologist, Head of the Raymond Escourolle Department of Neuropathology, and Director of the Academic and Medical Department of Neuroscience (DMU Neurosciences), APHP-Sorbonne University, Paris, France
Paris Brain Institute, Hôpital de la Pitié-Salpêtrière, Paris, France

Leroy R. Sharer, MD
Professor of Pathology (Neuropathology, ret.), Rutgers New Jersey Medical School, Newark, NJ, USA
Neuropathologist (ret.), University Hospital, Newark, NJ, USA

Colin Smith, MD, FRCPath
Professor of Neuropathology and Director, Centre for Clinical Brain Sciences, University of Edinburgh, Edinburgh, Scotland, UK

Isaac H. Solomon, MD, PhD
Assistant Professor of Pathology, Harvard Medical School, Boston, MA, USA
Neuropathologist, Brigham and Women's Hospital, Boston, MA, USA

Matthew Torre, MD
Assistant Professor of Pathology and Immunology, Baylor College of Medicine; Ben Taub Hospital, Texas Children's Hospital, and Baylor St. Luke's Medical Center, Houston, TX USA

Toshiki Uchihara, MD
Director, University of Hawaii Postgraduate Medical Education Program at Okinawa Chubu Hospital, Okinawa, Japan
Clinical Professor of Neurology, Tokyo Medical and Dental University, Tokyo, Japan
Guest Professor of Neurology, Juntendo University, Tokyo, Japan
Guest Researcher, RIKEN, Yokohama, Japan

Jean-Michel Vallat, MD
Professor of Neurology, Centre Hospitalier Universitaire Dupuytren, Service de Neurologie, Limoges, France

Chiara Villa, MD
Neuropathologist, Raymond Escourolle Department of Neuropathology, Academic and Medical Department of Neuroscience (DMU Neurosciences), APHP-Sorbonne University, Paris, France
Paris Brain Institute (ICM), Hôpital de la Pitié-Salpêtrière, Paris, France

Harry V. Vinters, MD
Professor of Pathology and Laboratory Medicine and Professor of Neurology, University of California–Los Angeles, UCLA Medical Center, Los Angeles, CA, USA

1

Basic Pathology of the Central Nervous System

DANIELLE SEILHEAN, MATTHEW TORRE, GABOR G. KOVACS, AND UMBERTO De GIROLAMI

AUTOPSY DIAGNOSIS in neuropathology is based on the macroscopic and microscopic study of the brain, brainstem, cerebellum, and spinal cord. Increasingly, the ability to reach greater diagnostic precision is buttressed by the new laboratory techniques of molecular biology and genetics. Three consecutive steps are involved in reaching a diagnosis, and these are, in fact, closely interrelated: (1) a morphological analysis of the lesions; (2) a topographical analysis of the lesions; and (3) a critical integration of these findings and their subsequent correlation with the clinical data and the general autopsy findings, thus permitting an etiological diagnosis to be established in most instances

1.1. MORPHOLOGICAL ANALYSIS OF CENTRAL NERVOUS SYSTEM LESIONS

Several disorders of the central nervous system (CNS) are characterized morphologically by the co-expression of multiple reactions to injury that may not necessarily be diagnostic in themselves. These reactions affect the cells of the nervous system (neurons, astrocytes, oligodendrocytes, and microglia) and/or the supporting structures (meninges, connective tissue, or blood vessels). Basic cellular reactions are demonstrable on microscopic examination, whereas tissue lesions associated with more extensive destructive or atrophic changes are recognized by the naked eye or with the help of a magnifying lens.

Although, for didactic purposes, the reactions to injury seen in the neurons, glia, connective tissue, and vascular structures are described separately in this chapter, there is a close functional interdependence of the various cellular elements of the nervous system. This is particularly important in the case of nerve cell alterations where, except for very acute injury, the possibility of artifactual change should be entertained whenever the reaction is not accompanied by a glial cell response.

1.1.1. Basic *cellular* reactions to CNS injury

1.1.1.1. NEURONAL LESIONS

Neuronal injury may be sufficiently severe to result in irreversible damage (cell death) or may be transient, or minimal, and cause reversible functional damage. Destruction of neurons may be focal or may involve many populations of neurons throughout the nervous system. In acute neuronal injury, when the tissue is examined stained with hematoxylin and eosin (H&E) at a relatively short time after a lethal insult to the cell (12–24 hours or somewhat longer), one observes eosinophilia of the cytoplasm, shrinkage and hyperchromasia of the nucleus, and disappearance of the nucleolus; after the disintegration of the cell, neuronophagia by scavenger cells is evident at a later time interval (days later). In chronic diseases, evidence of cell death is recognized morphologically as neuronal "cell loss" or alternately (as "atrophy") on macroscopic examination when the irreversible injury has occurred relatively slowly (months or years) and has progressively involved increasing numbers of cells. In some degenerative diseases of the nervous system where there is progressive neuronal injury over variable time periods, the affected cells have distinctive morphologic hallmarks (e.g., neurofibrillary degeneration, neuronal storage of metabolic products, and intracellular inclusions).

Nerve cell loss (i.e., reduction in the number of cell bodies in a given brain region as compared to normal), when it involves less than 30% of the normal cell population, may be difficult to ascertain in the absence of rigorous morphometric analysis. Furthermore, precise assessment depends on consideration of the thickness of the section and on the normal cytoarchitectonics of the area examined.

1.1.1.1.1. Nerve cell atrophy. Neuronal *atrophy* is the descriptive term given to a wide range of irreversible neuronal injuries that give rise to a relatively slowly evolving death of the cell. Neuronal atrophy is characterized morphologically by (1) retraction of the cell body with diffuse basophilia of the cytoplasm; and (2) pyknosis and hyperchromasia of the nucleus of the neuron in the absence of an inflammatory reaction. Neuronal atrophy occurs in degenerative disorders that involve several interconnected neuronal systems (i.e., multiple-system atrophy, Friedreich ataxia, and amyotrophic lateral sclerosis). It is also seen in anterograde and retrograde trans-synaptic degeneration, as may occur in the lateral geniculate body following a lesion of the optic nerve/tract.

Apoptosis, a type of programmed cell death, is an active, genetically controlled, energy-consuming process frequent in neurodegeneration. Initially, it affects the nucleus of the cell. Apoptosis proceeds via two main molecular pathways: (1) an intrinsic pathway that is largely mediated by the mitochondria and (2) an extrinsic pathway that can be induced by activation of transmembrane death receptors. Downstream of both pathways is the execution pathway, characterized by specific effector/executioner caspases (e.g., caspase 3). Neurons undergoing simple neuronal atrophy or apoptosis have similar morphologic features and may show positive in situ end labeling of internucleosomal DNA fragmentation (Fig. 1.1) or be demonstrable by activated caspase 3 immunostaining.

Nerve cell atrophy should not be mistaken with what is referred to as "dark neurons." This phenomenon is now recognized to be an artifactual change of the neuron cell body, seen particularly in brain biopsies fixed in formalin by immersion, and is characterized by shrinkage of the neuronal cytoplasm and a deeply stained, irregularly shaped nucleus, without other cellular alterations.

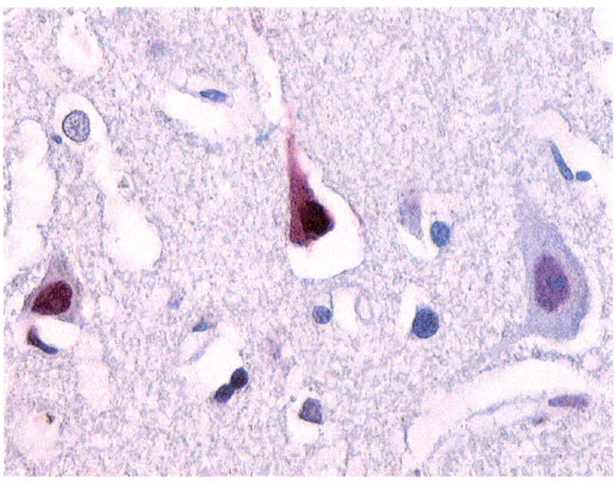

FIGURE 1.1 Two neurons undergoing apoptosis are positively stained by in situ end labeling to demonstrate internucleosomal DNA fragmentation. In one neuron, on the left, only the nucleus is stained, whereas in the other, which is at a later stage of the programmed cell death process, the entire cell body is stained. Compared to a normal neuron, on the right, both apoptotic neurons have similar morphological features and show a pyknotic nucleus and shrunken cytoplasm.

1.1.1.1.2. Acute neuronal necrosis (anoxic/ischemic neuronal change). Acute neuronal necrosis (anoxic/ischemic neuronal change) cell death occurs in not only a wide range of acute injuries, including anoxia and ischemia, but also many other acute pathological processes (e.g., hypoglycemia or exposure to excessive amounts of excitotoxic neurotransmitters). Unlike apoptosis, the predominant cellular changes in acute neuronal necrosis involve the cytoplasmic organelles and the cell membrane, which when ruptured leads to cell death.

In experimental animal studies and in carefully studied human tissue at postmortem, the following sequence of changes is noted by light and electron microscopy over the course of 12–24 hours after the insult: (a) cytoplasmic microvacuolization due to swelling of mitochondria and endoplasmic reticulum; (b) shrinkage of the cell body with retraction of the cellular outlines and disappearance of Nissl bodies with eosinophilic condensation of the cytoplasm ("red neuron"); (c) condensation of nuclear chromatin and nuclear pyknosis (Fig. 1.2); and (d) late disappearance of the nuclear chromatin, resulting in increased acidophilia of the nucleus, which appears to merge into the surrounding cytoplasm (karyorrhexis).

Occasionally, dead neurons, especially those adjacent to old, mostly hemorrhagic, infarcts or to traumatic scars, become encrusted with basophilic mineral deposits, chiefly iron and calcium salts. This condition is referred to as *mineralization* or *ferruginization* of neurons (Fig. 1.3).

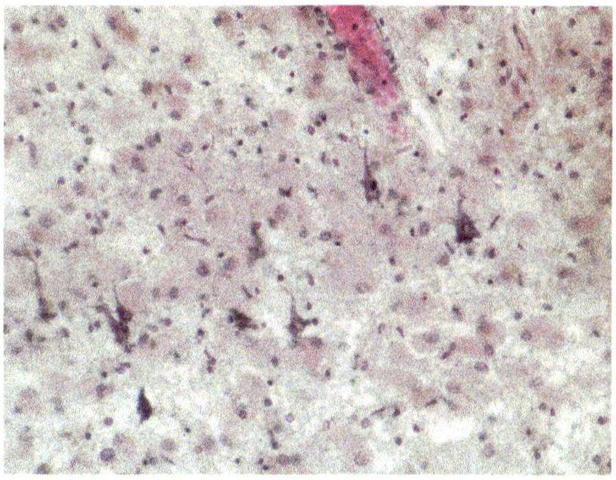

FIGURE 1.3 Ferruginization (mineralization) of the neurons at the edge of an old hemorrhagic infarct (H&E).

1.1.1.1.3. Central chromatolysis. Central chromatolysis is characterized morphologically by swelling of the cell body, disappearance of Nissl bodies beginning centrally and extending outward, and flattening and eccentric displacement of the nucleus to the periphery (Fig. 1.4). It is seen usually in lower motor neurons (anterior horns of the spinal cord, cranial nerve nuclei), where it represents a reparative reaction of the cell body to a lesion of the axon (retrograde degeneration or axonal reaction) (Fig. 1.5).

A confident diagnosis of central chromatolysis requires comparison with the normal morphology of the affected gray matter structure, because the nerve cell body in some nuclei (e.g., the mesencephalic nucleus of the fifth cranial nerve, Clarke's column) normally contains rounded neurons with marginated Nissl bodies.

Eccentric localization of the nucleus is seen in so-called ballooned neurons associated with

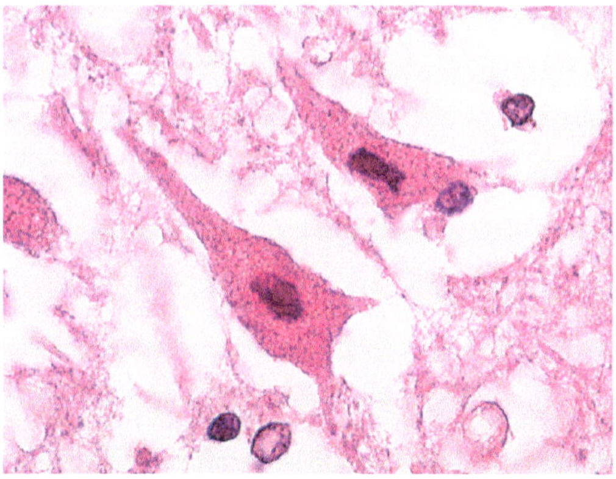

FIGURE 1.2 Acute ischemic nerve cell change (H&E). Eosinophilic, shrunken cytoplasm and hyperchromatic nucleus.

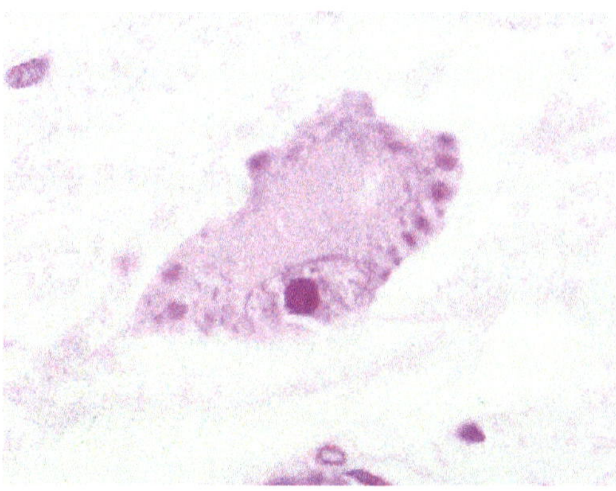

FIGURE 1.4 Central chromatolysis (Nissl stain). Note the cellular swelling, the eccentric displacement of the nucleus, and the margination of the Nissl bodies.

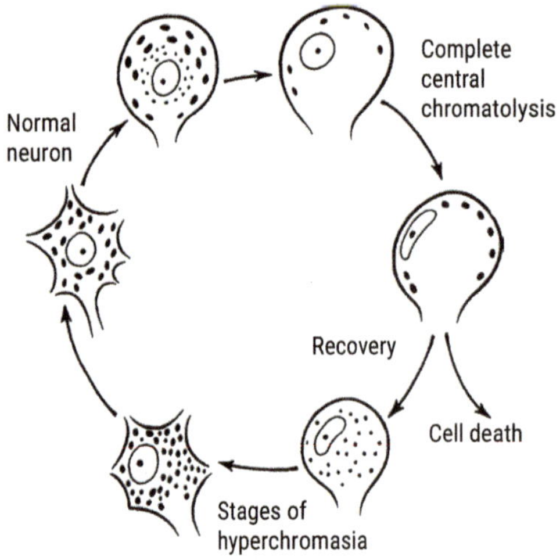

FIGURE 1.5 Nerve cell changes resulting from central chromatolysis.

various neurodegenerative diseases. For example, ballooned neurons occur in affected cortical areas in corticobasal degeneration (CBD) or in the amygdala in argyrophilic grain disease (AGD). Ballooned neurons in neurodegenerative disease are immunoreactive for αB-crystallin, in contrast to swollen ballooned-like neurons seen in pellagra encephalopathy in the cortex and basis pontis.

1.1.1.1.4. Vacuolated neurons and neuropil. Vacuolated neurons and/or vacuolated neuropil is observed typically in Creutzfeldt–Jakob disease (Fig. 1.6). In rare instances, swelling with vacuolization of the nerve cell may result from transsynaptic degeneration, such as occurs in the neurons of the inferior olive in olivary hypertrophy secondary to a lesion of the ipsilateral central tegmental tract or of the contralateral dentate nucleus; this phenomenon is also designated "fenestrated neurons" (Fig. 1.7). The spongiform change seen in Creutzfeldt–Jakob disease should not be mistaken for vacuolation seen in acute hypoxic/ischemic brain damage or brain edema, irregular vacuolation of superficial cortical layers in late stages of neurodegenerative diseases, and fixation-related shrinkage artifact with retraction spaces around neurons.

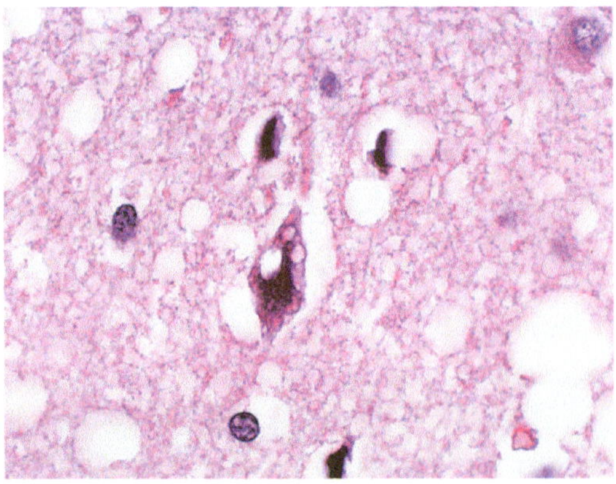

FIGURE 1.6 Vacuolated neuron in a case of Creutzfeldt–Jakob disease (H&E).

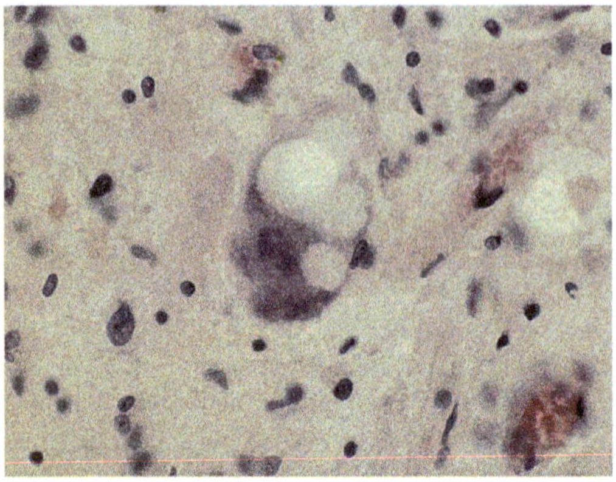

FIGURE 1.7 Fenestrated neuron in a case of hypertrophic olivary hypertrophy (Nissl stain).

1.1.1.1.5. Binucleated neurons. Binucleated neurons are seen rather infrequently, sometimes under normal circumstances, or otherwise at the edge of old focal destructive lesions, as a dysplastic/malformation phenomenon (e.g., tuberous sclerosis), or in certain neoplasms (e.g., ganglion cell tumors).

1.1.1.1.6. Neuronal storage. In some hereditary metabolic diseases related to enzymatic defects involving synthetic or degradative pathways for lipids or carbohydrates, interruption of the pathway leads to cytoplasmic accumulation of intermediate substrates or their by-products, resulting in swelling and distention of the cell body of nerve cells, with eccentric displacement of the nucleus (Fig. 1.8). In several neuronal storage disorders, the stored material has distinctive histochemical and ultrastructural features that may help characterize clinically suspected cases of a given storage disease. Biochemical tests on blood, leukocytes, and other body fluids are now particularly useful to diagnose more precisely many of these disorders.

Lipofuscin accumulation within the perikaryon of neurons and other cells in the nervous system is a characteristic aging change and may reflect

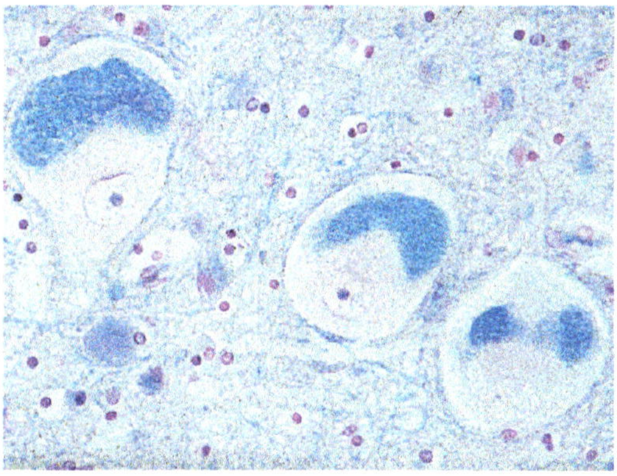

FIGURE 1.8 Distended nerve cell bodies in a case of neuronal storage disease (Luxol fast blue with Bodian silver impregnation).

oxidative stress and alterations in cellular metabolism. Lipofuscin accumulates in neurons diffusely throughout the brain in ceroid lipofuscinosis, a family of neuronal lysosomal storage disorders. In that disease, the neurons are distended by the accumulation of pigments and are described as "utricular." Increased accumulation of lipofuscin is also observed in several other neurodegenerative disorders, including Alzheimer disease and Parkinson disease. Lipofuscin is identified on H&E preparations as refractile yellow-brown pigment aggregates (Fig. 1.9). It is autofluorescent; rich in acid phosphatase; and consists of oxidized lipids, proteins, and metal ions. The pigment is periodic acid–Schiff (PAS)-positive and can be stained by Luxol fast blue. It has distinctive ultrastructural features (see Chapter 10).

1.1.1.1.7. Alzheimer neurofibrillary degeneration and granulovacuolar degeneration. *Alzheimer neurofibrillary degeneration* is characteristically seen in the brains of aged individuals and in patients with Alzheimer disease, but it has also been described in a variety of other cerebral disorders. This degenerative change is manifest by the formation of neurofibrillary tangles (NFTs), structures that are well demonstrated by silver impregnation and by immunohistochemical techniques; they consist of thickened and tortuous skeins within the neuronal perinuclear cytoplasm and contain both three- and four-repeat isoforms of tau. The configuration of the tangle may vary according to the anatomic site, the type of neuron affected, and the stage of formation (Fig. 1.10). A band-shaped perikaryal NFT can be seen in both large and small pyramidal cells and is perhaps an early stage of NFT development (Fig. 1.10A). A triangular flame-shaped perikaryal NFT is seen mainly in large pyramidal cells (Fig. 1.10B, C). Small compact globose perikaryal NFTs are typically seen in small cortical neurons (Fig. 1.10D). Large globose NFTs reminiscent of a ball of yarn are more common in the nucleus basalis of Meynert and in the brainstem (Fig. 1.10E). In the final stages of the disease, the cell outline disappears and only the distorted fibrils remain as "ghost NFT" (Fig. 1.10F). Globose NFTs that contain only four-repeat tau isoform are characteristic finding in progressive supranuclear palsy (PSP) in subcortical nuclei.

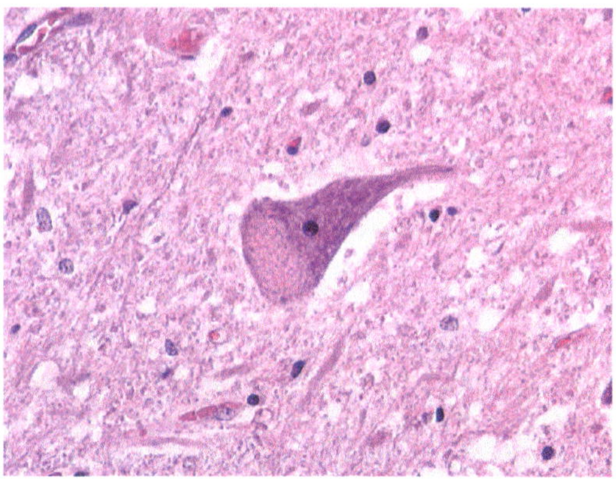

FIGURE 1.9 Lipofuscin in neuronal cell body (H&E).

The predominant biochemical component of NFTs is the microtubule-associated protein *tau*, which accumulates in an abnormally highly phosphorylated form. Tangles are particularly well demonstrated by tau immunohistochemistry, which is now used routinely in diagnostic work. NFTs may on occasion also be immunoreactive for ubiquitin and p62. By electron microscopy, most NFTs consist of paired helical filaments measuring approximately 20 nm across with a regular constriction to 10 nm occurring every 80 nm. In Alzheimer disease, they may also be associated with straight filaments. In PSP, tangles have been found to consist mainly of straight filaments measuring 15 nm in diameter. Whereas NFTs in chronic traumatic encephalopathy (CTE) show a paired helical filament ultrastructure, cryogenic electron microscopy demonstrates distinct protofilament folds of tau from those in Alzheimer disease.

Granulovacuolar degeneration is a neuronal alteration found in pyramidal cells of Ammon's horn; it is seen in normal aging as well as in Alzheimer disease and Pick disease. The abnormality consists of an accumulation of small, clear vacuoles measuring 4 or 5 µm in diameter and containing an argyrophilic granule

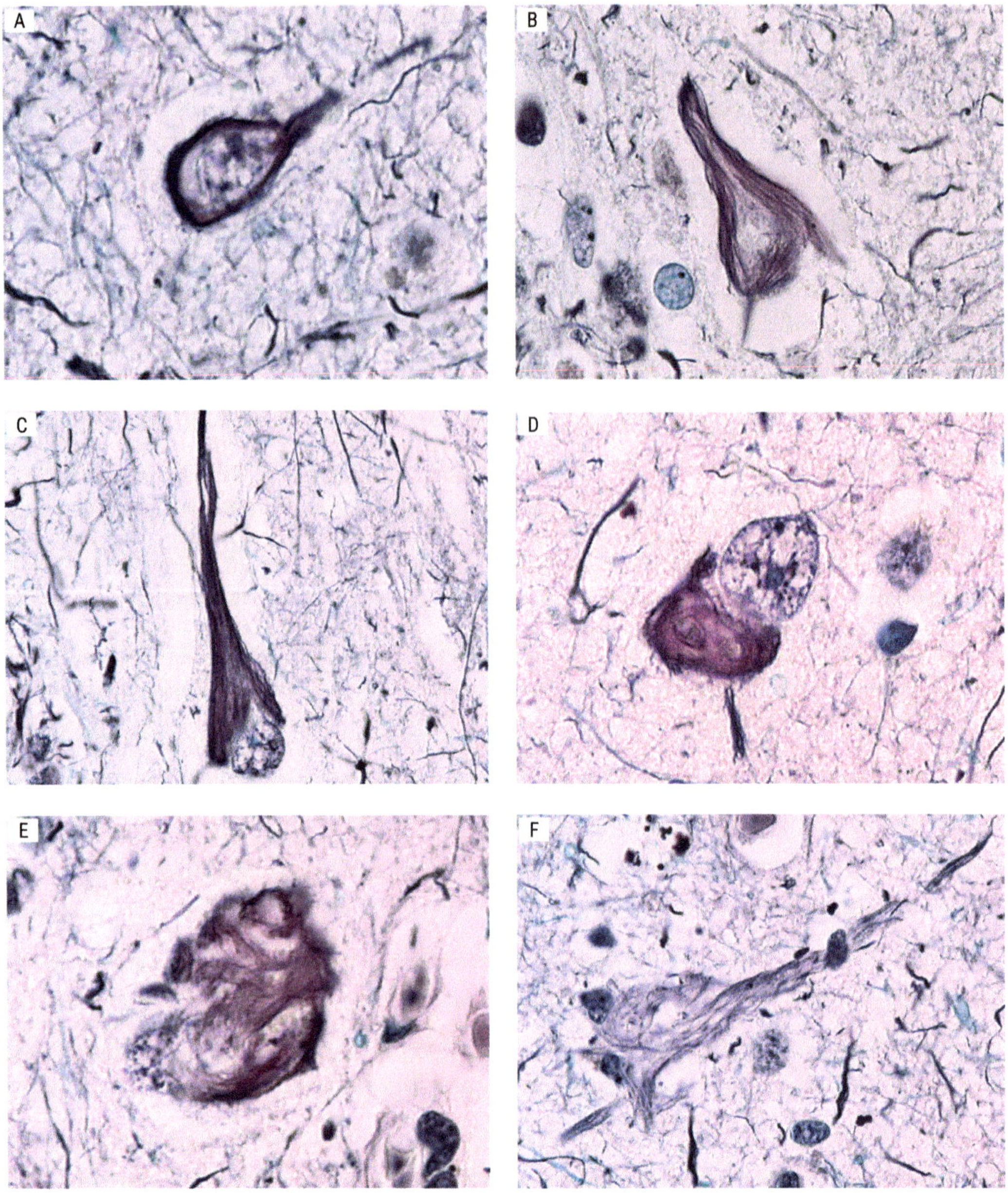

FIGURE 1.10 Different types of neurofibrillary tangles (Bodian silver impregnation combined with Luxol fast blue): band-shaped perikaryal NFT (**A**); triangular flame-shaped perikaryal NFT (**B**, **C**); small, compact, globose perikaryal NFT (**D**); large globose NFT (**E**); "ghost NFT" (**F**).

that is well stained by hematoxylin (Fig. 1.11). Some of the granules are immunoreactive for phosphorylated neurofilament, tubulin, tau, and ubiquitin, suggesting that the vacuoles are autophagic lysosomal structures in which cytoskeletal components are being degraded.

1.1.1.1.8. Intraneuronal inclusion bodies. Intracytoplasmic or intranuclear inclusion bodies are important indicators of neuronal injury. They occur in degenerative, metabolic, and viral diseases and often have diagnostic immunohistochemical and ultrastructural features. Some of these can be detected in H&E staining (summarized below), whereas in neurodegenerative proteinopathies, most can be visualized only by silver staining or specific antibodies and immunohistochemistry (see Chapter 8).

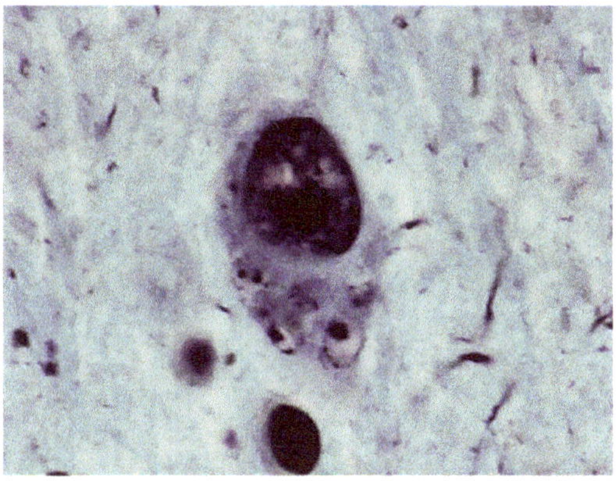

FIGURE 1.11 Granulovacuolar degeneration (Bodian silver impregnation).

Pick bodies are round eosinophilic homogeneous intracytoplasmic neuronal inclusions (Fig. 1.12) characteristic of Pick disease, where they may be seen in pyramidal neurons and dentate granule cells of the hippocampus, as well as in affected regions of the neocortex. The structure is intensely argyrophilic and immunoreactive for tau and the 3R-tau isoform. Pick bodies are also reactive for ubiquitin and tubulin. The ultrastructure of the body is characterized by poorly circumscribed masses of intermediate filaments, 15-nm straight filaments, and some paired helical filaments, as well as entrapped vesicular structures. Basophilic neuronal cytoplasmic inclusions can be seen in the rare *basophilic inclusion body disease* (i.e., FUS proteinopathy) in affected brain regions and in the hippocampus in limbic-predominant neuronal inclusion body disease, a recently described tauopathy.

Lewy bodies are neuronal cytoplasmic inclusions; their appearance varies depending on whether they are found in the perikaryon or in the nerve cell processes, cortex, brainstem, or sympathetic ganglia (Fig. 1.13). Typical (brainstem) Lewy bodies are roughly spherical with an eosinophilic core surrounded by a paler "halo." One or more of these structures may be present in the cytoplasm of a single neuron (Fig. 1.13A, B). They may also be oval or elongated structures, especially when they occur in axonal processes or in sympathetic ganglia (Fig. 1.13C, D). Cortical Lewy bodies are less clearly outlined and consist of a homogeneous zone of hypereosinophilia that usually lacks the characteristic surrounding halo (Fig. 1.13E, F). Lewy bodies are immunoreactive for α-synuclein as well as for ubiquitin and αB-crystallin. By electron microscopy, they consist of an amorphous electron-dense core surrounded by a halo of radiating filaments. Their presence defines several conditions termed *Lewy body disorders*; the most common disorder in this group is Parkinson disease. In these conditions, eosinophilic pale bodies not showing the classical morphology of Lewy bodies can also be seen in pigmented brainstem nuclei.

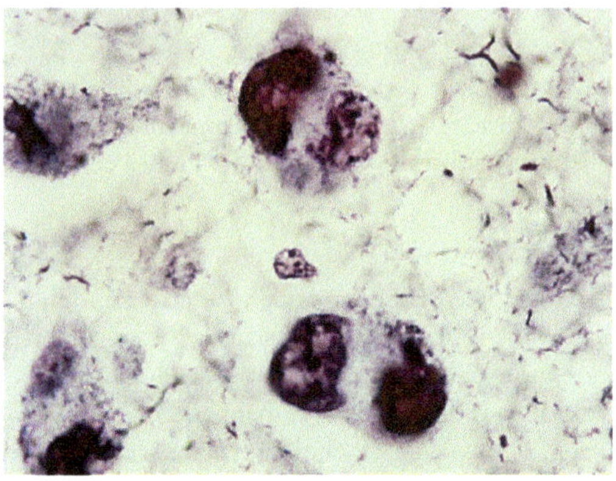

FIGURE 1.12 Neuronal argyrophilic inclusion in Pick disease (Bodian silver impregnation).

Hirano bodies are brightly eosinophilic rod-shaped or elliptical cytoplasmic inclusions that appear to overlap the cell border of a neuron cell body (Fig. 1.14). They are mostly found in the CA1 field of the hippocampus and are particularly numerous in Alzheimer disease and Pick disease and in patients with the Guam parkinsonism–dementia complex. They are immunoreactive for actin and actin-associated proteins. Ultrastructurally, they are highly characteristic and consist of parallel filaments 60–100 nm in length that alternate with a longer sheet-like material.

Bunina bodies are eosinophilic, nonviral intracytoplasmic inclusions found in motor neurons in cases of familial or sporadic amyotrophic lateral sclerosis (Fig. 1.15A, B). They are immunoreactive for cystatin C. Ultrastructurally, they appear as electron-dense, membrane-bound bodies.

Skein-like inclusions are abnormal ubiquitinated, p62-positive structures occurring in anterior horn cells in motor neuron diseases. They are linear, thread-like structures; in some instances, they occur as a single inclusion, and in other cases, they form networks of threads. Occasionally, the threads are aggregated to form larger and dense inclusions (Fig. 1.16). They contain TDP-43, ordinarily a nuclear protein, and accumulate within the cytoplasm of motor neurons in amyotrophic lateral sclerosis. Ultrastructurally, they consist of bundles of

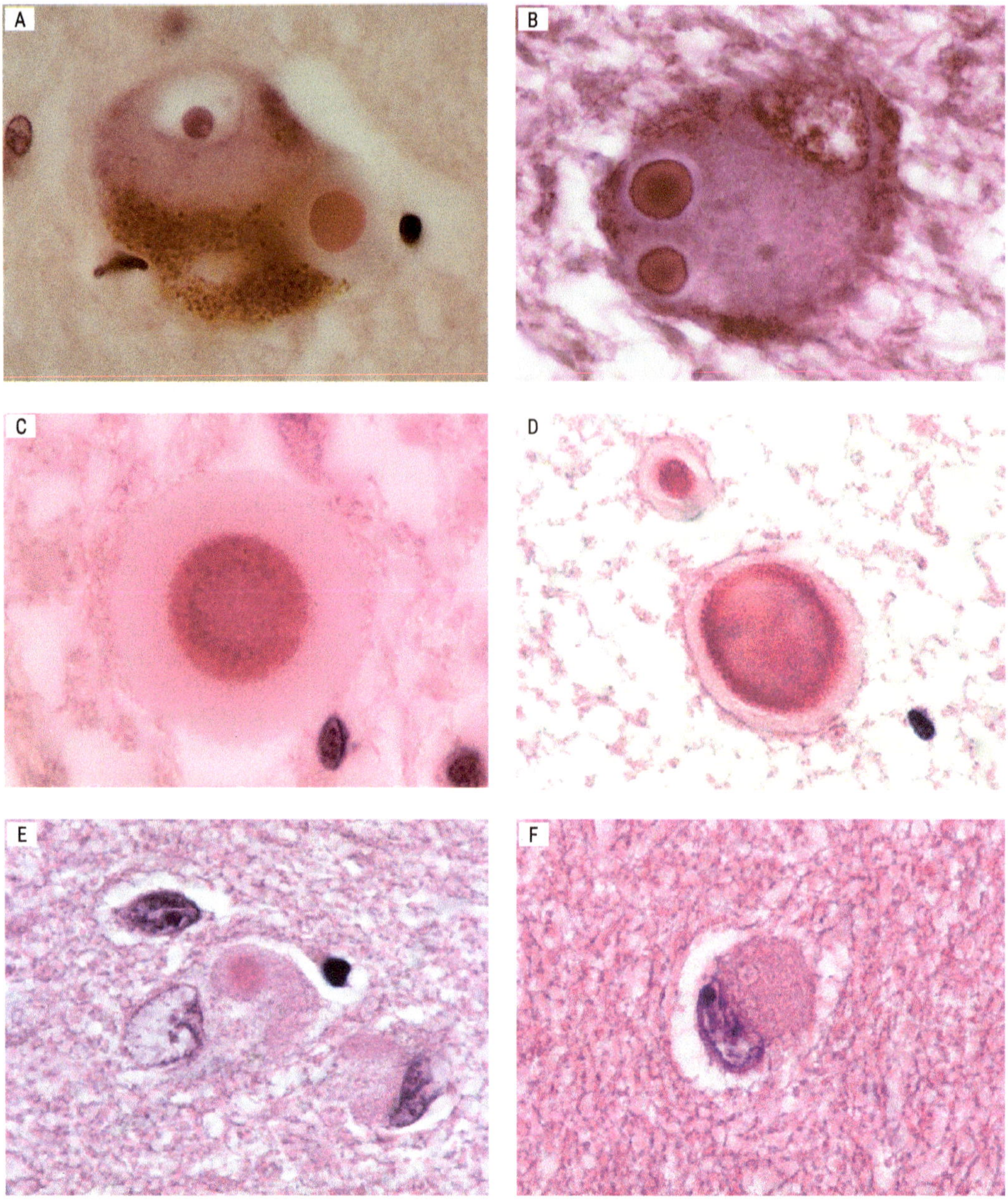

FIGURE 1.13 Lewy bodies (H&E). Single (**A**) and multiple (**B**) Lewy body (bodies) in the perikarya of pigmented neurons of the substantia nigra in a case of Parkinson disease. Lewy bodies in axonal processes (**C**, **D**), in the dorsal nucleus of cranial nerve X in a case of Parkinson disease. Cortical Lewy bodies (**E**, **F**) in the perikarya of cortical neurons in a case of Lewy body disease.

filaments 15–25 nm in diameter, with a tubular profile on cross section.

Marinesco bodies are small eosinophilic intranuclear inclusions located chiefly in melanin-containing brainstem neurons (Fig. 1.17A). They are strongly ubiquitin and p62 positive.

When ubiquitinated, intranuclear inclusions may occur in other regions of the brain and suggest other disorders. Small, round eosinophilic inclusions (about the same size of the nucleolus), immunoreactive for 1C2 anti-polyglutamine expansion antibody, are found in neurons of CAG repeat diseases (including spinal cerebellar ataxias, Huntington disease, or dentatorubral–pallidoluysian atrophy) (Fig. 1.17B). Larger eosinophilic, ubiquitinated, inclusions are found in CGG

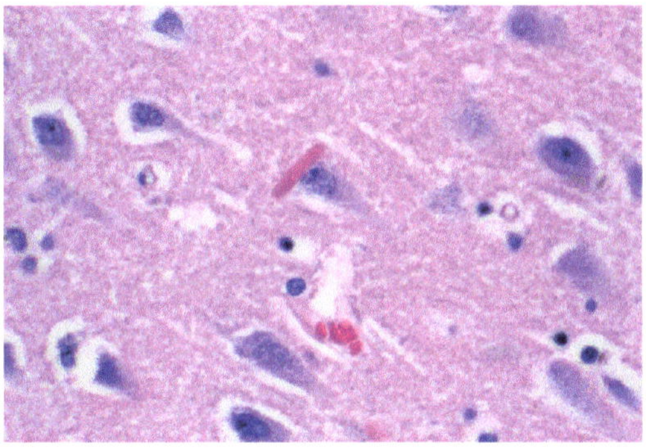

FIGURE 1.14 Hirano bodies are brightly eosinophilic and can be rod shaped, as illustrated, or elliptical (H&E).

repeats (X fragile) and *neuronal intranuclear inclusion disease.* Similar large intranuclear inclusions are found in *intranuclear inclusion body disease.*

Lafora bodies are neuronal intracytoplasmic rounded structures composed of polyglucosan (polymers of sulfated polysaccharides) and are similar to corpora amylacea (discussed later in the chapter) in composition and staining characteristics. They are found in large numbers in myoclonic epilepsy both in the CNS (chiefly in the dentate nucleus) and in certain tissues outside the CNS, including sweat glands, liver, and skeletal muscle. They usually have a dense, intensely PAS-positive core surrounded by filamentous, fainter PAS-positive structures (Fig. 1.18).

Viral inclusions are eosinophilic intranuclear inclusions that occupy a greater or a lesser proportion of the nucleus and may be surrounded by a clear halo; they are associated with some viral infections of the CNS (see Chapter 5). They are seen in

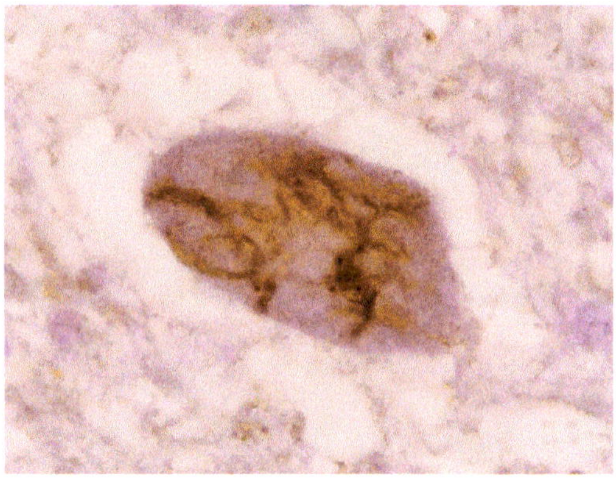

FIGURE 1.16 Skein-like inclusion in an anterior horn cell in a case of motor neuron disease (immunohistochemistry for ubiquitin).

herpes virus infections, particularly in necrotizing encephalitis caused by herpes simplex virus (Fig. 5.37C), and in subacute sclerosing panencephalitis (Fig. 5.31A). In rabies, the viral inclusions are intracytoplasmic and are referred to as *Negri bodies* (Fig. 5.30). In some instances (e.g., cytomegalovirus infection; Fig. 5.38), both intranuclear and intracytoplasmic inclusions may be seen. Viral inclusion bodies are immunoreactive with appropriate antivirus antibodies, allowing for a specific diagnosis. Electron microscopy may also be used to identify virions; however, it is now used less often in diagnostic work.

1.1.1.1.9. Axonal alterations. Following axonal lesions that acutely disrupt the integrity and continuity of the cell process, the distal part of the axon undergoes Wallerian degeneration, which

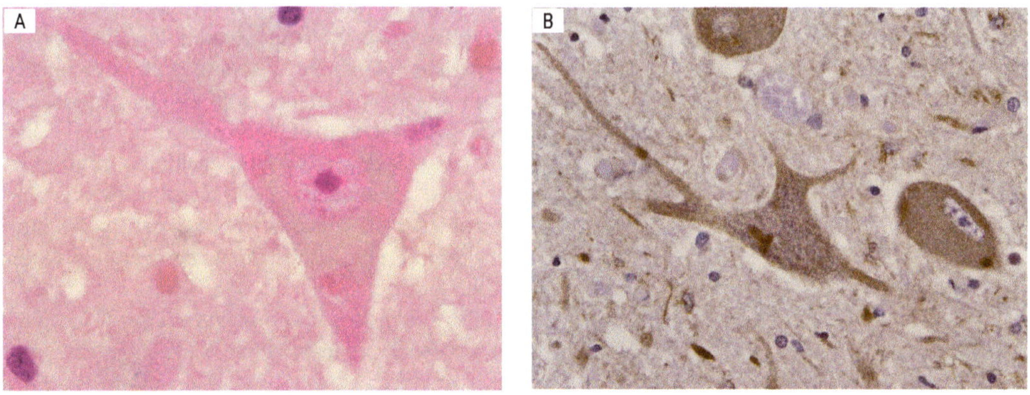

FIGURE 1.15 Bunina bodies in anterior horn cells of the spinal cord in a case of motor neuron disease (H&E) (**A**); immunocytochemistry for cystatin C (**B**).

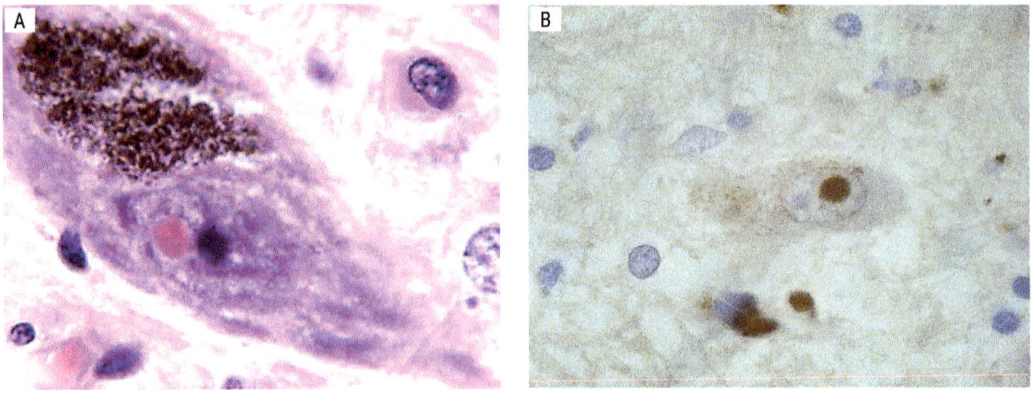

FIGURE 1.17 Intranuclear inclusions: (**A**) Marinesco bodies: small intranuclear inclusion in a pigmented neuron of the substantia nigra (H&E); (**B**) ubiquitin-positive intranuclear inclusion in a case of spinocerebellar degeneration with CAG repeat expansion. (Courtesy of Professor Francesco Scaravilli.)

is described further, elsewhere in this book (see basic lesions of the peripheral nervous system; Chapter 13).

In conditions associated with nerve cell "atrophy" as described previously, the damage of the cell body of the neuron results in degeneration of all its processes, including the dendrites and the axon, which becomes swollen, then fragmented, eventually involuting. This phenomenon, if widespread, as occurs in system degenerations, results in thinning out and rarefaction of the white matter, demonstrable with myelin and axon stains. In these diseases, the phenomenon seems to start at the most distal portions of the longest axons.

Axonal swellings or *spheroids* are localized eosinophilic enlargements along the length of the axon. At these sites, there is a collection of the neurofilaments, organelles, and other molecules that are normally conveyed along the axon by an anterograde transport system but accumulate focally when the transport system is impaired. Spheroid formation characterizes axonal damage by diverse extrinsic insults and occurs in trauma and ischemia. Spheroids are well demonstrated by either silver impregnation (Fig. 1.19A) or immunostaining with ubiquitin (Fig. 1.19B), neurofilament protein markers, and the precursor of the β-amyloid protein (β-APP) (Fig. 1.19C). The latter is transported by the axonal flow and accumulates when disrupted. The term *torpedo* is applied to Purkinje cell axonal swellings and occurs in a wide range of metabolic and degenerative cerebellar diseases. They are well demonstrated by silver impregnations and by the immunohistochemical methods mentioned. They are most notable in the initial portion of the axon, before the origin of the collateral branches (Fig. 1.19C).

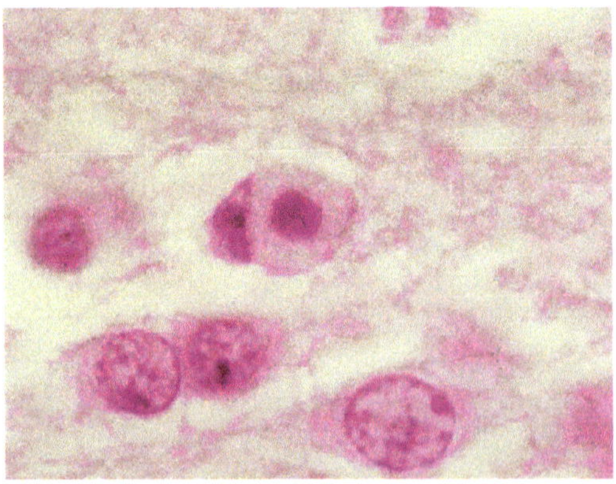

FIGURE 1.18 Lafora body in a case of myoclonic epilepsy (periodic acid–Schiff).

The axonal swellings that develop when axonal transport is disrupted by neuronal metabolic dysfunction are usually termed *dystrophic*. This occurs in some acquired (e.g., vitamin E deficiency) or inherited metabolic diseases. Extensive formation of axonal swellings is an important pathological manifestation of neuroaxonal dystrophy and of some leukodystrophies, including adult-onset leukoencephalopathy with axonal spheroids and pigmented glia, a rare late-onset rapidly progressive leukodystrophy associated with mutations in the *CSF1R* gene.

The term *dystrophic neurite* is used to describe a neuronal process within the gray matter that is distended by tau protein or other abnormal ubiquitinated material. This occurs in several neurodegenerative diseases.

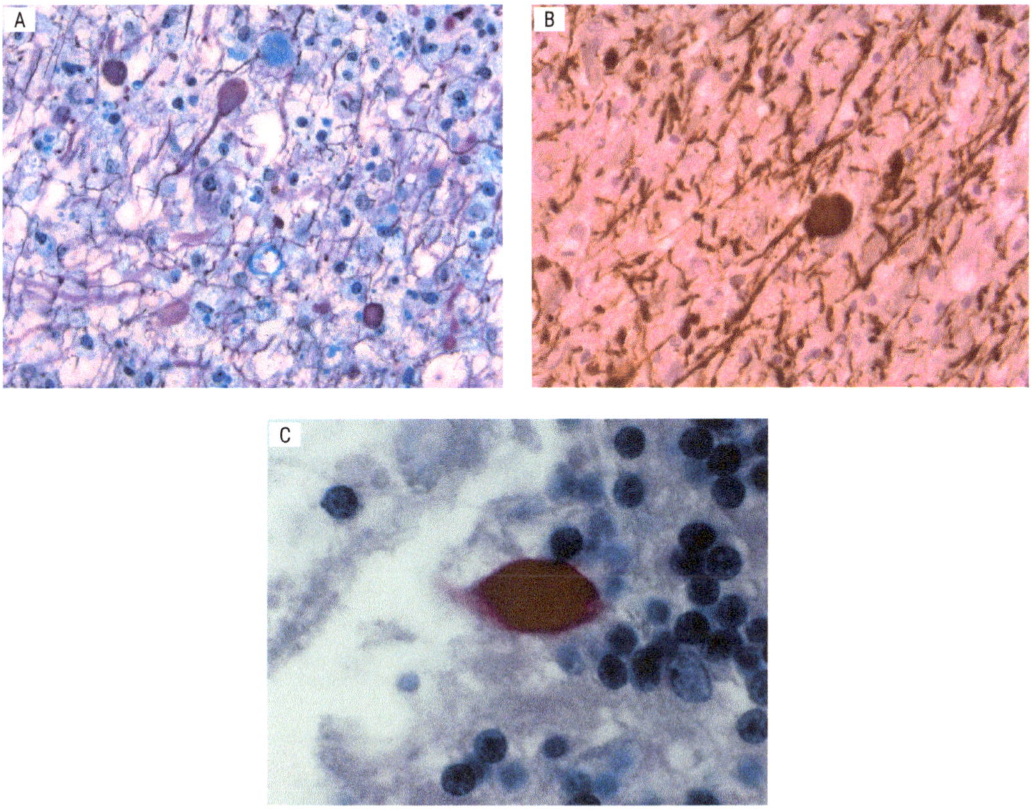

FIGURE 1.19 Axonal swellings in the white matter identified on silver impregnation (**A**) (Bodian stain) and on ubiquitin immunostain (**B**). Torpedo (axonal swelling) of a Purkinje cell axon identified by β-APP immunostaining (**C**).

1.1.1.2. ASTROCYTIC LESIONS

1.1.1.2.1. Gliosis (astrogliosis). The presence of gliosis (alternate term *astrogliosis*) is the most certain indication that an abnormality is of pathologic significance and not artifactual. This reactive process accompanies most instances of subacute or chronic injury of the CNS. The process of gliosis is the response of astrocytes to CNS tissue injury. Transcriptomic analyses of reactive astrocytes highlight a diversity of molecular states and functional alterations in response to different insults. For example, although likely an oversimplification, so-called A1 astrocytes are said to have a neurotoxic phenotype, whereas A2 astrocytes have a neuroprotective phenotype. The associated morphological changes associated with gliosis include an increase in the number of astrocyte nuclei per unit area, eosinophilia of the cytoplasm around the nucleus, and expansion and distortion of the astrocytic cytoplasmic arborization. Mitotic figures are only rarely identified in gliotic tissue, and techniques that bring out dividing cells (Mib-1/Ki-67) also confirm the slow turnover.

The morphologic aspects of the process of gliosis varies depending on the site, stage of evolution, and nature of the pathological process. The early stages are characterized by hypertrophy of the nucleus, which is often hyperchromatic and eccentrically placed in the perikaryon. As mentioned previously, the cytoplasm around the nucleus and cell processes become more extensive than normal (Fig. 1.20A) and are found to contain glycogen. Characteristically, at this stage, the cytoplasm is homogenized and eosinophilic in H&E preparations; these reactive astrocytes are referred to as *gemistocytic astrocytes* (Fig. 1.20B, C).

Over time, in chronic disease states and slowly evolving degenerative processes, astrocyte nuclei return to their resting size and shape, although their cytoplasmic network of cell processes is more extensive and can best be appreciated with

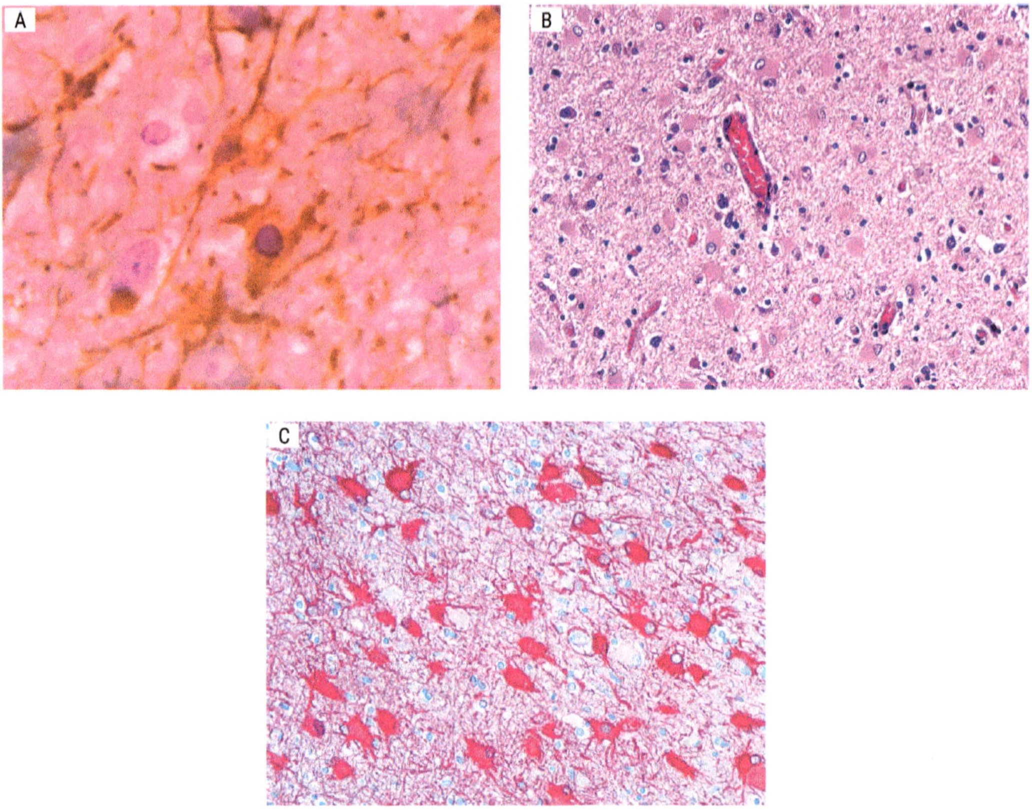

FIGURE 1.20 Gliosis. Fibrillary gliosis (**A**) with hypertrophy of nucleus and of cytoplasm and processes that are very visible on GFAP stain. Gemistocytic astrocytes with large homogenized and eosinophilic cytoplasm (H&E) (**B**), (GFAP) (**C**).

immunostaining for glial fibrillary acidic protein (GFAP).

An older term, *isomorphic fibrillary gliosis*, refers to the alignment of reactive astrocyte processes conforming to a degenerating fiber tract.

1.1.1.2.2. Creutzfeldt–Peters cells. Creutzfeldt–Peters cells are reactive enlarged astrocytes with multiple nuclei, abnormal fragmented nuclear DNA, and irregularly distributed chromosomes observed in multiple sclerosis (see Fig. 7.6D). Also referred to as Creutzfeldt cells, they may sometimes be seen in malignant gliomas.

1.1.1.2.3. Alzheimer type II glia. *Alzheimer type II glia* are observed in hyperammonemic states such as occur in Wilson disease and in liver failure from acquired or hereditary metabolic disease, but they can also occur in other systemic metabolic disorders (e.g., renal failure). This reaction of astrocytes is characterized by enlargement of the nucleus, reaching 15–20 μm in diameter, which appears irregular in shape and pale and empty looking because of the disappearance of chromatin granules (Fig. 1.21). One or two dense, rounded PAS-positive bodies resembling nucleoli are often

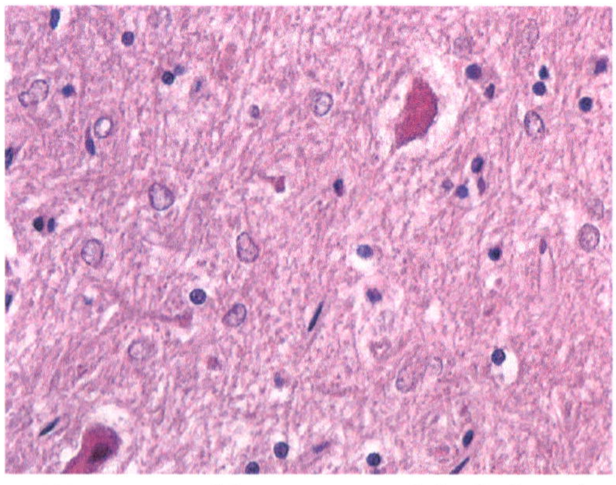

FIGURE 1.21 Alzheimer type II glial cells (H&E).

seen next to the nuclear membrane, which is sharply defined. The cell body is not usually visible on conventional preparations and stains poorly with GFAP. Alzheimer II glia are unrelated to Alzheimer disease; they tend to occur in the gray matter, involving particularly deep gray nuclei, especially the pallidum and the dentate nuclei, and also the cerebral cortex. Alzheimer type II glia are metabolically active cells engaged in the catabolism of toxic substances such as ammonia; on ultrastructural study, they are shown to contain numerous mitochondria.

1.1.1.2.4. Rosenthal fibers. By light microscopy, Rosenthal fibers are rounded, oval, or elongated beaded structures measuring 10–40 μm that appear homogeneous and brightly eosinophilic (see Fig. 2.5B). On electron microscopy, they consist of swollen astrocytic processes that are filled with electron-dense amorphous granular material and glial filaments. Peripheral labeling for GFAP, ubiquitin and αB-crystallin can be demonstrated with immunohistochemistry (IHC). Rosenthal fibers are seen in various pathological conditions that have in common intense fibrillary gliosis of long standing, as seen throughout the brain in multiple sclerosis plaques, in the spinal cord in syringomyelia, and in the hypothalamus around craniopharyngiomas. They are also characteristic of certain neoplasms (pilocytic astrocytoma, particularly of the cerebellum, but also elsewhere in the brain; see Chapter 2) and in Alexander disease (see Chapter 10).

Eosinophilic granular bodies are rounded hyaline droplet aggregates that occupy the cytoplasm of astrocytes and are seen in certain tumors, including pilocytic astrocytoma, pleomorphic xanthoastrocytoma, and ganglion cell tumors.

1.1.1.2.5. Clasmatodendrosis. *Clasmatodendrosis* refers to a beading or fragmentation of astrocytic processes, which can be highlighted by GFAP immunostaining. This process may be observed in the context of head trauma, seizure disorders, ischemia, cerebral edema, and various toxic exposures and encephalopathies, although it may also be a postmortem artifact.

1.1.1.2.6. Inclusions and storage material. Accumulation of *lipofuscin* occurs in astrocytes as part of aging as it does in neurons. Similarly, in lipid storage diseases, *glial lipid storage* may accompany neuronal storage.

Although various neurodegenerative disease-related proteins (e.g., α-synuclein, TDP-43) can be deposited in astroglia without showing argyrophilia, only the accumulation of *tau protein*, which is the main component of NFTs, is considered of diagnostic utility. This is of particular relevance for distinguishing PSP and CBD (see Chapter 8).

Tufted astrocytes are considered to be highly characteristic of PSP (Fig. 8.26A). The whole length of their processes contains tau protein, and they are often binucleated. They may be demonstrated by Gallyas stain or tau immunohistochemistry. In CBD, accumulation of tau protein in astroglia forms distinctive structures in gray matter areas termed *astrocytic plaques*: Tau protein accumulates at the distal end of the astrocytic processes, while the center of the astrocytic plaque is devoid of tau immunoreactivity (Fig. 8.30).

Thorn-shaped astrocytes have an argyrophilic cytoplasm with a few short processes (Fig. 8.26B) and often a small eccentric nucleus. They are commonly associated with non-argyrophilic granular-fuzzy astrocytes and seen in aging-related tau astrogliopathy. Thorn-shaped astrocytes are also observed in CTE. Globular astroglial inclusions that are not detectable on Gallyas staining can be detected in globular glial tauopathies. Ramified astrocytes can be seen in Pick disease.

Viral inclusion bodies may also be found in astrocytes, such as in subacute sclerosing panencephalitis and cytomegalovirus infection, and rarely also in progressive multifocal leukoencephalopathy (see Chapter 5).

Corpora amylacea are spherical, basophilic, PAS-positive inclusions, 10–50 μm in diameter, that are predominantly found in astrocyte processes, although they occasionally occur within axons. Ultrastructurally, they consist of densely packed 6- or 7-nm filaments that may be admixed with amorphous granular material and are not membrane bound. Corpora amylacea increase in number with aging, particularly in the subpial and subependymal regions (Fig. 1.22), around small blood vessels, and in the posterior columns of the spinal cord. Corpora amylacea are hypothesized to serve as containers for accumulated waste products to be cleared away by the immune system. Adult polyglucosan body disease (see Chapter 10) is characterized by diffuse accumulation of corpora amylacea, involving the cortex and white matter and associated with diffuse or focal myelin damage.

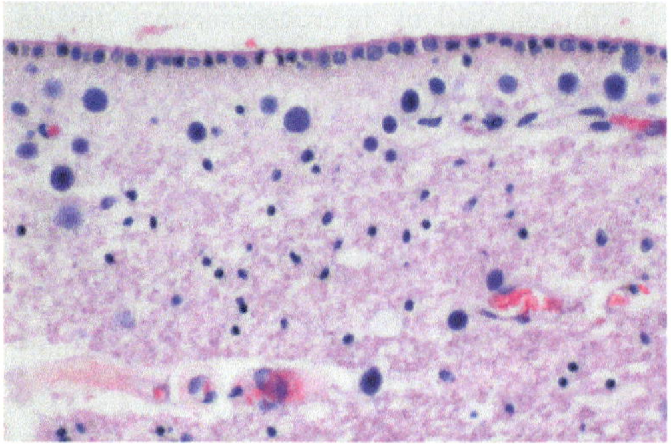

FIGURE 1.22 Numerous corpora amylacea in the subependymal region (H&E).

1.1.1.3. LESIONS OF OLIGODENDROCYTES

Like neurons and astrocytes, oligodendrocytes may be infected by virus and manifest intranuclear or intracytoplasmic inclusions (e.g., progressive multifocal leukoencephalopathy; see Chapter 5) or be affected by excess storage of lipid or glycogen in genetically determined enzymopathies (e.g., metachromatic leukodystrophy).

Cytoplasmic inclusions involving mainly oligodendrocytes have been shown to be a characteristic feature of certain neurodegenerative diseases, including multiple system atrophy (see Chapter 8). These inclusions are usually flame- or sickle-shaped; can be demonstrated by silver impregnation; and are immunoreactive for ubiquitin, p62, αB-crystallin, and α-synuclein.

Accumulation of tau protein in oligodendrocytes, known as "coiled body," may be found in PSP, CBD, and AGD (see Chapter 8). These consist of fibrillary structures "coiling" around the nucleus. Argyrophilic globular oligodendroglial inclusions are hallmark features of globular glial tauopathies. Tau-negative and p62- and TDP-43–positive coiled-body-like pathology can be seen in the brain and spinal cord in TDP-43–related frontotemporal degeneration and amyotrophic lateral sclerosis. Furthermore, in Lewy body disorders, α-synuclein immunoreactive coiled body-like pathology can be detected mostly in the substantia nigra and thalamic projections. Crystalloid inclusions in oligodendrocytes have been described in a rare form of hereditary spastic paraparesis.

Oligodendrocytes, along with oligodendrocyte precursor cells, may also be particularly vulnerable to a wide range of insults, including toxins and radiation exposure, and resulting in myelin injury.

1.1.1.4. MICROGLIAL LESIONS

Microglia are a distinctive family of cells of monocyte lineage. They have several important physiologic functions, playing important roles in brain development, synaptic pruning, phagocytosis, neuroinflammation, immune response modulation, and cell survival/repair. They can be demonstrated under the microscope by silver impregnation, lectin-binding techniques, and immunohistochemical techniques using antibodies against monocyte/macrophage markers (e.g., CD68, CD163, IBA-1, and Tmem119) (Fig. 1.23B).

In normal brain, microglia have been subdivided into (a) *resident microglia*, with little turnover and present throughout the CNS parenchyma; and

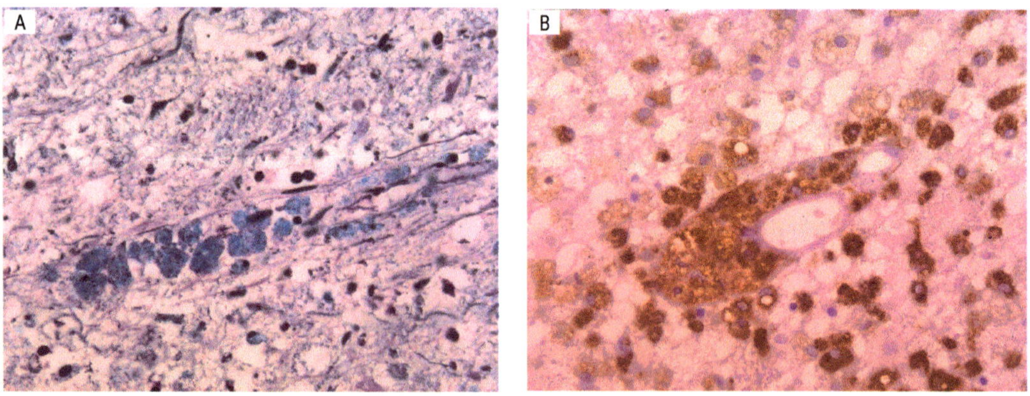

FIGURE 1.23 Perivascular lipid-laden macrophages (compound granular corpuscles, foam cells, or gitter cells) in a demyelinating lesion (**A**) with Luxol fast blue combined with Bodian silver impregnation and (**B**) with CD68 immunostaining.

(b) *perivascular microglia*, found within the perivascular basal lamina and with characteristic turnover as with hematogenous monocytes. Microglial activation occurs in inflammatory conditions of the CNS and involves (a) increased entry of hematogenous monocytes into the CNS; (b) proliferation of resident microglia; and (c) expression or secretion of a wide range of proteins, most of which are concerned with antigen presentation and inflammation.

The following are typical microglial reactive processes:

- *Macrophage proliferation and phagocytosis* (the cells are also known as compound granular corpuscles, foam cells, lipid phagocytes, or gitter cells). This is a frequent finding in many brain lesions, particularly those associated with demyelinating processes or with traumatic or ischemic tissue destruction. After a destructive or demyelinating insult, macrophages invade the damaged region within approximately 48 hours of injury. These are cells with a counted shape and distinct cytoplasmic borders, measuring 20–30 μm in diameter. They have small, darkly staining, and sometimes eccentric nuclei and a clear, granular cytoplasm that can contain lipid products, hemosiderin pigment, or other phagocytized material (Fig. 1.23A, B). Most scavenger cells derive from blood monocytes. Their number increases over a period of days and weeks, and they may still be present in injured tissue months after the injury. During demyelination, the cytoplasm of the macrophages contains myelin debris (see Chapter 7). Multinucleated giant cells that are derived from the microglia/macrophage lineage are one of the hallmarks of HIV infection of the CNS.
- *Rod cell proliferation* (Figs. 1.24 and 5.27C) is a microglial response to subacute parenchymal injury in the setting of minimal or absent necrosis. On H&E preparations, rod cells are elongated, spindle-shaped cells with an elongated nucleus. The best descriptions of this glial change are found in reports of cases of general paresis in the older literature (see Chapter 5). Rod cells are also seen in cases of subacute encephalitis and evolving ischemic lesions.
- *Microglial nodules* consist of clusters of microglial cells; they are typically found in subacute encephalitis in and around sites of neuronal destruction: *neuronophage nodules* (see Chapter 5).

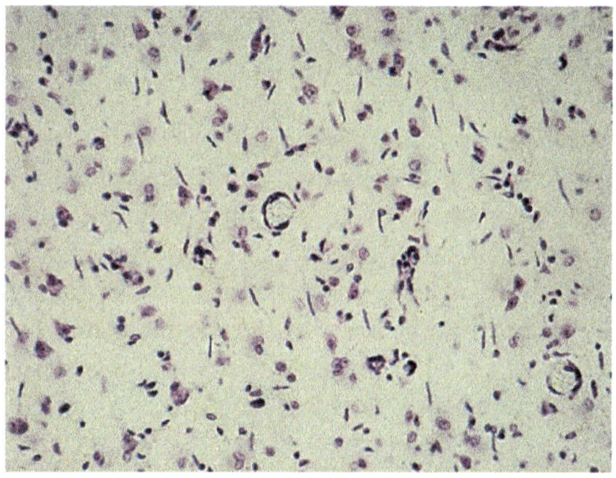

FIGURE 1.24 Rod-shaped microglia in a case of "general paresis of the insane" or syphilitic dementia (Nissl stain).

Activated microglia are sometimes categorized as having an "M1" (classic) phenotype or an "M2" (alternative) phenotype, although this binary classification is an oversimplification for the cellular phenotypes. M1 microglia secrete proinflammatory cytokines and chemokines, generate reactive oxygen species, and are neurotoxic. In contrast, M2 microglia secrete anti-inflammatory cytokines, growth factors, and neurotrophic factors, promoting cell survival and repair. Microglia may be involved in various neurodegenerative and neuropsychiatric diseases, and impaired microglia function may contribute to age-related changes in the brain.

1.1.1.5. EPENDYMAL CELLS

Ependyma have a limited range of reactions to injury. Along with neurons and other glial cells, ependymal cells may be infected in viral diseases such as cytomegalovirus infection (see Chapter 5). In the adult CNS, ependymal cells do not proliferate to any extent in response to injury. Their destruction leaves bare stretches of the ventricular lining; this is accompanied by proliferation of subependymal astrocytes, which form small hillocks along the ventricular surface: *ependymal granulations*. Occasionally, surviving ependymal cells may be overgrown by the astrocytic reaction and appear as clusters of tubules buried within the ependymal granulations (subventricular glial nodules). Rosette formation is mostly seen in neoplastic conditions but rarely noted in the subventricular region in normal brains, particularly at the terminal ends of the ventricles.

1.1.2. General *tissue* reactions of the CNS to injury and herniations

A set of general tissue reactions are known to occur in the CNS that stand apart from the reactions to specific pathological processes (i.e., vascular, infectious, inflammatory, demyelinating, metabolic, and degenerative). As described in other chapters of this book, these may accompany one or more of the specific pathologic processes described previously that are visible under the microscope or may result in more extensive changes that can be visible to the naked eye.

1.1.2.1. CEREBRAL ATROPHY

Cerebral atrophy is the end stage of a number of neurological diseases. The brain is lighter than a normal age-matched control. Macroscopically, there is narrowing of the gyri and widening of sulci. On section, the cortical ribbon is thinned, and ventricular dilation is often present (Fig. 8.10). The histological substratum consists of a variable loss of neurons often associated with gliosis, depending on the underlying illness, and a variety of neuronal alterations, which are discussed in subsequent chapters.

1.1.2.2. CEREBRAL EDEMA

Cerebral edema is defined as an increase in the brain volume associated with an increase in water and sodium content. Depending on its pathogenesis, brain edema has been classified as vasogenic, cytotoxic, or interstitial (hydrocephalic). A combination of these prototypes of edema is frequent.

- *Vasogenic edema*, probably the most common type of brain edema, complicates head injury, abscess, tumors, and hemorrhages. Both vasogenic edema and cytotoxic edema occur with ischemia. Vasogenic edema results from blood–brain barrier injury leading to increased permeability of the microcirculation to macromolecules, particularly to proteins. By radiologic imaging, sites of vasogenic edema are marked by contrast enhancement because the injected contrast medium leaks across the permeable vascular lining of the microcirculation. Biochemically, the edema fluid resembles a plasma filtrate. The fluid is located chiefly in the extracellular spaces of the white matter.
- In *cytotoxic edema*, excessive amounts of water enter one or more of the intracellular compartments of the CNS (neurons, glia, endothelial cells, or myelin sheaths) because the cellular concentration of osmotically active solutes is increased. This usually results from an injury impairing the capacity of the cell to maintain ionic homeostasis. It is also seen in association with systemic disturbances in fluid and electrolyte metabolism. Cytotoxic edema complicates hypoxia and ischemia because of failure of the adenosine triphosphate–dependent sodium pump in the affected cells. It also occurs in osmotic disequilibrium syndromes associated with hemodialysis or diabetic ketoacidosis and in acute plasma hypo-osmolality states, such as water intoxication and inappropriate secretion of antidiuretic hormone. Because the so-called cerebrovascular macromolecular barrier remains intact, disease processes that give rise to cytotoxic edema are not associated with radiologic enhancement after injection of contrast medium.
- *Interstitial* or *hydrocephalic edema* is the accumulation of cerebrospinal fluid (CSF) in the extracellular spaces of the periventricular white matter often resulting from obstructive hydrocephalus. As fluid collects within the obstructed ventricles, pressure increases, and the CSF is forced across the ependymal lining into the adjacent extracellular spaces.

Macroscopically, the edematous areas of brain are swollen and soft (Fig. 1.25). The swelling increases the volume of the intracranial contents, with consequent increased intracranial pressure (see Section 1.1.2.3). When the brain is cut, the surface appears wet and shiny. If the edema is diffuse, the ventricles are compressed; in severe cases, they are reduced to slit-like cavities.

Under light microscopy, myelin stains demonstrate pallor of the white matter. The cerebral tissue has a less compact appearance compared to normal and is interspersed by vacuoles of variable size. Glial cells are swollen; perivascular and pericellular spaces are dilated.

These macroscopic and microscopic features correspond to ultrastructural features that vary according to the etiological and pathogenetic mechanism. They include dilation of the perivascular and extracellular spaces, swelling of astrocytic

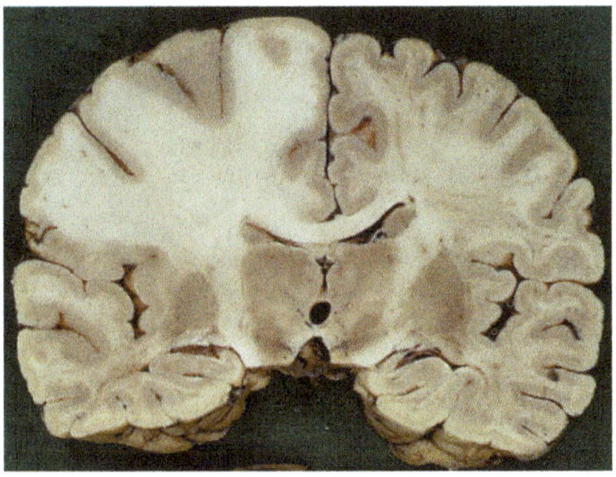

FIGURE 1.25 Cerebral vasogenic edema of the cerebral hemisphere (on left), with swelling of the parenchyma, which appears paler; flattening of the gyri; narrowing of the sulci; and compression of the lateral ventricles.

cell processes, and splitting of the myelin lamellae (Fig. 1.26).

1.1.2.3. HYDROCEPHALUS

Hydrocephalus is an abnormal increase in the intracranial volume of CSF associated with dilation of all or some portion of the ventricular system. It is secondary to a dysequilibrium between CSF formation and reabsorption. Rarely, it results from increased production of CSF (e.g., choroid plexus papilloma). More commonly, it is the consequence of altered flow and absorption of the CSF as a result of obstruction of CSF pathways within the ventricular system (noncommunicating hydrocephalus) or in the subarachnoid space (communicating hydrocephalus). Obstruction at "bottleneck" areas such as the foramina of Monro, the aqueduct of Sylvius, and the exit foramina of the fourth ventricle (lateral foramina of Luschka and midline foramen of Magendie) can occur when there is extension of blood or tumor into the ventricular system. Subarachnoid pathways most often become blocked over the cerebral convexities and around the rostral brainstem (incisural block) as a result of inflammation or hemorrhage. In the acute phases, the blood extravasation or inflammatory exudate forms a barrier to flow. Subsequently, organization of the clot or exudate leads to fibrous obliteration of the subarachnoid space.

Hydrocephalus is often associated with increased intracranial pressure. In children, in the absence of appropriate shunting procedures, the head can become enlarged when hydrocephalus develops before the cranial sutures close. When the progressive obstructive lesion causing the hydrocephalus is not severe, the hydrocephalic process may stabilize, and the CSF pressure returns to normal limits (the disputed entity "normal-pressure hydrocephalus").

Several alterations in the brain are common to all forms of hydrocephalus. These include dilation of the ventricular system; interstitial edema; reduction of the volume of the white matter; accentuation of the primary, secondary, and tertiary cerebral sulci (producing a prominent gyral pattern); and perforation of the septum pellucidum. Disruption and loss of the ependymal lining, with localized subependymal astrocytic proliferations protruding into the ventricular cavities, termed *ependymal granulations*, is frequent (see Section 1.1.1.5). Proliferation of the subependymal glia may bring about stenosis of the aqueduct, which is a cause of obstructive hydrocephalus in childhood.

1.1.2.4. INCREASED INTRACRANIAL PRESSURE AND BRAIN HERNIATION

After closure of the sutures, the volume of the cranial cavity is fixed by rigid bony walls and compartmentalized by partitions of bone and dura. The normal contents of the cranial cavity (blood, brain, and CSF) are relatively incompressible. Under these circumstances, an increase in the volume of the cranial contents will result in increased intracranial pressure.

The intracranial contents may expand because of diffuse brain edema; increased cerebral blood flow and blood volume; or the development of space-occupying lesions such as tumors, abscesses, hematomas, or large, recent infarcts accompanied by edema. The effects of space-occupying lesions on intracranial pressure are the result not only of the mass of the lesion but also of the accompanying edema and obstruction of venous or CSF pathways. In children with persistently open cranial sutures, increase in volume of intracranial contents can lead to splaying of the sutures, resulting in an increase in the size of the skull and in digital convolutional markings. In older children and in adults when bony skull can no longer expand, intracranial hypertension leads to compression of the brain surfaces against the inner table of the skull, with consequent flattening of cerebral gyri, narrowing of intervening sulci, and accentuation of foraminal and tentorial markings on the inferior cerebellar and medial temporal surfaces.

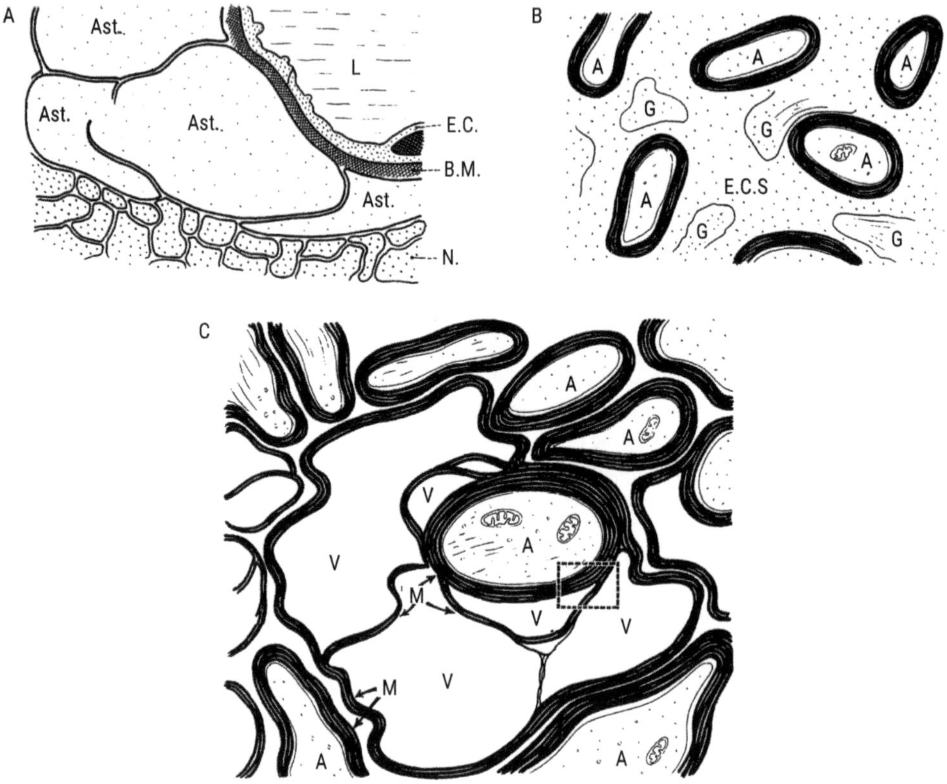

FIGURE 1.26 Cerebral edema: principal ultrastructural features. (**A**) Gray matter, vasogenic edema (as in traumatic and inflammatory etiologies). Swelling of astrocytic processes, especially near capillaries. Ast, astrocytic cell process; BM, basement membrane; EC, capillary endothelial cell; L, capillary lumen; N, neuropil. (**B**) White matter, vasogenic edema. Expansion of extracellular space. A, myelinated axons; ECS, extracellular space; G, glial cell process. (**C**) White matter, cytotoxic edema (due to triethyltin poisoning). Splitting of myelin lamellae at the intraperiod line. A, myelinated axon; M, myelin; V, vacuole.

The expanding cerebral mass will also insinuate itself into the anatomic openings that can accommodate it. These compensatory displacements of brain from one intracranial compartment to another, caused by an increase in the volume of intracranial contents, are referred to as *cerebral herniations*. They differ depending on whether the space-occupying lesion is supratentorial or infratentorial (Fig. 1.27).

1.1.2.4.1. Cerebral herniations in supratentorial lesions. *A unilateral lesion* (Fig. 1.28) that increases the hemispheric volume is likely to cause a herniation of the cerebral hemisphere through openings limited by the inferior border of the falx and by the free edge of cerebellar tentorium on the ipsilateral side of the lesion. Depending on the size and the site of the expanding lesion within the hemisphere, one of several forms of herniation will occur, sometimes in combination:

- Herniation of the cingulate gyrus under the falx (subfalcine herniation) with lateral displacement of the anterior cerebral arteries.
- Lateral displacement of the midline structures (i.e., the third ventricle, pineal gland, and vein of Galen).
- Downward herniation of the diencephalon through the tentorial notch with downward displacement of the floor of the hypothalamus and of the mammillary bodies (central, diencephalic herniation).
- Herniation of the hippocampal gyrus in the tentorial notch between the brainstem and the free edge of the tentorium cerebelli. The herniated temporal lobe can compress and stretch the third and sixth cranial nerves. When the *ipsilateral* cerebral peduncle is compressed directly, a hemiparesis contralateral to the lesion

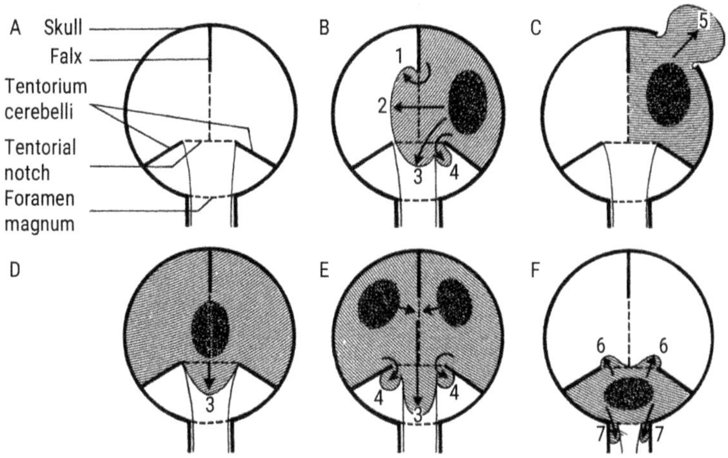

FIGURE 1.27 Localization of the principal types of cerebral herniation. (**A**) Normal aspect of rigid structures within the skull. (**B**) Unilateral hemispheric expanding lesions. (**C**) Herniation through bone flap. (**D**) Midline hemispheric expanding lesion. (**E**) Bilateral hemispheric expanding lesions. (**F**) Expanding infratentorial lesion. (1) Cingulate subfalcine herniation. (2) Lateral displacement of midline structures. (3) Central diencephalic herniation. (4) Temporal or transtentorial herniation. (5) External herniation (through bone flap). (6) Superior cerebellar herniation (through tentorial opening). (7) Cerebellar tonsillar herniation (through foramen magnum).

may ensue; when the *contralateral* peduncle is displaced and compressed against the free edge of the tentorium (Kernohan notch), an ipsilateral hemiparesis may follow; if the adjacent posterior cerebral artery is compressed, there can be secondary infarction anywhere along its territory of distribution.

- Compression due to temporal herniation and the downward thrust of central diencephalic herniation may result in stretching of the blood vessels, especially the veins that supply the midbrain and pons, which may be torn and cause potentially lethal brainstem hemorrhages; these are called *Duret hemorrhages.*
- External cerebral herniation through surgical or traumatic defects in the calvarium may also occur.
- *Bilateral cerebral lesion or circumstances that result in global increase of the volume of both hemispheres* will ordinarily result in central diencephalic herniation or bilateral temporal lobe herniation.
- *A midline expanding lesion* will likely result in central diencephalic herniation.

1.1.2.4.2. Cerebellar herniations in infratentorial lesions. Two types of herniations exist:

- *Upward herniation of the mesencephalon and cerebellum through the tentorial notch.* Direct mesencephalic lesions may result from this complication, as well as secondary lesions due to vascular compression.
- *Cerebellar tonsillar herniation* through the foramen magnum is the most frequent and most dangerous complication of an infratentorial expanding process, regardless of the nature of the insult or, in case of a neoplasm, the degree of malignancy. The result of increased intracranial pressure in the posterior fossa is the herniation of the cerebellar tonsils downward through the foramen magnum (Fig. 1.29), culminating in medullary compression with compromise of vital cardiorespiratory centers.

1.2. TOPOGRAPHIC ANALYSIS OF CENTRAL NERVOUS SYSTEM LESIONS

Topographic analysis of the lesions observed is just as important as the study of their morphologic aspects. It constitutes a crucial step in the attempt to arrive at an etiological diagnosis and necessitates a rigorous and systematic examination of all the neural structures. Systematic sampling of multiple anatomic levels is necessary, and wherever possible, techniques that allow for whole-brain sections provide invaluable material that permits the synchronous study of various areas of the CNS under the dissecting and light microscopes.

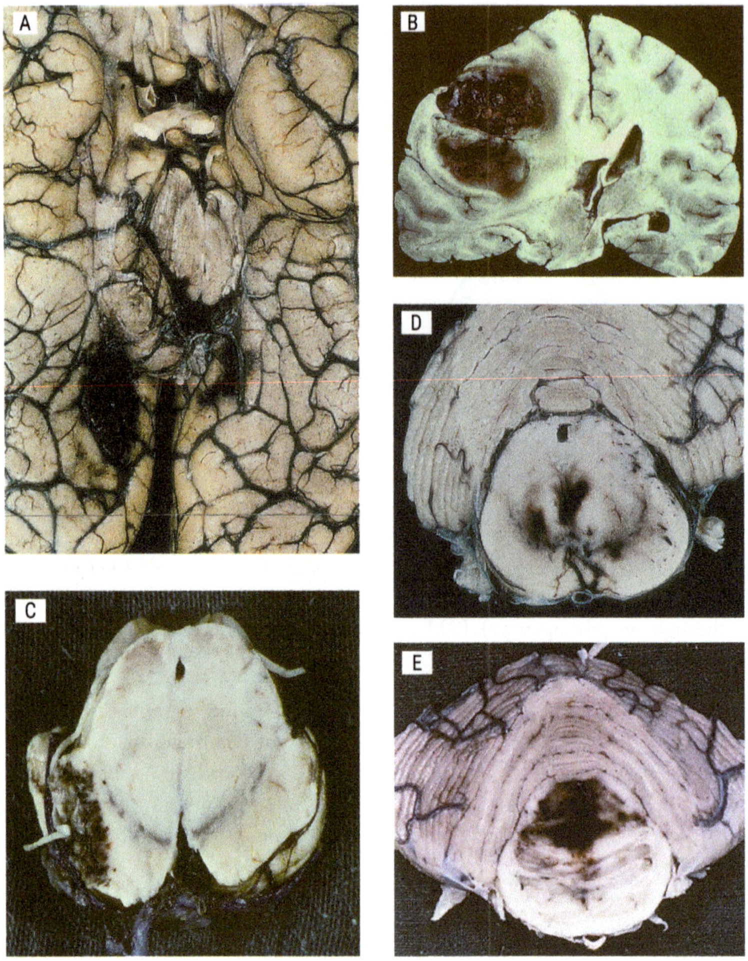

FIGURE 1.28 Cerebral herniations: (**A**) Inferior aspect of the cerebral hemispheres; note the herniated rim of the right hippocampal gyrus (on left) compressing the oculomotor nerve and displacing the brainstem. (**B**) Cerebral metastases causing temporal herniation; note displacement of the midline structures and cingulate herniation. (**C**) Midbrain; note hemorrhagic lesion in the crus of the cerebral peduncle contralateral to the temporal herniation (Kernohan notch). (**D, E**) Midbrain and pontine midline hemorrhages involving mostly the tegmentum, secondary to temporal herniation.

1.2.1. Diffuse distribution

Lesions that are diffusely distributed throughout the brain may be seen in systemic diseases, such as metabolic or circulatory disorders, or also can be the result of blood-borne infective processes. Some of the degenerative diseases may likewise cause diffuse lesions of the CNS. It is nevertheless important to emphasize that despite the diffuse character of these changes, lesions often show regional predominance.

1.2.2. Focal distribution

- Lesions may be localized to an anatomically well-defined area (lobe of the cerebral hemisphere, basal ganglia, brainstem), and certain preferential sites of involvement are linked to specific etiological entities (e.g., some cerebral tumors preferentially occur in certain locations of the brain).
- Lesions may be localized to a vascular territory. By definition, cerebral infarcts exemplify this type of focal lesion.

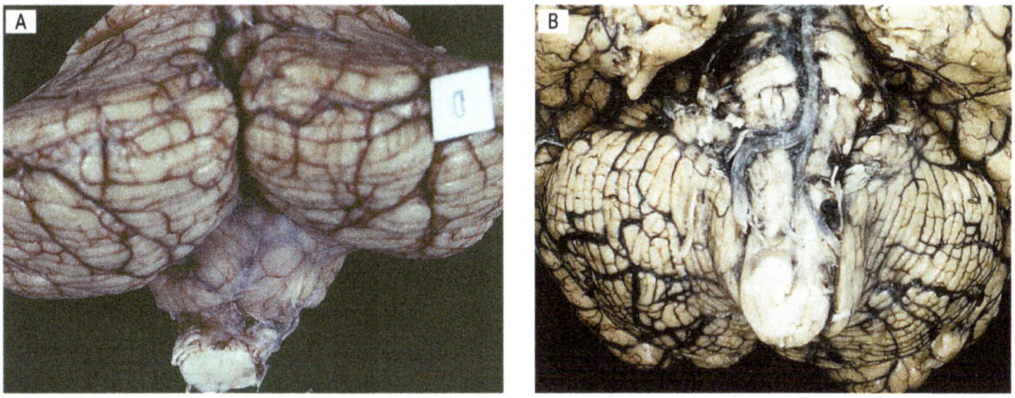

FIGURE 1.29 Cerebellar tonsillar herniation: (**A**) posterior view; (**B**) anterior view.

1.2.3. Disseminated distribution

Disseminated distribution is seen essentially in multifocal processes, of which multiple sclerosis is the most characteristic example.

1.2.4. Systematized distribution

A number of nervous system disorders, especially neurodegenerative diseases, cause changes that involve certain functionally related morphological systems, such as involvement of upper and lower motor neurons in amyotrophic lateral sclerosis, spinocerebellar involvement in Friedreich ataxia, and others.

1.3. SYNTHETIC INTEGRATION

The findings in the two aspects of neuropathological examination, artificially set apart as *morphologic* and *topographic* analyses, need to be integrated. Furthermore, and most important, correlation of these findings with the clinical data, laboratory and radiologic data, general autopsy findings, and all other available diagnostic data must occur to arrive at an accurate etiologic diagnosis.

Thus, for example, an understanding of cerebral infarcts is possible only after careful and complete postmortem examination of the vascular tree, heart, and lungs and after comparing the anatomical findings with information provided by the clinical picture, the chronology of the functional disturbances, and data from cerebral and vascular imaging.

Likewise, for example, the study of the lipidoses cannot be based solely on neuropathological findings. It necessitates detailed alignment with data from the general *postmortem* examination and neurochemical/genetic analysis.

Finally, the analysis of hereditary disorders of the CNS or peripheral nervous system and of diseases of skeletal muscles now requires correlation with molecular and genetic data.

2

Tumors of the Central Nervous System

FRANCK BIELLE, SANDRO SANTAGATA, AND KEITH L. LIGON

2.1. CLASSIFICATION

Traditionally, the classification of nervous system tumors has been based on the histological appearance of a particular neoplasm supplemented by immunohistochemical features. However, tumor classification and patient management now rely increasingly on the evaluation and incorporation of molecular and genetic information. The classification scheme established by the World Health Organization (WHO) in its 2021 Classification of Tumors of the Central Nervous System incorporates the recommendations provided by the International Society of Neuropathology—Haarlem Consensus Guidelines. These resources emphasize the new importance of pathologist generation of "integrated diagnoses," which formally encompass histologic diagnosis, histologic grade, and pertinent molecular information (including genetic alterations and profile of DNA methylation).

Tumors of the central nervous system (CNS) can be broadly classified into two main categories: *primary tumors* and *secondary tumors.* Primary tumors originate from cells that are intrinsic to the CNS or its coverings, such as the calvarium. These primary tumors include those of neuroepithelial origin as well as those of nonneuroepithelial origin. Secondary tumors arise from sites elsewhere in the body and primarily involve the brain or spinal cord through hematogenous dissemination (metastases) or, less frequently, contiguous extension.

CNS tumors can also be classified based on their location and their corresponding incidence according to age. In *adults,* approximately 70% of all brain tumors are *supratentorial,* meaning that they occur within the cerebral hemispheres or their coverings. The most common types, in order of frequency, are metastases, gliomas, meningiomas, and schwannomas. In *children,* approximately 70% of *brain* tumors are *infratentorial,* located within the cerebellum or brainstem, and are predominantly neuroepithelial in origin. The most common types in children, in decreasing order of frequency, are pilocytic astrocytoma, medulloblastoma, and ependymoma. *Spinal cord* tumors make up approximately 15% of all primary CNS tumors and include schwannoma, meningioma, and glioma such as ependymoma and astrocytoma in decreasing order of frequency.

2.2. PRIMARY NEOPLASMS

2.2.1. Tumors of neuroepithelial tissue

2.2.1.1. DIFFUSE GLIOMAS

Diffuse gliomas are characterized by the infiltration of normal brain tissue by tumor cells extending beyond the tumor core (i.e., they are not circumscribed). By contrast, other types of neuroepithelial neoplasms (medulloblastoma, pilocytic astrocytoma) have more clearly defined borders between the tumor and normal brain (i.e., they are circumscribed). Due to their diffuse growth, complete surgical resection of diffuse gliomas is generally not possible. As a result, clinical relapse is typically inevitable in adults with diffuse gliomas, and resistance to chemotherapy and radiotherapy eventually leads to disease progression. However, the outcomes of patients vary depending on various factors, such as the specific tumor type and the patient's age, with tumor progression observed after only a few months to as long as several decades.

Once the diagnosis of diffuse glioma is established through histological examination of cellular morphology, various tests are used to identify the molecular pathways that are activated or disabled by genetic or epigenetic mechanisms in each tumor, thereby generating the information necessary to formulate an "integrated diagnosis." Specific genetic and epigenetic alterations have been strongly linked to certain tumor cell phenotypes, such as the oligodendroglial or astrocytic lineage differentiation that is observed in tumors by inspecting cellular morphology or gene expression data. These molecular alterations have been found to form a reliable basis for the classification of most diffuse gliomas, especially when highly intermixed and dynamic lineage morphologies occur within individual samples.

The oncogenesis pathways of diffuse gliomas are strongly influenced by two key factors: patient age and tumor anatomic location. As a result, diffuse gliomas are classified into *adult-type* and *pediatric-type*. Tumors are first classified by histological criteria, and then the classification is integrated with molecular results. In cases in which molecular testing for a diffuse glioma cannot be obtained, tumor type can be designated based solely on histologic criteria. For example, a tumor may be histologically classified as oligodendroglioma, astrocytoma, or glioblastoma (GBM). When molecular testing results are not available, the designation "not otherwise specified" (NOS) is applied. Alternatively, if no definitive subclass criteria are present even after molecular testing, the designation "not elsewhere classified" (NEC) can be used.

Various grading schemes have been used to classify diffusely infiltrating gliomas based on morphologic criteria. The current WHO classification grading system incorporates morphological criteria adapted from the Sainte Anne/Mayo grading system. For example, for adult-type astrocytomas, high grades (3 or 4) are assigned to tumors based on an assessment of three histologic features: *frequent mitoses, microvascular proliferation,* and *necrosis.* Low-grade (2) astrocytomas lack these features. However, molecular alterations can also be used to guide tumor grading in the current WHO classification, such as a tumor with grade 2 histologic features that has TERT promoter mutation, or *EGFR* amplification, or other grade 4 molecular features (Table 2.1). Thus, although the prognostic value of morphological

Table 2.1 Integrated Diagnosis of Adult-Type Diffuse Gliomas

INTEGRATED DIAGNOSIS	OLIGODENDROGLIOMA, IDH MUTANT, AND 1P/19Q CO-DELETED	ASTROCYTOMA IDH MUTANT	GLIOBLASTOMA, IDH WILDTYPE
Present genetic alterations	*IDH1/2* mutation and 1p/19q whole arm co-deletion[a] *TERT* mutation	*IDH1/2* mutation[a] *ATRX* and *TP53* mutation	*TERT* mutation *EGFR* amplification Gain of 7, loss of 10
Absent genetic alterations	*ATRX, TP53*	Absence of 1p/19q co-deletion[a]	Absence of *IDH1/2* or histone H3 mutation[a]
Grade	2 or 3	2, 3, or 4	4

[a]These molecular alterations are mandatory to achieve the diagnosis.

criteria has been well established previously, it is currently being reevaluated in the context of molecular analysis and integrated diagnoses.

2.2.1.1.1. Adult-type diffuse gliomas. The clinical characteristics of patients with adult-type diffuse glioma typically include the following features: occurrence at any site throughout the CNS, diffuse infiltration of adjacent and often distant brain structures, and a tendency for progression to anaplasia over time.

2.2.1.1.1.1. Astrocytoma, IDH mutant. IDH-mutant astrocytoma commonly arises in one of the cerebral hemispheres, most frequently in the frontal lobes. Grade 2 tumors typically occur at a median age in the mid-30s, whereas grade 3 and 4 tumors arise in the mid-40s. Oncogenesis of IDH-mutant astrocytomas occurs over a long period of evolution, starting as low-grade tumors before spontaneous or post-treatment progression to a higher grade. Although most tumors are initially diagnosed at grade 2 and then later progress to grade 3 or 4, some tumors are identified as grade 3 or 4 at the time of initial diagnosis. The clinical symptoms experienced by patients depend on the specific area of the brain affected by the tumor. Seizures are a common presenting symptom. Imaging studies of grade 2 tumors typically reveal a poorly defined, homogeneous, low-density lesion that does not enhance with contrast and grows slowly. The development of focal contrast enhancement and/or rapid growth during the course of the illness indicates progression toward anaplasia and a higher histologic grade, with a more aggressive clinical course.

The macroscopic characteristics of IDH-mutant astrocytoma include the presence of a mass lesion with ill-defined boundaries, causing distortion of the surrounding brain structures, resulting in blurring of normal anatomical landmarks (boundary between gray and white matter). The tumor may exhibit cyst formation of varying sizes, which may give the tissue a spongy or gelatinous appearance.

The microscopic characteristics of IDH-mutant astrocytoma grade 2 include low to moderate tumor cell density with varying cytologic properties, resembling those of well-differentiated astrocytes and oligodendrocytes (Fig. 2.1A). The neoplastic cells express the glial markers OLIG2 and glial fibrillary acidic protein (GFAP). Nuclear irregularities such as altered size, contour, and chromatin organization, collectively termed nuclear atypia, are typically present, which helps distinguish neoplastic cells from nonneoplastic astrocyte nuclei. Mitotic activity is low, and microvascular proliferation or necrosis should be absent. The background matrix of the tumor may appear loose, vacuolated, or microcystic. The Ki-67/MIB-1 labeling index, a measure of cellular proliferation, is usually less than 10%. The tumor cells have nuclei associated with scant perikaryal cytoplasm and are surrounded by a fibrillary background on conventional hematoxylin and eosin (H&E) preparations. In some cases, the tumor contains abundant "gemistocytic" cells with eosinophilic cytoplasm and nuclei displaced toward the periphery; these are referred to as *gemistocytic astrocytoma*. Perivascular inflammation is commonly observed in this variant. In addition, certain cases may exhibit extensive mucoid degeneration and a cobweb-like appearance.

The key genetic alteration in IDH-mutant astrocytoma is a mutation in the isocitrate dehydrogenase 1 (*IDH1*) gene and, in rare cases, the *IDH2* gene. Co-deletion of 1p/19q is not observed in these tumors by definition. Mutations in the *TP53* tumor suppressor gene, which reduces degradation of the P53 protein and leads to its accumulation (Fig. 2.1B), and mutations in the *ATRX* gene, leading to the loss of ATRX protein expression (Fig. 2.1C), are commonly found in IDH-mutant astrocytoma. Although sequencing assays are optimal to identify mutations in *IDH1*, *TP53*, and *ATRX*, immunohistochemical reagents have been developed that serve as surrogate markers, providing practical tools for rapidly inferring the molecular status of these genes. One such antibody recognizes the most common *IDH1* mutation R132H, which is present in more than 90% of *IDH1* mutant cases (Fig. 2.1D).

Astrocytoma, IDH-mutant, grade 3, exhibits high cellular density, increased nuclear atypia, frequent mitoses, and a Ki-67 labeling index generally exceeding 10%. Astrocytoma, IDH-mutant, grade 4 tumors are a new entity in the WHO 2021 classification that exhibit any one of the features of vascular proliferation, necrosis, or homozygous deletion (loss of both copies) of the *CDKN2A* gene. These grading criteria may be present only focally, with one area of the tumor progressing to higher grade while the remaining tumor mass retains lower grade features. Importantly, these features are required to be absent from grade 3 tumors. Median survival rates for astrocytoma, IDH-mutant tumors vary significantly by grade, ranging from 3 years for tumors

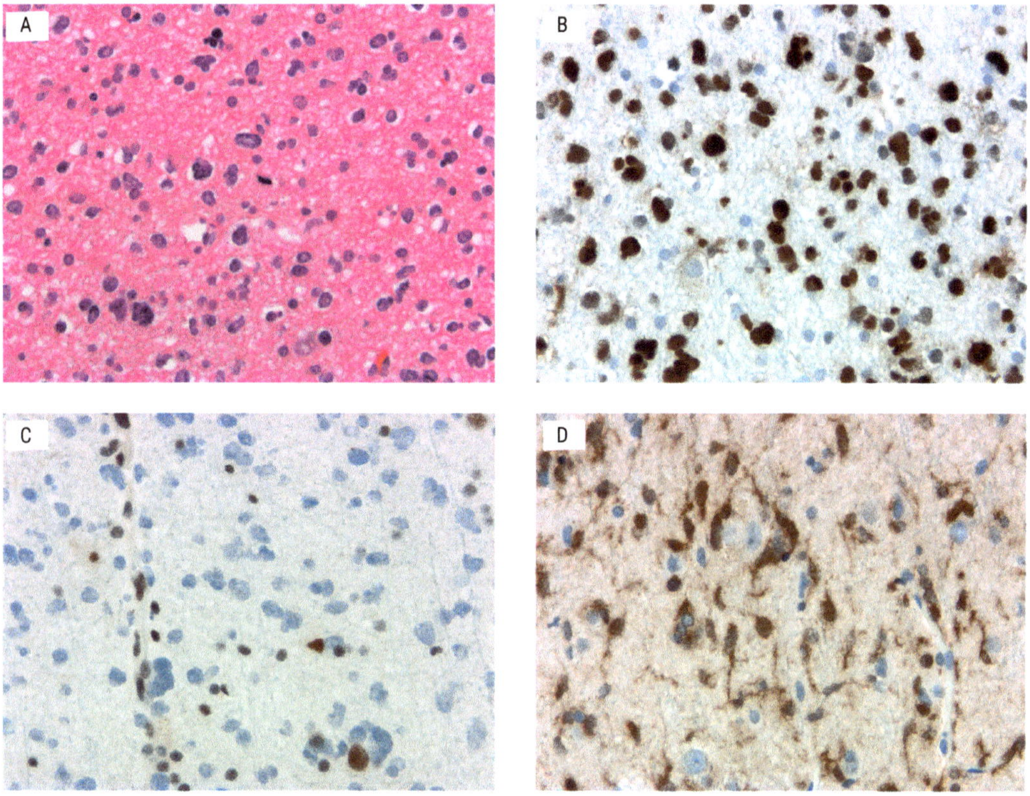

FIGURE 2.1 Astrocytoma IDH mutant: (**A**) Glial tumor cells with astrocytic (ovoid nuclei), oligodendroglial (round nuclei and clear perinuclear halo), and intermediate morphologic phenotypes. One mitosis in the center, marked nuclear atypia (H&E). (**B**) Pathological expression of p53 in tumor cells (p53 IHC). (**C**) Loss of ATRX expression in tumor cells versus retained expression in endothelial cells, neurons, and normal glial cells (ATRX IHC). (**D**) IDH1 R132H immunoreactivity of tumor cells (IDH1 IHC).

with *CDKN2A* homozygous deletion to more than 15 years for grade 2 tumors that have undergone complete surgical resection. Progression to higher grades is often associated with additional molecular changes, including increased number of copy changes, activating mutations in the PI3K pathway and MYC oncogenes, as well as mismatch repair mutations producing acquired resistance to treatment with the chemotherapy.

2.2.1.1.1.2. Oligodendroglioma, IDH mutant, and 1p/19q co-deleted (WHO grade 2 or 3). Oligodendroglioma is a type of diffusely infiltrating glioma characterized by tumor cells that resemble mature oligodendrocytes. The diagnosis of this tumor type is now based on genetic markers, specifically the presence of an IDH mutation and co-deletion of the chromosomal arms 1p and 19q. Oligodendroglioma account for approximately 5% of all intracranial gliomas, and grade 2 tumors predominantly affect adults between ages 30 and 60 years. Grade 3 tumors typically occur 5 or 6 years later. These tumors most commonly arise in the cerebral hemispheres, particularly the frontal lobes. These tumors are different than diffuse leptomeningeal glioneuronal tumors, which may also demonstrate oligodendroglioma-type morphology and co-deletion of 1p/19q but lack IDH mutations. Due to their slow-growing nature, patients with oligodendroglioma may have a long history of neurological symptoms, often characterized by seizures. Imaging studies usually reveal a well-defined mass with features such as calcifications, occasional intratumoral hemorrhage, and edema around the mass. Contrast enhancement may be present in some grade 2 tumors, and it is more common in grade 3 tumors.

The macroscopic appearance of oligodendroglioma WHO grade 2 is characteristically that of a variably well-circumscribed, grayish pink neoplasm including areas of mucoid change, which may result in a gelatinous consistency as well as zones of cystic degeneration, focal hemorrhage, and calcifications. Grade 3 tumors show a macroscopic appearance similar to grade 2 tumors except that areas of necrosis may be present.

The microscopic characteristics of oligodendroglioma are highly distinctive. In routine paraffin-embedded sections stained with H&E, the tumor cells appear closely packed with a small, round nucleus that is usually slightly larger than that of a normal oligodendrocyte and that is surrounded by a clear halo (Fig. 2.2A). However, this pattern is not apparent in smear preparations, frozen sections, and paraffin sections made from previously frozen material. The tumor stroma also contains a network of thin-walled branching capillaries (Fig. 2.2A). Occasional mitoses or nuclear atypia, which may be marked in some cases, are still compatible with WHO grade 2. Anaplastic transformation (WHO grade 3) is marked by elevated mitotic activity, microvascular proliferation, or necrosis. In most WHO grade 2 oligodendroglioma, the Ki-67 labeling index is less than 10%. Some tumors may contain nodules of increased cellularity, and careful examination of these areas may reveal other high-grade features within them. Small calcifications, known as calcospherites, are a characteristic histologic feature (Fig. 2.2B), but they are only seen in 20% of cases and are not specific for oligodendroglioma. Another diagnostically useful feature is the presence of perineuronal, perivascular, or subpial tumor aggregates when the tumor infiltrates cortex. It is not uncommon to find cells with well-differentiated GFAP-positive astrocyte morphology and visible cytoplasm admixed within the tumor. Microscopically, WHO grade 3 tumors share similar characteristics with grade 2 oligodendroglioma, but they also exhibit focal or diffuse evidence of high-grade features, including increased cellularity, cytologic atypia, frequent mitoses (≥6 mitoses per 10 high-power fields), and often microvascular proliferation or necrosis with or without palisading (Fig. 2.2C). Occasionally, mixed tumors with

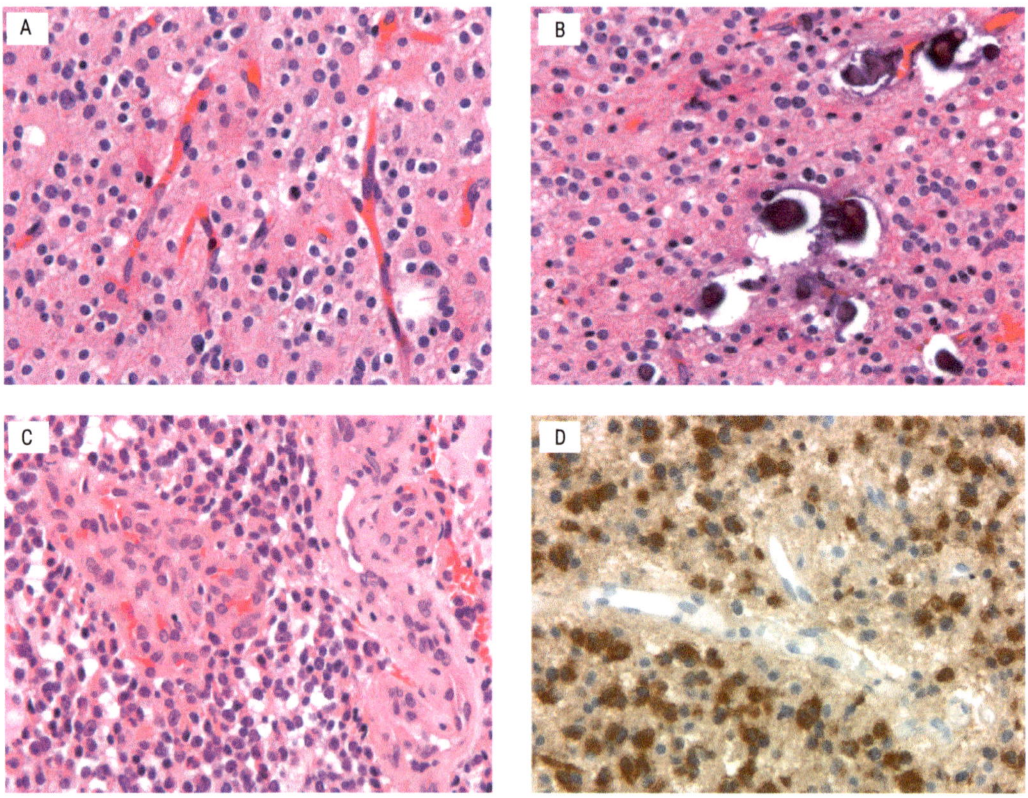

FIGURE 2.2 Microscopic appearance of oligodendroglioma, IDH mutant, and 1p/19q co-deleted: (**A**) uniform round cells with haloes and "chicken-wire" vascular pattern (H&E); (**B**) microcalcifications (H&E); (**C**) microvascular proliferation (H&E); (**D**) IDH1 R132H expressed in tumor cells (IDH1 R132H IHC).

oligodendroglioma and astrocytoma pattern are seen; in these cases, tumor classification is guided by molecular data.

Immunohistochemistry (IHC) can help further characterize oligodendroglioma using antibodies specifically recognizing the IDH1 R132H mutant protein (Fig. 2.2D). Sequencing can be used to detect other *IDH1* mutations in amino acid R132 or mutations in the *IDH2* gene. Although *IDH2* mutations are found in fewer than 10% of cases, their presence is more specific for oligodendrogliomas and is only rarely reported in IDH-mutant astrocytomas. Oligodendrogliomas exhibit a normal retained expression of ATRX and weak p53 expression typically in less than 10% of cells on IHC, which are not suggestive of underlying mutations and enable one to distinguish them from IDH-mutant anaplastic astrocytoma. In addition, OLIG2, an oligodendroglial lineage-restricted transcription factor, is expressed in more than 90% of tumor cells in oligodendroglioma, which is higher than typical for astrocytomas and glioblastomas, and also aids in the differential diagnosis with other round clear cell neuroepithelial tumors such as neurocytomas and ependymomas that often have minimal or no expression. Although some cases of oligodendroglioma may express GFAP, these cells often resemble small gemistocytic astrocytes.

The evaluation of the 1p and 19q chromosome arms is now a required part of the diagnostic workup of IDH-mutant diffuse gliomas. It can be performed using various methods such as DNA sequencing and different types of genomic array platforms or fluorescent in situ hybridization (FISH). The presence of concurrent whole-arm co-deletion of 1p and 19q, resulting from a translocation involving these chromosomes, is integral to the diagnosis of oligodendroglioma. It is important to note that partial deletions of 1p and 19q can be observed in up to 10% of astrocytomas and GBM. Therefore, FISH alone cannot distinguish between whole-arm and partial-arm deletions. Copy number microarrays or sequencing assays assessing the entire chromosome are therefore more reliable. More than 50% of oligodendrogliomas have loss-of-function mutations in the transcription factor *CIC* (located on 19q), and some tumors also harbor mutations in *FUBP1* (located on 1p). In these cases, 1p and 19q loss results in biallelic inactivation of these genes. Nearly all cases of oligodendroglioma have mutations in the promoter of the *TERT* gene, which encodes the polymerase that maintains telomere ends. This serves as an additional positive diagnostic marker to distinguish oligodendroglioma from astrocytoma IDH-mutant. These mutations lead to increased expression of the TERT protein. In addition, WHO grade 3 tumors may have gains and losses of various chromosomal arms, although no single copy number change appears to occur with high frequency. More than 90% of oligodendrogliomas display methylation of the *MGMT* promoter and are deficient in activity of MGMT protein. *CDKN2A* homozygous deletion or loss of heterozygosity is associated with grade 3 tumors and with worse prognosis. A smaller subset of cases have inactivation of *CDKN2C* or activating mutations in *PIK3CA*.

Patients diagnosed with oligodendroglioma IDH-mutant and 1p/19q co-deleted generally have the most favorable outcomes among adults with diffuse gliomas. The median survival exceeds 15 years for WHO grade 3 tumors. This positive prognosis is partly attributable to the tumor's favorable response to chemotherapy, which is based on temozolomide or combined procarbazine, CCNU (lomustine), and vincristine (PCV). Some patients, however, experience multiple recurrences, with eventual progression to frank anaplasia, and progression from grade 2 to grade 3 is often associated in *MGMT* methylated patients with acquired resistance to temozolomide and mutations in mismatch repair proteins MSH2, MSH6, MLH1, or PMS2. These mutations lead to unrepaired DNA damage and a hypermutation/high tumor mutation burden in tumors. Tumor dissemination through the cerebrospinal pathways may also occur during these transformation processes.

2.2.1.1.1.3. Glioblastoma, IDH-wildtype (WHO grade 4). Glioblastoma is a highly malignant and rapidly growing neoplasm classified as WHO grade 4. GBM differs from other adult-type diffuse gliomas due to the absence of mutation in the *IDH1* and *IDH2* genes. Therefore, it is referred to as glioblastoma IDH-wildtype (GBM hereafter) based on its histomolecular characteristics. GBM is the most common primary brain tumor, accounting for approximately 10–15% of all intracranial tumors and 40–50% of all glial tumors. GBM most often occurs in adults between ages 55 and 85 years and rarely in patients younger than age 40 years.

GBM may develop in any region of the CNS but most commonly arises in the subcortical white matter of the cerebral hemispheres, particularly the temporal, parietal, frontal, and occipital lobes in descending order of incidence. GBM can also occur in the thalamus or the basal ganglia, although it is rare in the brainstem and the spinal cord. When an IDH-wildtype high-grade glioma occurs in midline regions or in patients younger than age 40 years, it is important to exclude the presence of histone H3 mutations, which are hallmarks of other types of gliomas.

GBM can be identified by radiological imaging based on its characteristic features. Typically, GBM appears as an irregular mass with a central hypodense region of necrosis surrounded by a contrast-enhancing "ring" that represents the more cellular and vascularized portions of the tumor. A classic radiologic (and macroscopic) presentation is the "butterfly" pattern, which occurs when the tumor spreads across the corpus callosum to the contralateral hemisphere. In the tissue surrounding the tumor, considerable vasogenic edema can be observed. This edema is often visible as hyperintensity on a T2-weighted magnetic resonance imaging (MRI) scan.

Macroscopically, GBM often appears as a relatively well-defined mass lesion, although microscopic examination reveals extensive infiltration of tumor into the surrounding brain tissue. The tumor typically has a "variegated" appearance, with solid gray-pink tissue at the periphery and yellow zones of central necrosis (Fig. 2.3A). In some instances, there is evidence of both old and recent hemorrhage. Infiltration of tumor cells often extends along anatomic fiber tracts, sometimes at considerable distance from the main tumor mass. Consequently, patients may develop multiple foci distant from main

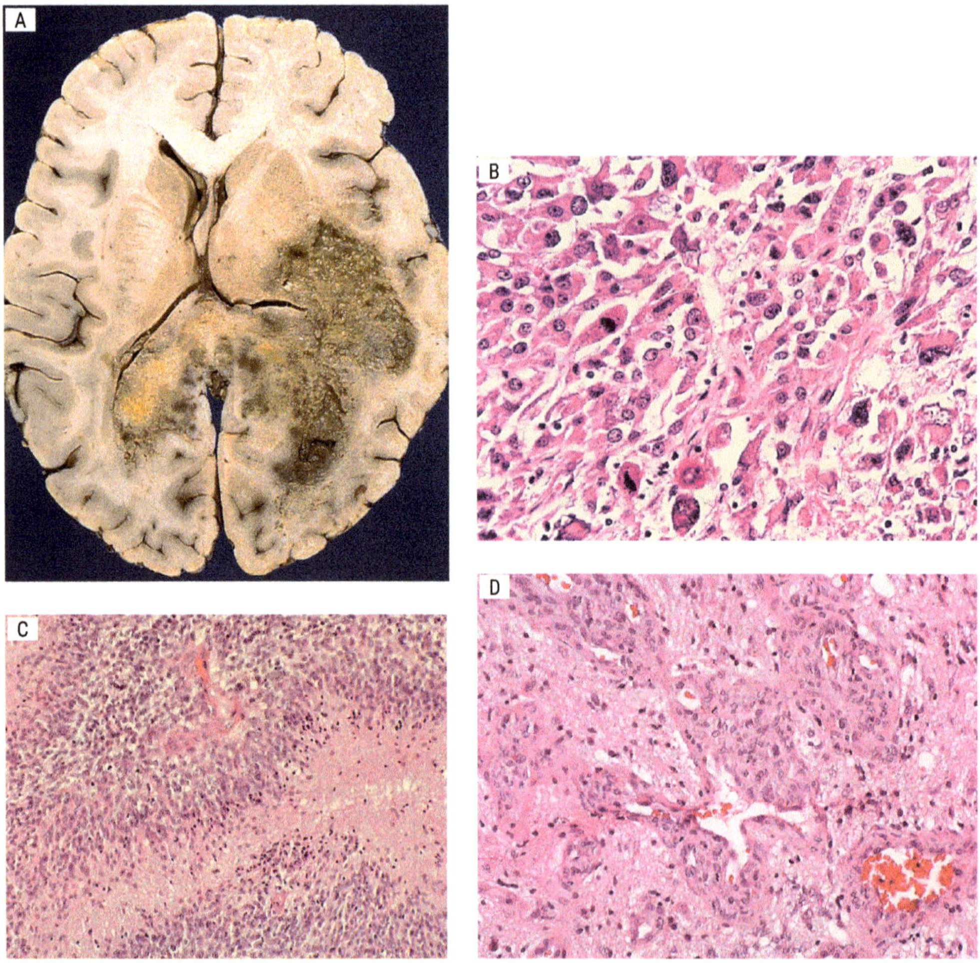

FIGURE 2.3 Glioblastoma, IDH-wildtype: (**A**) glioblastoma (macroscopic). *Microscopic features*: (**B**) cellular anaplasia, mitoses (H&E); (**C**) necrosis with pseudopalisading (H&E); (**D**) microvascular proliferation with glomeruloid structures (H&E).

tumor mass, creating the impression of a multifocal lesion on neuroimaging. However, molecular analysis shows that these cases represent a single clonal tumor with regional variation in tumor density. In some instances, the tumor may extend into the subarachnoid space or ventricles, which infrequently leads to dissemination of tumor cells into the cerebrospinal fluid (CSF). Extracranial extension and hematogenous dissemination are very rare, typically observed only in patients who have undergone prior surgery.

The clinical course of GBM is highly aggressive, comparable to that of the most malignant human tumors. The median survival for patients with GBM after standard treatment is 18 months; less than 5% of patients survive beyond 5 years. The typical microscopic features of GBM include high cellular density, mixed lineage morphologies of astrocytic and oligodendroglial cells, marked nuclear atypia, mitoses (Fig. 2.3B), and both microvascular proliferation and necrosis. The presence of even small foci of microvascular proliferation or necrosis is sufficient for a diagnosis of GBM, and microvascular proliferation is invariably present in enhancing tumors. However, it is important to note that the microscopic appearance of GBM can be highly variable, displaying considerable regional heterogeneity. In some cases, GBM cells may exhibit considerable nuclear and cytoplasmic pleomorphism, including multinucleated giant cells. In other cases, the tumor may primarily consist of small "undifferentiated" cells with limited cytoplasm, as seen in small-cell GBM. Although many GBMs contain zones with better differentiated fibrillary and gemistocytic astrocytes, they also contain numerous oligodendroglial tumor cells. In addition, other cell types may be present in GBM, including cells with glandular or epithelioid features, granular cells, heavily lipidized cells, and densely packed bundles of sarcomatous cells.

In GBM, there is prominent proliferative activity with frequent mitoses present, including atypical mitoses that deviate from the typical appearance of mitoses present in normal cells. The Ki-67 labeling index, which marks cells in the cell cycle, is likewise high, commonly averaging 15–20%. The expression of OLIG2 and GFAP in GBM is heterogeneous. Necrosis is a characteristic feature of GBM and can be present as either large confluent zones of coagulative necrosis or *palisading necrosis* with a densely packed band of tumor cells arranged around necrotic foci (Fig. 2.3C). *Microvascular proliferation* is defined as an abnormal thickening of the vessel walls in the tumor microcirculation, involving two or more layers of endothelial cells, some of which may be mitotically active. In some instances, these vessels can cluster to form distinct structures resembling glomeruli referred to as *glomeruloid vascular proliferation* (Fig. 2.3D). Microvascular proliferation is frequently associated with thrombosis of the affected vessels.

In recent years, the pathogenesis and molecular genetics of GBM have been an area of intense investigation. Most evidence from human and animal studies suggests that GBMs likely arise from proliferative neuroepithelial progenitor cells, including oligodendroglial progenitor cells or neural stem cells of the subventricular zone.

GBM is one of the most well-characterized cancers at the molecular level and was one of the first cancers to be studied using large-scale integrative genomic approaches. Collectively, these molecular studies have identified three primary signaling pathways that are altered in GBM. First, GBM frequently exhibits increased activation of receptor tyrosine kinases/RAS/phosphatidylinositol 3-kinase signaling. This pathway is activated in 88% of GBMs, primarily due to amplification of the *EGFR* gene, along with rearrangements and overexpression of mutant EGFRvIII and extracellular domain mutants. Activation of these pathways can occur through amplification of *PDGFRA, MET,* or *AKT*; through *PIK3CA* activating mutations; and through aberrations that lead to loss of function for the *PTEN* tumor suppressor gene. Second, *TP53* signaling exhibits a higher rate of mutation and inactivation in GBM than previously believed. *TP53* is now recognized as the most frequently mutated gene in GBM, occurring in at least 42% of adult tumors. Third, the retinoblastoma (RB) pathway is targeted through various mechanisms. Genomic losses and mutation in the *RB* gene, along with genomic losses affecting the *CDKN2* family of genes, and amplification of the negative regulators of the RB pathway, such as *CDK4*, can disrupt normal functioning of this pathway.

In some GBM cases, samples may be classified as infiltrating gliomas without the histological criteria typically associated with GBM, such as microvascular proliferation and necrosis. This can occur when the biopsy can only be obtained from the periphery of the tumor mass or because the biopsy is performed at an early stage of tumorigenesis, before angiogenesis and necrosis have occurred. Current guidelines enable samples to be classified as GBM based on molecular criteria. These criteria include the absence of *IDH1* and *IDH2* mutations, along with the presence of at least one the following three alterations: *TERT* promoter mutation, gain of chromosome 7 and loss of chromosome 10, or *EGFR* amplification. A genetic profile with only a *TERT* promoter mutation has low specificity for GBM and requires active consideration of other potential differential diagnoses.

The prognostic evaluation of patients with GBM is a common clinical challenge, and genetic testing has emerged as a reliable means for predicting patient outcomes. Numerous studies have demonstrated that increased methylation of the promoter of the *MGMT* gene is predictive of improved progression-free survival in GBM when treated with alkylator chemotherapy. *MGMT* promoter methylation and decreased expression of MGMT protein are detected in nearly 50% of GBMs. *MGMT* encodes a DNA repair protein that removes alkyl groups from the O6 position of guanine, thereby reducing the therapeutic efficacy of DNA alkylating agents such as temozolomide.

2.2.1.1.1.4. Glioblastoma variants. Glioblastoma IDH-wildtype, grade 4 (GBM), can display different histological variants. Their prognosis is similar to those of other GBMs.

2.2.1.1.1.4.1. Giant cell GBM. This is a rare variant of GBM that accounts for less than 5% of all cases of GBM. It shares a similar clinical presentation to typical GBMs. Radiologically and macroscopically, giant cell GBM tends to be better circumscribed compared to conventional GBM. Microscopically, giant cell GBM is characterized by the presence of giant and multinucleated cells, which may display variable expression of GFAP. These features can pose a challenge in differential diagnosis, as they are also observed in high-grade pleomorphic xanthoastrocytoma (PXA), although a frequent BRAF V600E mutation and a specific DNA methylation profile distinguish PXA. Giant cell GBMs exhibit a high frequency of *TP53* mutations. In some cases, a DNA repair deficiency is present. However, amplification of *EGFR* and deletion of *CDKN2A* are relatively uncommon in this variant of GBM.

2.2.1.1.1.4.2. Gliosarcoma. This tumor is characterized by the presence of both neoplastic glial and mesenchymal tissue elements, exhibiting an intermixed or biphasic growth pattern. It accounts for approximately 2% of all cases of GBM and can either be present at the time of initial diagnosis or develop during relapse. Typically, the tumor is located in the cerebral hemispheres, but it can invade skull bone and surrounding soft tissues. The radiographic appearance of gliosarcoma can be similar to that of typical GBM. However, if the sarcomatous component predominates, it may manifest as a hyperdense, circumscribed, uniformly contrast-enhancing mass mimicking a meningioma. To establish the diagnosis, it is important to identify unequivocally malignant glial and mesenchymal elements. The sarcomatous regions usually consist of malignant spindle cells arranged in fascicular or storiform patterns. In some cases, other types of mesenchymal differentiation, including cartilage, bone, skeletal, and smooth muscle, can be observed. IHC for GFAP and smooth muscle actin is valuable in distinguishing between the glial and mesenchymal components, respectively. Reticulin stain reveals abundant reticulin fibrils in the sarcomatous component but not in the glial component. Gliosarcoma appears to have a monoclonal origin of both the glial and mesenchymal components of the tumor, with the mesenchymal component representing an advanced form of glial–mesenchymal transition analogous to epithelial–mesenchymal transition in carcinomas. Distinction from vigorous proliferative fibrous reaction resulting from superficial GBMs invading the meninges is important for these tumors.

2.2.1.1.1.4.3. Epithelioid GBM. This variant of GBM is characterized by densely packed collections of malignant epithelioid cells that strongly express GFAP. These cells exhibit abundant cytoplasm and distinct cell boundaries. Histologically, epithelioid GBM shares similarities with high-grade PXA, including similar histology, CD34 expression by tumor cells, the presence of a reticulin network, and the occurrence of BRAF V600E mutations in approximately half of the cases. DNA methylation profiling, which is a profiling technique used to discriminate tumor types based on different patterns of DNA methylation, can be helpful in distinguishing epithelioid GBM and PXA from each other. Identification of BRAF mutant gliomas is of important therapeutic significance due to recent approval of combination BRAF/MEK inhibitor therapy for adult and pediatric gliomas based on significant responses to treatment in these patients.

2.2.1.1.1.4.4. Other GBM subtypes. A GBM with primitive neuronal component contains regions of discrete nodules resembling the "small blue cells" found in medulloblastoma. The undifferentiated foci express neuronal markers such as synaptophysin, but they lack astrocytic markers such as GFAP. They also demonstrate very high Ki-67 labeling index exceeding 30% and often reaching above 80%. Homer Wright rosettes or large cell/anaplastic histology may be present in these areas. Patients with this variant are more prone to tumor dissemination through the CSF. A subset of these tumors has amplification of *MYCN* or *MYC*, and some astrocytomas IDH-mutant grade 4 share a similar histology.

All categories of diffuse gliomas may have mismatch repair deficiency (MMRD) either constitutionally (CMMRD and Lynch syndrome patients with germline mutations) or acquired during treatment with chemotherapy with temozolomide. MMRDs are most reliably detected indirectly by the presence on sequencing assays of a high tumor mutation burden (e.g., >15 mutations/Mb) or by loss of expression of MSH2, MSH6, MLH1, or PMS2 proteins. The presence of MMRD and these findings most commonly result from inactivating mutations in one of the MMR genes or less commonly through promoter methylation or structural/copy inactivation of the genes. The presence of MMRD in gliomas has important therapeutic implications because such tumors are thought to be resistant to standard treatment with temozolomide. Furthermore, some CMMRD/Lynch glioma patients may respond well to checkpoint blockade immunotherapies (e.g., PD1 inhibitors).

2.2.1.1.1.5. Other adult-type diffuse gliomas. Adult patients with tumors that resemble diffuse gliomas but lack IDH mutations and do not meet the histological and molecular criteria of GBM exhibit a broad range of clinical outcomes and genetic alterations. These tumors are rare, and some have been shown to correspond to pediatric-type high-grade glioma types with dismal prognosis, and others to pediatric-type low-grade diffuse glioma types that typically do not progress to higher grade lesions and have favorable long-term survival. Other diffuse gliomas that lack IDH mutations are also encountered and require in-depth characterization to understand their specific features.

2.2.1.1.2. High-grade pediatric-type diffuse gliomas. Patients with high-grade pediatric-type diffuse gliomas typically display specific clinical features that distinguish them from those with adult-type diffuse gliomas. These include de novo occurrence, anatomic origin-related genetic alterations, and diffuse infiltration of adjacent and often distant brain structures. Although classified as "pediatric-type" gliomas, these tumors also frequently occur in young adults as well as adults of all ages. The genetic alterations and DNA methylation profiles of these tumors are distinct from those of adult-type diffuse gliomas (Table 2.2).

Table 2.2 Integrated Diagnosis of High-Grade Pediatric-Type Diffuse Gliomas

INTEGRATED DIAGNOSIS	DIFFUSE MIDLINE GLIOMA, H3 K27 ALTERED	DIFFUSE HEMISPHERIC GLIOMA, H3 G34-MUTANT	DIFFUSE PEDIATRIC TYPE HIGH-GRADE GLIOMA, H3-WT AND IDH-WT	INFANT-TYPE HEMISPHERIC GLIOMA
Location of the primary site	Midline (thalamus, pons, spinal cord)	Cerebral hemispheres	Cerebral hemispheres > midline	Cerebral hemispheres
Present genetic alterations	Loss of H3 K27 trimethylation[a] Histone H3.3 or H3.1 K27M mutation	Histone H3.3 G34R or G34V mutation[a]	Not constant: *PDGFRA*, *MYCN* or *EGFR* amplification	Not constant: gene fusions in *NTRK*, *ROS1*, *ALK*, or *MET*
Absent genetic alterations	*IDH1/2* mutation	*IDH1/2* mutation	*IDH1/2* and histone H3 mutation[a]	*IDH1/2* and histone H3 mutation[a]
Grade	4	4	4	4

[a]Fulfilled molecular criteria by definition.

2.2.1.1.2.1. Diffuse midline gliomas, H3 K27-altered, WHO grade 4. Diffuse midline gliomas, H3 K27-altered, are also known as H3 K28 in different nomenclature systems but represent the same mutation. These tumors most commonly occur in the pons and thalamus, although they can also arise in the spinal cord, pineal gland, and cerebellum. Microscopically, they exhibit an infiltrative growth pattern with variable astrocytic and oligodendroglial differentiation not unlike the morphology seen in GBM (Fig. 2.4A). Mitotic activity and proliferation are commonly high, but low levels of proliferation are also observed. Microvascular proliferation and necrosis may vary. The infiltrative pattern of tumor growth can be highlighted by IHC for neurofilament protein, which marks residual axons admixed between tumor and helps discriminate these tumors from others that display circumscribed growth, such as ependymoma. IHC for OLIG2 marks a majority of tumor cells and is also helpful in the differential diagnosis with ependymoma, which exhibits a low percentage of cells expressing OLIG2.

A characteristic feature of diffuse midline gliomas, H3 K27-altered, is a significant reduction in the levels of trimethylation of lysine 27 of histone H3 proteins (H3 K27me3) within tumor cells. This decrease, which can be assessed using IHC (Fig. 2.4B), results from the inhibition of the methyltransferase EZH2 that results from K27M mutations in histones *H3.1* or *H3.3* or by overexpression of EZHIP. An antibody that recognizes the mutant H3 K27M protein assists with rapid diagnosis through IHC (Fig. 2.4C). Although H3 K27M is the hallmark mutation of this tumor class, they also harbor co-occurring mutations in *NF1*, *PIK3CA/PIK3R1*, *FGFR1*, and the *BRAF* V600E mutation. Cases occurring in the pons (previously called diffuse intrinsic pontine gliomas) often have mutations in *ACVR1* co-occurring with K27 mutations in *HIST1H3C*. Patients with these tumors have a dismal prognosis, with a 2-year survival rate of less than 10% in children and less than 50% in adults.

2.2.1.1.2.2. Diffuse hemispheric gliomas, G34-mutant, WHO grade 4. Diffuse hemispheric gliomas, G34-mutant, primarily occur in the cerebral hemispheres of teenagers and young adults. The hallmark of this tumor type is the presence of mutant histone H3.3 G34R/V. Microscopically, these gliomas exhibit an infiltrative growth pattern, and they frequently display microvascular proliferation and necrosis. Tumor cells have a poorly differentiated astrocytic phenotype characterized by high nuclear:cytoplasmic ratio and hyperchromasia resembling embryonal tumors. Giant multinucleated tumor cells may also be present. An unusual feature among these diffuse gliomas is the absence of expression of OLIG2 by tumor cells. These tumors also frequently harbor mutations in *TP53* and *ATRX* and can have amplification of *PDGFRA* and *CDKN2A* homozygous deletion. Unlike adult GBM, amplification of *EGFR* is rare.

2.2.1.1.3. Low-grade pediatric-type diffuse gliomas. The clinical characteristics of children with the low-grade pediatric-type diffuse gliomas typically include the following features: stable or

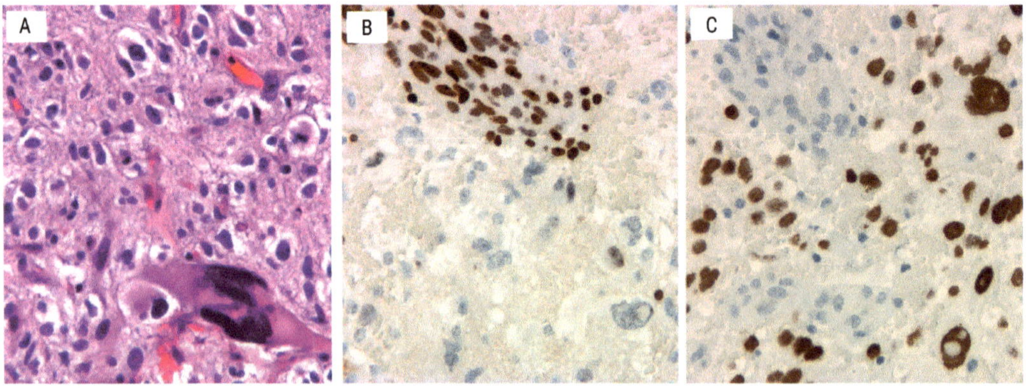

FIGURE 2.4 Diffuse midline glioma, H3 K27-altered: (**A**) astrocytic tumor cells with major nuclear atypia (H&E); (**B**) loss of immunoreactivity for trimethylation of lysine 27 of histone H3.3 within the tumor cells (H3K27me3 IHC); (**C**) immunoreactivity of tumor cells for histone H3.3 p.K27M mutant protein.

slowly growing tumor volume with occasional progression to anaplasia over time, and frequent occurrence at the cerebral cortex responsible for drug-resistant epilepsy. These tumors are grade 1, and some exhibit an overlap of histological and genetic features with circumscribed gliomas and glioneuronal tumors.

Diffuse astrocytoma MYB- or MYBL1-altered, WHO grade 1, is typically a cortical/subcortical tumor with low cell density, monomorphic glial cells scattered in the neuropil, or a fibrillary matrix. The molecular hallmark is a gene fusion involving *MYB* or *MYBL1*.

Angiocentric glioma, WHO grade 1, is typically a cortical/subcortical diffuse glioma with a pseudo-ependymal histological morphology: the perivascular tumor cells are organized into pseudorosettes perpendicularly to the vessel axis and are often negative for OLIG2, positive for GFAP, and exhibit a punctiform labeling for Epithelial Membrane Antigen (EMA). The genetic hallmark in almost all cases is a *MYB::QKI* gene fusion.

Polymorphous low-grade neuroepithelial tumor of the young (PLNTY), WHO grade 1, is typically a cortical/subcortical tumor. The microscopic appearance is highly variable but with diffuse growth and moderate cellularity and an oligodendroglial phenotype or fusiform astrocytic phenotype, organized into vague pseudorosettes. Often, they contain branched capillaries and microcalcifications and express CD34. Sequencing detects molecular alterations activating the mitogen-activated protein kinase (MAPK) pathway: gene fusion involving *FGFR2* is most common, with alterations in *FGFR3* or the mutation BRAF V600E, but there is a high degree of genetic and histological overlap with other tumors.

Diffuse low-grade gliomas MAPK pathway-altered are pediatric tumors that do not fit within the three previous types. Their classification is still provisory. These tumors are described throughout the craniospinal axis but most frequently in the cerebral hemisphere. They can have an astrocytic or oligodendroglial phenotype. Tumors with mutations activating FGFR1 typically have a histological appearance of low-grade oligodendroglioma and were previously called *pediatric oligodendroglioma*. These overlap with dysembyoplastic neuroepithelial tumors. In contrast with adult oligodendrogliomas, they do not harbor IDH mutations and rarely undergo anaplastic progression, similar to other low-grade pediatric-type diffuse gliomas.

2.2.1.2. CIRCUMSCRIBED ASTROCYTOMAS

2.2.1.2.1. Pilocytic astrocytoma (WHO grade 1). The pilocytic astrocytoma (WHO grade 1) in its classic form is a well circumscribed, slow growing, and often cystic tumor which predominantly occurs in children and young adults (Fig. 2.5A). It is by far the most common glioma in children but does occur in adults, although much less frequently; it is rare after age 50 years. The most common sites of occurrence are the cerebellum and cerebral midline structures, such as the hypothalamus/third-ventricular region, optic nerves, or brainstem, but the tumor may also originate in the cerebral hemispheres and spinal cord. The patient's clinical signs and symptoms at presentation are dependent on the anatomic location of the tumor. Clinical progression is in keeping with the slow growth rate of the tumor. Imaging studies show a circumscribed, cystic, or (less often) solid mass with contrast enhancement in most cases. In the cystic examples, contrast enhancement is restricted to a nodular mass of tumor within the cyst wall ("mural nodule").

The microscopic features of pilocytic astrocytoma are highly distinctive in their classic form within the posterior fossa tumors. These consist of a biphasic pattern of compact and loose ("spongy") tissue (Fig. 2.5B, C). The compact zones consist of dense aggregates of elongated bipolar astrocytes with variable numbers of strongly eosinophilic irregular Rosenthal fibers, whereas the loose or spongy areas consist of small, round, multipolar astrocytes in association with *microcysts* and, less commonly, *eosinophilic granular bodies*. The proportion of these two characteristic patterns may vary within a given tumor, and some cases (especially when only a small biopsy amount is available for study) may show a predominance of one pattern. Adding to the diagnostic difficulty is the presence of other tissue patterns (e.g., foci of oligodendroglioma-like cells) that can form part of the histologic spectrum of pilocytic astrocytoma. In pilocytic astrocytoma, microscopic examination may also reveal features that could be mistaken as evidence of anaplasia; these include frequent definitive microvascular proliferation (including glomeruloid vessels); nuclear atypia; extension into the subarachnoid space; and, occasionally, bland (infarct-like) areas of necrosis. Mitoses are rare, and most examples have a very low Ki-67 labeling index (usually <1%). A variant histological pattern formerly named *pilomyxoid astrocytoma*

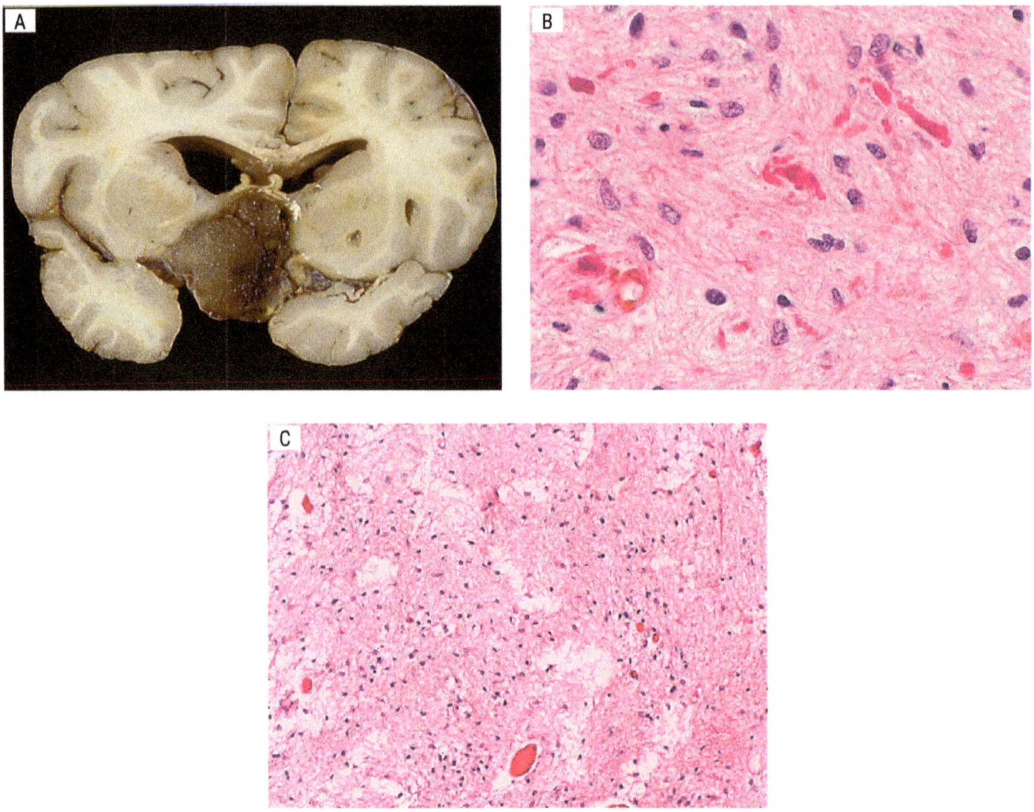

FIGURE 2.5 Pilocytic astrocytoma: (**A**) optic glioma (macroscopic). *Microscopic features*: (**B**) Rosenthal fibers (H&E); (**C**) microcystic change (H&E).

consists of a monomorphous population of bipolar cells with fibrillary GFAP-positive processes within a loose myxoid background; they often have an angiocentric arrangement.

In most patients with pilocytic astrocytoma, the clinical course is indolent; the treatment of choice is surgical excision, with excellent long-term survival. However, when the tumor is localized to the hypothalamus, optic pathways, or brainstem, clinical management will differ, and the clinical course is variable depending on recurrences and progression. Malignant transformation of a pilocytic astrocytoma is very rare, and most case reports have occurred in patients following radiotherapy.

Pilocytic astrocytomas are characterized by the presence of *BRAF* rearrangements or alterations in MAPK signaling genes. The most common alteration is a tandem duplication/fusion event involving the gene *KIAA1549* and the gene encoding the serine/threonine kinase BRAF. This alteration leads to loss of a negative regulatory domain in the BRAF fusion protein and constitutive activation of the MAPK/ERK (extracellular signal-related kinase) signaling pathway. Such alterations can be identified in more than 90% of cerebellar pilocytic astrocytomas but are found to a lesser degree in gliomas with piloid features in the supratentorial regions (~50%). A small subset of cases have fusions of *BRAF* to other genes, all characterized by an intact BRAF kinase domain and a deleted BRAF N-terminal regulatory domain. Additional MAPK pathway alterations described in a small percentage of cases are inactivation of *NF1*, activating mutations in *KRAS* or mutation/fusions of *FGFR1*, and fusions involving *NTRK* family members. BRAF V600E mutation is rarely seen and generally raises the possibility of a ganglioglioma or other tumor. Notably, pilocytic astrocytoma within the optic nerve is the brain tumor most commonly found in patients with neurofibromatosis type 1, a disorder that occurs in approximately 1 in 3,000 individuals with germline mutations in *NF1*.

2.2.1.2.2. High-grade astrocytoma with piloid features. The high-grade astrocytoma with piloid features tumor type is unique in that diagnosis of this glioma relies on the genome-wide profiling of DNA methylation. It has no typical histological feature or specific genetic markers. The tumor can be sporadic or occur in the context of neurofibromatosis type 1. The preferential anatomic localizations are the cerebellum and the midline. In contrast with pilocytic astrocytoma, the peak incidence is in the fourth decade, with few pediatric cases. The prognosis is very heterogeneous, with a median survival of 4 years. The histological aspect is highly variable from a well-circumscribed to a diffuse glioma and can mimic a pilocytic astrocytoma, a GBM, or a PXA. It most often corresponds to astrocytic tumor cells with an increased mitotic activity. The piloid features (piloid tumor cells and Rosenthal fibers) are inconstant (<50%). Loss of ATRX expression, the presence of a MAPK pathway-activating alteration (*KIAA1549::BRAF* fusion; *NF1* or *FGFR1* mutations), and *CDKN2A* homozygous deletion are frequent but lack enough specificity to support the diagnosis.

2.2.1.2.3. Pleomorphic xanthoastrocytoma (WHO grades 2 and 3). Pleomorphic xanthoastrocytoma is a glioma that occurs primarily in children and young adults, often presenting with a chronic seizure disorder. Almost all of these tumors are located above the tentorium, with a preponderance originating in the temporal lobes. The tumor is most often WHO grade 2 and slow growing. PXA characteristically involves the superficial cortex, with extensive involvement of the leptomeninges, and may be solid or cystic (sometimes with a mural nodule).

The microscopic features of PXA include a variable mixture of cell types: typical astrocytoma cells with fibrillary processes, strikingly bizarre giant cells with single or multiple pleomorphic nuclei, and xanthomatous change in the cytoplasm of some tumor cells. In cases of WHO grade 2 PXA, mitoses are infrequent, and necrosis and microvascular proliferation are lacking. The Ki-67 proliferative index in such tumors is usually less than 5%. These low-grade features stand in marked contrast to the alarming cytologic pleomorphism. IHC analysis of the tumor cells shows consistent but variably intense GFAP immunoreactivity, whereas OLIG2 immunoreactivity may be low. Some examples also express "neuronal" markers, including synaptophysin and neurofilament protein, and CD34, a marker of prenatal neural progenitors. Other characteristic but not invariable histologic features include the presence of a conspicuous reticulin network (possibly reflecting a putative origin from subpial astrocytes), lymphocytic infiltrates, and eosinophilic granular bodies similar to those found in ganglioglioma. WHO grade 3 PXA are defined by an increased mitotic activity of five or more mitoses per 10 high-power fields and may exhibit necrosis and/or microvascular proliferation. The prognosis for patients with WHO grade 2 PXA is excellent, with a 5-year overall survival of nearly 90% compared with 55% for patients with grade 3 tumor. Some grade 2 PXA become grade 3 at recurrence. Cases of high- or low-grade PXA typically harbor a *CDKN2A* homozygous deletion (94%) and a *BRAF* V600E point mutation (80%). The identification of BRAF mutations in PXA is therapeutically important because such patients may respond to BRAF/MEK combination targeted therapy, particularly patients with grade 2 tumors.

2.2.1.2.4. Subependymal giant cell astrocytoma (WHO grade 1). Subependymal giant cell astrocytoma (SEGA) is a benign, slow-growing tumor arising in the wall of the lateral ventricle close to the foramen of Monro, where SEGA can cause blockage of CSF. This tumor is characteristically associated with tuberous sclerosis syndrome, occurring in up to 20% of patients with this genetic disorder. In some cases, SEGA may be the presenting feature of this disease and is one of the major clinical diagnostic criteria. Most cases arise during the first two decades of life, and patients present with worsening of a seizure disorder or symptoms of increased intracranial pressure. Some sporadic SEGAs also exist.

The tumor is composed of relatively large cells resembling gemistocytic astrocytes with prominent nucleoli (Fig. 2.6) or spindle-shaped cells with elongated fibrillar processes. Some tumor cells may show considerable nuclear pleomorphism, and occasional mitoses, necrosis, and microvascular proliferation may be present; however, these features, as well as intratumoral hemorrhage, do not indicate anaplastic change. Immunohistochemically, the tumor cells may express either or both glial and neuronal-associated antigens, which may reflect their putative origin from dysplastic bipotential cells in the subependymal region. The transcription factor TTF-1 is typically positive, suggesting that the tumor derives from the medial ganglionic eminence.

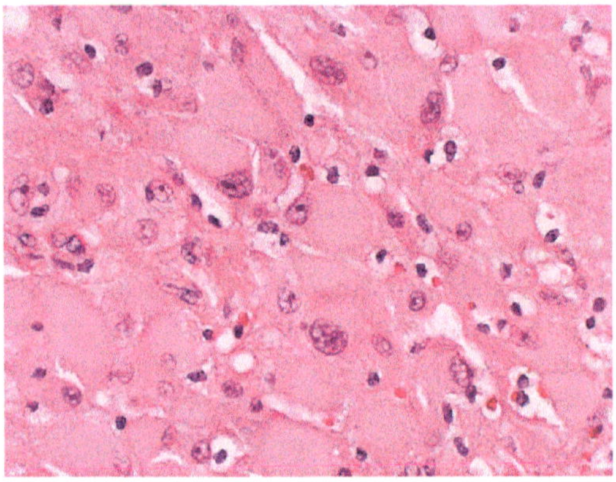

FIGURE 2.6 Microscopic appearance of subependymal giant cell astrocytoma (H&E).

Most genetic alterations in SEGA relate to the two genes implicated in tuberous sclerosis: the *TSC1* gene on chromosome 9q that encodes the hamartin protein and the *TSC2* gene on 16p that encodes the tuberin protein. SEGAs are treated by surgical excision alone and rarely recur. The mammalian target of rapamycin (mTOR) inhibitor everolimus is a therapeutic option for managing patients with SEGA who are poor surgical candidates.

2.2.1.2.5. Astroblastoma MN1-altered. Astroblastoma is a rare glial neoplasm of uncertain histogenesis. The peak incidence is in adolescence, with a striking female predominance, but some cases have also been reported in children and adults. These tumors have been characterized histologically by perivascular pseudorosettes composed of GFAP-positive tumor cells with processes radiating to a central blood vessel, which often has a thickened hyalinized wall. The tumor cell processes are usually shorter, thicker, and less variable in diameter and lack the fibrillar characteristic of ependymomas. Although both low- and high-grade features can be seen, the tumor has not been assigned a WHO grade due its variable biologic behavior and insufficient clinical–pathologic data for analysis. Recurrent genetic alterations include gene fusions of *MN1* (meningioma disrupted in balanced translocation 1) with *BEND2* (BEN domain containing 2) or *CXXC5* (CXXC-type zinc-finger protein 5).

2.2.1.2.6. Chordoid glioma (WHO grade 2). This rare glioma exclusively occurs adjacent to the lamina terminalis on the anterior wall of the third ventricle. It consists of nests and cords of OLIG2-negative, strongly GFAP-positive cells within a mucinous stroma, often containing lymphoplasmacytic infiltrates. Tumor cells also express CD34 and TTF-1. The tumor has little or no mitotic activity and a very low Ki-67 labeling index. It is a relatively circumscribed, slow-growing tumor, but because of its location, it is difficult to treat surgically. When incompletely resected, the tumor tends to regrow. A putative origin from specialized ependymal cells of the circumventricular organs has been proposed on the basis of ultrastructural and transcriptome studies. A recurrent kinase domain mutation in *PRKCA* p.D463H has been described as a common aberration in these tumors, in the same gene that is involved in a fusion event in papillary glioneuronal tumors.

2.2.1.3. EPENDYMAL TUMORS

2.2.1.3.1. Introduction. Based on recent molecular findings, the classification of ependymoma has been substantially revised. Ependymal tumors are now categorized based on a combination of histologic and molecular features, as well as the location of the tumor within the brain and spine. In the supratentorial region of the brain, ependymomas are split into two groups characterized by gene fusions either involving the *ZFTA* (C11orf95) gene or involving the *YAP1* gene. In the posterior fossa, ependymomas are divided into two groups known as posterior fossa group A (PFA) and posterior fossa group B (PFB). The classification is determined either by methylation profiling or by IHC to assess the presence of trimethylation at histone lysine 27 (H3K27me3), which is lost in the PFA ependymoma. Spinal ependymomas are classified into myxopapillary ependymoma and classic ependymoma, and a small fraction have *MYCN* amplification. Furthermore, each of the three anatomic locations (supratentorial, posterior fossa, and spinal) can also give rise to subependymomas. Previously recognized histologic subtypes such as clear cell, tanycytic, and papillary ependymoma are no longer considered distinct subtypes. Instead, they are now recognized as growth patterns observed within classic ependymomas. In addition, anaplastic ependymoma is no longer designated as a separate subtype. However, ependymomas can be classified as WHO grade 2 or grade 3 based on certain histologic features, albeit the clinical significance of the grading of ependymoma is uncertain.

2.2.1.3.2. Supratentorial ependymoma. Supratentorial ependymomas arise in the cerebral hemispheres and can occur in both children and adults. They tend to be more common in the frontal and parietal lobes. These gliomas are typically well circumscribed and lack diffuse infiltration. The tumor cells are relatively small and uniform, with round nuclei present in a fibrillary matrix. Pseudorosettes, regions that lack nuclei around blood vessels, are generally present, although they may be infrequent in some cases. True ependymal rosettes are less commonly observed. Supratentorial ependymomas show GFAP and S100 positivity, which is most distinct around blood vessels, whereas OLIG2 is only expressed in a small subset of cells. EMA IHC typically reveals paranuclear dot-like staining in most tumors. Molecular analysis can further subclassify these tumors into "supratentorial ependymoma, ZFTA fusion-positive" or "supratentorial ependymoma, YAP1 fusion-positive."

In supratentorial ependymoma, ZFTA fusion-positive, *RELA* is generally the fusion partner for *ZFTA*, resulting from chromothripsis on chromosome 11. This fusion leads to the nuclear accumulation of the p65 protein encoded by *RELA* and activation of the Nuclear Factor-κB pathway. L1CAM is a useful marker of ZFTA-fused ependymoma. Branching capillaries and clear cell features are often present in this subtype. These tumors make up more than 70% of supratentorial ependymoma and have the worst prognosis of the supratentorial molecular subgroups. Loss of *CDKN2A* and/or *CDKN2B* is associated with poor outcome in this molecular subtype.

In supratentorial ependymoma, YAP1 fusion-positive, the fusion partner for the *YAP1* gene is *MAMLD1*. These tumors tend to occur near or in the lateral ventricles in girls younger than age 3 years. Despite presenting as relatively large tumors with necrosis, they are associated with favorable outcome. A distinctive histologic feature is the presence of periodic acid–Schiff (PAS)–positive eosinophilic granular bodies, which can be focal or rather conspicuous. Unlike *ZFTA*-fused ependymoma, *YAP1*-fused ependymoma is negative for L1CAM. For fusion-negative tumors, the differential diagnosis should include *BCOR*-altered tumors and *MN1*-altered astroblastomas.

Grading of supratentorial ependymomas as WHO grade 2 or 3 is based on high-grade features such as brisk mitotic activity and microvascular proliferation. The importance of necrosis and nuclear pleomorphism in grading is less clear. Tumors with abundant high-grade features may be considered grade 3, although the grade does not consistently correlate with patient outcomes and distinction between grade 2 and 3 is subjective.

2.2.1.3.3. Posterior fossa ependymoma. Posterior fossa ependymomas are well-circumscribed gliomas that arise in the area of the fourth ventricle (Fig. 2.7A). Although they can occur in all age groups, they most commonly develop in young children. These tumors can grow on all surfaces of the fourth ventricle and may extend through the foramina of Luschka to involve the cranial nerves or through the foramen of Magendie into the cisterna magna. In some cases, they can also arise in the cerebellopontine angle. Similar to ependymoma in the supratentorial region, posterior fossa ependymomas exhibit uniform small cells with round nuclei embedded in a fibrillary matrix. Pseudorosettes are frequently present (Fig. 2.7B), whereas ependymal rosettes are less commonly observed (Fig. 2.7C). Many tumors display variable cellularity with interspersed cellular nodules. Focal papillary or pseudopapillary architecture can also be seen. Although clear cell change can occur, it is less common than in supratentorial ependymoma. Occasionally, a tanycytic growth pattern may be observed, characterized by elongated cells organized in fascicles. Similar to supratentorial ependymomas, most posterior fossa ependymomas express S100 and GFAP, with distinctively increased signal in the pseudorosettes. OLIG2 expression is present in only a small subset of cells, and EMA staining reveals paranuclear "dots" (Fig. 2.7D). Methylation profiling can be used to classify these ependymomas into two molecular subgroups: posterior fossa group A (PFA) and posterior fossa group B (PFB). IHC provides a practical surrogate marker, with PFA ependymomas identified by the loss of nuclear H3K27me3 expression.

PFA ependymomas occur primarily in infants and young children, whereas PFB ependymomas are uncommon in this age group. In adolescents, the frequency of PFA and PFB ependymomas is roughly equal, and in adults, PFB ependymomas constitute the great majority. The median age of initial diagnosis is approximately 6 years for PFA ependymomas and approximately 30 years for PFB ependymomas. Methylation profiling studies have revealed that PFA ependymomas exhibit hypermethylation of CpG islands and global DNA hypomethylation. A common feature in PFA ependymomas is the overexpression of EZHIP, which binds to EZH2 and inhibits the function

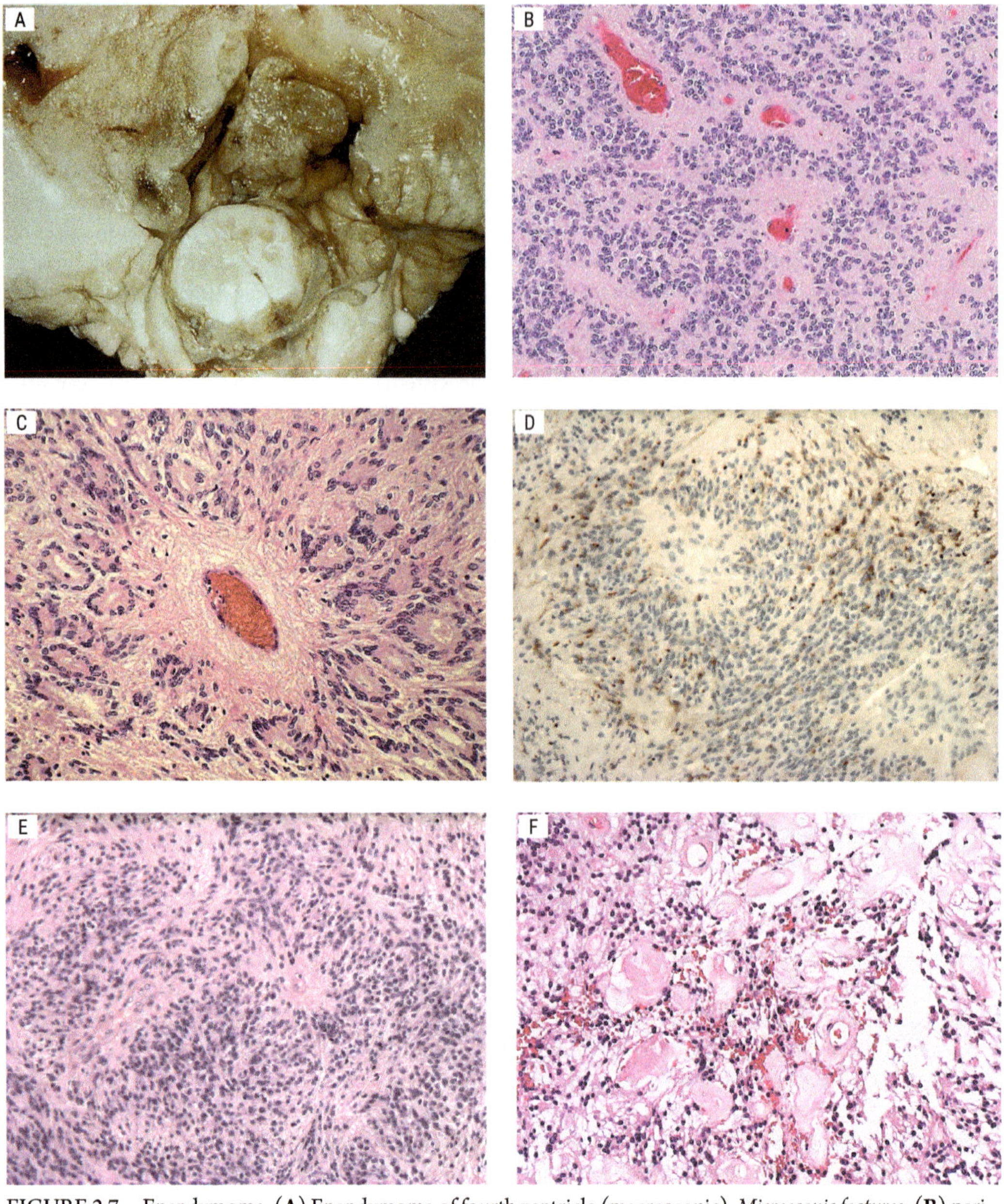

FIGURE 2.7 Ependymoma. (**A**) Ependymoma of fourth ventricle (macroscopic). *Microscopic features*: (**B**) perivascular pseudorosettes (H&E); (**C**) ependymal tubules (H&E); (**D**) dot-like EMA positivity; (**E**) ependymoma with increased cellularity and brisk mitotic activity (H&E). (**F**) Myxopapillary ependymoma (H&E).

of the polycomb repressive complex 2 (PRC2). A small fraction of PFA ependymomas have mutations in the *EZHIP* gene or the H3 K27M mutation, which is characteristic of midline gliomas.

PFA ependymomas generally have a less favorable prognosis compared with PFB ependymomas. Unfavorable clinical outcomes in posterior fossa ependymomas have been associated with gain of chromosome 1q and incomplete surgical resection. Posterior fossa ependymomas are assigned a WHO grade 2 or 3 based on an assessment of high-grade features such as mitotic activity and microvascular proliferation (Fig. 2.7E). However, it is important to note that the grade of the tumor does not consistently predict patient outcomes.

2.2.1.3.4. Spinal ependymoma. Spinal ependymomas are gliomas that are localized within the spinal cord (referred to as intramedullary tumors). They most commonly occur in the cervical or cervicothoracic spine and account for approximately one-fifth of all spinal cord tumors. These tumors share similar histologic and immunohistochemical features with posterior fossa ependymomas and are distinct from myxopapillary ependymomas and subependymomas. Mitotic activity in spinal ependymomas is typically low. A tanycytic growth pattern is more frequently observed in spinal ependymomas compared to ependymomas arising in other anatomic locations. This growth pattern can sometimes lead to confusion with schwannomas and pilocytic astrocytomas. However, unlike these tumors, spinal ependymomas do not express SOX10. Most spinal ependymomas are classified as WHO grade 2, indicating a relatively low-grade tumor. Overall, spinal ependymomas have very good clinical outcomes, particularly for tumors with gross total resection, although these tumors can have late recurrences. A small subset of spinal ependymomas is designated as grade 3 due to high mitotic activity and dense cellularity. Having neurofibromatosis type 2 (NF2) is a risk factor for developing spinal ependymomas. Up to half of patients with NF2 may develop these tumors, although many are asymptomatic. Sporadic spinal ependymomas, which occur in patients without NF2, frequently have a somatic *NF2* mutation and monosomy 22.

A rare form of ependymoma is "spinal ependymoma, MYCN-amplified." Although these tumors share some histologic characteristics with other ependymomas, such as the presence of pseudorosettes and ependymal rosettes, these features can be less prominent. Instead, these tumors exhibit high cellularity, a high nuclear to cytoplasmic ratio, frequent mitoses, microvascular proliferation, and necrosis. They may also display a pseudopapillary architecture. Testing should be used to distinguish these tumors from diffuse midline glioma, H3 K27-altered that can also have *MYCN* amplification. Spinal ependymoma, MYCN-amplified tumors have a tendency to spread within the neuroaxis, and the prognosis for patients with this subtype is poor.

2.2.1.3.5. Myxopapillary ependymoma (WHO grade 2). Myxopapillary ependymoma (grade 2) is a distinct subtype of ependymoma that occurs in the conus medullaris and filum terminale of the spinal cord, with rare cases found in subcutaneous sacrococcygeal or presacral regions. These tumors occur at all ages but primarily affect adults. Patients typically present with chronic lower back pain and symptoms related to spinal cord involvement. Imaging studies reveal a circumscribed ovoid mass with strong contrast enhancement, occasionally showing cystic changes and hemorrhage. Histologically, myxopapillary ependymoma has a characteristic appearance (Fig. 2.7F). It consists of GFAP-positive cuboidal to elongated tumor cells surrounding vascularized and hyalinized stromal cores. There is accumulation of perivascular myxoid material that can be highlighted by PAS or Alcian blue stains. Microcystic areas can also be observed. The tumor is slow growing, with very few or no mitotic figures and a low Ki-67 labeling index that is usually less than 3%. Anaplastic features are not present. Overall, myxopapillary ependymoma has a relatively favorable prognosis. However, many patients have persistent disease, with local recurrence necessitating repeated surgical resection. Pediatric patients have a higher risk of dissemination and seeding of the thecal sac and other areas of the spinal cord. Tumors originating in the conus medullaris are more challenging to remove completely, leading to an increased risk of recurrence compared to those in the cauda equina.

2.2.1.3.6. Subependymoma (WHO grade 1). Subependymoma is a benign (grade 1) tumor characterized by well-defined borders and slow growth. These tumors consist of clusters of cells resembling subependymal glia. Typically, the tumors are firm, gray, and well circumscribed. They adhere to the walls of the ventricles and protrude into the lumen. Although these tumors can occur in various locations of the supratentorial, posterior fossa, and spinal regions, more than half arise in the fourth ventricle and one-third in the lateral ventricles. Other less common locations include the third ventricle and the cervicothoracic spine. In most cases, subependymomas do not cause noticeable symptoms and remain clinically silent. However, in some instances, they can become symptomatic by causing ventricular obstruction and increased intracranial pressure. Microscopically, these tumors are composed of small nests and clusters of glial cells surrounded by a hypocellular fibrillary matrix that stains positive for GFAP. The tumors may have calcifications, and the tumor cells generally lack perivascular pseudorosettes.

Microcystic changes are frequent, most commonly in subependymomas arising in the lateral ventricles. Mitoses are generally absent. Subependymomas have an excellent prognosis, and they rarely recur after surgery. Some tumors exhibit mixed features of both subependymoma and ependymoma; these mixed tumors, when located in the posterior fossa, have an increased risk of relapse.

2.2.1.4. CHOROID PLEXUS TUMORS

Choroid plexus tumors (papilloma and carcinoma) account for 0.5% of all brain tumors and for 2% of the tumors of the glioma group. The tumor occurs most frequently in the first decade, with 10–20% of cases occurring in the first year of life. The incidence ratio of choroid plexus papilloma (CPP) to choroid plexus carcinoma (CPC) is approximately 5:1; furthermore, 80% of cases of CPC arise in children. Both of these neoplasms involve the sites of the ventricular system where the choroid plexus is normally found. They occur, in order of decreasing frequency, within the lateral ventricles, the fourth ventricle, and the third ventricle. They rarely occur in the spinal cord. Most lateral ventricle tumors occur in individuals younger than age 20 years, whereas those in the fourth ventricle are more evenly age distributed. Patients present clinically with signs of hydrocephalus and increased intracranial pressure. Only rarely is there convincing evidence of excessive CSF production by the tumor. Imaging studies show them to be hyperintense, contrast-enhancing, intraventricular tumors. Choroid plexus tumors are treated primarily by surgical excision. The prognosis is excellent for CPP (nearly 100% 5-year survival) but much less favorable (40% 5-year survival) for CPC.

2.2.1.4.1. Choroid plexus papilloma (WHO grade 1) and atypical choroid plexus papilloma (WHO grade 2). Choroid plexus papilloma is a histologically benign tumor whose structure recapitulates that of normal choroid plexus except for having slightly more crowded and elongated papillae (Fig. 2.8A, B). The papillae consist of vascular connective tissue cores lined by a simple columnar or cuboidal epithelium. Prominent mitotic activity, necrosis, and brain invasion are absent. In the majority of cases, the tumor is immunoreactive for transthyretin as well as for FOXJ1, vimentin, pancytokeratin, and S-100 protein but not EMA. Focal staining for GFAP may also be present (25–55% of cases). The distinction between atypical CPP (WHO grade 2) and CPP WHO grade 1 rests primarily on the demonstration of an elevated mitotic index (defined as two or more mitoses per 10 consecutive high-power fields corresponding to 2.3 mm^2) in the atypical tumor, which is also associated with a somewhat greater likelihood of recurrence. In some cases of atypical CPP, the architectural pattern of the tumor is more complex and approaches choroid plexus carcinoma (CPC).

2.2.1.4.2. Choroid plexus carcinoma (WHO grade 3). Choroid plexus carcinoma is a tumor showing clear histologic features of malignancy. At least four of the five following features must be present: increased cellular density, frequent mitoses, nuclear pleomorphism, solid growth pattern, and necrotic areas. In comparison to the other choroid plexus tumors, CPC often shows brain invasion. The diagnosis of CPC is most commonly made in the pediatric age group, whereas in adults the differential diagnosis is broader and more likely to include

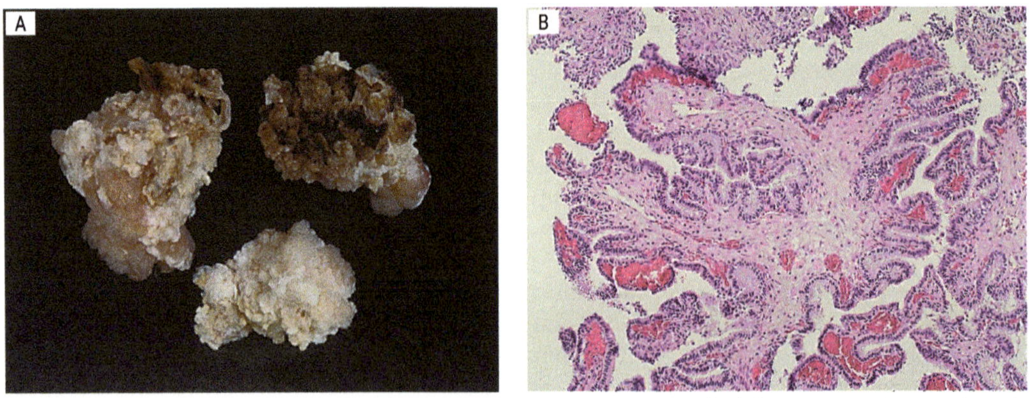

FIGURE 2.8 Choroid plexus papilloma: (**A**) surgical specimen (macroscopic); (**B**) microscopic features (H&E).

metastatic carcinoma. IHC may be helpful, especially if the tumor expresses markers that are considered more characteristic of the choroid plexus; however, some of these markers (e.g., transthyretin, FOXJ1) are not always expressed in CPC or, conversely, may also be expressed by some metastatic carcinomas. In some cases of CPC, the histologic features may include prominent rhabdoid morphology, which can lead to confusion with atypical teratoid/rhabdoid tumors (AT/RTs); however, unlike the latter, CPCs will show normal nuclear immunoreactivity for INI-1/SMARCB1. Comparable to carcinomas elsewhere in the body, the molecular alterations of CPC can be complex; mutations in *TP53* have been found to be present in a subset of these tumors, including familial variants.

The genomic profile of choroid plexus tumors shows considerable overlap between CPP and atypical CPP, both demonstrating numerous recurrent chromosome-wide gains and sharing similar RNA and methylation profiles, suggesting that these are a similar molecular entity. Nearly 90% of CPCs show aneuploidy, with one subset with frequent gains (hyperdiploid) and others hypodiploid. Somatic mutations in *TP53* occur in approximately 60% of cases but are enriched in hyperdiploid tumors. The hyperdiploid tumors with concurrent *TP53* mutations frequently have uniparental disomy, particularly of chromosome 17. Approximately one-third of CPC have two copies of mutant *TP53*, with nearly all having complete inactivation of *TP53*. The number of copies of mutant *TP53* appears to correlate with patient outcome, with the best outcome seen in patients with wild-type *TP53* and the worst in patients with complete inactivation of *TP53*.

2.2.1.5. NEURONAL AND GLIONEURONAL TUMORS

Neuronal and glioneuronal tumors are less common than pure glial tumors and are made up either entirely or partially by cells having neuronal morphologic features. These cells may be evident at the light microscopic level and may range from small "blue" cells reminiscent of neuroblasts to differentiated neurons or "ganglion cells" with vesicular chromatin, prominent nucleoli, and even cytoplasmic Nissl substance. It is not unusual, however, for neuronal features to be appreciated only after immunostaining for neuronal epitopes (e.g., chromogranin A, synaptophysin). Tumors with neuronal elements tend to occur preferentially in children and young adults and can be located adjacent to focal cortical dysplasia.

2.2.1.5.1. Gangliocytoma and ganglioglioma. Gangliocytoma and ganglioglioma are tumors that occur most commonly in the temporal lobe; however, they can arise in almost any region of the neuraxis, including the spinal cord. The tumor is mostly well circumscribed and homogeneous and has an even, granular cut surface, although small cysts or calcifications can be encountered. Alternately, there can be a cyst with a mural nodule (similar to pilocytic astrocytoma and PXA).

2.2.1.5.1.1. Gangliocytoma (WHO grade 1). Gangliocytoma is a rare tumor, consisting entirely of mature, readily recognized, ganglion cells, some of which may be binucleated or have unusual bizarre shapes (Fig. 2.9A). By definition, a neoplastic glial component should be absent. A fine reticulin network may be identified around individual cells, particularly in cases in which the tumor extends superficially along the isocortex. Mitoses and necrosis are absent, and although conspicuous in number, vessels do not have multilayered walls. A variant is seen rarely in a sellar or suprasellar location, with concurrent pituitary adenomas in some instances.

2.2.1.5.1.2. Ganglioglioma (WHO grade 1). These tumors are characterized by having both glial and neuronal elements, and more than half harbor BRAF p.V600E mutations. The glial elements can have an astrocytic or, less commonly, an oligodendroglial phenotype (Fig. 2.9B). In most cases, the ganglionic neuronal component is focal and may be overshadowed by the glial component, requiring immunostaining with neuronal markers for confirmation. Care must be taken that "entrapped" normal neurons (e.g., in a portion of cortex infiltrated by a diffuse glioma) are not mistakenly identified as neoplastic. When present, binucleated or bizarre forms serve to distinguish neoplastic from entrapped ganglion cells. NeuN is often negative in ganglionic tumor neurons and preserved in normal infiltrated neurons. Furthermore, this distinction can be aided with immunostains for CD34 when positive in the neuronal component or when stellate cells are demonstrable in the peritumoral area. Classic histologic features include eosinophilic granular bodies, a unique spindled fibrillar background, and prominent perivascular lymphoid cuffs and stromal fibrosis. The features of these tumors commonly

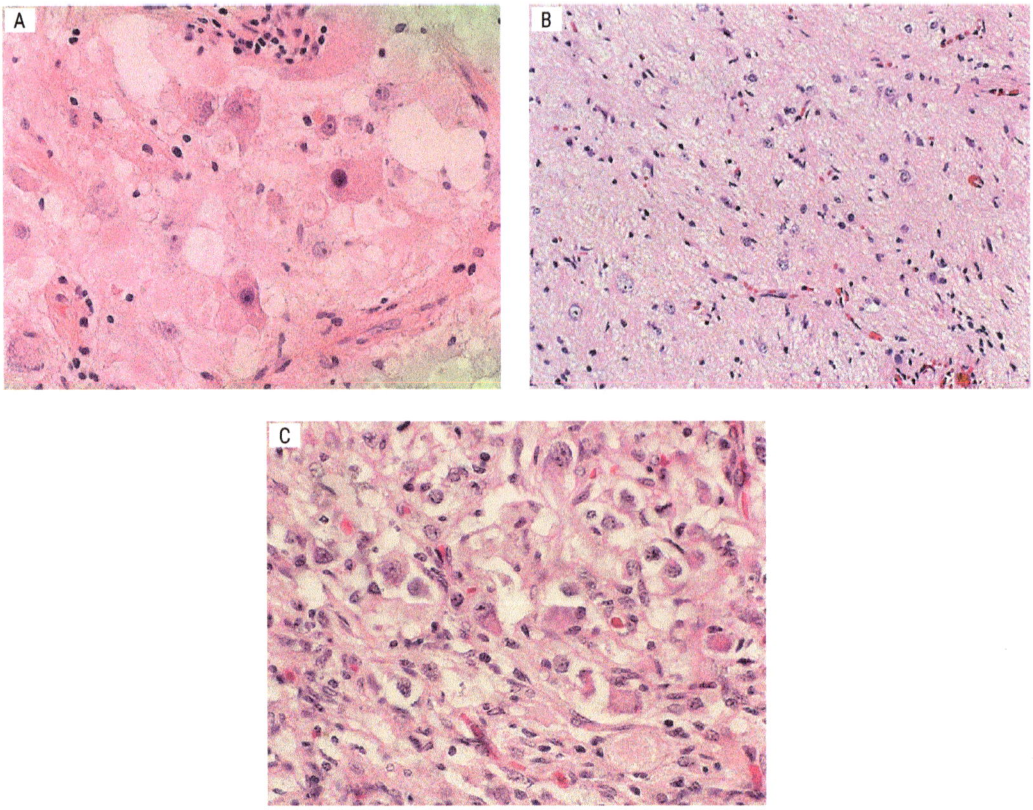

FIGURE 2.9 Neuronal–glial tumors (microscopic appearance): (**A**) gangliocytoma (H&E); (**B**) ganglioglioma (H&E); (**C**) desmoplastic infantile ganglioglioma (H&E).

overlap with pilocytic astrocytoma, and diagnostic distinction is often difficult if the neuronal component is not prominent, although Rosenthal fibers are rarely present in gangliogliomas.

The tumor is slow growing and best treated by excision. A histological aspect of ganglioglioma with anaplastic features should raise differential diagnoses such as diffuse glioma or PXA. Former "*anaplastic gangliogliomas*" are no longer recognized by WHO classification. Given more than half of cases of ganglioglioma have BRAF V600E point mutations and have activation of the RAS/MAPK signaling pathway, therapeutic responses to BRAF/MEK targeted therapy combinations are seen.

2.2.1.5.1.3. Dysplastic gangliocytoma of the cerebellum (Lhermitte–Duclos disease; WHO grade 1). This is a distinctive lesion that is characterized by grossly visible expansion of the cerebellar folia, usually in only one hemisphere. The centers of the affected folia contain large, bizarre ganglion cells, with morphologic and focal immunohistochemical resemblance to Purkinje cells, and some small granular neurons, whereas the surface is covered by aberrant white matter bundles—a configuration sometimes referred to as "inverted cerebellar cortex." In the latest WHO classification, this lesion is considered a grade 1 tumor, but biologically it tends to behave more like a hamartoma than a true neoplasm. Local recurrences after surgical resection are not uncommon.

Approximately half of all cases of Lhermitte–Duclos disease are associated with *Cowden syndrome*, which is a constellation of multiple verrucous skin lesions, facial trichilemmomas, fibromas of the oral mucosa, and hamartomatous polyps of the gastrointestinal tract, as well as thyroid and breast tumors (both benign and malignant). Cowden syndrome arises from mutations in the *PTEN* gene on chromosome 10q, and protein loss of function is involved in Lhermitte–Duclos pathogenesis.

2.2.1.5.1.4. Desmoplastic infantile ganglioglioma/astrocytoma (WHO grade 1). These are rare tumors that occur in neonates and infants up to age 2 years and most often involve the superficial aspect of the frontal and parietal lobes, often with an accompanying cyst. Histologically, the tumor may have both astrocytic and neuronal components (Fig. 2.9C) or, in some cases, only an astrocytic component. Additional characteristic histologic features include the presence of abundant connective tissue (desmoplasia) and a tendency to adhere to overlying meninges. Both types of tumors are slow growing and treatable by surgery. They are caused by genetic alterations activating the MAPK pathway (e.g., *BRAF* mutation).

2.2.1.5.2. Neurocytic tumors

2.2.1.5.2.1. Central neurocytoma (WHO grade 2). This is a low-grade neuronal tumor that usually arises in the third or lateral cerebral ventricle in the region of the foramen of Monro, most commonly in older children and young adults. It is composed of small, well-differentiated neurons with uniform round nuclei, fine chromatin, and occasional nucleoli in a loose neuropil-like background (Fig. 2.10A). Immunostainings positive for NeuN and synaptophysin and negative for OLIG2 confirm the neuronal nature of the lesion and distinguish neurocytoma from oligodendroglioma. The prognostic value of the presence of microvascular proliferation, necrosis, elevated mitotic activity, and Ki-67 proliferation index in some cases is uncertain.

2.2.1.5.2.2. Cerebellar liponeurocytoma (WHO grade 2). Cerebellar liponeurocytoma is composed of neurocytoma-like cells admixed with lipidized neuroepithelial cells (not true adipocytes). The tumor arises in the cerebellar hemispheres of adults, but it can also occur in the cerebellopontine angle, vermis, or fourth ventricle. "Atypical" histologic features are usually absent. Although the clinical behavior of this tumor is generally favorable following surgical excision, a high rate of recurrence is observed.

2.2.1.5.2.3. Extraventricular neurocytoma (WHO grade 2). In contrast with central neurocytoma,

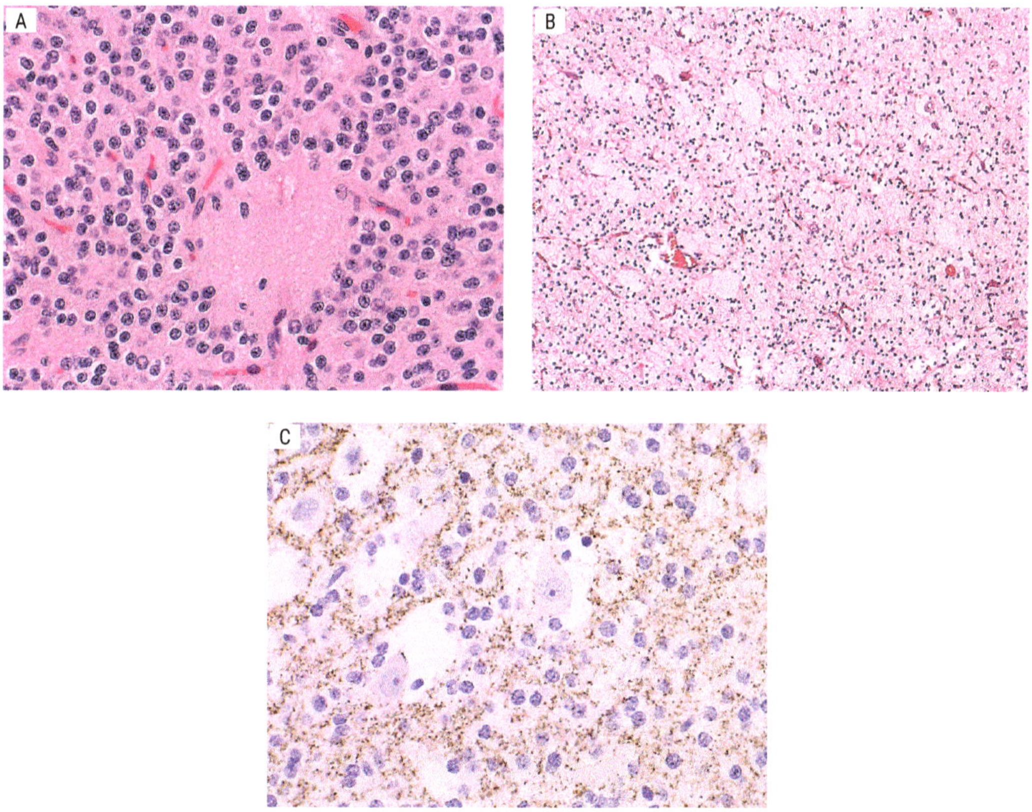

FIGURE 2.10 Neuronal–glial tumors (microscopic appearance): (**A**) central neurocytoma (H&E); (**B**) dysembryoplastic neuroepithelial tumor (DNT) (H&E); (**C**) DNT (synaptophysin IHC).

extraventricular neurocytomas occur in any location in the CNS (including occasional tumor protruding in the ventricles), with a peak incidence in the third and fourth decades of life. They exhibit a various range of histological aspects with intratumoral heterogeneity in comparison with the stereotypical and monomorphous aspect of central neurocytoma. They generally contain a neurocytic component (small round monomorphic tumor cells associated with neuropil islands) and a glial component (astrocytic or oligodendroglial). They often express both neuronal markers (synaptophysin) and glial (OLIG2, GFAP) markers. *FGFR1::TACC1* fusion is frequently detected and overlaps other categories such as PLNTY.

2.2.1.5.3. Other glioneuronal tumors

2.2.1.5.3.1. Dysembryoplastic neuroepithelial tumor (WHO grade 1). The dysembryoplastic neuroepithelial tumor (DNT) is a low-grade glioma containing oligodendroglial cells similar to oligodendroglioma. However, unlike oligodendrogliomas, these tumors have a multinodular architecture and intracortical location, resulting in a multicystic "bubbly" radiological aspect, and they are focally circumscribed on imaging. Most DNTs are revealed during the first two decades by a drug-resistant epilepsy without neurological deficit. A histologic hallmark of DNT is the microarchitectural association of the round oligodendroglial-like cells diffusely infiltrating and arranged along axon bundles bounding microcystic spaces in which larger preexisting normal cortical neurons lie ("floating neurons") (Fig. 2.10B, C). The cortex adjacent to the tumor nodules can show an altered lamination, suggesting that tumorigenesis occurred during cortical development and caused the adjacent cortical dysplasia. Calcifications and cysts are also observed frequently. Mitoses are usually absent or rare. Microvascular proliferation or focal necrosis may very rarely occur, and neither appears to have a negative prognostic effect. Surgical excision is considered curative. The frequent presence of activating mutations in *FGFR1* and the constant absence of mutation in *IDH1/2* support the diagnosis of DNT against adult-type oligodendroglioma. DNTs are typically very localized despite their diffuse intermingling with normal cells, and as such the presence of extensive diffuse infiltration involving large areas of brain should raise suspicion of other diffuse glioma types.

2.2.1.5.3.2. Papillary glioneuronal tumor (WHO grade 1). This is a rare low-grade glioneuronal tumor that most often arises in the deep white matter of cerebral hemispheres of young adults. The usual radiologic appearance is that of a contrast-enhancing, circumscribed solid or cystic mass with hemorrhagic changes. Histologically, the tumor is characterized by pseudopapillary structures consisting of a central hyalinized blood vessel surrounded by spindle-shaped to cuboidal GFAP-positive glial cells with an intervening synaptophysin-positive neurocytic component. The tumor is designated as WHO grade 1, and the clinical course is favorable after surgical resection. A *SLC44A1::PRKCA* gene fusion has been reported in these tumors.

2.2.1.5.3.3. Rosette-forming glioneuronal tumor (WHO grade 1). The rosette-forming glioneuronal tumor is a rare low-grade glioneuronal tumor often arising in the midline along the wall of the third ventricle, cerebral aqueduct, and fourth ventricle or in the cerebellum, preferentially in young adults. The tumor is a circumscribed solid mass that shows focal contrast enhancement. Histologically, two components characterize the tumor: uniform, OLIG2-expressing, neurocytic cells forming rosettes around a synaptophysin-expressing fibrillary core and astrocytic cells resembling pilocytic astrocytoma, a close differential diagnosis. The clinical course in these patients is generally benign after complete resection, whereas despite WHO grade 1, some cases with incomplete surgical resection may gradually grow and become a source of major disabilities or even life-threatening. The tumor typically harbors combined mutations in *FGFR1* and *PIK3CA*, whereas pilocytic astrocytomas lack this combination of alterations.

2.2.1.5.3.4. Myxoid glioneuronal tumor (WHO grade 1). This low-grade circumscribed tumor is typically located in the septum pellucidum region. It exhibits small and monomorphic oligodendroglial OLIG2-positive tumor cells in a myxoid stroma. Floating neurons and synaptophysin-positive neuropile organized into neurocytic rosettes or perivascular pseudorosettes may be present. A mutation of lysine 385 in the *PDGFRA* gene is typically found.

2.2.1.5.3.5. Diffuse leptomeningeal glioneuronal tumor (no WHO grade). This neoplasm mostly affects children and has a striking extraparenchymatous and diffuse anatomic location along spinal and intracranial leptomeninges and in ventricles. Occasional concurrent intraparenchymal lesions may also exist.

The biopsy shows an infiltration of leptomeningeal spaces by diffuse sheets or small nests of monomorphic oligodendroglial-like tumor cells with a clear perinuclear halo. Islands of neuropil and ganglion cells may be present, whereas histological features of anaplasia are rarely present. Immunostainings show a diffuse positivity for OLIG2, a focal positivity for GFAP, and a frequent expression of synaptophysin. These tumors harbor multiple genetic drivers but most commonly have *KIAA1549::BRAF* fusion and loss of 1p; however, IDH mutations are never detected.

2.2.1.5.3.6. Multinodular and vacuolating neuronal tumor (WHO grade 1). This is a low-grade neuronal tumor located in the juxtacortical white matter and the adjacent cerebral cortex. The radiological diagnosis of MVNT is incidental or in the context of epilepsy and shows no mass effect and no growth during follow-up. Neuronal tumor cells are organized into nodules on a neuropil-like α-internexin–positive background. They have round nuclei with visible nucleoli and eosinophilic cytoplasm. They express OLIG2 and HuB/HuC/HuD but not NeuN, phosphorylated neurofilament, or chromogranin. A prominent vacuolization of tumor cell cytoplasms and of the neuropil-like background is a hallmark. Mitoses and features of anaplasia must be absent. A genetic alteration activating the MAPK pathway is typically found in *MAP2K1*, *BRAF* (excluding the V600E variant), or *FGFR2* (gene fusion).

2.2.1.5.3.7. Diffuse glioneuronal tumor with oligodendroglioma-like features and nuclear clusters (no WHO grade). This recently described rare tumor mimics oligodendroglioma with a diffuse pattern of oligodendroglial tumor cells exhibiting frequent multinucleated glial cells expressing OLIG2. The range of atypia and histological features is wide. This tumor has a specific DNA methylation profile and harbors recurrent monosomy of chromosome 14 but lacks IDH mutations and 1p/19q co-deletion.

2.2.1.6. PINEAL PARENCHYMAL TUMORS

Pineal region tumors are rare and comprise less than 1% of all CNS tumors. They are grouped into three major categories: *germ cell tumors* (most common), *pineal parenchymal tumors*, and *gliomas*. Other nonglial tumors (e.g., meningioma) may rarely occur in this region. This section only discusses the pineal parenchymal tumors, which are derived from pinealocytes (or their precursors). Pinealocytes have phenotypic characteristics of both neuroendocrine cells and retinal photoreceptors, with which they share a common embryonic lineage. Pineal parenchymal tumors may be well differentiated and difficult to distinguish on biopsy from normal pineal gland (*pineocytoma*), or they may be poorly differentiated, small "blue" cell tumors (*pineoblastoma*). Tumors with histologic features that fall between these two extremes are currently designated as *pineal parenchymal tumors of intermediate differentiation* (PPTIDs). All demonstrate neural and photosensory characteristics on IHC (synaptophysin, neuron-specific enolase, neurofilament protein, rhodopsin, S-arrestin, and CRX). CRX has emerged as a highly specific and useful clinical transcription factor marker for positive lineage identification of all types and grades of pineal parenchymal tumors, albeit expression in poorly differentiated pinealoblastoma may be reduced. Ultrastructurally, synaptic vesicles and microtubules confirm neural differentiation; cytoplasmic annulate lamellae are further reminiscent of retinal differentiation.

2.2.1.6.1. Pineocytoma (WHO grade 1). Pineocytoma is a tumor that occurs in young to middle-aged adults and represents approximately 45% of all pineal parenchymal tumors. The component cells are uniform, with round to oval nuclei and occasional fine nucleoli, and they have fibrillary or club-shaped eosinophilic processes that may converge in the center of pineocyte rosettes. The tumor has a lobular architecture recalling the normal structure of the pineal gland; however, the lobules are separated by delicate fibrovascular septa (Fig. 2.11A, B). Variable amounts of neuropil may be present in the background. The tumor is histologically low grade and lacks mitotic activity; pleomorphism may rarely be manifest. The tumor is well circumscribed and slow growing but not easily accessible to surgical removal because of its anatomic location. Nonetheless, a 5-year survival higher than 90% may be expected.

2.2.1.6.2. Pineal parenchymal tumor of intermediate differentiation (WHO grade 2 or 3). The PPTIDs (WHO grade 2 or 3) occur in both children and adults but are relatively rare. Architecture is diffuse or lobulated. Tumor cells have round nuclei with moderate atypia and salt-and-pepper chromatin

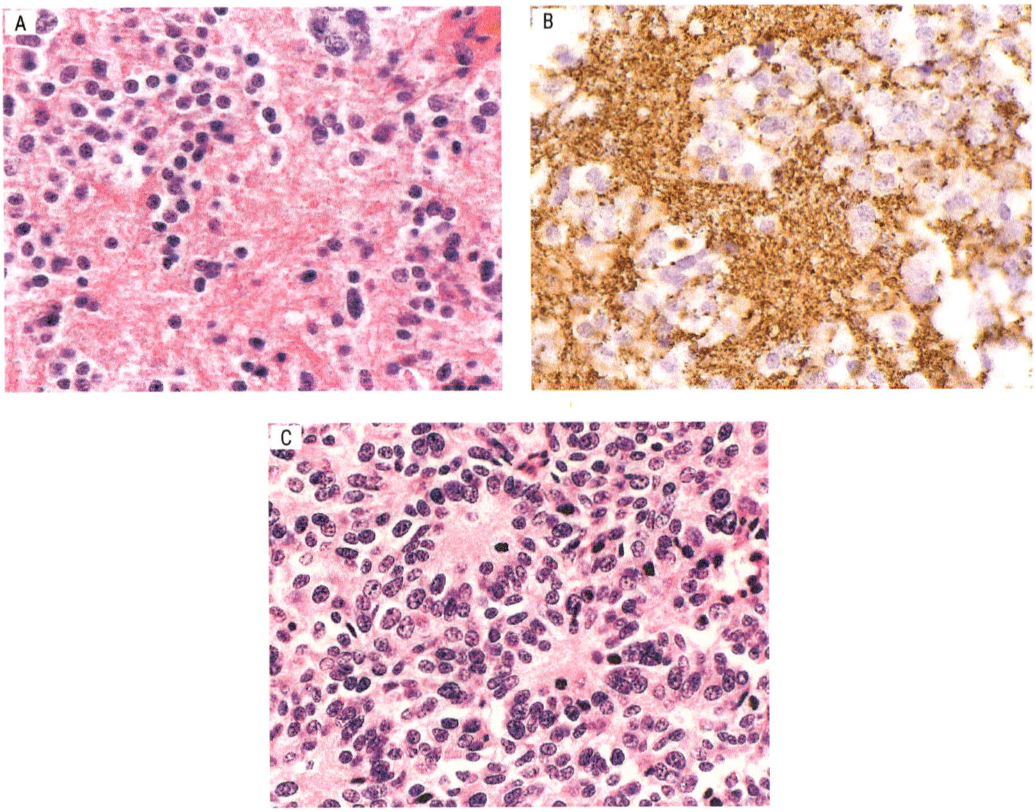

FIGURE 2.11 Pineal parenchymal tumors: (**A**) pineocytoma (H&E); (**B**) pineocytoma (synaptophysin IHC); (**C**) pineoblastoma with Homer Wright rosettes (H&E).

and a distinguishable cytoplasm. Biologic behavior and clinical survival in affected individuals are intermediate between those of the more aggressive pineoblastoma and more indolent pineocytoma. Risk of recurrence is higher in PPTID cases showing high mitotic activity (≥6 mitoses/10 high-power fields), but no consensus criteria are defined to draw grades with firm prognostic conclusions. Transformation of PPTID into pineoblastoma is infrequent. Small in-frame insertions in *KBTBD4* are characteristic.

2.2.1.6.3. Pineoblastoma (WHO grade 4). Pineoblastoma is a tumor that occurs mostly in children and young adults and has a rapid rate of growth. The tumor is heterogeneously contrast enhancing on neuroimaging, and macroscopic features include a tendency toward hemorrhage, necrosis, and cystic degeneration. Histologically, it is a densely cellular small blue cell tumor made up of oval, hyperchromatic nuclei with little visible cytoplasm, resulting in molding of nuclear contours. Some cells may have recognizable eosinophilic processes or form rosettes of Homer Wright or Flexner–Wintersteiner type (Fig. 2.11C). Invasion of adjacent brain structures, high mitotic activity, and necrosis are evidence of malignancy. Leptomeningeal dissemination is present in one-third of patients. Distinct molecular subtypes related to microRNA processing (mutations in *DICER1*, *DROSHA*, and *DGCR8*), retinoblastoma 1 (*RB1*), and *MYC/FOXR2* identify distinct prognoses. *DICER1* and *RB1* mutations may correspond to a hereditary cancer syndrome.

2.2.1.6.4. Papillary tumor of the pineal region (WHO 2 or 3). The papillary tumor of the pineal region (WHO 2 or 3) is a rare neuroepithelial tumor that primarily occurs in the pineal region of both children and adults. Although it is not considered a true pineal parenchymal tumor derived from pinealocytes, it is included in this section because the growth pattern is similar to that of pineocytoma. This tumor is first manifest as a well-circumscribed and occasionally cystic mass that on MRI exhibits a low T1 signal, increased T2, and contrast enhancement. Histologically, this tumor has epithelial features and papillary architecture with solid areas that show occasional ependymal-like differentiation with true rosettes and tubes. The tumor shows immunoreactivity for cytokeratins and focally GFAP; it is negative for neurofilament protein but may be weakly positive for synaptophysin and chromogranin. Proliferative activity (mitotic index, Ki-67/MIB-1 labeling) has been described as moderate. Necrosis may be present, but microvascular proliferation is usually absent. Because of its immunohistochemical and ultrastructural features suggestive of ependymal, secretory, and neuroendocrine differentiation, a possible origin from specialized ependymal cells of the subcommissural organ has been proposed. The biological behavior of this tumor is variable and may correspond to either WHO grade 2 or 3; however, precise histological grading criteria remain to be defined. The 5-year overall survival is approximately 75%.

2.2.1.7. EMBRYONAL TUMORS

The embryonal tumor category comprises neoplasms of immature cells resembling the primitive neuroepithelium, the origin of the precursor cells of the nervous system. Tumors of this type may retain the capability to differentiate along both neural and glial lines, as detected by immunohistochemical or ultrastructural means. As a group, the tumors have a rapid growth rate and a marked tendency to extend into the subarachnoid space, resulting in "seeding" along CSF pathways. Metastatic dissemination to extraneural sites such as bone, lymph nodes, and, rarely, other organs has been described, often as a late complication following treatment or recurrence.

2.2.1.7.1. Medulloblastoma (WHO grade 4). Medulloblastoma is the most common and prototypical embryonal tumor of the CNS, representing a notable proportion of primary brain tumors in children. A second peak age incidence occurs in early adulthood. The tumor by definition arises in the cerebellum (Fig. 2.12A). Frequently encountered signs and symptoms in affected patients include ataxia of gait, headache, and vomiting. Neuroimaging studies typically demonstrate an enhancing, lobulated mass. At presentation, as many as one-third of patients show evidence of leptomeningeal enhancement, indicative of CSF seeding.

Medulloblastoma is currently defined by both histologic and molecular criteria. The major histologic variants of medulloblastoma include the following:

1. *Classic* medulloblastoma is a densely cellular small blue cell tumor that may contain Homer Wright rosettes with central neurofibrillary processes (only seen in approximately 40% of cases) (Fig. 2.12B). Cell death occurs both in single cells (apoptosis) and in confluent fields of necrosis. Mitotic activity is conspicuous.
2. *Desmoplastic/nodular medulloblastoma* is characterized by broad reticulin-free nodules of tumor cells separated by reticulin-rich internodular zones occupied by densely arranged tumor cells. The nodules exhibit neuronal differentiation (abundant neuropil and synaptophysin expression) and decreased mitotic activity and Ki-67 proliferation index compared to internodular zones.
3. *Medulloblastoma with extensive nodularity* ("cerebellar neuroblastoma"; Fig. 2.12C) differs from the desmoplastic subtype by less conspicuous collagenous stroma and greater evidence of neural differentiation in the form of neurocytoma-like broad areas and, rarely, mature ganglion cells, especially following radio-/chemotherapy thought to induce differentiation of tumor cells.
4. *Anaplastic medulloblastoma* shows marked nuclear pleomorphism and molding, cell–cell "wrapping," high rates of single cell apoptosis, and high mitotic activity, often with atypical forms; these features must be the predominant pattern within the tumor.
5. *Large cell medulloblastoma* closely resembles classic medulloblastoma, but the tumor cells have a larger vesicular nucleus, prominent nucleoli, and, in many cases, unusually intense immunohistochemical staining for synaptophysin. The cytologic features of this tumor often overlap with those found in the anaplastic variant; for this reason, the tumor has sometimes been termed *large cell/anaplastic medulloblastoma*. Large cell/anaplastic tumors have a poor prognosis and are considered high risk.
6. *Medulloblastoma with myogenic differentiation* or *medullomyoblastoma* is a variant that includes evidence of "strap" cells, representing immature rhabdomyoblasts.

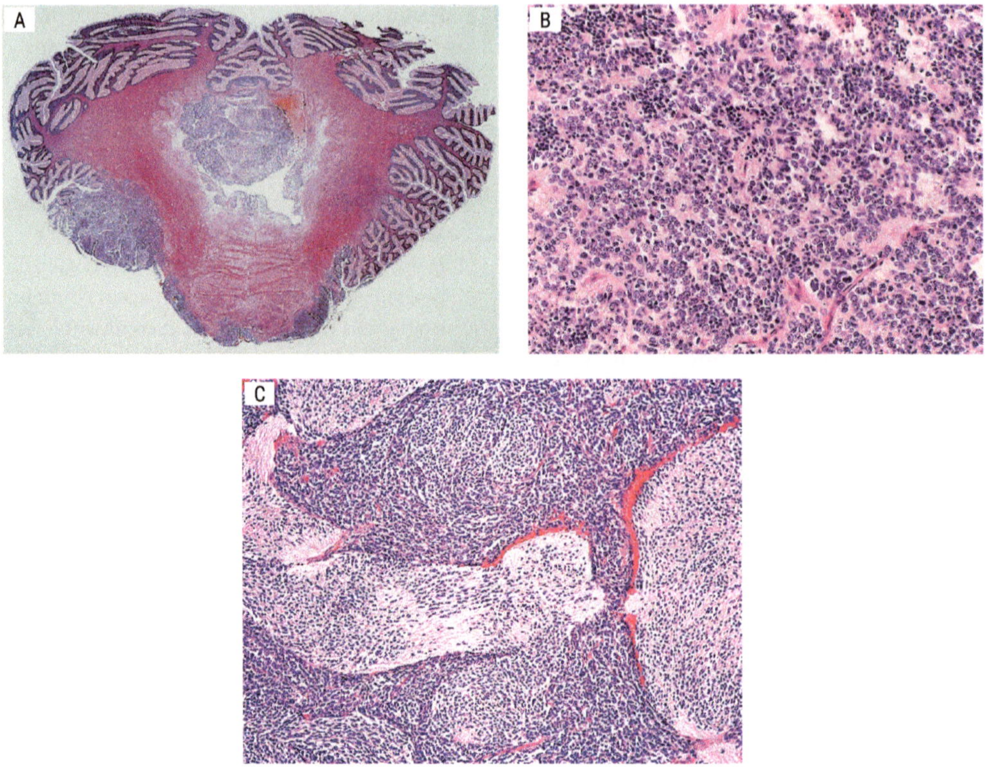

FIGURE 2.12 Medulloblastoma: (**A**) medulloblastoma of cerebellar vermis with ependymal and leptomeningeal spread (H&E whole mount). *Microscopic features*: (**B**) Homer Wright rosettes (H&E); (**C**) nodular architecture (H&E).

7. *Medulloblastoma with melanotic differentiation* is characterized by scattered tubular clusters of pigmented, melanosome-laden tumor cells.

The last two variants are extremely rare.

Remarkable progress has been made in the characterization of medulloblastoma at the molecular level. Three clinically relevant classes of medulloblastoma are now recognized through genetic and/or methylation profiling methods. These classes include WNT-activated tumors, which account for approximately 10% of all medulloblastomas. WNT-activated tumors most often occur in children and are defined genetically by the presence of monosomy 6 and mutations in *CTNNB1*, the gene that encodes β-catenin. Focal nuclear expression of β-catenin on IHC can be used to help identify cases, but genetic or methylation confirmation is generally required. In this class, the histologic appearance of the tumor is the classic variant, and the tumor can arise in patients with germline APC mutations.

A second class includes the Sonic hedgehog (SHH)–activated tumors, which have aberrations in components of the SHH pathway; this class accounts for 30% of all medulloblastoma. In this class, the tumor can occur in all age groups. The cases can be further subdivided by whether they harbor *TP53* mutations. SHH-activated–TP53 wild-type tumors generally have inactivating mutations in *PTCH1* and a deletion of *PTCH1* on 9q. These tumors display desmoplastic/nodular morphology. SHH-activated–*TP53*-mutant tumors can have *MYCN* or *GLI2* amplification and one copy loss of 17p, the region where *TP53* resides. Histologic features in these tumors often include large cell/anaplastic morphology.

The third class includes the non-WNT/non-SHH tumors, which can have either classic or large cell/anaplastic morphology and account for 60% of all medulloblastoma. These types of tumors can occur in all age groups and frequently have isochromosome 17q. They are subclassified into group 3 tumors, which frequently have *MYC* amplification, and group 4 tumors, which frequently have *MYCN* amplification.

Nearly all patients with WNT-activated tumors survive following surgery and adjuvant therapy. The 5-year survival is approximately 75% in patients with SHH-activated tumors and wild-type *TP53*, but the survival is much shorter in patients with SHH-activated tumors that also harbor *TP53* mutations. Patients with non-WNT/non-SHH tumors have the worst outcome, with a large subset presenting with metastatic disease. Genetic counseling and testing are indicated for patients with WNT-activated and SHH medulloblastomas because these individuals have a high prevalence of tumor predisposition syndromes. All medulloblastomas are considered malignant (WHO grade 4), biologically aggressive tumors and require an intensive treatment, including wide surgical approaches, craniospinal radiation, and adjuvant chemotherapy. Children who survive medulloblastoma face long-term toxicities of the treatments, including neurological disabilities and the risk of radiation-induced meningiomas and gliomas.

2.2.1.7.2. Atypical teratoid/rhabdoid tumor (WHO grade 4). The AT/RT is a highly malignant embryonal tumor that primarily occurs in infants within either the supra- or infratentorial compartments. It is histologically characterized by the presence of distinctive *rhabdoid cells*, which have an eccentric nucleus with a prominent nucleolus and "inclusion-like" pink cytoplasm. These cells often exhibit positive immunostaining for vimentin, EMA, smooth muscle actin, and sometimes desmin or cytokeratin. The rhabdoid cell component is frequently admixed with undifferentiated small blue cells resembling medulloblastoma. Some AT/RTs may express widely divergent differentiation along neuronal, glial, and mesenchymal lines. The AT/RT generally has few genomic changes and is nearly always associated with biallelic inactivation of the *SMARCB1* (*INI1*) gene, a tumor suppressor gene that encodes a component of the mammalian SWI/SNF complex on chromosome 22.

The diagnosis of AT/RT and its distinction from other histologically similar tumors have been facilitated by immunohistochemical staining for the INI1 protein, which is normally expressed within the nucleus of normal cells and most other CNS tumors but is absent in AT/RTs. Rare cases of AT/RT have intact INI1 expression and are found to have mutations in another gene, *SMARCA4*, that also encodes a component of the SWI/SNF complex. DNA sequencing can be helpful in the evaluation of the AT/RT with equivocal INI1 immunohistochemistry or in establishing the presence of a germline mutation. Familial cases of AT/RT can arise in the rhabdoid tumor predisposition syndrome due to germline mutations in SMARCB1 or SMARCA4. Importantly, INI1 loss of expression is not specific for AT/RT and is found in other tumors along the neuraxis: some chordoma, schwannoma, malignant peripheral nerve sheath tumor (MPNST), cribriform neuroepithelial tumors, and rare mesenchymal tumors of meninges.

2.2.1.7.3. Other embryonal tumors of the CNS. Other embryonal tumors (ET) of the CNS constitute a heterogeneous group of tumors that arise mainly in children and adolescents and can occur almost anywhere along the neuraxis. They are biologically aggressive tumors. Histologically, they share in common a population of relatively undifferentiated neuroepithelial cells (small blue cell component) variably admixed with more differentiated neuroepithelial cells of neuronal or glial phenotype.

2.2.1.7.3.1. Embryonal tumor with multilayered rosettes (WHO grade 4). The embryonal tumor with multilayered rosettes (ETMR) characteristically is biphasic with small primitive embryonal cells forming multilayer rosettes and differentiated neuropil-like areas with neoplastic neurocytic cells. This group comprises some tumors that were previously diagnosed as embryonal tumor with abundant neuropil and true rosettes (ETANTR), ependymoblastoma, and medulloepithelioma. This tumor arises in the cerebral hemispheres but can occur infratentorially. Occasionally, multiple lobes are involved. Ninety percent of these tumors have a fusion of the *TTYH1* gene with the *C19MC* microRNA cluster on chromosome arm 19q. This results in high-level focal amplification of a 0.89-Mb region that includes the *C19MC* cluster. Although not specific for ETMR, IHC for the RNA-binding protein LIN28A can be used to support the diagnosis. ETMRs are very aggressive, leading to an overall patient survival of approximately 1 year.

2.2.1.7.3.2. Other CNS embryonal tumors. Many embryonal tumors remain difficult to distinguish from one another due to a lack of histologic or genetic markers and lack of testing available to identify specific alterations in tumors. They may be found throughout the CNS but most often occur in the cerebral hemispheres in a periventricular location. In general, these are all aggressive tumors with poor prognosis. New entities are defined by recurrent molecular alterations and DNA methylation profile: CNS neuroblastoma; FOXR2-activated, cribriform neuroepithelial tumor; and CNS tumor with BCOR internal tandem duplication.

2.2.2. Peripheral nerve sheath tumors

The peripheral nerve sheath tumors are defined as tumors that clearly arise from an identifiable peripheral nerve or those whose component cells show evidence (by IHC or electron microscopy) of nerve sheath cell differentiation (i.e., Schwann or perineurial cells). The four major categories of nerve sheath tumors are schwannoma, neurofibroma, perineurioma, and MPNST.

2.2.2.1. SCHWANNOMA (WHO GRADE 1)

Schwannoma is a benign encapsulated tumor that is composed entirely of Schwann cells. The tumor may occur in all age groups, with a peak incidence in the fourth to sixth decades, and is rare in children. Because the tumor arises wherever Schwann cells are present, it may be found to involve cranial nerves (III–XII), spinal nerve roots, peripheral nerve trunks, and even nerve endings and autonomic nerves/ganglia, leading to cutaneous, subcutaneous, or, less often, visceral tumors. Intracranial schwannomas most often involve the vestibular branch of cranial nerve VIII, where the tumor is referred to as a *vestibular schwannoma* (Fig. 2.13A). Most are situated in the cerebellopontine angle and, when reaching a critical size, can cause clinical symptoms due to changes on neighboring structures, which include enlargement and erosion of the internal auditory meatus and compromise of the auditory branch of the nerve, vestibular dysfunction, stretching of other neighboring cranial nerves, and cerebellar or brainstem compression. Schwannomas of cranial nerves V, IX, and X are much less common. Motor cranial nerves are involved only rarely.

Spinal schwannomas are situated most frequently on dorsal sensory nerve roots, but some have also been described on the ventral motor nerve roots. The thoracic segments are most often implicated, but cervical and lumbar schwannomas are not rare. They may also be situated in the cauda equina. The tumor is usually restricted to the subdural space but may sometimes extend through the intervertebral foramen, resulting in an hourglass appearance to the mass lesion as seen on imaging studies. Intraparenchymatous (intracerebral or intraspinal) or intraosseous schwannomas have been reported but are rare.

Macroscopically, schwannoma is a firm, well-circumscribed, encapsulated tumor of variable size. Small tumors are spherical white or slightly translucent and have an elastic consistency. Larger examples are irregularly lobulated and may be cystic. On section, some may show hemorrhages and yellowish foci. The tumor displaces rather than invades the affected nerve. As a general rule, these are solitary tumors; however, in NF2, multiple schwannomas, especially bilateral vestibular schwannomas (which are pathognomic of NF2), may be found. Multiple schwannomas in the absence of other features of NF2 are seen in schwannomatosis. The clinical evolution is slow, and the tumors remain histologically benign but may recur locally if incompletely surgically excised.

Microscopically, schwannomas consist of two characteristic tissue types, which are often intermingled within the same tumor: (1) *dense fibrillary (Antoni A) tissue*, which consists of elongated bipolar cells having scant cytoplasm and cylindrical nuclei arranged in elongated drifts, whorls, or characteristic palisades (Verocay bodies) (Fig. 2.13B); and (2) *loose reticulated (Antoni B) tissue*, which is less densely cellular and consists of small, round nuclei randomly arranged in a matrix containing microcysts and vacuolated cells, imparting a finely honeycombed appearance (Fig. 2.13C). Reticulin fibers are present in both tissue types.

Antoni A tissue usually predominates in intracranial schwannomas. A moderate degree of nuclear pleomorphism may be seen (Fig. 2.13D). Mitotic figures are often absent, but increased mitotic activity does not rule out the diagnosis if both other histological criteria and strong S100 expression are maintained. Many examples show hyaline thickening of vessel walls and sometimes thrombosis, necrosis, and evidence of prior hemorrhage. Unlike neurofibroma, nerve fibers are usually not present within a schwannoma but are displaced and compressed against the surrounding fibrous capsule. Ultrastructurally, schwannomas are composed solely of Schwann cells ensheathed by a continuous

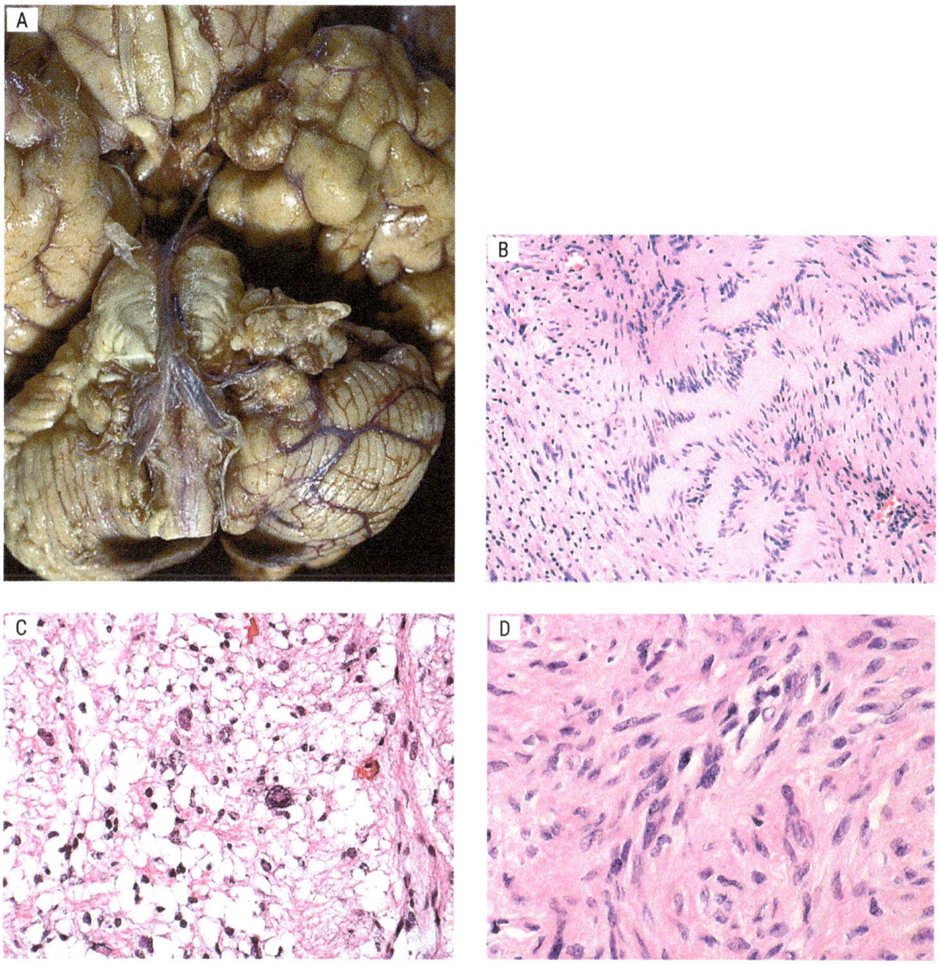

FIGURE 2.13 Schwannoma: (**A**) vestibular schwannoma (macroscopic). *Microscopic features*: (**B**) Antoni A tissue with palisading (Verocay bodies) (H&E); (**C**) spongy Antoni B tissue (H&E); (**D**) Pleomorphic nuclei (H&E).

basal lamina in association with a variable proliferation of collagen fibers. Virtually all cases show strong immunoreactivity for S100 protein and for SOX10 transcription factor; some examples may also show variable GFAP expression.

More than half of schwannomas have a deletion of the long arm of chromosome 22 and a mutation or a deletion of the *NF2* gene on the remaining allele. Total inactivation of the *NF2* gene, with subsequent loss of merlin (schwannomin) expression, is demonstrated by immunocytochemistry or Western blotting, which seems to be a crucial step in the tumorigenesis of schwannomas. Genomic analysis has also revealed mutations in the ARID1A and ARID1B components of SWI/SNF chromatic remodeling complex in 30% of cases. In addition, approximately 10% of schwannomas have an in-frame fusion of the *SH3PXD2A* and *HTRA1* genes on 10q.

2.2.2.1.1. Plexiform schwannomas. The plexiform schwannomas are most often dermal or subcutaneous in location and occur on the trunk or upper extremities. Histologically, the tumors consist of multiple nodules of varying sizes embedded in fibrous connective tissue. Some may be locally aggressive and recur but are not considered overtly malignant. Plexiform schwannomas may be associated with NF2; they must be distinguished from *plexiform neurofibromas*, which are almost always associated with NF1.

2.2.2.1.2. Cellular schwannoma. The cellular schwannoma is a tumor composed exclusively or predominantly of an Antoni A pattern of spindle-shaped Schwann cells without Verocay bodies. The tumor is characteristically located near the vertebral column in the mediastinum or retroperitoneum. Occasionally, bone destruction and neurological symptoms develop. The high cellular density, fascicular pattern, moderate nuclear pleomorphism, and elevated mitotic count can lead to the erroneous diagnosis of a soft tissue sarcoma. Cellular schwannomas always have a benign course and show distinctive schwannian differentiation by electron microscopy and IHC.

2.2.2.2. NEUROFIBROMA (WHO GRADE 1)

Neurofibromas constitute a spectrum of benign nerve sheath tumors that include (1) localized or diffuse cutaneous lesions, (2) solitary or plexiform intraneural lesions, and (3) massive soft tissue tumors. Multiple and plexiform neurofibromas (involving multiple nerve fascicles) are a hallmark of NF1. All ages and both sexes may be affected. Histologically, neurofibromas contain a variable mixture of Schwann cells, perineurial-like cells, fibroblasts, and cells with intermediate features. More cellular central zones containing fibroblasts and Schwann cells with dense collagen bundles and myelinated or unmyelinated nerve fibers are often seen (Fig. 2.14), as well as a less dense peripheral zone devoid of nerve fibers. The Schwann cells and fibroblasts are embedded in a clear, often myxoid-appearing, matrix. Some cases may show numerous atypical nuclei (*atypical neurofibromas*) or increased cellularity (*cellular neurofibromas*), but mitoses are typically absent. Large diffuse neurofibromas may contain tactile-like structures ("pseudo-Meissnerian" corpuscles) and occasionally melanotic cells. Malignant change, including mitotic activity, may develop in a neurofibroma, resulting in a *malignant peripheral nerve sheath tumor* (see Section 2.2.2.4). Such an evolution is frequently associated with NF1 and is seen particularly in plexiform neurofibroma and neurofibroma of major nerves; *atypical neurofibroma/atypical neurofibromatous neoplasm of uncertain biological potential* is a premalignant or early malignant step between neurofibroma and MPNST and is characterized by cytological atypia, hypercellularity, loss of neurofibroma architecture, and increased mitotic activity.

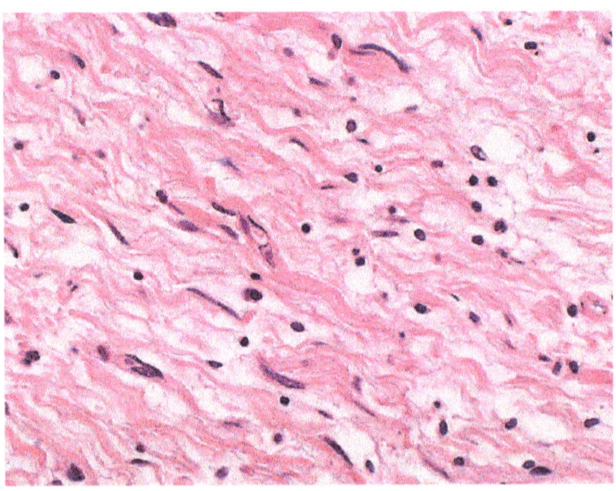

FIGURE 2.14 Microscopic appearance of neurofibroma (H&E).

2.2.2.3. INTRANEURAL PERINEURIOMA (WHO GRADE 1)

An intraneural perineurioma (WHO grade 1) is a rare neoplasm most often presenting in adolescence or early adulthood; it shows no sex preference. It mainly affects peripheral nerves of the extremities and presents as a localized segmental or tubular enlargement of the nerve. Multiple fascicles may be involved, although the lesion does not have a "plexiform" growth pattern. Microscopically, the tumor is characterized by proliferations of perineurial cells in the form of concentric layers ("pseudo-onion bulbs") around nerve fibers within the endoneurium. Although the histology of intraneural perineurioma may resemble the onion-bulb formations seen in the various forms of hypertrophic neuropathy (e.g., some forms of Charcot–Marie–Tooth disease), the tumor lacks the multiplicity of nerve involvement or genetic background of those conditions. Electron microscopy and IHC of the cells forming the pseudo-onion bulbs support the perineurial differentiation: they are immunoreactive for EMA and negative for S100 protein. These are benign tumors with no tendency toward recurrence or metastasis.

Although the intraneural perineurioma is not specifically related to NF1 or NF2, alterations of the long arm of chromosome 22 have been documented in the tumor and probably involve the *NF2* gene. A closely related but histologically distinct tumor also composed of perineurial cells is the *soft tissue perineurioma*, which is very rarely associated with a nerve.

2.2.2.4. MALIGNANT MELANOTIC NERVE SHEATH TUMOR

This relatively rare, grossly pigmented tumor consists of Schwann cells with melanosomes and exhibits immunoreactivity for melanocytic markers such as HMB-45 and MART-1. Representative cases can be divided into two subtypes—nonpsammomatous and psammomatous forms—with the former having a propensity for posterior spinal nerves and ganglia, and the latter frequently involving autonomic ganglia and viscera as part of the *Carney complex* (a multi-endocrine autosomal dominant disorder). Loss of expression of PRKAR1A, *PRKAR1A* mutation, or DNA methylation profile confirms the diagnosis. Patients with malignant melanotic nerve sheath tumor generally have a favorable course after surgical treatment, although approximately 25–45% of cases may have more aggressive or frankly malignant behavior, including local recurrence and metastases.

2.2.2.5. MALIGNANT PERIPHERAL NERVE SHEATH TUMOR (WHO GRADES LOW OR HIGH)

The MPNST is defined as a malignant tumor that either arises from or within a peripheral nerve or occurs in a patient with NF1 syndrome or with a preexisting neurofibroma. Several terms (e.g., malignant schwannoma, neurogenic sarcoma, and neurofibrosarcoma, which are more or less synonymous with MPNST) are misleading and should be avoided. Tumors derived from epineurial elements or blood vessels are excluded.

The MPNST is a tumor that primarily occurs in adults and represents approximately 5% of all soft tissue sarcomas. The tumor can occur de novo or from a preexisting tumor, usually a neurofibroma. The MPNST is very closely associated with NF1, with 25–65% occurring during the course of NF1; approximately 4% of patients with NF1 will develop a MPNST. The most common location is along the main nerve trunks of limbs (sciatic nerve, brachial plexus, sacral plexus), on the trunk, and in the head and neck. An MPNST involving cranial nerves is rare. The clinical course in most cases is poor, with a 10-year survival rate of approximately 23%.

Histologically, the MPNST is a highly cellular malignant spindle cell tumor with nuclear atypia, numerous mitoses, and frequent "geographic" necrosis. Invasion through the peri- and epineurium into adjacent soft tissues may occur. Subtypes of MPNST can be further subdivided into *low-grade* (WHO grade 2) and *high-grade* (WHO grade 3 or 4) tumors, which are distinguishable by high mitotic activity or necrosis. The majority of cases have a high Ki-67/MIB-1 labeling index. Various forms of divergent differentiation may be observed, which may include elements of osteosarcoma, chondrosarcoma, liposarcoma, angiosarcoma, or rhabdomyosarcoma (malignant Triton tumor). Epithelial components (epithelioid, epidermoid, or glandular), melanocytes (melanotic malignant schwannoma), or perineurial cells may also be encountered.

Immunohistochemistry is useful for the diagnosis of MPNSTs, particularly for making the distinction from other different spindle cell tumors with a similar histologic appearance. However, in keeping with the overall poor differentiation of the MPNST, only 50–70% of cases will show only focal S100 and SOX10 protein immunoreactivity supporting schwannian differentiation. For the same reason, electron microscopy has generally limited diagnostic utility.

Sporadic and NF1-associated MPNSTs have complex numerical or structural karyotypic abnormalities. More common ones include triploidy, loss of the *NF1* locus (17q11), and loss of the band containing the tumor suppressor gene *TP53* (17p13). The genetic evolution of the tumor appears to be a multistep process initiated by mutations in one or both copies of the *NF1* gene, leading to subsequent loss or mutation of the *TP53* tumor suppressor gene. Alterations in other genes involved in cell cycle regulation are also observed.

Inactivation of PRC2 due to inactivating mutations in either of two of its components, *SUZ12* or *EED1*, occurs in 70–90% of MPNSTs. Inactivation of PRC2 leads to loss of histone H3K27 trimethylation (H3K27me3). IHC for H3K27me3 can help discriminate it from other spindle cell lesions, as can the absence of *SS18::SSX* fusion, which is a hallmark of synovial sarcoma. Loss of H3K27me3 is frequent in sporadic, NF1-associated, and radiation-induced MPNSTs and more commonly occurs in higher grade MPNSTs. Loss of INI1 expression is present in 50% of epithelioid MPNSTs.

2.2.2.6. CAUDA EQUINA NEUROENDOCRINE TUMOR (WHO GRADE 1)

This neuroendocrine tumor is typically located in the cauda equina region as a circumscribed nodule in the filum terminale or spinal nerves. It was previously named paraganglioglioma. It is made up of cell nests or "zellballen" of plump neuroendocrine cells separated by fine fibrovascular septa. Tumor cells are chromogranin and synaptophysin positive and sometimes express cytokeratins, whereas interspersed sustentacular cells are S100 positive. Focal ganglion cell differentiation may occur in some examples. Unlike paragangliogliomas of the autonomic nervous system, cauda equina neuroendocrine tumors do not express GATA3 but, rather, express HOXB13, a transcription factor that defines the molecular identity of the embryonic caudal spinal cord.

2.2.3. Tumors of the meninges

2.2.3.1. TUMORS OF MENINGOTHELIAL CELLS: MENINGIOMAS

Meningiomas are tumors that generally develop attached to the inner surface of the dura mater. They are the most common primary brain tumor in adults, comprising more than one-third of all CNS tumors. However, they are rare in children. The median age at the time of initial diagnosis is approximately 65 years. Grade 1 meningiomas arise more often in women (2.3-fold), whereas the incidence of atypical (grade 2) and anaplastic (grade 3) meningiomas is slightly higher in men than in women. With the widespread use of computed tomography and MRI scans, small meningiomas are frequently discovered incidentally. Several well-established risk factors for the development of meningioma are ionizing radiation (particularly during childhood), high body mass index, and familial predisposition syndromes. Progestin and its agonists can stimulate the growth of meningiomas.

Meningiomas can arise wherever arachnoidal cells are present. The most common intracranial site is over the convexity of the brain including parasagittal areas in association with the falx cerebri as well as the lateral convexities, accounting for approximately 50% of cases. The next most common location is the skull base, which includes the olfactory groove, intraorbital region, lesser wing of the sphenoid bone, pterion, and para- or suprasellar regions, comprising approximately 40% of cases. Meningiomas in the posterior fossa including the tentorium and foramen magnum are less common, accounting for only 10% of cases. Intraventricular meningiomas are very uncommon. Spinal meningiomas occur most commonly in the thoracic segments and are usually located in the lateral compartment of the subdural space, adjacent to the motor roots.

Macroscopically, the typical meningioma is a spherical or lobulated, well-circumscribed mass that is firmly and broadly attached to the dura (Fig. 2.15A, B), displacing the underlying brain parenchyma without invading it. However, higher grade meningiomas can be broadly adherent to the brain and invasive. Some meningiomas can invade the dural sinuses, whereas others invade bone that results in hyperostosis. Most meningiomas are firm and rubbery, whereas psammomatous meningiomas, which typically arise in the spine, have a gritty texture resulting from calcifications. Meningiomas are usually solitary, but multiple tumors may occur either sporadically or in patients with NF2.

Meningiomas exhibit a wide range of microscopic appearances, encompassing 15 different histologic subtypes. However, except for some poorly differentiated anaplastic tumors, virtually all meningiomas demonstrate morphologic features consistent with their arachnoid origin. The current WHO classification system categorizes meningiomas into three grades. Grade 1 meningiomas represent benign tumors, typically associated with a low risk of recurrence or aggressive growth. By contrast, patients with grade 2 (atypical) meningiomas have a higher probability of recurrence, and grade 3 (anaplastic) meningiomas display aggressive behavior. The assignment of the WHO grade to a meningioma is primarily based on its histologic appearance, along with the evaluation of specific biomarkers that have been associated with aggressive tumor behavior.

2.2.3.1.1. WHO grade 1 meningiomas. The WHO grade 1 meningioma is a benign tumor that manifests the following histological properties: (1) the mitotic index is less than four mitoses per 10 high-power fields (×40 objective; 1.6-mm^2); (2) fewer than three of the "atypical" histologic features associated with grade 2 or 3 tumors (see Sections 2.2.3.1.2 and 2.2.3.1.3, respectively) are evident; (3) the tumor does not belong to one of the defined grade 2 or 3 subtypes; and (4) there is no evidence of true brain invasion. The tumor has a low Ki-67 proliferation index (usually less than 4% or 5%). The well-recognized meningioma subtypes discussed next are ordinarily classified as WHO grade 1.

2.2.3.1.1.1. Meningothelial meningioma. This meningioma subtype is composed of monomorphic cells resembling arachnoid cap cells. They

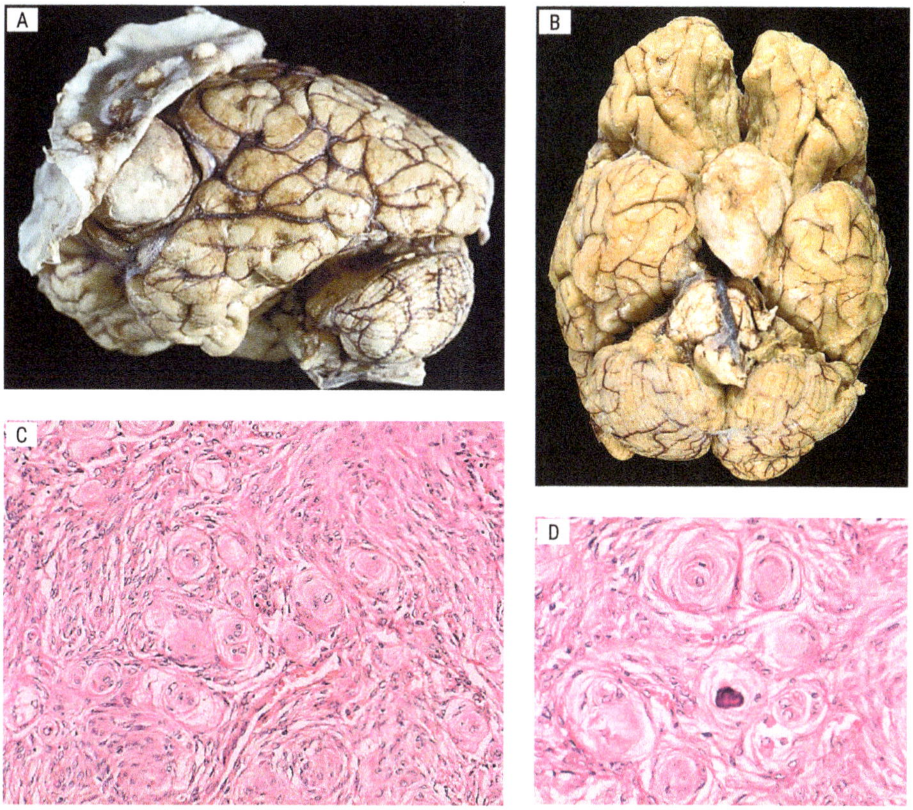

FIGURE 2.15 Meningioma: (**A**) left frontal convexity meningioma (macroscopic); (**B**) meningioma of skull base (macroscopic). *Microscopic features*: (**C**) cellular whorls (H&E); (**D**) whorls and psammoma body (H&E).

have pale cytoplasm and a spherical nucleus that occasionally has a large pseudoinclusion—a clear, well-defined intranuclear vacuole ("hole") that does not represent a true cellular inclusion but is rather an invagination of the cytoplasm. The tumor cells are arranged in lobules separated by scant vascular connective tissue septa. The tumor cell borders are often difficult to visualize, imparting a "syncytial" pattern to the tumor. Psammoma body calcifications are infrequent. These tumors commonly arise in the skull base. This meningioma subtype frequently has a diploid genome lacking gains and losses of chromosomes and has mutations in *AKT1*, *PIK3CA*, and *TRAF7*. Olfactory groove meningiomas commonly have mutations in *SMO*.

2.2.3.1.1.2. Fibrous meningioma. Fibrous meningioma is characterized by the presence of elongated fusiform cells arranged in wavy interlacing fascicles and a storiform pattern. Between the individual cells, there may be a well-developed network of collagen and reticulin fibers. When extensive, the possibility of a solitary fibrous tumor should be considered, which can be identified by the presence of nuclear STAT6 using IHC. Fibrous meningiomas frequently arise over the convexities.

2.2.3.1.1.3. Transitional meningioma. The transitional meningioma is a commonly encountered subtype characterized by the presence of mixed histology, comprising both meningothelial and fibrous elements, as well as transitional features. A distinctive and diagnostically useful pattern is the formation of cellular *whorls* (Fig. 2.15C) in which tumor cells wrap tightly around one another. These whorls can hyalinize and undergo calcification, giving rise to structures known as *psammoma bodies* (Fig. 2.15D). Fibrous meningiomas and transitional meningioma typically arise from the dural convexities and have monosomy 22 and pathogenic mutations of *NF2*.

2.2.3.1.1.4. Psammomatous meningioma. This subtype is characterized by the presence of numerous psammoma bodies, which can sometimes merge to form confluent masses with sparse tumor cells. The tumors display fibrous and transitional histology, and they are frequently develop in the thoracic spinal region, primarily affecting middle-aged to elderly women. These meningiomas have monosomy of chromosome 22 and inactivation of *NF2*.

2.2.3.1.1.5. Angiomatous meningioma. Angiomatous meningioma is distinguished by an abundant vasculature, comprising densely packed blood vessels that frequently have hyalinized walls. Although tumor cells can have large and irregular nuclei, this feature is not associated with aggressive behavior and is termed "degenerative atypia." The histologic features of this variant often overlap with those of microcystic meningioma, and they share similar molecular genetic features such as polysomies of multiple chromosomes, including 5, 13, and 20.

2.2.3.1.1.6. Microcystic meningioma. A microcystic meningioma has tumor cells with thin elongated (cobweb-like) processes that form multiple small "microcystic" spaces.

2.2.3.1.1.7. Secretory meningioma. The secretory meningioma is a variant characterized by the presence of small eosinophilic PAS-positive globular inclusions within gland-like spaces bordered by cells that are immunoreactive for carcinoembryonic antigen and cytokeratin (in addition to EMA). This subtype is characterized by mutation of both *KLF4* and *TRAF7*.

2.2.3.1.1.8. Lymphoplasmacyte-rich meningioma. This subtype is rare and demonstrates prominent chronic inflammation (including macrophages and lymphocytes and variable, often limited numbers of plasma cells) that can overshadow the tumor component. A differential diagnosis is the Rosai–Dorfman syndrome (see Section 2.3.2.2).

2.2.3.1.1.9. Metaplastic meningiomas. Metaplastic meningiomas include tumors that show (1) *lipomatous* change, (2) *myxomatous* change characterized by an abundant homogeneous stroma separating the individual cells, (3) *cartilage or bone* within the tumor, or (4) *melanin pigment* within the connective tissue trabeculae (pigmented meningiomas).

2.2.3.1.2. WHO grade 2 meningiomas. A meningioma is classified as WHO grade 2 if it falls into either of the following two groups: (1) *atypical meningioma*, which is determined by specific histologic criteria as explained in the following section; or (2) *chordoid* or *clear cell* subtype. Meningioma that exhibits histologic characteristics resembling a benign (WHO grade 1) tumor but *shows true brain invasion* must be tested for the absence of molecular criteria of grade 2 or 3 in order to remain grade 1.

2.2.3.1.2.1. Atypical meningioma. An atypical meningioma is characterized by either *increased mitotic activity (four or more mitoses per 10 high-power fields)* or the presence of *three or more of the following histologic features*: (1) increased cellularity, (2) small cells with a high nuclear:cytoplasmic ratio, (3) prominent nucleoli, (4) uninterrupted patternless or sheet-like growth, or (5) foci of spontaneous necrosis that does not result from therapeutic interventions such as embolization. The presence of "cytologic atypia" (enlarged or bizarre-appearing hyperchromatic nuclei) is not a required or defining feature for classifying a tumor as an atypical meningioma. The Ki-67 labeling indices of WHO grade 2 meningiomas are moderately high (usually >4% and <10%) but can vary. Some cases may overlap with grade 1 tumors, whereas others may approach the range of anaplastic meningioma.

2.2.3.1.2.2. Chordoid meningioma. This is an uncommon meningioma subtype in which the majority of the tumor resembles chordoma, with epithelioid (and less often spindled) cells that form cords or trabeculae which are embedded in a mucin-rich matrix that can be visualized using an Alcian blue histochemical stain. The tumor cells are variably vacuolated, and inflammatory cell infiltrates may be prominent. The genetic profile of these tumors is similar to those of other grade 2 meningiomas.

2.2.3.1.2.3. Clear cell meningioma. This is a rare meningioma subtype characterized by a patternless proliferation of polygonal cells with clear cytoplasm (which is positive for PAS due to its glycogen content) and prominent perivascular and interstitial collagen. The tumor generally lacks other histologic features typical of meningioma. It tends to localize in the spinal cord and the cerebellopontine angle. This subtype is most commonly observed in children and young adults. The biologic behavior of the tumor is aggressive, with frequent recurrence and occasional seeding of the CSF. These tumors are characterized by inactivation of *SMARCE1*.

2.2.3.1.3. WHO grade 3 meningiomas. A meningioma is classified as WHO grade 3 if it falls into one of the following two groups: (1) *anaplastic meningioma* based on specific histologic criteria described in the following section or (2) *papillary* or *rhabdoid* subtype with anaplastic features.

2.2.3.1.3.1. Anaplastic meningioma. An anaplastic meningioma is characterized by either *histologic features that resemble frank malignancy* (e.g., carcinomas, sarcomas, or melanomas) or the presence of *20 or more mitoses per 10 high-power fields* (*1.6 mm*^{2}), or a *TERT* promoter mutation, or a *CDKN2A/B* homozygous deletion. Generally, the distinction between atypical and anaplastic meningioma is clear-cut, although there are some borderline cases that pose challenges for classification. Tumors displaying diffusely anaplastic histology can be diagnostically difficult and may require evidence of evolution from a lower grade meningioma at the same site or compelling immunohistochemical or molecular data. The Ki-67 labeling index is typically greater than 15–20%.

Anaplastic meningiomas exhibit aggressive biologic behavior, with a median survival of approximately 2 years. Although invasion of the brain parenchyma is commonly observed in these tumors, it is not solely sufficient for the diagnosis of anaplastic meningioma because lower grade meningiomas can also exhibit brain invasion. In rare cases, the tumor may spread within the CNS along CSF pathways or present with metastatic disease outside the nervous system.

2.2.3.1.3.2. Papillary meningioma. This is a rare meningioma subtype characterized by the presence of a perivascular pseudopapillary growth pattern. In some cases, the tumor cells lining the papillary structures exhibit rhabdoid cytomorphology. These tumors are aggressive and are often invasive, recurrent, and even metastatic.

2.2.3.1.3.3. Rhabdoid meningioma. A rhabdoid meningioma is an uncommon tumor characterized by the presence of discohesive aggregates or sheets of cells that resemble classic rhabdoid cells. These cells have plump eccentric nuclei with macronucleoli and prominent pink cytoplasmic inclusions. Despite their resemblance to rhabdoid cell tumors found in other locations, the tumor cells in rhabdoid meningioma exhibit *normal* nuclear immunoreactivity for the INI1 protein. Rhabdoid meningioma can have inactivation of the *BAP1* gene and then have aggressive evolution. Initially, the cohorts describing this rhabdoid subtype consisted of highly aggressive tumors with grade 3 histology. More recent cohorts have shown that some meningiomas with rhabdoid features lack other malignant characteristics. These tumors demonstrate less aggressive behavior and should be graded according to the standard criteria used for grading meningiomas (grade 1 or 2), as described above. Tumors having both rhabdoid and papillary architecture may occur.

2.2.3.1.4. Familial predisposition syndromes. Genetic factors that predispose to meningioma development are now well established. The risk of developing a meningioma is significantly increased in individuals with NF2, an autosomal dominant disease resulting from germline mutation of the *NF2* gene. Individuals with NF2 may also develop schwannomas, particularly bilateral vestibular schwannomas, and also spinal ependymomas. Another genetic link exists between pathogenic germline variants in *SMARCE1* and the development of clear cell meningiomas in the spine and, less frequently, in the cranium. Schwannomatosis characterized by multiple cutaneous, spinal, and cranial schwannomas may develop in individuals with germline pathogenic variants in *SMARCB1* or *LZTR1* coupled with inactivation of the *NF2* gene that occurs within the tumor cells but not in the germline. These individuals can also develop cranial and spinal meningiomas. Aggressive meningiomas including ones with rhabdoid and rhabdoid–papillary histology can occur in patients with the BAP1 tumor predisposition syndrome, resulting from pathogenic variants in the *BAP1* gene. Family members of these individuals may have other BAP1-related tumors, including uveal melanoma, cutaneous melanoma, renal cell carcinoma, and mesothelioma. Assessing familial risk is important in each of these tumor predisposition syndromes.

2.2.3.1.5. Molecular changes associated with aggressive behavior. Recurrent cytogenetic abnormalities are found in meningiomas, generally in accordance with the tumor grade. More than 50% of WHO grade 1 meningiomas have loss of one copy of chromosome 22 (monosomy 22). However, many other grade 1 meningiomas lack any recurrent copy number changes. By contrast, grade 2 and 3 meningiomas frequently exhibit additional recurrent copy number aberrations, such as loss of chromosome 1p; gain of chromosome 1q; or monosomies of chromosomes 6, 10, 14, and 18. Loss of 1p is the most commonly observed copy number alteration associated with unfavorable clinical outcomes. Meningiomas with loss of chromosome 1p, along with co-occurring monosomy of 22q and/or *NF2* mutation, are now considered to represent grade 2 tumors, even if they appear histologically benign. Grade 3 meningiomas often present with a one or two copy loss of *CDKN2A* on chromosome 9p21, which is associated with very poor prognosis. In addition, mutations in the *TERT* promoter (C228T and C250T) and somatic intragenic deletions of the *DMD* gene, located on the X chromosome, are associated with aggressive behavior in meningiomas.

2.2.3.2. NONMENINGOTHELIAL MESENCHYMAL TUMORS

2.2.3.2.1. Solitary fibrous tumor (WHO grade 1, 2, or 3). Solitary fibrous tumors are much less frequent than meningioma, accounting for less than 1% of all CNS tumors. Macroscopically, the tumors are often firm and well circumscribed and attached to the dura, thereby resembling meningiomas. The microscopic characteristics can vary. At one end of the histologic spectrum are tumors that consist of ovoid monomorphic tumor cells with admixed conspicuous bands of collagen fibers and prominent dilated thin-walled and hyalinized branching ("staghorn") blood vessels. At the other end are cellular tumors with densely packed round to ovoid cells that have limited stroma and less obvious vasculature. Most of these tumors have an inversion involving chromosome 12q13 that results in fusions of the *NAB2* and *STAT6* genes, resulting in strong expression of STAT6 in the nucleus of tumor cells that can be detected by IHC. In the CNS, a three-tier grading system is currently used. Grade 1 tumors have less than five mitoses per 10 high-power fields. They are generally hypocellular and highly collagenized. Grade 2 or 3 tumors have five or more mitoses per 10 high-power fields, but grade 3 tumors also have necrosis. Both grades 2 and 3 are generally densely cellular tumors.

2.2.3.2.2. Hemangioblastoma (WHO grade 1). Hemangioblastoma accounts for approximately 1–2.5% of all intracranial tumors and 7% of the primary tumors originating in the posterior fossa. It may also occur within the parenchyma of the spinal cord, the medulla oblongata, and, rarely, the supratentorial compartment. The tumor can occur at any age.

Although hemangioblastoma is most often a solitary tumor, in approximately 25% of cases there may be multiple tumors, especially in the setting of von Hippel–Lindau (VHL) disease. This inherited autosomal dominant condition is caused by mutations of the *VHL* tumor suppressor gene located on chromosome 3p. The diagnosis of VHL disease is based on the presence of a CNS or retinal hemangioblastoma or association with a known family history, pheochromocytoma, clear cell renal carcinoma, pancreatic tumor, or endolymphatic sac tumor of the inner ear.

Macroscopically, the tumor is well circumscribed and very often cystic, sometimes consisting solely of a small mural nodule attached to the wall of a large cyst. The characteristic yellow color of the tumor is due to its abundant lipid content. The rich vascularization of the tumor is drained by well-developed vascular pedicles and accounts for the frequency of bleeding within the tumor.

The histological picture of hemangioblastoma is highly characteristic, consisting of numerous capillary blood vessels of different sizes separated by trabeculae or sheets of clear cells (*stromal cells*) with round or elongated nuclei (Fig. 2.16). These stromal cells, which are considered the neoplastic component of the tumor, often have a spongy appearance due to an abundance of intracytoplasmic vacuoles

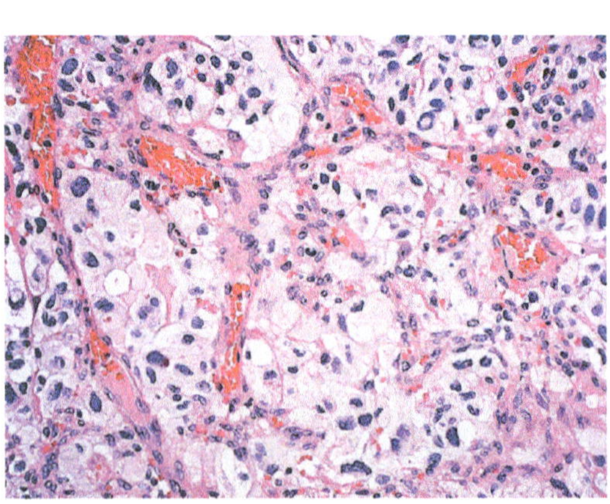

FIGURE 2.16 Hemangioblastoma: microscopic appearance (H&E).

that have been emptied of their lipid contents as a result of the embedding procedure. Mitoses are rare. A fine network of reticulin fibers surrounds the capillary blood vessels and individual stromal cells. The endothelial cells express factor VIII, CD31, CD34, and vascular endothelial growth factor (VEGF) receptor. The stromal cells do not express endothelial cell markers, GFAP, EMA, or cytokeratin, but they do express vimentin, inhibin, S100, and VEGF. In some cases, these immunohistochemical characteristics may be helpful in distinguishing between hemangioblastoma and metastatic clear cell renal carcinoma. Approximately 10% of cases of hemangioblastoma will have foci of extramedullary hematopoiesis, most likely due to erythropoietin production by the stromal cells.

From the molecular standpoint, a complex including VHL targets the transcription factor hypoxia-inducible factor (HIF) to proteasomal degradation after polyubiquitination. Loss of function of VHL results in abnormal accumulation of HIF, which in turn leads to overexpression of several hypoxia-inducible genes, including VEGF, erythropoietin, and platelet-derived growth factor, which have been related to the development of various angiogenic tumors.

Hemangioblastoma is a histologically benign tumor (WHO grade 1) with a low Ki-67 proliferation index (<2%), but postoperative recurrences occur if incompletely resected. The prognosis in patients with VHL is somewhat less favorable due to the occurrence of multiple tumors.

2.2.3.2.3. Mesenchymal tumors of uncertain differentiation. Regarding intracranial tumors of uncertain differentiation, the phenotype of the tumor cells is not related to a normal cell type, and the definition of tumor types involves molecular alterations. *Intracranial mesenchymal tumor FET::CREB fusion-positive* exhibits a wide spectrum of histological aspects with collagenous or myxoid stroma and frequent dense lymphoplasmacytic infiltrates at the periphery of the tumor. This tumor type is defined by a fusion of a FET RNA-binding protein family gene with a member of the CREB family of transcription factor. *CIC-rearranged sarcoma* is composed of sheets of small round hyperchromatic tumor cells. It contains a fusion of the CIC transcriptional repressor with various partners (most often DUX4). *Primary intracranial sarcoma DICER1-mutant* is caused by somatic or germline mutation of *DICER1*, which encodes a microRNA processing enzyme. It is composed of spindle or pleomorphic cells with myogenic or cartilaginous differentiation. *Ewing sarcoma* contains a gene fusion between a FET RNA-binding protein family member and an ETS transcription factor, most frequently *EWSR1::FLI1*. It is composed of sheets of monomorphic, small round hyperchromatic tumor cells.

2.2.3.2.4. Other mesenchymal nonmeningothelial tumors. Various other benign and malignant tumors of mesenchymal origin may arise within the CNS; their histologic appearance is essentially identical to their extra-CNS counterparts arising from soft tissue and bone. These are rare tumors (<0.5% of all intracranial tumors) and may occur at any age. Many of these tumors are localized to the skull, vertebral column, or meninges but can also occur within the brain or spinal cord (e.g., lipoma). The etiology is largely unknown, although some malignant examples (sarcomas) have been related to prior cranial radiation; more recently, Epstein-Barr virus (EBV) has been implicated in the pathogenesis of cranial and spinal smooth muscle tumors in immunocompromised patients.

2.2.3.2.4.1. Tumors of adipose tissue. *Lipomas* are rare benign growths. In the cranial cavity, they favor midline sites: corpus callosum (often associated with partial or complete agenesis of that structure), quadrigeminal plate, and cerebellopontine angle. Most intraspinal lipomas are discovered in childhood and are congenital lumbosacral lipomas associated with spinal dysraphism (spina bifida occulta) or "tethered cord" (abnormally low-lying conus tethered by the lipomatous mass). In adults, intraspinal intradural lipomas are isolated tumors, composed of normal-appearing adipose tissue and most frequently located at the thoracic level; they represent less than 1% of all spinal cord tumors. Rare complex lipomas containing bundles of nerve fibers associated with muscle fibers have been described. They have been referred to as neuromuscular hamartomas, suggesting a possible relationship with peripheral nerve fibrolipomatous hamartomas. A differential diagnosis of spinal localizations is spinal epidural lipomatosis associated with Cushing syndrome or induced by long-term corticosteroid therapy.

2.2.3.2.4.2. Muscle tumors. *Leiomyoma* and *leiomyosarcoma* are very exceptional tumors, corresponding microscopically to their well-known soft-tissue counterpart. They are composed of fascicles of spindle cells and are desmin and smooth muscle actin positive by IHC. *Epstein–Barr virus-associated smooth muscle tumor* is a distinct entity occurring in the settings of congenital or acquired immunodeficiency (HIV, transplantation, long-term corticosteroid therapy). EBV infection of smooth muscle cell is driving the tumor transformation. These tumors are often located in the meninges or, if not, in the CNS parenchyma. The presence of multiple nodules along the neuraxis is considered as an independent event of tumor transformation by EBV rather than a metastatic process. The prognosis is related to the treatment of the immunodeficiency rather than histological features of anaplasia.

Rhabdomyosarcoma may arise within the meninges or CNS parenchyma, and virtually all are histologically of the embryonal type, consisting primarily of small cells that show little or no myogenic differentiation on H&E staining. Thus, IHC (tumor cells reactive for myoglobin, desmin, and muscle-specific actin) is usually required for diagnosis. Primary CNS rhabdomyosarcoma should be distinguished from other tumors that may occasionally show skeletal muscle differentiation, such as medulloblastoma with myogenic differentiation.

2.2.3.2.4.3. Osteocartilaginous tumors. Chondroma, osteoma, and *osteochondroma* are benign osteocartilaginous tumors, commonly arising from the bones of the skull base or spine. Their histology is similar to that of their more frequent systemic counterparts.

Chondrosarcomas are preferentially located in the petrosal, occipital, or sphenoid bone. The hyaline pattern is composed of polyhedral cells in lacunar spaces within a dense basophilic chondroid matrix. The myxoid pattern is composed of stellate cells on loose basophilic matrix. Both patterns exist in most tumors. Grades 1–3 depend on the degree of cellularity, cytological atypia, and mitotic activity. Most skull base chondrosarcomas are grade 1. Examples located at the skull base must be distinguished from *chordomas* (especially so-called chondroid chordomas); thus, IHC is of paramount importance. S100 protein is expressed in both tumors, but chordomas are vimentin negative and EMA positive, brachyury positive, and cytokeratin positive; chondrosarcomas are vimentin positive and EMA negative, brachyury negative, and cytokeratin negative.

Mesenchymal chondrosarcoma is a biphasic tumor associating an undifferentiated highly cellular component and a well-differentiated chondroid component. The presence of a *HEY1::NCOA2* fusion and the negativity of STAT6 immunostaining allow its identification compared to solitary fibrous tumor, its differential diagnosis.

2.2.3.2.4.4. Blood vessel tumors. Hemangiomas of either the capillary or cavernous type are benign neoplastic vascular lesions in spine or skull. They are composed of multiple vessels separated by a loose fibrous stroma and bone trabeculae. *Angiosarcoma* may rarely occur as a primary CNS malignancy, often requiring immunohistochemical studies for a definitive diagnosis. Cerebral involvement by *Kaposi sarcoma* is metastatic, probably from primary foci in the lungs.

2.2.4. PRIMARY MELANOCYTIC LESIONS

Primary melanocytic lesions are relatively rare tumors that originate from melanocytes located within the leptomeninges. They can present as either circumscribed or diffuse tumors and may be benign or malignant. Four major categories are thus recognized: *diffuse meningeal melanocytosis* and *melanomatosis*; and, for circumscribed tumors, *melanocytoma* and *melanoma*. The *diffuse* category is associated with a rare childhood phakomatosis known as *neurocutaneous melanosis*, which in addition to the CNS lesion is characterized by numerous large congenital cutaneous nevi. It is caused by postzygotic somatic mutation of *NRAS* or rarely *BRAF*. Unlike melanomas arising in the skin, which frequently harbor *BRAF* mutations, the *circumscribed* primary melanocytic tumors of the CNS have hotspot mutations in the *GNAQ* and *GNA11* genes that encode two closely related G-proteins of the Gq family as well as secondary alterations such as mutations of *SF3B1* or *EIF1AX* or *BAP1* inactivation.

The histologic diagnosis of all these lesions rests on confirmation of their melanocytic nature, which is most easily achieved by demonstrating immunohistochemical reactivity for S100 protein or the transcription factor SOX10 and one of the melanocytic markers, HMB45 or MART-1 (Melan A). The differential diagnosis of a primary CNS melanocytic lesion must also include (1) metastatic melanoma from another primary site (which may be occult) and (2) occasional primary CNS tumors (e.g., schwannoma, meningioma, medulloblastoma) that may show melanocytic differentiation.

2.3. LYMPHOMAS AND HEMATOPOIETIC NEOPLASMS

2.3.1. Lymphomas

2.3.1.1. PRIMARY CNS LYMPHOMAS

Primary CNS lymphomas (PCNSLs) are, by definition, confined to the brain, spinal cord, eyes, or leptomeninges without evidence of lymphoma outside the CNS. They occur in two distinct clinical populations: *immunocompetent* and *immunosuppressed* patients. In immunocompetent patients, PCNSL is uncommon, accounting for approximately 4% or 5% of all primary CNS tumors and 1% or 2% of all non-Hodgkin lymphomas. In this group, they tend to occur in older adults, with a slight male preponderance. PCNSL in immunodeficient patients occurs in the setting of HIV infection, transplant recipients, autoimmune disorders, and congenital immunodeficiency syndromes. For unexplained reasons, the incidence of PCNSL in older immunocompetent patients has been increasing.

PCNSLs may occur as either single or multiple masses and can rarely infiltrate the cerebral parenchyma in a diffuse manner (*lymphomatosis cerebri*). PCNSLs can occur almost anywhere in the CNS, including the spinal cord (very rare) and leptomeninges, but their most frequent site is supratentorially in the deep periventricular region (Fig. 2.17A). PCNSLs contiguous with the subarachnoid space or ventricles can lead to CSF dissemination.

The vast majority of the lymphomas arising in the CNS (nearly 95%) are *diffuse large B-cell lymphomas* (DLBCLs), with the remaining 5% being T-cell lymphomas, low-grade B-cell lymphomas, and Burkitt lymphomas (rare). The

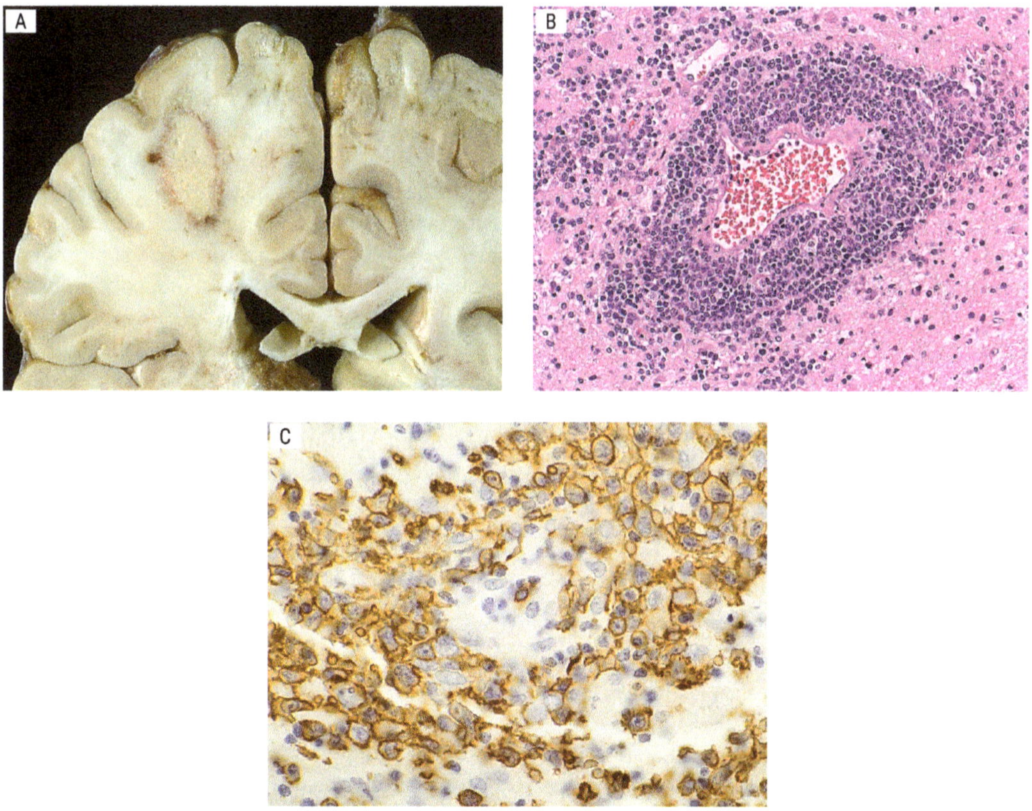

FIGURE 2.17 Primary CNS lymphoma: (**A**) tumor in periventricular white matter (macroscopic). *Microscopic features*: (**B**) perivascular localization of tumor cells (H&E); (**C**) immunoreactivity of neoplastic lymphoid cells for B-cell marker (CD20 IHC).

CNS is involved in approximately one-third of cases of *intravascular lymphoma*, most of which are large B-cell lymphomas. Histologically, the diffuse large B-cell variant of PCNSL consists of dense aggregates of relatively large atypical lymphoid cells (mainly centroblasts with variable numbers of immunoblasts), which are frequently centered on blood vessels (Fig. 2.17B, C). The parenchyma adjacent to the main tumor may show variable numbers of reactive T cells, macrophages, and gliosis. The administration of corticosteroid before the biopsy may lead to a massive cell death of the tumor cells resulting in a nondiagnostic biopsy or in the presence of ghost tumor cells revealed by CD20 immunostaining.

DLBCL confined to the CNS at presentation is classified according to a cell-of-origin system into two distinct molecular subtypes: germinal center B-cell–like (GCB) and non germinal center B-cell–like (non-GCB). Patients with GCB DLBCL have a significantly better 5-year overall survival. The subgroups were first defined by gene expression profiling, but in clinical practice they are often evaluated by IHC according to the Hans algorithm using stains for CD10, BCL6, and IRF4/MUM1 and in some laboratories by methods that evaluate RNA transcript levels. Double expression of BCL2 and MYC is also commonly evaluated by IHC and rearrangements of these genes by FISH. Almost all cases of PCNSL in immunocompromised patients show expression of the EBV genome in tumor cells.

The origin of PCNSL remains uncertain. Lymphoid cells are normally quite sparse in the CNS, and it is unclear whether neoplastic transformation of these cells occurs within the CNS or before they enter the CNS. It has been suggested that the CNS as a relatively immune-privileged organ could provide a "safe haven" for circulating neoplastic lymphoid cells, or alternatively, lymphoid cells existing within the CNS as part of a chronic inflammatory reaction could become transformed. Demyelinating inflammation can be a "sentinel" lesion preceding a PCNSL.

Patients who present with a CNS lymphoma must have it staged to exclude systemic lymphoma with secondary CNS involvement, given systemic lymphoma is more common than primary CNS lymphoma. Ophthalmologic examination is key due to the high frequency of concurrent ocular involvement in PCNSL, and spinal fluid examination must be undertaken for possible CSF dissemination of lymphoma.

2.3.1.2. SECONDARY CNS INVOLVEMENT BY SYSTEMIC LYMPHOMAS AND LEUKEMIAS

Secondary involvement of the CNS by systemic non-Hodgkin lymphoma is more common than PCNSL, with an incidence ranging from 2% to 27% (usually approximately 5%). Leukemias (especially acute lymphoblastic leukemia/lymphoma) also involve the CNS relatively frequently. The propensity for CNS involvement by these hematopoietic neoplasms is most often a function of the specific tumor type and stage of the disease. *DLBCLs* are the most likely lymphoma subtype (>80%) to secondarily involve the CNS and usually manifest as *dural* or *leptomeningeal* disease, with occasional superficial cortical involvement, in contrast to PCNSLs, which more often present as deep periventricular lesions. Hodgkin lymphoma rarely involves the CNS and most often occurs in the setting of a relapse with concurrent systemic disease.

2.3.2. Histiocytic tumors

The common histologic feature of the relatively heterogeneous group of histiocytic tumors is the presence of histiocytes, which occurs primarily as dendritic Langerhans cells (Langerhans cell histiocytosis [LCH]) or as conventional macrophages in the non-LCH tumors. The histopathologic features of these tumors in the CNS generally mimic those of their systemic counterparts. As a group, histiocytic tumors involving the CNS most often occur in children and are rare, with a 0.5% incidence of involvement by LCH; the other types are distinctly rarer. The findings of oncogenic mutation in some entities of histiocytosis revealed their tumoral etiology, whereas abnormal immune regulation abnormalities may underlie other entities.

2.3.2.1. LANGERHANS CELL HISTIOCYTOSIS

Langerhans cell histiocytosis involving the CNS occurs most often in children and may present in several ways: bone involvement (skull base, craniofacial bones); intracranial extra-axial involvement of pituitary–hypothalamus, meninges, or choroid plexus; and intracranial intra-axial involvement of the brain. Histologically, the LCH lesions consist of variable numbers of eosinophils, macrophages, lymphocytes, plasma cells, and Langerhans cell histiocytes. The diagnosis of LCH requires identification of the characteristic Langerhans cells by IHC (reactivity for CD1a and langerin/CD207). Molecular studies have identified a mutation in the serine/threonine kinase *BRAF* (V600E) in LCH tumors, and clinical responses to BRAF inhibition have been observed in patients with multidrug-resistant forms of LCH.

2.3.2.2. NON-LANGERHANS CELL HISTIOCYTOSES

The non-LCH somewhat diverse group of diseases arising from mononuclear phagocytes includes intracranial Rosai–Dorfman syndrome (lymphocyte-rich meningioma-like unique or multiple dural mass harboring large pale histiocytes with emperipolesis—i.e., intracytoplasmic vacuoles containing preserved leucocytes), Erdheim–Chester disease, hemophagocytic lymphohistiocytosis, juvenile xanthogranuloma and xanthoma disseminatum, and the usually asymptomatic cases of choroid plexus xanthoma and xanthogranuloma. CNS involvement by malignant histiocytic tumors (e.g., histiocytic sarcoma, follicular dendritic cell sarcoma) is extremely rare.

2.4. SECONDARY (METASTATIC) NEOPLASMS

Metastatic tumors are the most common intracranial and intraspinal tumors, occurring in approximately 25% of patients who die of cancer. This category includes any tumor that originates outside the CNS and spreads secondarily to the CNS either via the hematogenous route (metastasis) or by direct spread from adjacent tissues. Their incidence increases with age. They may occur in virtually any region of the cranial cavity or spinal canal, including the central neuraxis (cerebral hemispheres, cerebellum, brainstem, or, less often, spinal cord), spinal or cranial nerve roots, choroid plexus, or meningeal coverings (e.g., meningeal carcinomatosis, spinal epidural metastases, dural metastases at skull base or convexity) (Fig. 2.18A–D).

In adults, the most common primary sources of brain metastases are lung adenocarcinoma and small cell neuroendocrine carcinoma, breast cancer, melanoma, renal cancer, and colon cancer. In children, the most common sources are leukemia, lymphoma, osteosarcoma, rhabdomyosarcoma, and Ewing sarcoma. Prostate, breast, and lung cancer are the most common sources of spinal epidural metastases. Direct extension of a tumor to the CNS is relatively uncommon by contrast, and most are head and neck tumors, such as squamous cell carcinoma, olfactory neuroblastoma, and salivary gland tumors.

Macroscopically, CNS metastases may be solitary but are most often multiple. Their size ranges from less than a millimeter to more than several centimeters. In the brain parenchyma, they are generally well-circumscribed masses, either firm or soft, and may have hemorrhage, necrosis, or cystic degeneration within the tumor. Hemorrhagic metastases are especially frequent in choriocarcinoma, melanoma, and renal cell carcinoma. Meningeal involvement (carcinomatosis) may cause diffuse meningeal opacification or present as discrete nodules, which can conspicuously involve the spinal nerve roots of the cauda equina. Dural involvement can manifest as diffuse plaque-like lesions or discrete nodules.

In most cases, the histopathologic appearance and immunophenotype of the metastatic tumor resemble those of the primary source. However, determination of a primary site of origin can be challenging in poorly differentiated or undifferentiated tumors or in cases with scant tissue, hemorrhage, or extensive necrosis. IHC that identifies cell lineage markers such as transcription factors can prove especially useful in these situations. Some tumors lose expression of lineage markers, and the primary source of these tumors can remain elusive even despite an appropriate analysis. It is especially important to discriminate such "cancers of unknown primary" from poorly differentiated or epithelioid primary brain tumor such as a morphological variant of GBM: The shared expression of neuroendocrine markers and TTF-1 in both variant of GBM and metastasis may be misleading. Up to 10% of people with a prior diagnosis of a peripheral malignancy who present with a mass lesion in the CNS actually have a GBM. Moreover, 10% of GBMs can present as multicentric lesions, further complicating diagnostic evaluations.

Even when the primary site is well established, immunohistochemical and genetic testing of a cerebral metastatic tumor for important treatment/prognosis-associated markers (e.g., estrogen and progesterone receptors and HER2/neu in metastatic breast carcinoma) is indicated because many primary targeted therapies are highly effective against brain metastasis lesions. FISH and molecular analysis (Sanger or next-generation sequencing) are

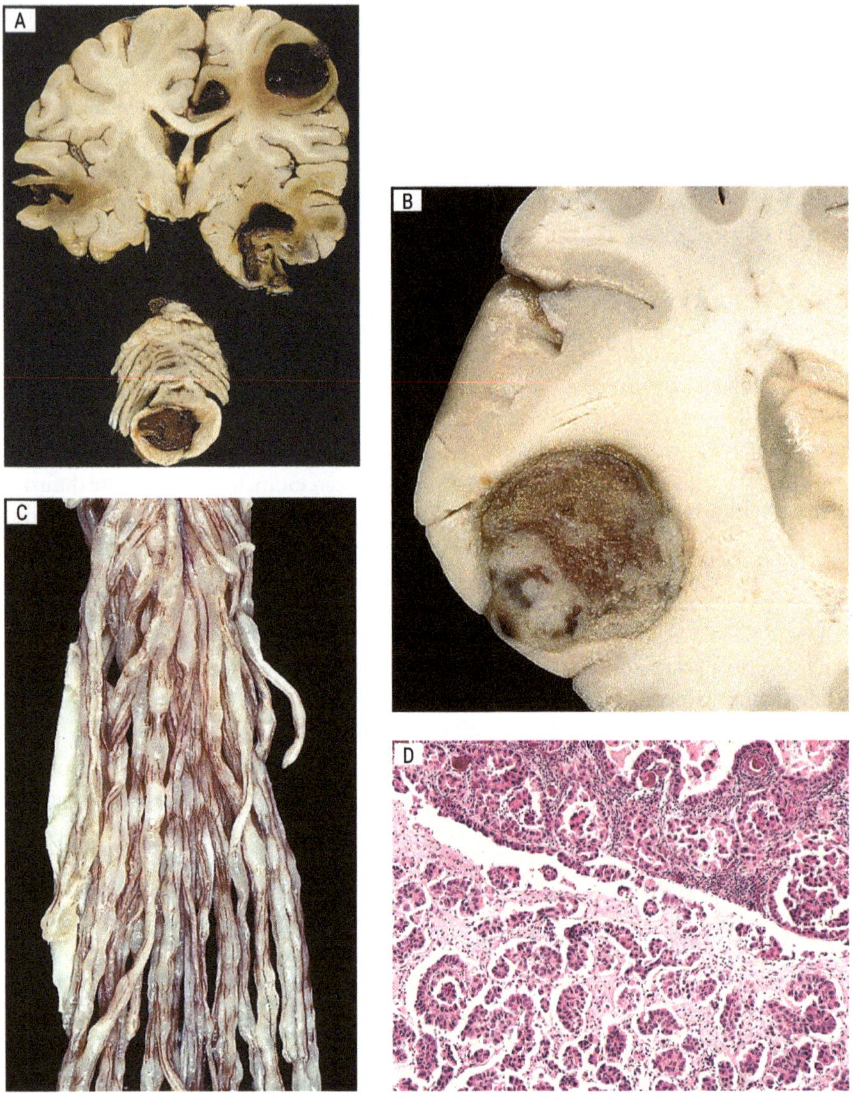

FIGURE 2.18 Metastatic tumors: (**A**) multiple hemorrhagic metastases from melanoma (macroscopic); (**B**) lung carcinoma metastatic to cerebrum (macroscopic); (**C**) meningeal carcinomatosis involving cauda equina as diffuse nodularity (macroscopic); (**D**) metastatic adenocarcinoma (lung) involving parenchyma and leptomeninges (H&E).

currently used to detect therapeutic targets and predictive biomarkers in metastatic neoplasms (e.g., lung adenocarcinoma, melanoma). Although not yet routine, methylome profiling and expression profiling are showing promise for diagnostically aiding determination of the site of origin for metastatic tumors. In addition, genomically guided clinical trials are emerging to test the value of selecting therapeutics based on the genomic aberrations identified in the tumor. Some studies have shown that surgically resecting brain metastases may be indicated in some situations because metastases to the brain may carry genetic alterations that are not detected by the analysis of the primary lesion.

3

Central Nervous System Trauma

COLIN SMITH AND R. ROSS REICHARD

3.1. EPIDEMIOLOGY AND CLASSIFICATION OF TRAUMATIC BRAIN INJURY

Traumatic brain injury (TBI) is a major cause of morbidity and mortality worldwide, yet in many cases it is entirely avoidable, particularly as occurs in road traffic accidents and assaults. Estimates by the World Health Organization indicate 57 million people throughout the world are hospitalized with one or more episodes of TBI. In the United States, statistics from the National Center for Injury Prevention and Control document that approximately 2.8 million cases of TBI-related emergency department visits were recorded in 2013 and that approximately 8% of emergency room visits require hospitalization with about 56,000 TBI-related fatalities per annum. This study also recorded a decline in road traffic–related TBI deaths compared to 2007 data but an increase in mortality related to falls due, at least in part, to accidental injury in the aged.

No single classification of TBI encompasses all the features of the complex series of processes that occur in these cases. In practice, the different classification systems proposed have employed clinical, pathological, or mechanistic parameters or have utilized various components of these in combination. A workshop convened by the National Institute of Neurological Disorders and Stroke in 2007 developed recommendations for classifications to support translational research and targeted therapies.

The most widely used clinical classification of TBI in adults considering altered mental status is the Glasgow Coma Scale (GCS). The GCS summarizes the numerical evaluation of three clinical parameters—eye response, verbal response, and motor response—resulting in a score between 3 and 15, with 3 the worst score and 15 the best score. In general, patients with mild head injury have a score of 13–15. Moderate head injury leads to a score of 9–12, and severe head injury to a score of 8 or less. The GCS is less useful in assessment of pediatric patients, and specific modifications have been made for evaluation of affected children at different stages of development, including the establishment of neonatal, infant, and childhood scales. The GCS is also less useful in assessing the extent of milder head

Table 3.1 Mechanisms of Traumatic Brain Injury

MECHANISM	MAIN PATHOLOGY
Contact (impact)	Vascular (hemorrhages) Traumatic axonal injury
Inertial loading	Traumatic axonal injury
Penetrating	Local tissue necrosis
Blast	Brain swelling

Table 3.2 Classification of Traumatic Brain Injury

FOCAL	DIFFUSE
Scalp lacerations Skull fractures Contusions/lacerations Intracranial hemorrhage Focal lesions secondary to raised intracranial pressure	Global ischemic injury Diffuse traumatic axonal injury/diffuse vascular injury Brain swelling

injuries, and specific criteria are being developed to determine the severity of concussive injury.

Mechanistic classifications of TBI describe contact, inertial (acceleration–deceleration), penetrating, and blast injuries (Table 3.1).

- *Contact* (impact) brain injury applies to circumstances in which the head makes contact with an object, or an object contacts the head, with the forces being transmitted to the brain. In contrast, *inertial* (acceleration–deceleration) brain injury results from situations associated with unrestricted movement of the head that leads to shear and compressive strains, which may be either linear or nonlinear (rotational). With rotational injury, the brain can twist within the cranial cavity, adding additional stress to brain tissues, particularly those in the midline. Focal lesions associated with impact are likely to be sustained from a fall or an assault. Diffuse lesions are more often due to road traffic accidents. In a given patient, the distribution of lesions is related to many associated factors. Elements of both contact and inertial forces acting on the brain are often in effect; therefore, the interpretation of the physical circumstances leading to the brain damage may be complex.
- *Penetrating* injuries produce brain damage when an object passes through the skull and extends directly into the underlying brain, causing direct parenchymal damage, known as *the permanent wound track/cavity*. In the case of firearm injuries, there is an additional component of tissue damage caused by the pressure cavities produced when the projectile passes through brain tissue, temporarily expanding the wound track (*temporary wound cavity*).
- *Blast injuries* are less well described and are seen particularly in the context of military or terrorist situations; it is suggested that the shock waves from an explosive device can result in injuries to the brain parenchyma in the absence of contact or inertial injuries, although definitive confirmatory data are currently lacking. Further complicating the understanding of blast injuries is the fact that affected individuals often also sustain blunt force injuries during the same event, which are referred to as primary and secondary injuries, respectively.

The description of the neuropathology of TBI presented in this chapter considers traditional categories from the perspective of anatomic pathology: focal or diffuse tissue injuries (Table 3.2). The discussion also considers penetrating and blast injuries, as well as specific issues as they apply to affected children and those relating to long-term problems associated with TBI.

3.2. FOCAL INJURY

3.2.1. Scalp and skull lesions

3.2.1.1. SCALP LESIONS

The scalp and skull may be directly damaged by contact injury. The presence of scalp contusions is indicative of contact injury and in some situations may provide clues to the possible intracranial lesions; occipital bruising is typically associated with a backward fall and indirect “contrecoup” contusions (see Section 3.2.2) involving the frontal and temporal lobes. Sharp and blunt force wounds are usually managed routinely in hospital emergency departments; these types of injury may result in serious blood loss, hypotension, and secondary brain damage.

3.2.1.2. SKULL LESIONS

The prevalence of skull fractures is directly related to the severity of the head injury and is mostly influenced by a combination of impact velocity, impact surface characteristics, cortical bone thickness, and cortical bone density. In general, impact against a flat surface, as may be seen in a fall, with distribution of the force over a large area, will produce linear fractures, which can be extensive. Impact against smaller objects, such as a club or hammer, tends to cause localized fractures that are often depressed fractures but may be associated with fragmentation of the bone (comminuted fractures). Compound fractures are associated with scalp laceration(s). In one autopsy study, skull fracture was found in 80% of subjects with fatal head injury. Clinical series indicate that skull fractures occur in 3% of patients with mild head injury at the time of presentation in the emergency room and in 65% of patients requiring admission to a neurosurgery inpatient service.

A description and classification of skull fractures, including linear, depressed, and basilar fractures, is given in Table 3.3.

- Fractures of the cranial vault are usually linear (Fig. 3.1) and situated between the bony ridges of the skull.
- Fractures of the skull base (basilar skull fractures) also include fractures of the vault, where the fracture lines radiate toward the base involving the anterior fossa, the middle fossa (Fig. 3.2), or the posterior fossa. The lesion is of clinical importance because the impact necessary to cause the fracture is much greater than that required for other fractures. In these cases, there may be severe brain damage in addition to the bone injury with contusions of the cerebellum, brainstem, and diencephalic structures. Furthermore, the cranial nerves and blood vessels are also particularly vulnerable in cases of fracture involving the floor of the skull. Finally, patients who survive these injuries may develop complications such as ascending infection or pneumocephalus.
- In neonates and infants, "ping-pong" fractures can be seen. These are depressed smooth fractures, their name reflecting the similarity in appearance to the defect produced when pushing a finger into a ping-pong ball. The lesion is not associated with a break in the inner table of the skull, and rarely is it associated with underlying parenchymal damage. Other types of fractures occurring in childhood include *growing fractures* and *diastatic fractures*. Growing fractures may occur when dural and arachnoid tissue is trapped between the edges of the fracture, preventing healing. Diastatic fractures are fractures that extend along and separate one or more sutures in the skull and can occur in both infants and adults.

No direct correlation can be drawn between the presence or absence of a skull fracture and the likelihood of an underlying parenchymal brain injury, unless the fracture is depressed and the broken

Table 3.3 Types of Skull Fracture

TYPE	DESCRIPTION
Linear	Break in bone extending through both the outer and the inner tables of the skull. No bone displacement.
Depressed	Fragments of the inner table of the skull are displaced inward.
Compound	A depressed skull fracture with associated scalp laceration. Complex, or penetrating, fractures are associated with additional dural tearing.
Hinge (basilar)	Linear fracture extends across the base of the skull.
Diastatic	A fracture line extending along skull bone sutures, causing widening of the suture.
Growing	In infancy, meninges extend through a fracture, preventing fracture healing.

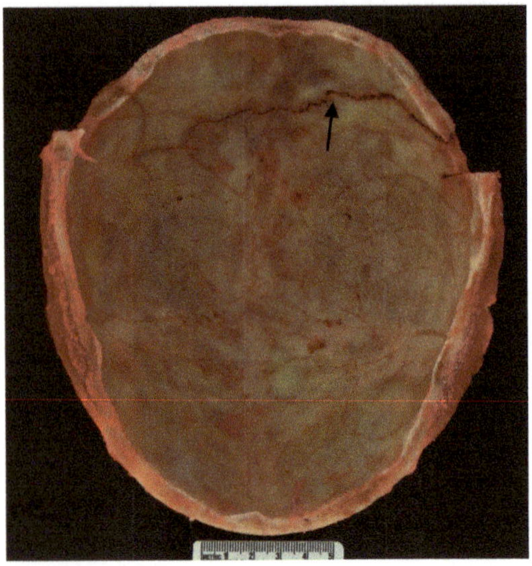

FIGURE 3.1 A linear skull fracture (*black arrow*) extending through the cranial vault.

bone makes direct contact with the underlying brain tissue. Also, there is a direct correlation between the presence of a skull fracture and the development of intracranial hemorrhages (described in Section 3.2.3).

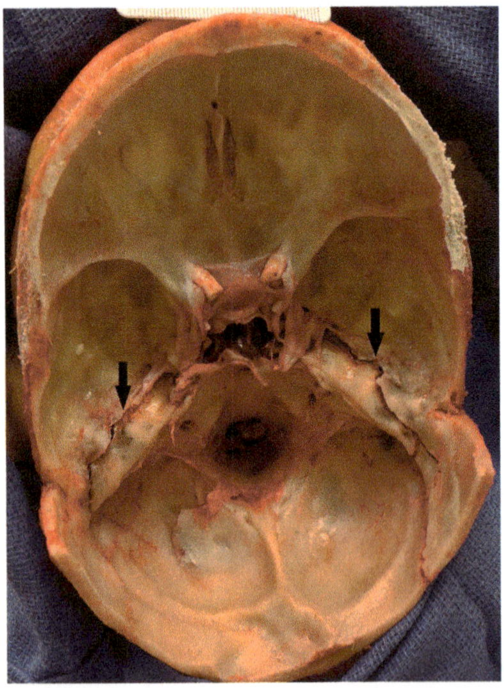

FIGURE 3.2 A typical basilar skull fracture that extends across the skull base and is referred to as a hinge fracture (*black arrows*).

3.2.2. Contusions and lacerations

Contusions are bruises on the surface of the brain and indicate direct contact between the brain surface and the skull bone. By definition, the overlying pia mater is intact in the case of contusions, but it is torn in lacerations.

Although it is not possible to infer the site of impact from the pattern of the contusions, two prototypical types of contusions are recognized: *coup contusions* and *contrecoup contusions.* In *coup* contusions, the damaged brain tissue occurs beneath the point of impact, such as when scalp bruising is over the forehead and the brain contusions involve frontal and temporal lobes. In *contrecoup* contusions, on the other hand, structural damage on the surface of the brain occurs in a region opposite the point of external impact (Fig. 3.3). Regardless of the site of impact, the frontal and temporal lobes are the most common location of brain contusions.

The size of a contusion may increase over time, some hours after the initial head injury. This phenomenon of delayed traumatic intracerebral hemorrhage usually becomes apparent within 48 hours after the head injury. The precise mechanism of this delayed injury is uncertain, but it is thought to be the result of increased blood flow or pressure through a vascular capillary network that is focally damaged by local vasoregulatory failure, possibly aggravated by post-traumatic coagulopathy.

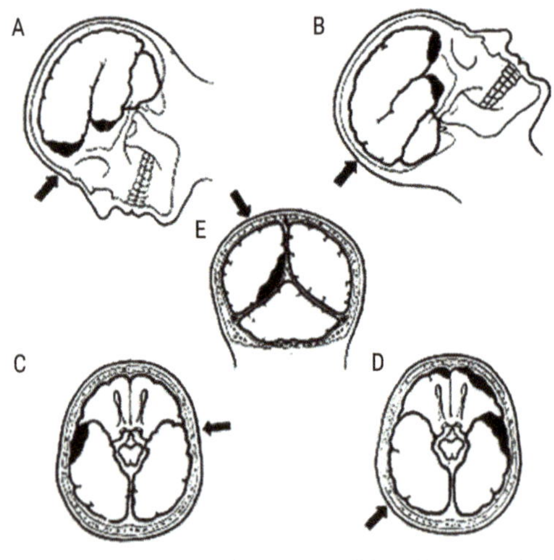

FIGURE 3.3 Typical patterns of distribution of contusions following inertial impact (*arrow*), showing contusions related to the site of impact ("coup") and contusions away from the impact ("contrecoup"). (From Courville CB. *Pathology of the Central Nervous System*. 1937.)

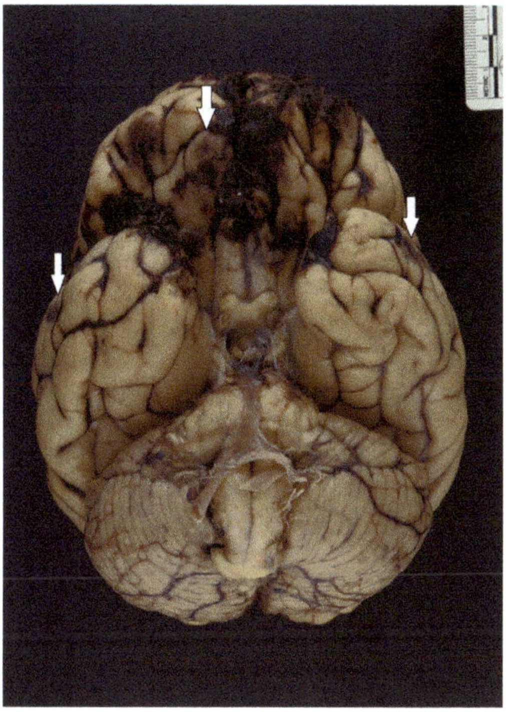

FIGURE 3.4 Acute contusions involving the cortex of the frontal and temporal lobes. The hemorrhages noted with *white arrows* demonstrate the typical punctate hemorrhages on the crests of gyri typical of contusions.

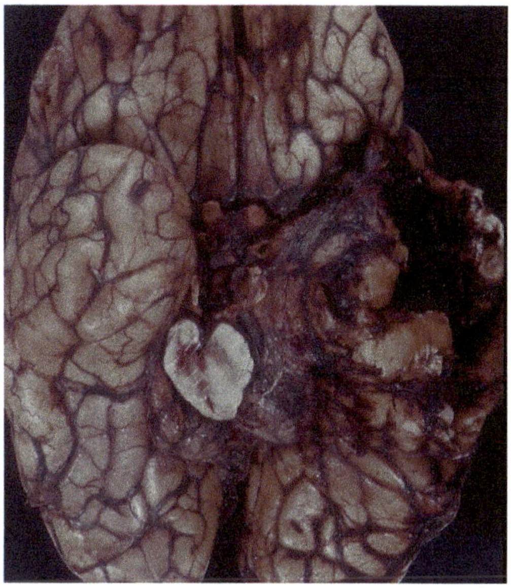

FIGURE 3.5 Inferior view of the brain showing a burst temporal lobe. There is laceration of the cortical surface and the blood clot extends through the disrupted brain tissue. There was an associated acute subdural hemorrhage adjacent to this lesion. There is also evidence of swelling around this lesion, with bilateral transtentorial herniation and brainstem compression. Duret hemorrhages are seen within the cut surface of the midbrain.

Topography. Cortical contusions are produced when there is relative motion of the brain in relation to the skull, with brain impact against the bony projections of the skull. Intracranial pressure gradients can develop, possibly resulting in cavitation bubbles, which can accentuate local tissue damage. Contusions typically involve the frontal poles; the inferior frontal lobe, including the gyrus rectus and medial and lateral orbital gyri; the temporal poles and lateral and inferior aspects of the temporal lobes; and the cortex above and below the Sylvian fissure (Fig. 3.4). Fracture contusions may be seen at atypical sites in direct relationship to a skull fracture. Contusions involving the occipital lobes and cerebellum are rare, perhaps in part because the adjoining smooth inner surface of the posterior fossa of the skull offers less attrition compared with the irregular bony ridges of the anterior and middle fossae. These lesions are usually associated with an adjacent skull fracture.

Contusions typically involve the crests of gyri and are often superficial, involving the gray matter only. However, the lesion may extend into underlying white matter and develop into a hematoma. In severe cases, extensive laceration injury with underlying parenchymal hemorrhage may be associated with subdural hemorrhage (SDH), forming a so-called burst lobe (Fig. 3.5). This type of injury most often involves the temporal lobes.

On neuropathologic examination, the smallest contusions are merely collections of minute perivascular hemorrhages in the cortex, often only a few millimeters in diameter, without appreciable edema. Larger contusions contain areas of tissue destruction as well as hemorrhage and are often associated with focal swelling. Several weeks following an injury, on macroscopic examination the affected brain appears abnormally pigmented and is shrunken (Fig. 3.6). Over time, the hemorrhage and the dead tissue are removed by macrophages, and there are foci of gliosis, often with associated hemosiderin deposition. Old contusions may create epileptogenic foci, and posttraumatic epilepsy accounts for approximately 5% of all causes of epilepsy. Old contusions are not infrequent incidental autopsy findings, particularly in at-risk groups, such as patients with chronic alcoholism.

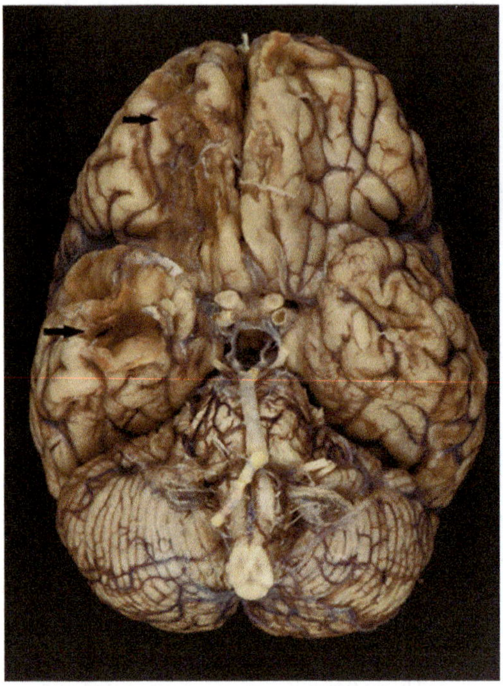

FIGURE 3.6 View of base of the brain with old contusions (*black arrows*). There is loss of cortical tissue and cystic degeneration involving the inferior frontal lobes bilaterally and right temporal tip.

The traumatic lesion can usually be distinguished from an old infarct because the topographic distribution is typically on the ventral surface of the frontal and temporal lobes and ordinarily occurs in multiple vascular territories. In addition, the conformation of the traumatic lesion is also characteristically wedge-shaped, with the base on the crest of the cortical gyri and apex in white matter, and there is often evidence of associated hemorrhage.

3.2.3. Intracranial hemorrhage

Intracranial hemorrhages are classified according to the anatomical compartment in which they develop.

3.2.3.1. EXTRADURAL (EPIDURAL) HEMORRHAGE

An extradural hemorrhage (EDH) is an extravasation of blood between the inner table of the skull and the dura. It is composed of clotted blood that tends to adhere early and firmly to the outer surface of the dura.

EDH is ordinarily limited in size; the bleeding remains localized and does not spread throughout the cranial cavity. EDH most commonly (approximately 50%) is the consequence of a fracture of the squamous temporal bone that causes contact damage (laceration) of the underlying middle meningeal artery and/or vein. As the hematoma expands, the dura (periosteum) is stripped from the inner table of the skull to form a circumscribed ovoid mass, producing a mass in the extradural space that is filled by blood. Other sites of involvement include the anterior cranial fossa (damage to the anterior meningeal artery), parasagittal region (superior sagittal sinus), and occipital lobe and posterior fossa (damage to the occipital meningeal artery or transverse or sigmoid sinuses). EDH has also been described in relation to the internal carotid artery before it enters the intracranial dura. Posterior cranial fossa EDH may occur in infants and young children from damage of a sinus in the absence of an overlying skull fracture. Spontaneous EDH has been described in association with vascular malformation, infections, and rarely as a complication of metastatic disease and anticoagulation therapy.

In up to 30% of cases, EDH may be associated with a "lucid interval." This clinical phenomenon characterizes some patients in whom there may be a period of variable duration after the head injury without clinical manifestations prior to the development of an often rapid decline in neurologic function. This syndrome has been presumed to be the consequence of the rapid volumetric expansion of the EDH.

In the absence of surgical evacuation of the hematoma, enlargement of the EDH results in a "space-occupying" lesion with concave deformation of the underlying brain (Fig. 3.7); midline shift and axial displacement; and, finally, raised intracranial pressure and brain herniation (Fig. 3.8).

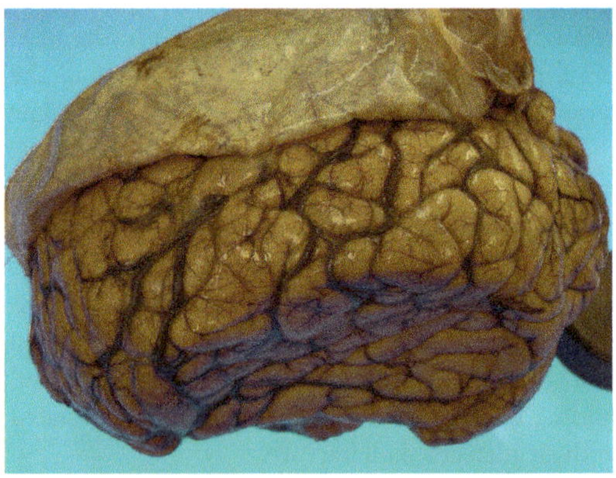

FIGURE 3.7 Concave deformation of one cerebral hemisphere secondary to overlying extradural hematoma (hematoma not shown).

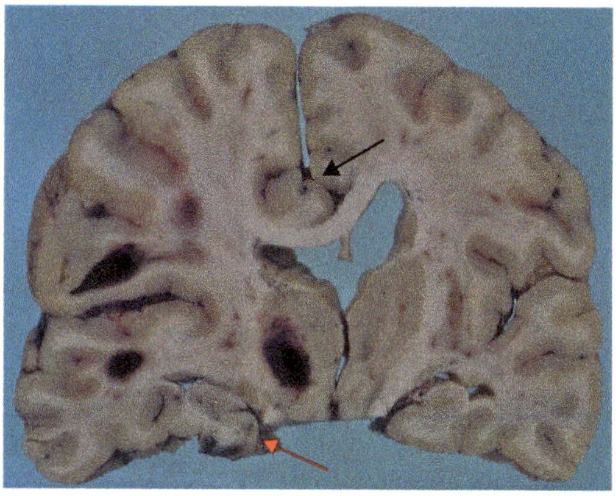

FIGURE 3.8 Secondary effects of a space-occupying lesion, such as an acute extradural or subdural hematoma. The lesion was on the left side of the image, resulting in subfalcine herniation (*black arrow*) and tentorial herniation (*red arrow*). The axial displacement has resulted in thalamic hemorrhage near the midline.

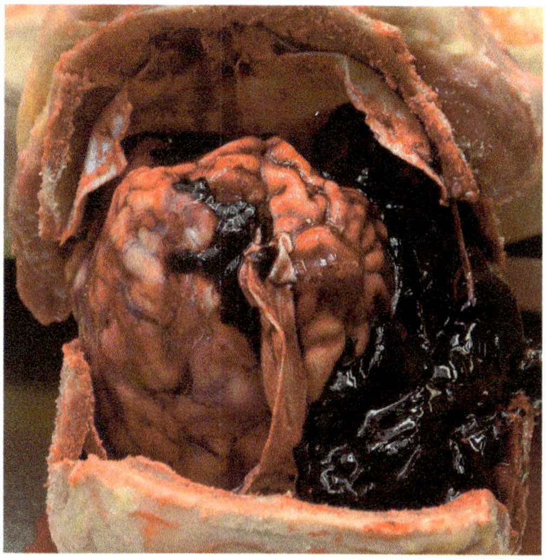

FIGURE 3.9 A large acute subdural hematoma overlying the right cerebral hemisphere.

3.2.3.2. SUBDURAL HEMATOMA

Subdural hemorrhage develops within a region of the dura called the dural border cell layer, at the interface between dura and arachnoid. This is a potential space, not an anatomical space, inasmuch as during life the two layers are apposed. However, with bleeding (or gentle handling by a neurosurgeon during surgery), this layer dissects, forming a subdural space.

After blunt force head injury, acute SDH (ASDH) may be due to either rupture of a bridging vein (cortical vein traversing the subarachnoid space, from the cortical surface to a dural sinus) or secondary to contusions with damage to cortical veins or arteries and the overlying leptomeninges. In the latter situation, there may be an associated intracerebral hemorrhage (ICH), and the term *burst lobe* is applied.

Experimental studies in nonhuman primates have demonstrated that, biomechanically, ASDHs secondary to torn bridging veins occur in a setting of rapid acceleration–deceleration injuries—that is, the movement stops or starts very quickly. This is consistent with the recognized association between SDH and falls or assaults in human beings, both situations in which there is a rapid acceleration or deceleration of the head on impact. Patients who develop an SDH may also show clinical evidence of a lucid interval as defined above.

ASDH may follow an episode of relatively trivial head injury, and in some cases there is no history of trauma. This is particularly the case in individuals with brain atrophy, such as elderly patients with neurodegeneration or children with metabolic brain disorders such as glutaric aciduria, in whom the bridging veins of the atrophic brain are presumably stretched out and are therefore potentially more vulnerable to tearing. Medical conditions associated with SDH include anticoagulation therapy; intracranial shunting procedures; ICH associated with amyloid angiopathy; epilepsy; alcohol abuse; and, rarely, intracranial tumors or a ruptured cerebral saccular aneurysm.

The neuropathology of SDH can be descriptively classified into acute, subacute, and chronic forms (Figs. 3.9 and 3.10). Notwithstanding this empiric subdivision, it is often most difficult to be absolutely certain of the exact age of a hematoma using radiological, intraoperative, or even histological criteria. The reasons for this predicament are multiple and complex. In the first place, although clinically it may be possible to give the time of onset of an episode of ASDH, radiologic imaging studies have demonstrated that in many patients, the ASDH involutes spontaneously and does not evolve into a chronic lesion. Mixing of blood with cerebrospinal fluid (CSF) can also result in difficulties in establishing the age of an SDH by radiologic analysis.

An SDH is regarded as chronic (chronic subdural hematoma [CSDH]) when still present 3 weeks after an injury. However, the pathologic entity CSDH should not be considered the end point of an organizing ASDH; rather, CSDH appears to be a specific entity in itself, and its relationship

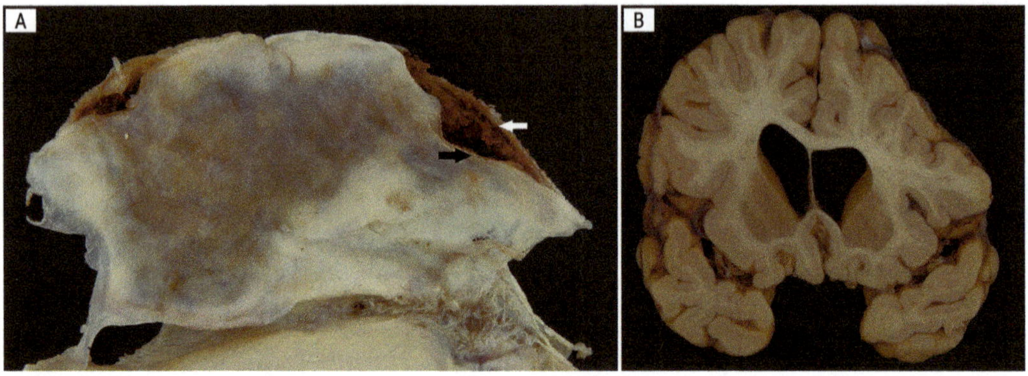

FIGURE 3.10 Chronic subdural hematoma: (**A**) Central blood clot surrounded by inner and outer neomembranes (*black* and *white arrows*, respectively); (**B**) subdural hematoma on the right, after removal, with residual deformation of the hemisphere.

with ASDH is not clear. CSDH appears to be an inflammatory angiogenic disorder and should not be considered to be a part of the typical evolution of an ASDH; most patients who survive an ASDH will show resorption of the hematoma with minimal residual membrane formation.

At postmortem examination of ASDH, the blood extends within the subdural space; the dura is tense, and blood can be seen underneath the dura. This fresh blood spills out when the dura is incised at surgery or autopsy. In subacute lesions, the blood clot shows at least focal attachment to the dura, and there may be a faint golden-brown color discoloration due to hemosiderin deposits. The designation CSDH applies to a clot that is encapsulated in fibrous membranes, containing blood products of different ages, including areas of fresh bleeding and older organized blood clot. Inner and outer neomembranes are seen surrounding the organizing blood clot (Fig. 3.10A), and new vessels extend from these neomembranes into the organizing blood clot. These new vessels are friable and liable to bleed, and subsequently, the slow expansion can lead to compression of the brain (Fig. 3.10B).

3.2.3.3. SUBDURAL HYGROMA

A subdural hygroma is a collection of CSF or serum, rather than blood, in the subdural border cell layer, creating a fissure (space) similar to the anatomical location of an ASDH. Current guidelines suggest that the term *subdural hygroma* be replaced by extra-axial CSF or proteinaceous collection. Subdural hygroma may be associated with trauma, often mild, and with infection in infants or may be seen after ventricular shunting. In the majority of these cases, the lesion is not clinically significant; however, some patients develop acute neurologic deficits after a traumatic injury that may mimic an ASDH. The two types of lesions can be distinguished by magnetic resonance imaging. At surgery or autopsy, subdural hygroma fluid is clear or xanthochromic and is not associated with a fibrous membrane.

3.2.3.4. TRAUMATIC SUBARACHNOID HEMORRHAGE

Within the setting of blunt force head injury, subarachnoid bleeding is commonly observed and typically associated with damage to cortical veins located in the subarachnoid space or related to sites of contusions. In general, subarachnoid bleeding, in itself, is not necessarily of clinical/prognostic significance. Massive basal traumatic subarachnoid hemorrhage (SAH) is typically seen in the setting of vertebral artery injury, with traumatic damage occurring to the artery at the craniocervical junction.

In these cases, the clinical manifestations associated with extensive basal hemorrhage can mimic those associated with a ruptured berry aneurysm (see Chapter 4). This possibility should be excluded at postmortem by careful examination. SAH resulting from vertebral artery injury has been described following a blow to the under aspect of the jaw, with associated external rotation and hyperextension of the head resulting in tearing of the vertebral artery. The clinical picture is one of sudden collapse and coma, usually with a short survival period. At postmortem examination, the site of origin of the massive bleeding may be difficult to identify.

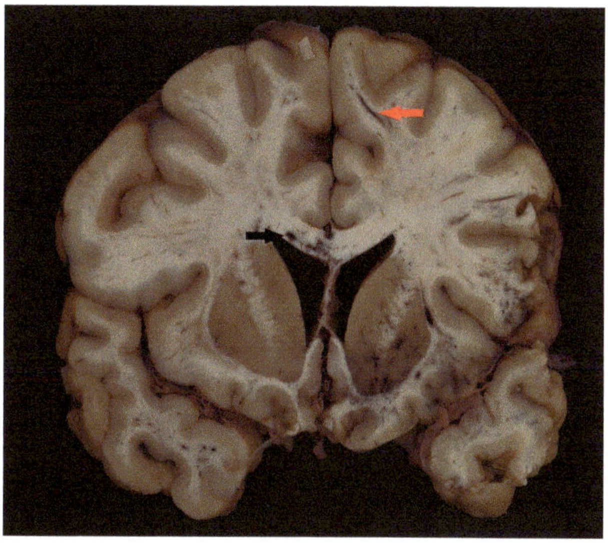

FIGURE 3.11 Basal ganglia hemorrhages secondary to rotational head injury (road traffic accident). In addition, there are parasagittal white matter hemorrhages (*red arrow*) and a hemorrhagic lesion laterally placed in the corpus callosum (*black arrow*), typical of traumatic diffuse axonal injury.

However, postmortem angiography and careful dissection of the vertebral arteries from the point at which they enter the foramina transversaria at the lower cervical vertebrae and followed up to the point where they leave the vertebrae and enter the base of the skull may be necessary to identify the arterial injury. The site of traumatic rupture is found in most cases and is typically at the site where the vertebral artery passes through the dura into the intracranial compartment.

3.2.3.5. INTRACEREBRAL HEMORRHAGE

Intracerebral hemorrhage, when it occurs in association with contusions, may attain sufficient size to cause mass effect with associated shift of midline structures. As discussed previously, in some cases hemorrhagic expansion of a contusion may develop some time after the initial traumatic insult, and this phenomenon may be witnessed clinically when a patient is observed to deteriorate several hours after the initial head injury.

Deep-seated basal ganglia ICH may be seen in a high-velocity, blunt force head injury, such as road traffic accidents. They are typically small parenchymal hemorrhages in the region of the diencephalic structures (Fig. 3.11). The lesions are part of the spectrum of rotational injuries, including diffuse traumatic axonal injury (TAI) and diffuse vascular injury, and do not lead to a significant mass effect but, rather, are an indication that severe parenchymal damage has occurred.

Parasagittal white matter lesions—historically, and rather inaccurately, known as *gliding contusions*—are hemorrhagic lesions seen predominantly in frontal parasagittal white matter. As with traumatic basal ganglia hemorrhages, they are secondary to rotational forces and seen in severe head injury. These lesions are often symmetrical, and when the interval of time between the initial injury and postmortem examination is prolonged, they evolve into a gliotic scar with surrounding hemosiderin containing macrophages.

3.2.3.6. INTRAVENTRICULAR HEMORRHAGE

Intraventricular hemorrhage is relatively uncommon in blunt force head injury, but when present, it carries the risk of acute obstructive hydrocephalus. Blood within the ventricular system may be a consequence of direct extension of a parenchymal hemorrhage into the ventricular system or of retrograde flow from SAH. In rare cases, there is isolated intraventricular hemorrhage with no obvious source of primary bleeding, and these lesions are also considered to be part of rotational TBI, often associated with parasagittal white matter hemorrhages, corpus callosum hemorrhage, and basal ganglia hemorrhage. In these cases, the hemorrhage is considered to arise from tears in subependymal veins, choroid plexus, or damage to the septum pellucidum and associated forniceal vessels.

3.2.4. Other focal lesions

3.2.4.1. VASCULAR

As discussed previously, a vertebral artery tear is a cause of massive basal traumatic SAH. However, a more common trauma-associated injury of the vertebral artery is dissection. Vertebral artery dissection develops when there is disruption of the intima of the vessel, allowing thrombus to form, which can lead to interruption of blood flow and to infarction of part of relevant territories of distribution in the brainstem (clinical manifestations include the lateral medullary syndrome) or, rarely, the spinal cord. Dissection can follow relatively minor trauma; can develop over a period of many hours; and can also involve other large arteries, including the internal carotid artery.

Post-traumatic pseudoaneurysms may involve both the external and internal carotid arteries and are thought to be a consequence of stretching of the blood vessel after neck injury. Arteriovenous fistulae can develop, particularly between the internal carotid artery and the cavernous sinus. Death from total transection of the internal carotid artery has been described in rare case reports.

3.2.4.2. BRAINSTEM LESIONS

A number of brainstem lesions are described in the setting of blunt force head injury. The most severe example is a pontomedullary rent, a lesion that is incompatible with life. The tear occurs at the junction between the lower pons and medulla, and its forensic validity can be confirmed by the demonstration of tissue damage on microscopic examination. This lesion is rare; it is associated with high-velocity lesions causing extreme hyperflexion- or hyperextension-type injuries of the head, such as falls from a height or motorcycle accidents.

Hemorrhages within the brainstem are secondary to axial displacement causing secondary midline flame-shaped hemorrhages in the midbrain and pons (Fig. 3.12) (Duret hemorrhages) or are part of diffuse TAI with a dorsolateral localization (Fig. 3.13) (see Section 3.3).

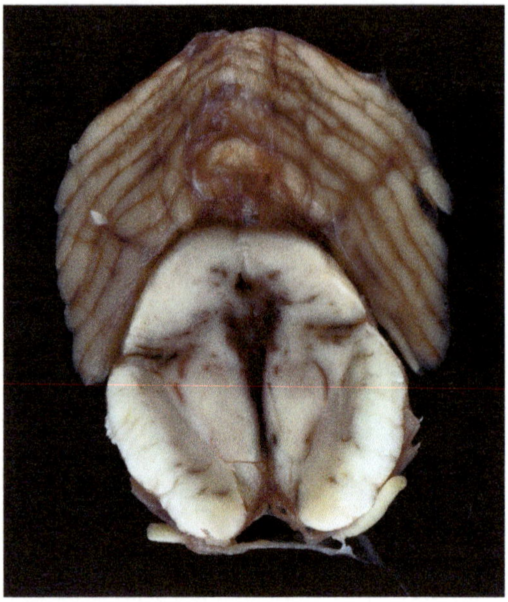

FIGURE 3.12 Midline (Duret) hemorrhage in the brainstem secondary to downward axial displacement caused by a large acute subdural hematoma.

3.2.4.3. SPINAL CORD TRAUMA

Traumatic spinal cord injuries (SCIs) are common and are most commonly the result of localized cord contusional injury secondary to a displaced vertebral fracture. Bleeding is initially petechial, but the lesions coalesce to form more extensive hemorrhages, usually situated centrally within the spinal cord. Ischemia develops, resulting in central infarction of the cord (Fig 3.14). Tissue damage

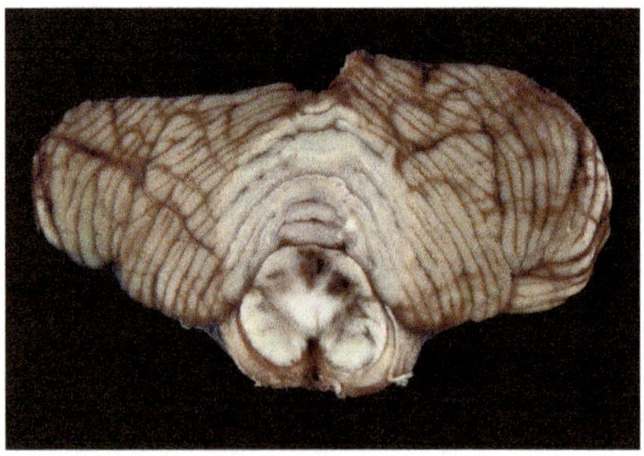

FIGURE 3.13 Dorsolateral brainstem hemorrhages that may be present in diffuse TAI.

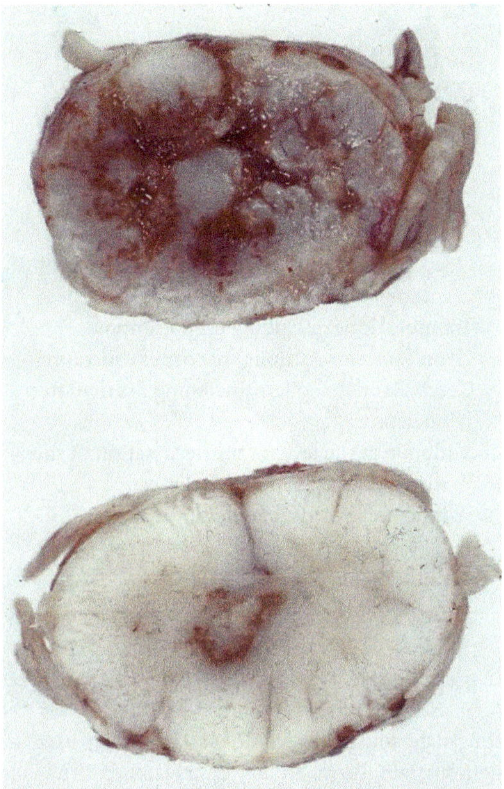

FIGURE 3.14 Spinal cord contusion. The upper image shows extensive tissue necrosis with hemorrhage, corresponding to the site of a fracture dislocation impinging on the cord; the lower image, taken from a lower level of the cord, shows central necrosis only. The injury can extend over several levels of the spinal cord and is not exclusively localized to the area of vertebral fracture.

extends for several levels above and below the site of direct injury.

It is now recognized that some patients, particularly children with traumatic SCI, may have no demonstrable evidence of a radiologic or structural lesion (SCI without radiographic abnormality); the hypothesis in these instances is that the patient's symptoms are the result of spinal cord "concussion."

3.3. DIFFUSE BRAIN INJURY

Diffuse lesions in TBI include diffuse ischemia, diffuse TAI, and diffuse brain swelling. In the absence of a demonstrable mass lesion, persistent coma after head injury can be supposed to be a consequence of TAI, diffuse ischemia, or a combination of both.

3.3.1. Ischemia

Ischemic brain injury, both focal and diffuse, is a common finding in fatal TBI and was found to be present in 91% of brains studied in one autopsy study. Ischemia remains an important factor in determining clinical outcome after head injury. Early stabilization of patients reduces the incidence of focal hypotensive brain injury but not of diffuse ischemic injury. There are a number of causes of ischemia after head injury (Table 3.4), and many types of lesions may be seen, including neuronal injury within selectively vulnerable areas documented on microscopic examination, watershed infarcts, and infarcts within major arterial territories.

3.3.2. Diffuse traumatic axonal injury

The term *diffuse axonal injury* (DAI) was a clinicopathological entity introduced to apply to structural lesions of axons that follow severe traumatic injury and are found at autopsy examination, in the absence of focal lesions, in fatal cases of progressively severe coma, or in patients surviving head injury who manifest severe disability, eventually evolving into vegetative state. However, the current terminology used to describe the neuropathologic substrate of DAI is TAI. TAI contributes to at least 35% of the mortality and morbidity of TBI cases without associated space-occupying lesions and contributes to the mortality and morbidity in focal brain injuries. In addition, along with diffuse ischemic injury, TAI is considered to be an important cause of severe disability and vegetative state in survivors of head injury. In cases of diffuse TAI, there is typically clinical documentation of a period of unconsciousness, although this period may be short or the patient may have lapsed into prolonged coma. Increasingly, however, TAI is thought to underlie a spectrum of clinical states, extending from "concussion" at one end to immediate and prolonged coma (severe diffuse TAI) at the other. Current practice reserves the designation DAI as a clinical diagnosis in patients with immediate prolonged coma and supportive neuroradiologic findings; focal TAI should apply to the histopathologic assessment of localized trauma-induced axonal injury; diffuse TAI should

Table 3.4 Patterns and Causes of Ischemic Brain Damage After Traumatic Brain Injury

PATTERN	CAUSE
Diffuse	Cardiorespiratory arrest
	Raised intracranial pressure
	Vasospasm
	Hypotension
Focal	Embolism
	Penetrating injuries

> **Box 3.1 Microscopic Examination if Diffuse Brain injury Is Suspected**
>
> **Recommended Minimum Sample for a Diagnosis of Diffuse TAI**
>
> Corpus callosum with adjacent parasagittal cortex and white matter
> Deep gray matter, including posterior limb of internal capsule
> Temporal lobe, including hippocampus
> Genu (anterior sections) of corpus callosum
> Cerebellar hemisphere, including the dentate nucleus
> Midbrain at the level of the decussation of the superior cerebellar peduncles
> Pons at the level of the middle cerebellar peduncles
> Medulla

be reserved for the histopathologic description of diffuse trauma-induced axonal injury.

Experimental studies have shown that TAI is primarily a non-impact phenomenon, resulting from angular or rotational acceleration. This formulation is in keeping with the circumstances in which TAI primarily occurs in human injuries, namely road traffic accidents and falls from a height. In such situations, TAI is primarily the result of inertial phenomena, and in these cases there is a lower incidence of impact lesions and skull fractures. TAI also occurs occasionally in fatal cases following accelerated falls from standing, notably assaults, but in these cases, impact phenomena play an important role, and a skull fracture is a much more usual associated finding.

3.3.2.1. MACROSCOPIC ASPECTS OF TAI

In the most severe cases of TAI, hemorrhagic lesions are seen in the lateral aspects of the corpus callosum and dorsolateral quadrant of the brainstem. Three grades of TAI have been described. In Grade 1 lesions, there are only microscopic changes in the white matter of the cerebral cortex, corpus callosum, brainstem, and cerebellum. In Grade 2 lesions, macroscopically visible focal hemorrhagic lesions are present in the corpus callosum only (Fig. 3.11), and in Grade 3 lesions, additional focal hemorrhagic lesions are seen in the dorsolateral quadrants of the rostral brainstem.

3.3.2.2. MICROSCOPIC ASPECTS OF TAI

A recommended sampling protocol is outlined in Box 3.1. On routine histologic preparations (e.g., stained with H&E), the damaged axons can be seen as eosinophilic swellings (Fig. 3.15). Several special histological techniques have been used to demonstrate them to better advantage. The abnormal axons can be detected by silver stains, and, in affected long white matter tracts, using the appropriate stains, the demonstration of myelin breakdown products identifies the lesions. The relative disadvantage of these techniques is that the abnormal axons can only be demonstrated after a survival period of at least 12–18 hours.

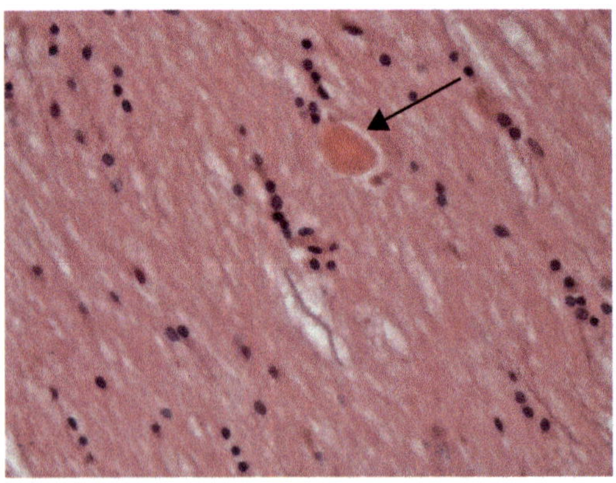

FIGURE 3.15 Eosinophilic axonal swellings (*arrow*) seen within the corpus callosum 24 hours after a road traffic accident. β-APP immunohistochemistry highlights many more damaged axons (H&E).

Immunostaining for β-amyloid precursor protein (β-APP), which is able to detect axonal flow disruption, is the most sensitive and widely used method. β-APP, a membrane-spanning glycoprotein and a normal component of neuronal cells, is transported along axons by fast transport mechanisms. When there is axonal transport interruption, β-APP has been shown to accumulate, indicative of dysfunction or possibly rupture of the axon. β-APP accumulation has been demonstrated in subjects who have survived for a period as short as 35 minutes from the time of injury. This phenomenon is thought to result from mechanoporation with axonal degeneration; where there is immediate axonal transection (e.g., after decapitation), β-APP may accumulate almost immediately.

It is apparent that β-APP is demonstrable only in axons with perturbation of axonal flow and is, in itself, not indicative of irreversible axonal damage. β-APP expression has been assessed alongside a proteolytic fragment of α-II spectrin (SNTF), a marker of neurofilament loss of phosphorylation (SMI-32), and a marker of neurofilament compaction (RMO-14), all processes associated with different aspects of axonal disruption. Using these markers, there is considerable overlap of expression, but there are also axonal populations identified by only one of the markers. This suggests that to fully evaluate axonal damage, a panel of antibodies should be applied.

Accumulation of β-APP is well known to occur in many other conditions that cause axonal damage (e.g., ischemia). In the context of TBI, the topographic pattern of axonal injury is rather distinctive. The corpus callosum, internal capsule, cerebellar peduncles, and descending long tracts in the brainstem are particularly vulnerable in TBI (Fig. 3.16). In ischemia, axonal injury and β-APP accumulation does not follow this pattern of white matter damage; rather, it involves all fiber tracts within the ischemic regions (Fig. 3.17). Often, a zigzag pattern can be seen in ischemic injury. In some cases, the degree of ischemic axonal injury may be so severe that it is not possible to comment on the presence or absence of TAI.

There is a sequence of cellular responses that evolves over time following TAI. In general, at 5- to 10-day survival after injury, microglial activation is first noted and followed by the formation of microglial "clusters" or "stars" around degenerating axons. Eventually, the swellings are no longer detectable by any technique; the microglial nodules remain as the only sign of damage. In some long-term survivors after diffuse TAI, long tract degeneration can be detected immunohistochemically using a macrophage marker (e.g., CD68; Fig. 3.18). With time, glial scarring occurs in the central white matter and long tracts.

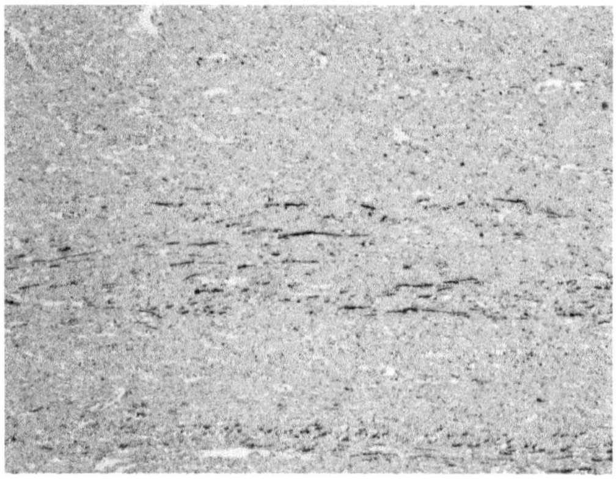

FIGURE 3.16 Traumatic axonal injury. Damaged axons, within the internal capsule from a case of severe diffuse TAI with a survival period of several hours, highlighted by β-APP immunohistochemistry (IHC). The orientation of the fiber bundles determines their susceptibility to traumatic rotational forces, unlike ischemic axonal injury (β-APP IHC).

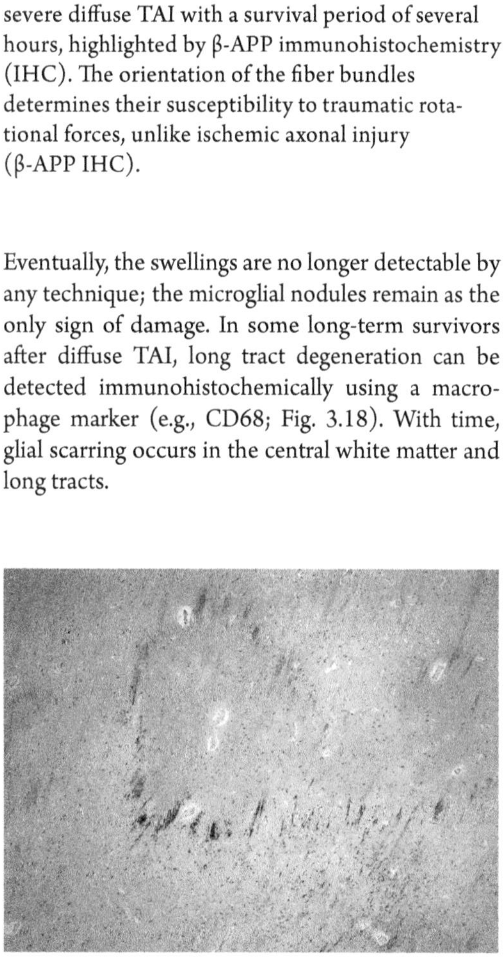

FIGURE 3.17 A diffuse pattern of axonal damage typical of ischemic injury highlighted with β-APP. The axonal damage is not defined by white matter bundle orientation but involves multiple axons in adjacent white matter bundles of different spatial orientation (β-APP IHC).

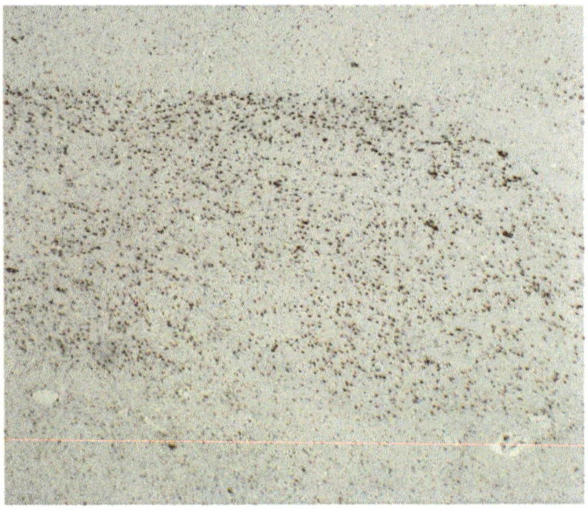

FIGURE 3.18 CD68 immunohistochemistry highlighting white matter damage consistent with axonal tract degeneration after diffuse traumatic axonal injury. The deceased was assaulted 16 months prior to death and never regained consciousness before succumbing to bronchopneumonia. The original admission magnetic resonance imaging was reported to show diffuse axonal injury (CD68 IHC).

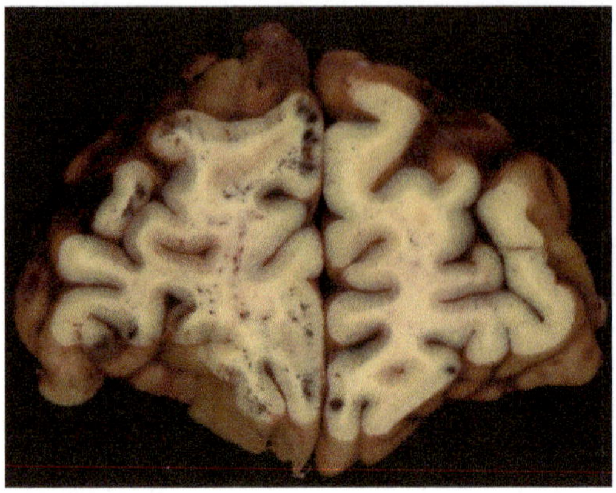

FIGURE 3.19 Coronal section through the frontal lobes showing the typical pattern of predominantly, but not exclusively, white matter petechial hemorrhages in diffuse vascular injury. The individual fell from a height.

3.3.2.3. AXONAL INJURY IN MILD HEAD INJURY

After mild head injury, axonal pathology has been detected in patients who have died from unrelated causes relatively soon after the insult. In these cases, the axonal injury was seen in the corpus callosum and fornices; it has been suggested that the forniceal pathology may be particularly relevant to post-traumatic amnesia.

Focal TAI is characterized by scattered foci of damaged axons in various parts of the neuraxis; in the context of TBI, its significance is currently uncertain. Focal TAI within the brainstem occurs in hyperflexion and hyperextension type injuries but is rare. In adults, this abnormality may be seen in fatal falls or in motorcycle accidents; in children, it is described in abusive head trauma (AHT). Focal TAI has been described within the corpus callosum in the absence of any diffuse process, and its significance is currently uncertain. It may be associated with concussive syndromes.

3.3.3. Diffuse vascular injury

Diffuse vascular injury is a severe form of rotational injury seen in fatal head injury and is associated with only short survival. Perivascular petechial hemorrhages are seen throughout the brain, particularly in the frontal parasagittal white matter (Fig. 3.19), basal ganglia, and brainstem.

3.3.4. Brain swelling

Brain swelling is a common finding in fatal TBI. The swelling may be focal, in relation to contusions; diffuse within one cerebral hemisphere; or diffuse involving both cerebral hemispheres.

The swelling may be congestive, secondary to an increase in the cerebral blood volume or due to edema. The edema with trauma is mostly cytotoxic (i.e., intracellular), with only a small component of swelling due to vasogenic edema from increased permeability of the microcirculation. Adjacent to contusions, there is physical disruption of the tissues, including the blood–brain barrier, and loss of the normal autoregulation within the local vasculature. Focal brain swelling may be seen in mild TBI (mTBI), but diffuse brain swelling is ordinarily only associated with severe head injury.

3.4. PENETRATING INJURIES

Penetrating injuries are injuries in which an object enters the cranial cavity. In strict terms, a penetrating injury is one in which the missile enters the cranial cavity but does not exit, whereas a perforating

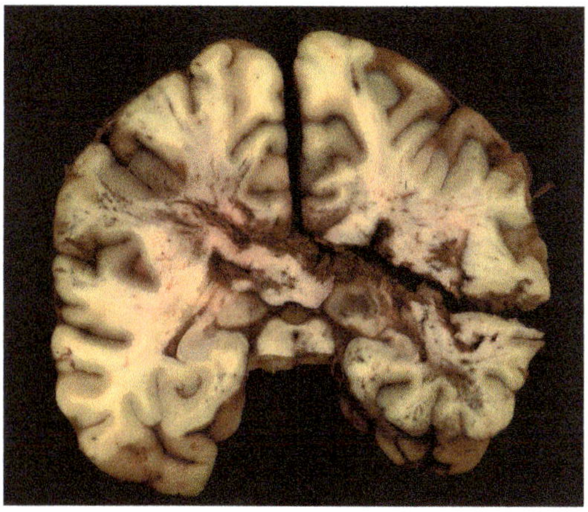

FIGURE 3.20 Perforating injury by a bullet producing a hemorrhagic tract through the two cerebral hemispheres into which the missile extended.

injury is one in which the missile also exits. The actual damage to the brain is extremely variable and depends on the nature of the missile. Sharp objects, such as knives, long nails, or metal poles, may pierce the skull and extend into the underlying brain parenchyma, causing local damage, such as a hemorrhagic tract ("permanent wound track") through the regions of parenchyma into which the missile extends. In contrast, high-velocity missiles, such as bullets (Fig. 3.20), cause considerably more damage because of the marked tissue displacement. The extent of the damage from high-velocity missiles is related to the velocity of the missile, with the missile producing pressure cavities that lead to tissue damage. High-velocity military weapons will cause greater tissue damage than small firearms. Infection is an important complication of almost all penetrating injuries.

3.5. BLAST INJURIES

Traditionally, the study of blast injuries has focused on the damage caused by blast waves to air-filled viscera, such as the lungs in the thoracic cavity. However, increasingly, attention has focused on the possibility of injury to solid viscera as well, particularly the brain. It has been suggested that the abrupt pressure changes associated with a blast can lead to mild head injury, particularly concussion. The current understanding of the pathophysiology of human blast injury is limited, and analysis of data is complicated because blast injury is often associated with blunt force TBI.

The cellular events that occur in this type of injury are poorly defined. Microscopic examination of brain tissue has shown microglial and astrocytic activation, particularly at the interface between brain parenchyma and fluids (periventricular region) and between gray and white matter.

3.6. CHRONIC TRAUMATIC ENCEPHALOPATHY

In recent years, there has been an increasing interest in evaluating the long-term complications of TBI, both in the setting of contact sports and also regarding the long-term complications associated with a single head injury. It has been known for many years that repetitive head injury is linked with neurodegeneration. The "punch-drunk" state was first described in 1928 and was later renamed *dementia pugilistica*, as it applied to professional boxers. Neurodegeneration as a sequela within the context of certain contact sports is now being carefully assessed throughout the world, and the current terminology has been adjusted to reflect this interest. The designation now used to apply to these cases is chronic traumatic encephalopathy (CTE).

The original clinical descriptions of dementia pugilistica described a degree of intellectual deterioration of variable severity, often with an associated movement disorder, usually Parkinsonism but in some cases patients exhibited predominantly ataxia. Currently, this clinical syndrome of dementia pugilistica is considered to be uncommon, although mild cognitive and movement disorders are still known to occur in some professional boxers.

The risks associated with repetitive mTBI are being considered in other contact sports, including soccer, rugby union and Australian rules football, American football, and ice hockey. In the absence of large prospective studies and difficulties in defining CTE clinically (the syndrome known as traumatic encephalopathy syndrome is still being defined), the absolute risk of cognitive impairment and development of movement disorders secondary to repetitive mTBI sustained in these contact sports remains unknown. Epidemiological studies do support an increased incidence of neurodegenerative disorders in professional contact sports, particularly amyotrophic lateral sclerosis and Parkinson disease.

The tauopathy associated with repetitive head injury was first reported in 1999, with neurofibrillary tangles and neuropil threads

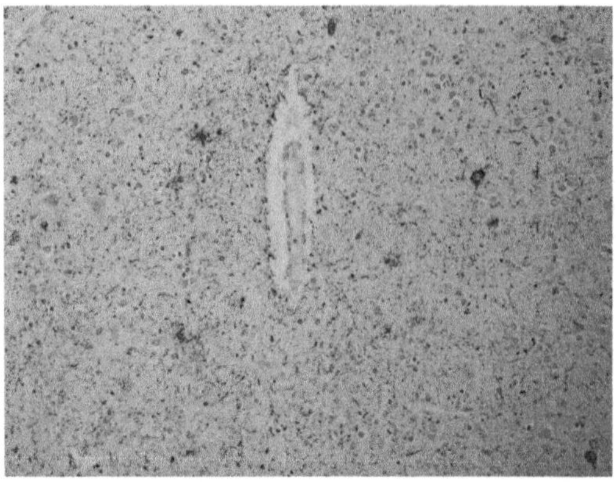

FIGURE 3.21 Immunohistochemistry for p-tau showing neuronal and glial tau inclusions in a perivascular distribution from a case of chronic traumatic encephalopathy (p-tau IHC).

immunoreactive to phosphorylated tau (p-tau), particularly around blood vessels (Fig. 3.21). A consensus statement defining the neuropathological criteria for CTE was published in 2016 and updated in 2021. The updated criteria recognize the difficulties in differentiating CTE from other tau proteinopathies, especially ARTAG and PART (see Chapter 8). There is a need for an algorithmic approach that starts with a case being diagnosed as CTE based on a pathognomic lesion and graded as low CTE or high CTE based on the severity of pathologic findings. The distribution of p-tau in CTE differs from that in Alzheimer disease, with CTE showing subpial clusters of astrocytic tangles; neurofibrillary tangles, predominantly within superficial cortical layers and within the depths of sulci; and perivascular distribution of both astrocytic and neuronal pathology.

TAR DNA-binding protein 43 (TDP-43) immunoreactivity has been described in 85% of CTE cases, predominantly neuritic, but in advanced CTE, intraneuronal and intraglial inclusions are also described. The concurrence of CTE with other neurodegenerative pathologies supports the concept that repetitive mTBI results in widespread cellular protein dysfunction at least in some cases.

At this stage, the diagnosis of CTE is a pathologic diagnosis, and there is a clear need to better define the association between neurodegenerative pathology and clinical phenotype through longitudinal cohorts and to demonstrate an association between repetitive mTBI/concussion and a specific pattern of neurodegenerative pathology.

3.7. PEDIATRIC HEAD INJURY

3.7.1. Perinatal nonabusive head injury

Perinatal head injuries can develop as a result of excessive molding of the cranial bones or excessive force applied to the skull during delivery. Hyperextension of the neck during delivery may result in craniocervical injuries.

Asymptomatic perinatal ASDH is common. However, life-threatening perinatal ASDH is rare and is traumatic in etiology. Tentorial laceration results in massive infratentorial SDH and may involve combinations of the vein of Galen, straight sinus, or transverse sinus. Laceration of the falx is less common than laceration of the tentorium cerebelli, and usually the tear is close to the junction of the falx and tentorium cerebelli. Finally, ASDH may be due to bridging vein rupture over the convexity of the brain and can be bilateral.

3.7.2. Accidental childhood head injury

Fatal head injury is not common in young children. Pediatric head injury after the age of 9–12 months reflects adult patterns of head injury; there are focal and diffuse injuries determined by the force and direction of the impact. Most injuries in this age group are due to falls or road traffic accidents.

Low-level falls are common events in childhood, and most household falls are benign. Witnessed fatal short falls are associated with skull fracture, usually linear, and EDH or SDH, the cause of death being the hemorrhage acting as a space-occupying lesion. Age and fall height influence the types of head injuries seen; infants sustain skull fractures more commonly than toddlers, and low-level falls (<3 feet) can cause intracranial injury in the absence of soft tissue injury or skull fracture.

3.7.3. Abusive head trauma

In the infant population, inflicted ("nonaccidental") injury, also called *abusive head trauma,* is an important cause of TBI. AHT may occur after the age of 9–12 months, but it is more common in younger infants, and in this group, head injury is rather different, presumably because of the anatomic and

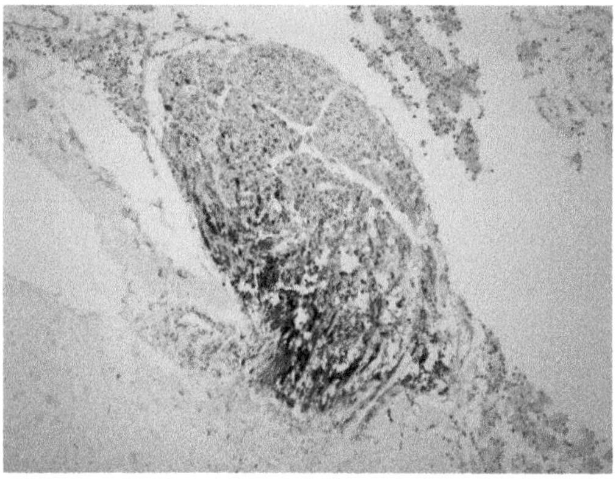

FIGURE 3.22 Immunohistochemistry of β-APP highlighting nerve root damage from a case in which an individual was convicted of a crime in association with abusive head trauma. The damaged axons were seen in nerve roots from the cervical region to the cauda equine (β-APP IHC).

physiologic immaturity of the infant's nervous system. Infants younger than age 9 months believed to have been shaken show a thin film of subdural bleeding or subdural hematoma, often midline; brain edema, potentially from global brain ischemia; and retinal hemorrhages. This "triad" is often considered "diagnostic" of abusive injury. Although the triad is not, in itself, pathognomonic of AHT, when this pattern of pathology (thin film SDHs, extensive, multi-layered retinal hemorrhages, and encephalopathy) is seen in the setting of a previously healthy infant who has sustained a sudden and catastrophic collapse in the absence of any natural disease, AHT is really the only diagnosis. In the world literature, there is not a single, independently witnessed accidental fatal head injury with the same pathology as seen in AHT. Therefore, despite the controversies associated with AHT, the diagnosis is usually straightforward.

Diffuse TAI is rare in AHT cases unless there is an obvious associated head impact. However, a significant number of cases do show focal TAI in the cervicomedullary region. In addition, β-APP immunostaining in spinal nerve roots (Fig. 3.22), often involving the full length of the spinal cord or accentuated in the lumbosacral region, is commonly seen in alleged AHT cases. It has been suggested that the thin-film SDH may sometimes have a "congestive" or hypoxic, rather than a traumatic, etiology and that retinal hemorrhages may result from the rapid rises in intracranial pressure aggravated by hypoxia. However, there is no convincing literature to support this hypothesis. SDH is not seen in independently witnessed choking events, or other potentially congestive etiologies, and is not seen in the setting of hypoxic ischemic encephalopathy, except in the perinatal and neonatal period where the bleeding most likely represents normal benign subdural bleeding associated with the compressive forces of uterine contraction during labor.

If shaking is the mechanism causing sudden collapse in these infants, an exaggerated "whiplash-type" injury in an infant with weak neck muscles may induce respiratory arrest (similar to impact brain apnea seen in adults), damage the thin bridging veins causing low-volume subdural bleeding, and damage retinal vessels.

4

Vascular Disease

JEAN-JACQUES HAUW, HARRY V. VINTERS, PIERRE AMARENCO, AND UMBERTO De GIROLAMI

FOR CONVENIENCE of presentation, we divide the discussion in this chapter into four broad categories: (1) hemorrhage, (2) infarction, (3) other disorders, and (4) mixed pathologic processes. Within these subdivisions, it is also possible to consider brain lesions that result from stenosis of large arteries and those that primarily involve arterioles or just components of the microcirculation; overlaps across these arbitrary subdivisions regularly occur.

4.1. INTRACRANIAL HEMORRHAGE

This section discusses brain hemorrhages that most often result in strokes (a term commonly used in clinical practice although not defined pathologically): nontraumatic *intracerebral hemorrhage* (ICH) and *subarachnoid hemorrhage* (SAH). An ICH is an extravasation of blood into the brain; a SAH is an extravasation of blood into the subarachnoid space (the space between the arachnoid membranes and the pia mater). ICH and SAH in the setting of traumatic injury are discussed in Chapter 3. Also excluded from consideration in this portion of the discussion are hemorrhagic infarcts (see Section 4.2.1.2), hemorrhages within neoplasms, and brainstem hemorrhages secondary to herniation (see Chapter 1).

- In SAH, bleeding primarily takes place in the leptomeningeal spaces and can extend within the subarachnoid space; rarely, it is localized as a subarachnoid hematoma. A SAH may also penetrate the brain parenchyma, extending into the cortex and white matter, and may ultimately burst into the ventricular cavities.
- In an ICH, or *intraparenchymal hemorrhage*, bleeding occurs first within the brain parenchyma. The hemorrhage may remain entirely within the brain substance, or it may also extend into the ventricular cavities and subarachnoid space. Extensive outpouring of blood into the ventricles eventually makes its way to the subarachnoid space via the foramina of Luschka and Magendie. In ICHs that involve the

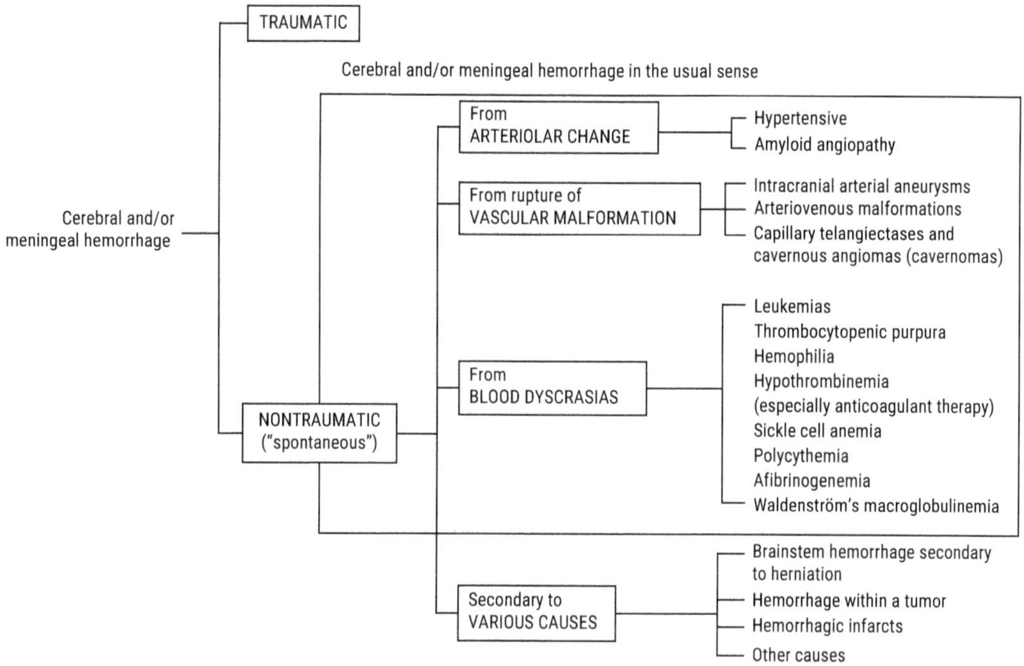

FIGURE 4.1 The principal causes of cerebral and/or meningeal hemorrhage.

superficial portions of the cerebral hemispheres, there may be direct extension of bleeding into the subarachnoid space (cerebromeningeal hemorrhage).

Although consideration of hemorrhage into various intracranial compartments provides an anatomic approach to assess different pathophysiologic mechanisms (Figs. 4.1 and 4.2), these classifications are somewhat arbitrary. For example, some causative agents and risk factors that lead to SAH are also important in ICH.

4.1.1. Subarachnoid hemorrhage

Hemorrhage into the subarachnoid space is an important cause of morbidity and mortality in all age groups of patients. *Primary SAH* most often results from rupture of an arterial berry or saccular aneurysm (localized dilation of an artery), usually on a branch of the circle of Willis. It may also complicate a vascular malformation within brain parenchyma adjacent to the subarachnoid space. SAH may also be seen in other settings, including cerebral amyloid angiopathy (CAA), reversible cerebral vasoconstriction syndrome, systemic hemorrhagic diatheses (e.g., severe thrombocytopenia), mycotic aneurysms, and other vasculitides.

4.1.1.1. BERRY/SACCULAR ANEURYSMS

An aneurysm is a localized pathologic dilation of an artery that results from the giving way of components of the arterial wall. *Saccular* or *berry aneurysms* are localized sac-like dilations of intracranial arteries. The aneurysmal outpouching is usually connected to the artery by a segment or *neck* that is narrower than the dome; the sac wall is formed by thin fibrous tissue with patchy interruption and attenuation of the elastic laminae, typically with thinning of the media (Fig. 4.3). Saccular aneurysms usually occur at major bifurcation points of the circle of Willis (Figs. 4.4 and 4.5). Most are found in the anterior circulation and involve the following sites: junction of the anterior cerebral artery and anterior communicating artery, junction of the internal carotid artery (ICA) and posterior communicating artery, ICA–ophthalmic artery, ICA–anterior choroidal artery, and the middle cerebral artery (MCA) bi-/trifurcation in the Sylvian fissure. Ten percent of all aneurysms are found in the vertebrobasilar territory, mainly at the top of the basilar artery. Berry aneurysms in older individuals may have superimposed atherosclerotic change.

Patients with a saccular aneurysm often come to medical attention between the ages 40 and

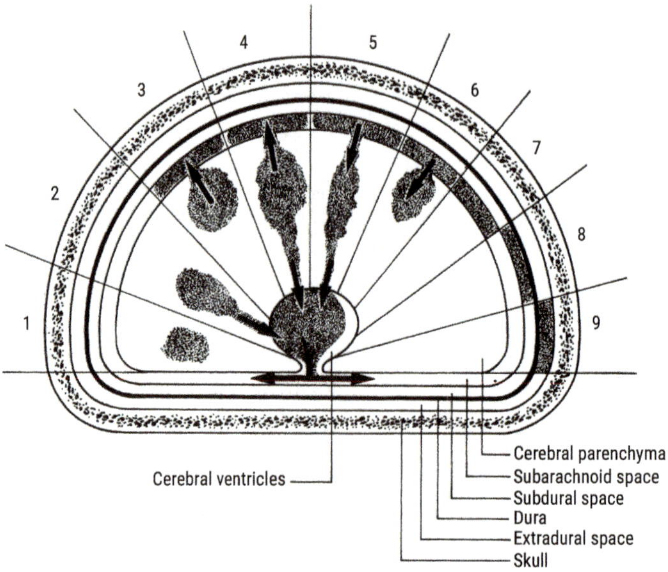

1. Pure cerebral hemorrhage (or cerebral hematoma)
2. Cerebral hemorrhage with ventricular rupture
3. Cerebromeningeal hemorrhage
4. Cerebromeningeal hemorrhage with ventricular ruputre
} Cerebral hemorrhages

5. Meningocerebral hemorrhage with ventricular rupture
6. Meningocerebral hemorrhage
7. Pure meningeal (subarachnoid) hemorrhage
8. Subdural hematoma
} Meningeal hemorrhages

9. Extradural (epidural) hematoma

FIGURE 4.2 Distribution of bleeding sites in the various forms of intracranial hemorrhage.

70 years. Saccular aneurysms are approximately 1½ to 2 times as common in women as in men; 10–30% of patients have multiple aneurysms. Aneurysms attributable to an identified genetic disorder, such as autosomal dominant polycystic kidney disease, are rare; however, the prevalence of aneurysms is 7–20% in first- or second-degree relatives of patients who have suffered an aneurysmal SAH. Although often referred to as congenital, saccular aneurysms are almost never encountered in children or infants. Rather, they are thought to develop as the result of degenerative changes within cerebral blood vessel walls, possibly secondary to abnormal smooth muscle and connective tissues. There is an increased incidence of intracranial aneurysms in some systemic diseases, including autosomal dominant polycystic kidney disease, Ehlers–Danlos syndromes, pseudoxanthoma elasticum, fibromuscular dysplasia, sickle cell disease, and coarctation of the aorta. Their association with Marfan syndrome has been questioned by recent data.

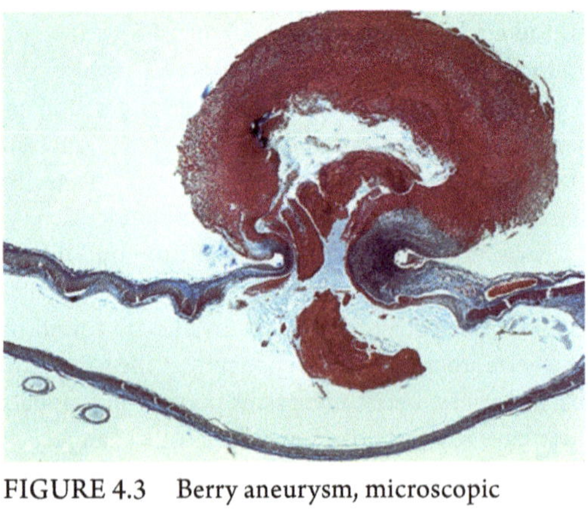

FIGURE 4.3 Berry aneurysm, microscopic appearance.

The clinical course of patients with saccular aneurysms depends most importantly on whether the lesion goes on to rupture (Fig. 4.6).

- Rupture of an aneurysm may lead to a life-threatening SAH (Fig. 4.7). Bleeding within the subarachnoid spaces spreads rapidly through the cerebrospinal fluid (CSF), causing multiple neurologic manifestations, including sudden

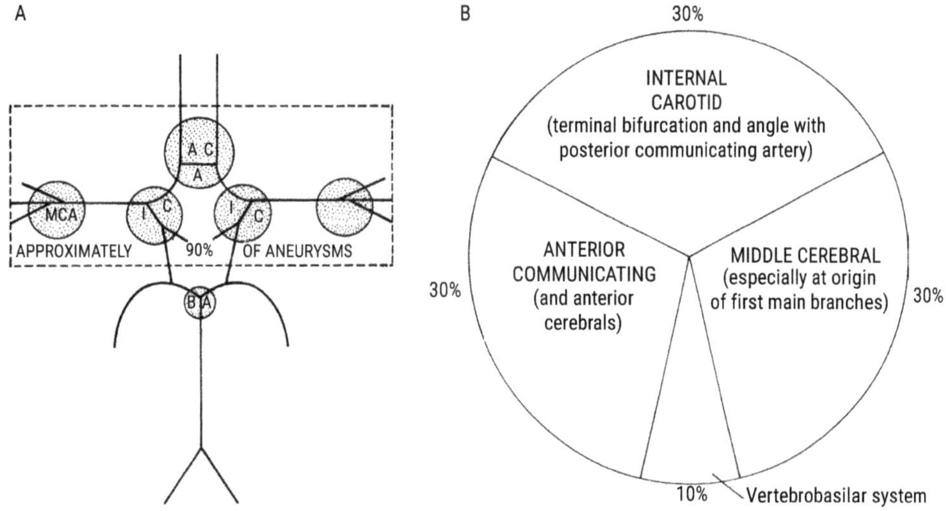

FIGURE 4.4 Distribution and frequency of arterial aneurysms. ACA, anterior communicating artery; BA, basilar artery; IC, internal carotid artery; MCA, middle cerebral artery.

onset of extremely severe headache, neck stiffness, and irritation of cranial nerves. Blood products elicit vasospasm in subarachnoid arteries, which may lead to multifocal infarcts or anoxic–ischemic change. Extensive SAHs may also result in rapidly increasing intracranial pressure, leading to death. Rebleeding may occur within 1 or 2 weeks after the initial event. The spread of hemorrhage in the SAH may be contained by the development of a subarachnoid hematoma. In many cases, the bleeding extends into the adjacent cerebral parenchyma (meningocerebral hemorrhage) (Figs. 4.8 and 4.9). Bleeding of a ruptured aneurysm may also occur directly into brain parenchyma, especially if the site of rupture on the dome of the aneurysm is embedded within brain substance. Over time, the blood in the CSF and parenchyma undergoes resorption, which is often incomplete (i.e., hemosiderin-laden macrophages may persist in it).

- Cerebral infarcts associated with aneurysmal rupture are frequent. Although their pathogenesis is uncertain, possible causes include arterial vasospasm, vascular compression from a subarachnoid hematoma, thrombosis of the affected vessel, embolization arising from a thrombus within the aneurysmal sac, microcirculatory dysfunction, and cortical spreading depression.
- Furthermore, patients with aneurysms, especially large ones, may develop symptoms due to compression of structures adjacent to the aneurysmal sac, particularly cranial nerves.
- Survivors of SAH may develop late post-bleed morbidity, often associated with hydrocephalus (secondary to fibrosis of the meninges resulting from accumulation of leptomeningeal blood products) or because of an associated cerebral infarction. A rare sequela of repeated episodes of a smoldering SAH is subpial siderosis. This phenomenon is the result of seepage of breakdown products of red blood cells, including iron pigment, into the molecular layer of the cerebral or cerebellar cortex (crests of folia) with secondary central nervous system (CNS) toxic injury and associated clinical manifestations.
- In many instances the aneurysm remains asymptomatic, and unruptured aneurysms are a relatively common incidental finding on imaging studies or at autopsy.

Surgical procedures to prevent aneurysm rupture or recurrent rupture include open surgical clipping; endovascular placement of coils to induce thrombosis within the aneurysm; and endovascular diversion procedures, such as placement of pipeline stents, to optimize flow dynamics and lower risk of rupture.

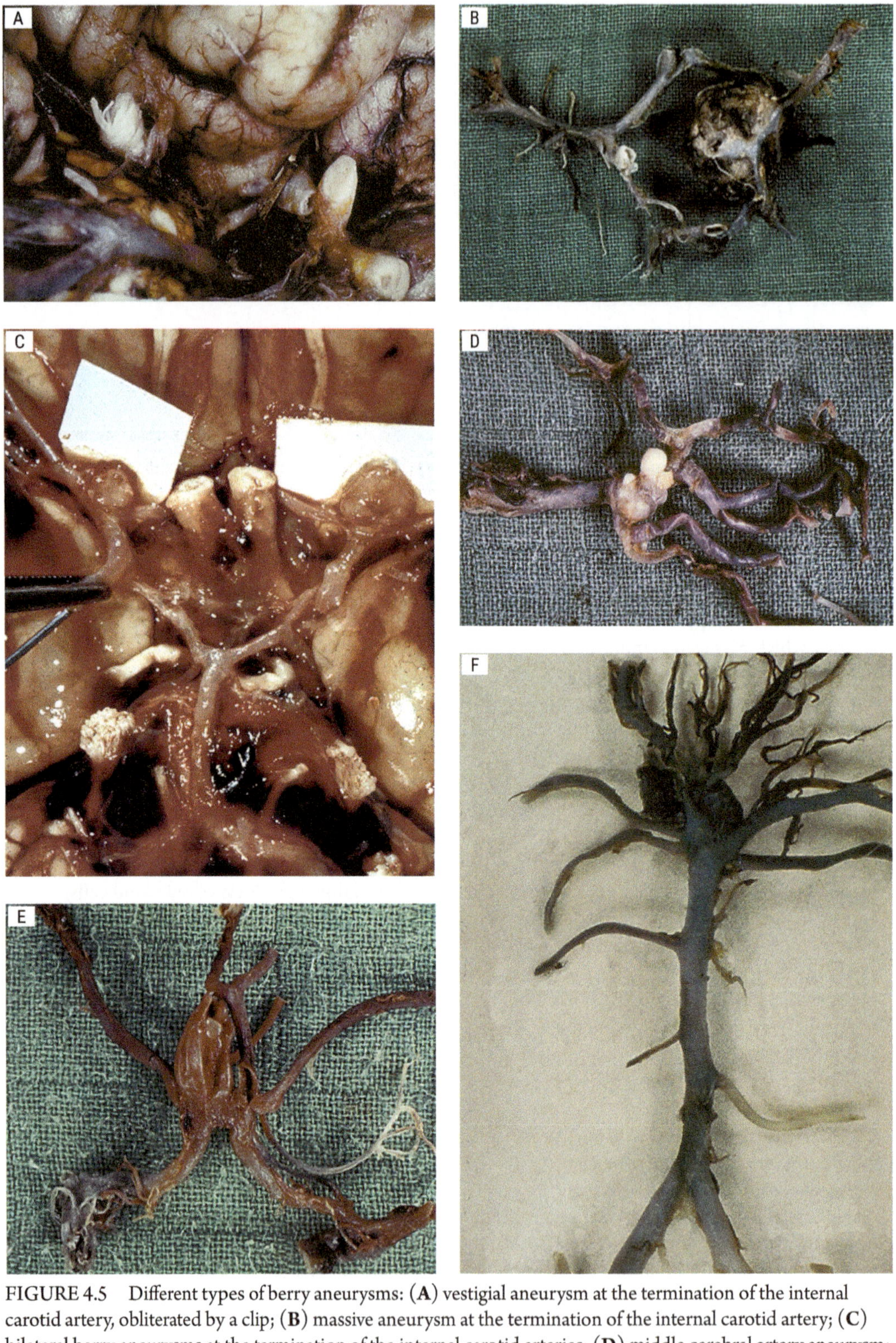

FIGURE 4.5 Different types of berry aneurysms: (**A**) vestigial aneurysm at the termination of the internal carotid artery, obliterated by a clip; (**B**) massive aneurysm at the termination of the internal carotid artery; (**C**) bilateral berry aneurysms at the termination of the internal carotid arteries; (**D**) middle cerebral artery aneurysm; (**E**) aneurysm of the anterior communicating artery; (**F**) aneurysm of the bifurcation of the basilar artery.

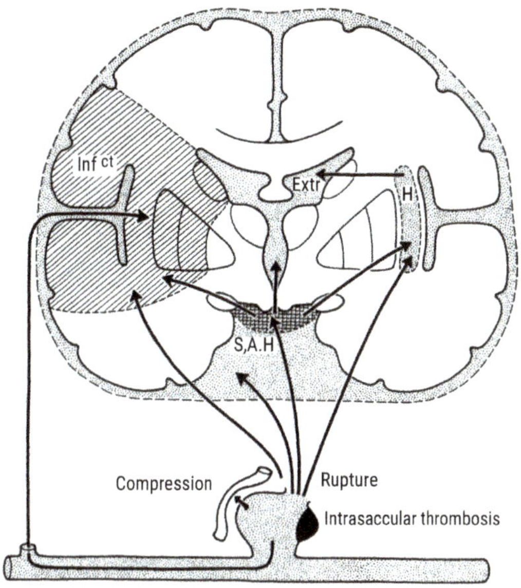

FIGURE 4.6 Representation of the principal complications resulting from arterial intracranial aneurysms. Inf^{ct}, infarction; Extr., ventricular extravasation; H, intracerebral hematoma; S.A.H., subarachnoid hematoma.

4.1.1.2. INFLAMMATORY/INFECTIVE ANEURYSMS ("MYCOTIC" ANEURYSMS)

The inflammatory/infective lesions ("mycotic" aneurysms), which account for 1–4% of all intracranial aneurysms, are usually seen with subacute or acute infective endocarditis. Less commonly, they may be seen with spread of infection from a contiguous site (e.g., osteomyelitis and meningitis) into the vessel wall. The microorganisms causing endocarditis are multiple, frequently of low virulence. Most infections are bacterial. Fungi, viruses, and parasites less commonly may be causative, particularly in immunocompromised patients and persons who use intravenous illicit drugs. Unlike berry aneurysms, infective mycotic aneurysms often occur in distal branches of the arterial tree and are almost always multiple. Rupture may result in subarachnoid or intraparenchymal bleeding.

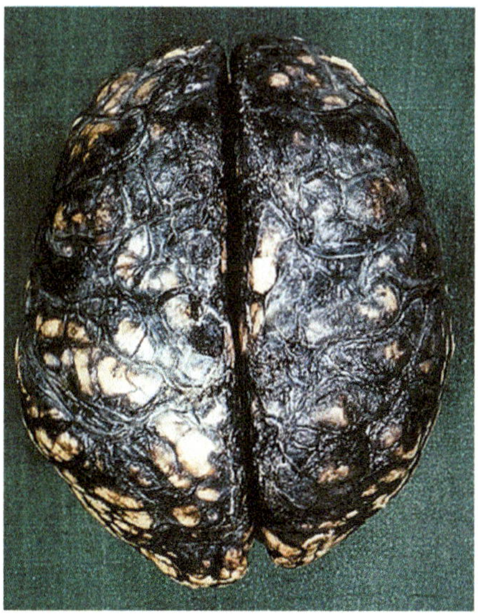

FIGURE 4.7 Diffuse subarachnoid hemorrhage over convexities, gross appearance.

Infective "mycotic" aneurysms due to endocarditis result from septic emboli that lodge within a branch of a cerebral artery with subsequent invasion of microorganisms from the emboli into the adjacent vessel wall. Emboli in individuals with infective endocarditis may lead to ischemic (bland) infarcts that may undergo hemorrhagic transformation, or they may cause pyogenic arteritis, leading to aneurysm, intracerebral hematoma, ischemic infarct, or cerebral abscess. The pathogenesis of the newly described GRE (gradient echo) or SWI (susceptibility-weighted imaging) magnetic resonance imaging (MRI) pattern of multiple microdeposits of hemosiderin in patients with infective endocarditis is yet to be fully elucidated (see Section 4.3.2.1 on cerebral microbleeds [CMBs]).

Postmortem examination of an intracerebral blood clot should include a search for an infectious ("mycotic") aneurysm, friable and weakened because of polymorphonuclear leukocytes in the vessel wall.

4.1.1.3. DISSECTING PSEUDOANEURYSMS (ARTERIAL DISSECTIONS)

Pseudoaneurysms resulting from arterial dissection are abnormities seen in young and middle-aged patients (<60 years); these lesions may be associated with infarcts or SAH. Dissection may occur in extracranial or intracranial branches of the carotid or vertebrobasilar system. When *intracranial* dissection occurs in the anterior circulation, the site of dissection is usually between the internal elastic lamina and the media, with resultant intravascular thrombosis. When dissection occurs in the posterior circulation, transmural dissection often results in SAH.

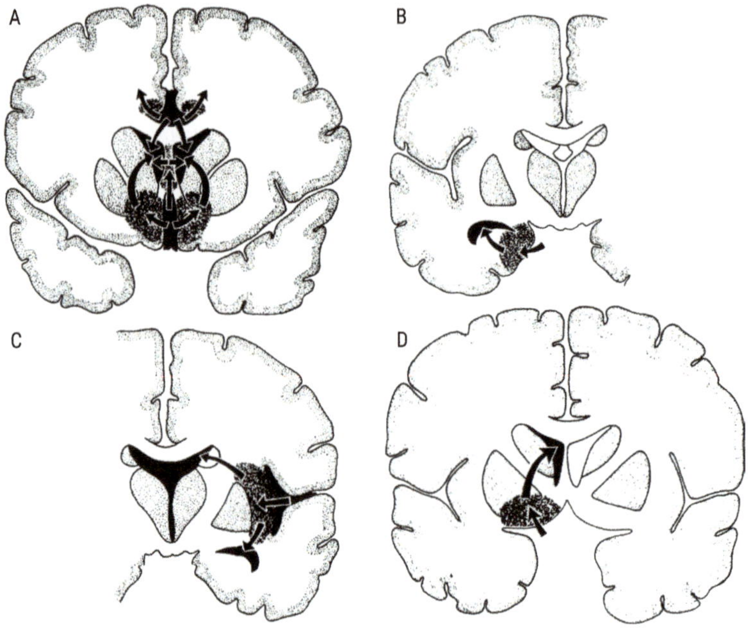

FIGURE 4.8 The sites of hematomas secondary to rupture of an arterial aneurysm: (**A**) aneurysm of the anterior communicating artery (and of the anterior cerebral artery); (**B**) aneurysm of the posterior communicating artery; (**C**) aneurysm of the middle cerebral artery; (**D**) aneurysm of the bifurcation of the internal carotid artery.

The aneurysmal swellings that occur are termed *pseudoaneurysms* because they form at the site of a tear in the vessel wall contained by adventitia rather than the full three-layer vessel wall seen with saccular aneurysms.

Specific vasculopathies associated with dissection include fibromuscular dysplasia and connective tissue disorders, including Marfan syndrome and Type IV (vascular) Ehlers–Danlos syndrome. Dissection of cervical arteries may also occur following frank trauma to the neck; minimal neck trauma, as from cervical manipulation or exercise; or seldom in association with heparin treatment or in the setting of disorders of connective tissue not related to specific syndromes. In most cases, the pathological substrate is undefined.

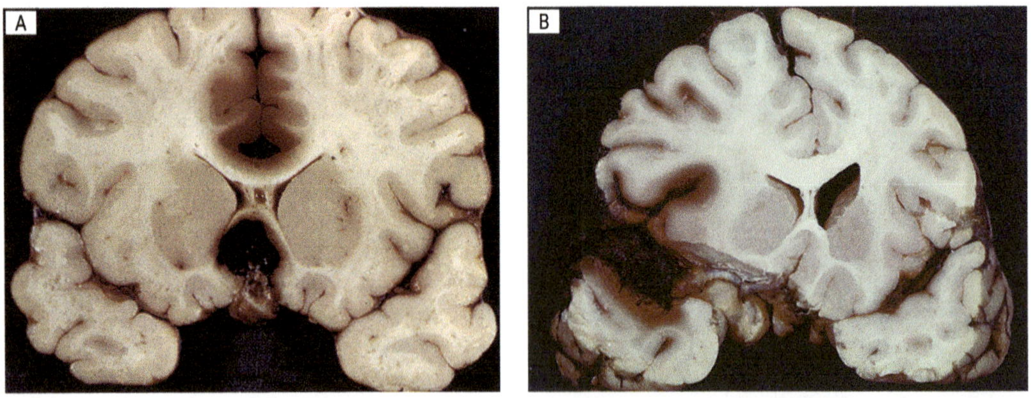

FIGURE 4.9 Hematomas resulting from the rupture of an arterial aneurysm: (**A**) bifrontal hematoma with ventricular rupture, following rupture of an aneurysm of the anterior communicating cerebral artery; (**B**) hematoma at the Sylvian fissure following rupture of an aneurysm of the middle cerebral artery.

4.1.1.4. FUSIFORM ANEURYSMS

A fusiform aneurysm (dilative arteriopathy or arterial dolichoectasia) in the brain occurs with an increase in the length and diameter of a large intracranial artery. An abnormally large external diameter (arbitrarily >2.5 cm) may reach giant proportions (Fig. 4.10A). These unusual lesions are most frequently found in geriatric patients. Dilative arteriopathy may be a systemic process involving several arterial beds simultaneously, such as the intracranial and/or coronary arteries and the aorta. It may be related to a dysfunction of matrix metalloproteinases. Dilative arteriopathy is also frequently associated with small vessel disease. Although not believed to be caused by atherosclerosis, it is often associated with it.

Fusiform aneurysms most commonly involve the basilar artery (Fig. 4.10B), causing brainstem displacement and compression, resulting in cranial nerve deficits among other neurological signs and symptoms. At autopsy, fusiform aneurysms have been associated with disruption of the arterial muscularis and internal elastic lamina. Laminated thrombi are often found within the lumen of the affected vessel (especially the aneurysmal segment), the result of severe complicated atherosclerosis. Platelet–fibrin or atheromatous thromboemboli may travel distally in the circulation to produce transient ischemic attacks or infarcts in branches of the vertebrobasilar circulation. They have been associated with ischemic events, even in the absence of concomitant atherosclerotic lesions. Slow blood flow in ectatic vessels may promote thromboembolic phenomena.

4.1.2. Intracerebral hemorrhage

The site and mechanisms of ICH vary depending on etiology. The most common causes of ICH are hypertension, CAA, coagulopathies (including hemorrhagic diathesis and as a complication of therapeutic anticoagulation), primary or secondary brain neoplasms, arteriovenous malformations (AVMs) and aneurysms, and *recreational* drug use (e.g., cocaine and heroin).

4.1.2.1. HYPERTENSION AND HYPERTENSIVE CEREBROVASCULAR DISEASE

Arterial hypertension is the most common cause of intraparenchymal hemorrhage; however, given the patient response to recommended decrease in salt intake and the increasingly effective medical treatment of hypertension, the incidence of hypertensive hemorrhage has markedly declined in many areas of the world. As the world population ages, CAA may become an increasingly important cause of ICH-related microvasculopathy.

4.1.2.1.1. Mechanisms. Intraparenchymal hemorrhage resulting from hypertension is usually attributed to hypertensive cerebral microvascular disease, also described as *arterio-* or *arteriolosclerosis (AS)* (depending on the diameter of the affected vessel) or *lipohyalinosis* in arteriolosclerosis, the latter describing a now conceptually disputed lesion in the arterioles of patients with severe hypertension. By comparison with large vessel atherosclerosis, the molecular pathogenesis of microvascular

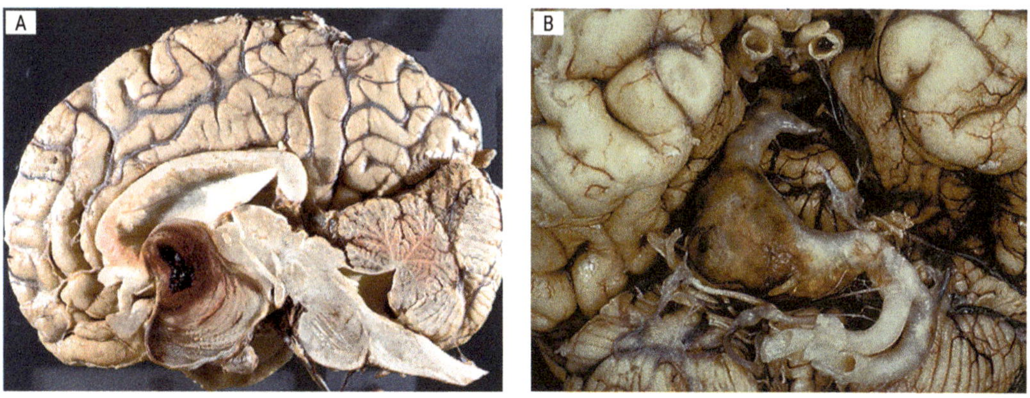

FIGURE 4.10 Giant atherosclerotic aneurysm (**A**) of the anterior cerebral artery and (**B**) of the basilar artery.

AS is poorly understood. The evolution of AS has been strongly associated with a documented history of hypertension. However, despite effective prophylactic treatment of severe and moderate hypertension in many countries, arteriosclerotic microvascular disease is still seen commonly in autopsy brain specimens, especially in the elderly.

Microscopic histopathologic features of AS include hyaline thickening (sometimes with degeneration of the internal elastic lamina), intimal fibromuscular hyperplasia, variable degrees of luminal narrowing, thinning of the media, concentric "onion-skin"–type smooth muscle cell proliferation, and the presence of foamy macrophages in the arterial wall (Fig. 4.11). Fibrinoid necrosis of the vascular wall occurs in malignant hypertension. These microvascular lesions may lead to occlusion of arterioles and to lacunar infarcts (see Section 4.3.2.2.1) or to weakening of the vessel, leading to rupture and intraparenchymal hemorrhage. Therefore, both arterial hypertension and inflammatory processes may lead to small artery rupture. This concept is under evaluation in trials using low-dose colchicine to reduce inflammation.

Hypertensive intraparenchymal hemorrhages are thought to be due to the rupture of small intracerebral arterioles 50–200 μm in diameter, the walls of which have been weakened by replacement of the normal media (muscular and elastic components) by collagenous fibrous tissue. Charcot–Bouchard aneurysms (also known as miliary aneurysms or microaneurysms) may sometimes be found in affected arterioles (Fig. 4.12), although they are often difficult to demonstrate, even when brain parenchyma around a putative hypertensive hemorrhage is extensively and carefully sampled. Although first described in association with high blood pressure, Charcot–Bouchard aneurysms are now known to occur with other types of microvascular disease (e.g., CAA).

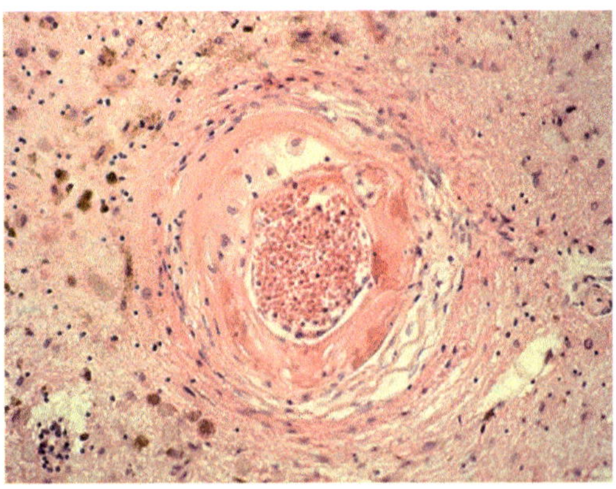

FIGURE 4.11 Arteriolosclerosis: narrowing of the lumen, concentric smooth muscle cell proliferation, and the presence of foamy macrophages in the arterial wall.

4.1.2.1.2. Evolution. The morphologic appearance of the hematoma varies depending on the time elapsed between its onset and the time of examination.

Initially, the intraparenchymatous bleeding results in a collection of blood that is under pressure, contains little parenchymatous debris, and displaces the cerebral structures (Fig. 4.13A, C, D). The edges of the hematoma are irregular, and small petechial hemorrhages are present along its borders. The bleeding may remain localized, but it may expand rapidly, resulting in increased intracranial pressure and brain herniation. The hematoma may also rupture into the ventricles, with subsequent extension of blood into the subarachnoid spaces. Less often, it may burst directly into the subarachnoid space through the cerebral cortex. This direct extension of ICH into the subarachnoid space more commonly occurs with CAA-related bleeding.

Over the course of 2–4 days, a phagocytic process begins to evolve. The focal hemorrhage is cleared by activated microglia/macrophages and macrophages derived from blood monocytes.

Hematomas that are months to years old appear as cystic cavities representing the remnants of resorbed blood; the cavities have an orange-yellow margin and gliotic brain tissue (Fig. 4.13B). Microscopic sections around the edges of the hematoma show hemosiderin-laden macrophages, reactive astrocytes, and often granular eosinophilic bodies.

4.1.2.1.3. Topography. Approximately 80% of hypertensive intraparenchymal hemorrhages are situated in the cerebrum, mostly in the basal ganglia (Fig. 4.13). Deep hemorrhages into the basal ganglia and thalamus are the most common. These hemorrhages can be divided into four groups based on location:

1. Putamen and external capsule (lateral basal ganglia) hemorrhages may extend superiorly and medially into the internal capsule and lateral ventricle.
2. Medial basal ganglia hemorrhages always extend into the internal capsule and usually the globus pallidus and frequently into the third ventricle;

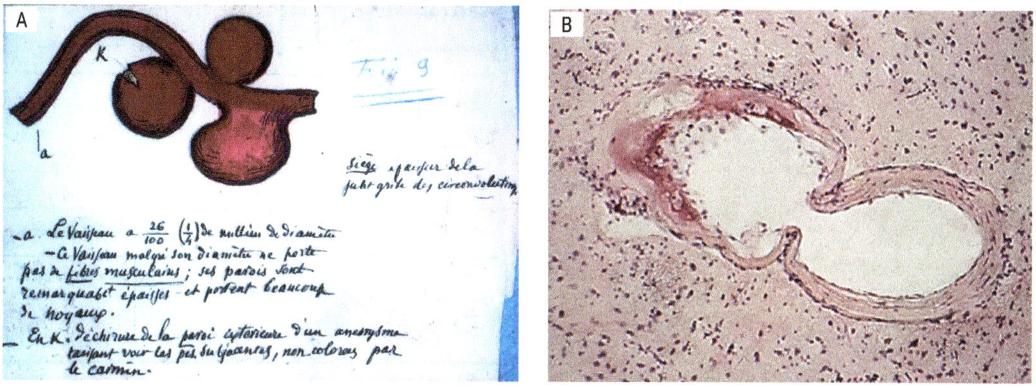

FIGURE 4.12 Miliary aneurysm (Charcot–Bouchard): (**A**) Charcot–Bouchard microaneurysms as drawn by J.-M. Charcot. "Location: Hemispheric gray matter. The vessel is 26/100 (1/4) mm wide; despite its size, the wall is devoid of a muscle layer and is thickened"; (**B**) microscopic appearance (hematoxylin and eosin [H&E]).

they may also involve the white matter of the superior temporal gyrus.

3. Thalamic hemorrhages are less common, accounting for 10–20% of hypertensive intraparenchymal hemorrhages. These can involve the internal capsule and caudate nucleus and rarely the subthalamic nucleus and midbrain. Extension into the third ventricle is seen in more than 50% of cases.
4. Massive hemorrhages destroying most of the structures mentioned are relatively infrequent. Increased intracranial pressure with herniation

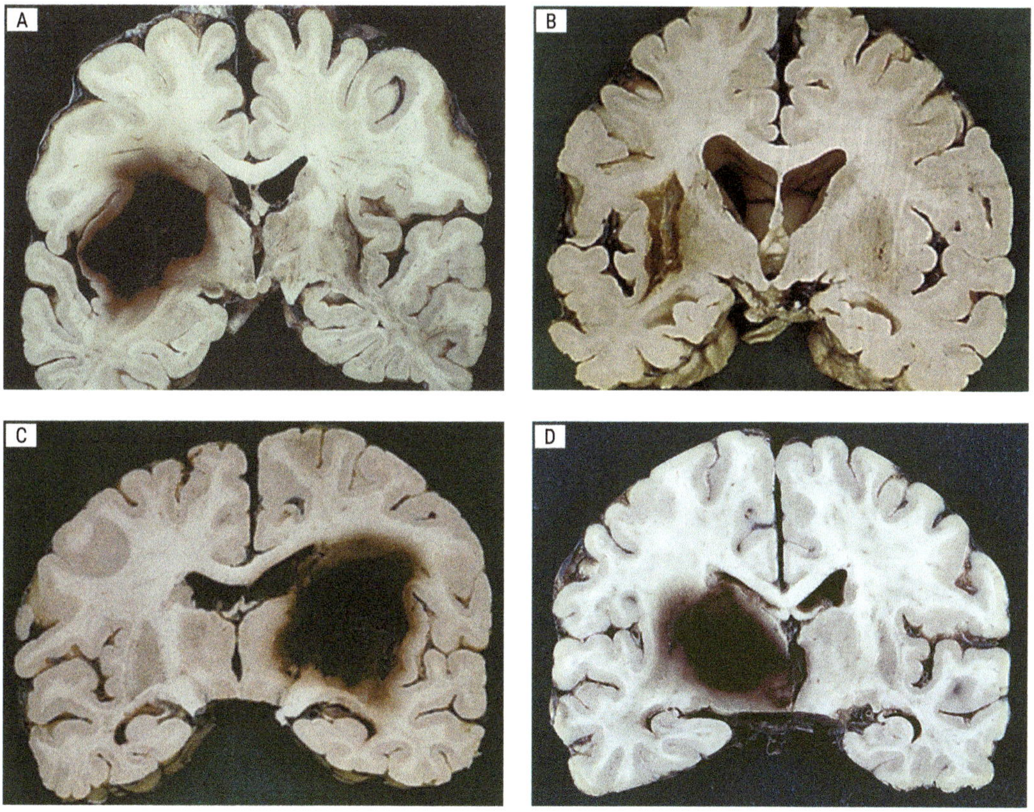

FIGURE 4.13 Basal ganglia hemorrhages: (**A**) lateral basal ganglia hemorrhage; (**B**) cystic scar of an old capsulo-lenticular hemorrhage; (**C**) massive hemorrhage; (**D**) medial thalamic hemorrhage.

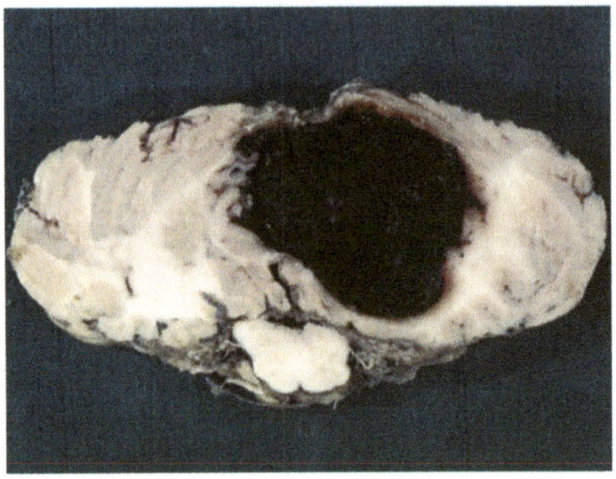

FIGURE 4.14 Intracerebellar hemorrhage.

is commonly seen in massive hemorrhages; this is uncommon in hemorrhages originating in the thalamus.

Hypertensive hemorrhage may also develop in the subcortical white matter. The lesions may be massive ("lobar") or localized small extravasations at the junction of the cortex and white matter ("slit hemorrhages").

Intracerebellar hemorrhages (Fig. 4.14) account for approximately 10% of all hypertensive intraparenchymal hemorrhages. The clinical course in these patients follows what is typical of a space-occupying mass in the posterior fossa; the hemorrhage may rupture into the fourth ventricle. Neurosurgical removal of a cerebellar hemorrhage may lead to clinical improvement.

Brainstem hemorrhages (Fig. 4.15) account for approximately 10% of hypertensive intraparenchymal hemorrhages and most often occur in the pontine tegmentum and basis pontis.

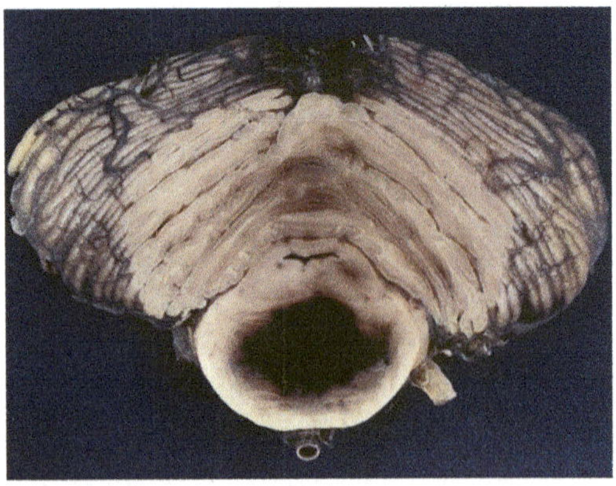

FIGURE 4.15 Pontine hemorrhage.

4.1.2.2. CEREBRAL AMYLOID ANGIOPATHY

Cerebral amyloid angiopathy is more commonly associated with cerebral hemorrhage than with ischemia. The lesion is characterized by the deposition of amyloid within the media or adventitia of small parenchymal and leptomeningeal vessels. The term *amyloid* refers to proteinaceous material that tends to aggregate into clumps due to the unique physicochemical structure of β-pleated sheets, giving it specific staining and optical properties. The deposits produce green fluorescence under ultraviolet light following staining with thioflavin T. Amyloid stains red with Congo red (congophilic angiopathy) and gives apple-green birefringence under polarized light (Fig. 4.16A). Immunohistochemical methods are now most often used to demonstrate the various types of amyloid deposits. Viewed by electron microscopy, the deposits have a characteristic ultrastructural fibrillary appearance. The biochemical composition of the amyloid varies, depending on the biochemical nature of the protein (see next section).

4.1.2.2.1. Etiology. The most common form of CAA is associated with deposition of Aβ protein, a small, 4.2-kDa peptide cleaved from the amyloid precursor protein (APP) and encoded by a gene on chromosome 21. CAA has a strong association with Alzheimer disease and aging. These conditions are associated with excessive deposition of Aβ in both the brain gray matter (as senile plaques and diffuse deposits) and vessel walls (as CAA) to variable extents in different patient populations (see Chapter 8). (Fig. 4.16B, C) Brains with moderate to severe CAA show a statistically significantly higher prevalence of hemorrhagic (and sometimes ischemic) lesions than do those without CAA.

Relatively rare familial forms of CAA have also been found in various countries throughout the world:

- In a circumscribed coastal region of the Netherlands, an autosomal dominant form of severe CAA (*hereditary cerebral hemorrhage with amyloidosis, Dutch type* [*HCHWA-D*]) is attributed to a unique *APP* gene mutation (at codon 693). Massive Aβ deposition occurs within the media of cerebral arterioles, and fatal cerebral parenchymal hemorrhages frequently result.

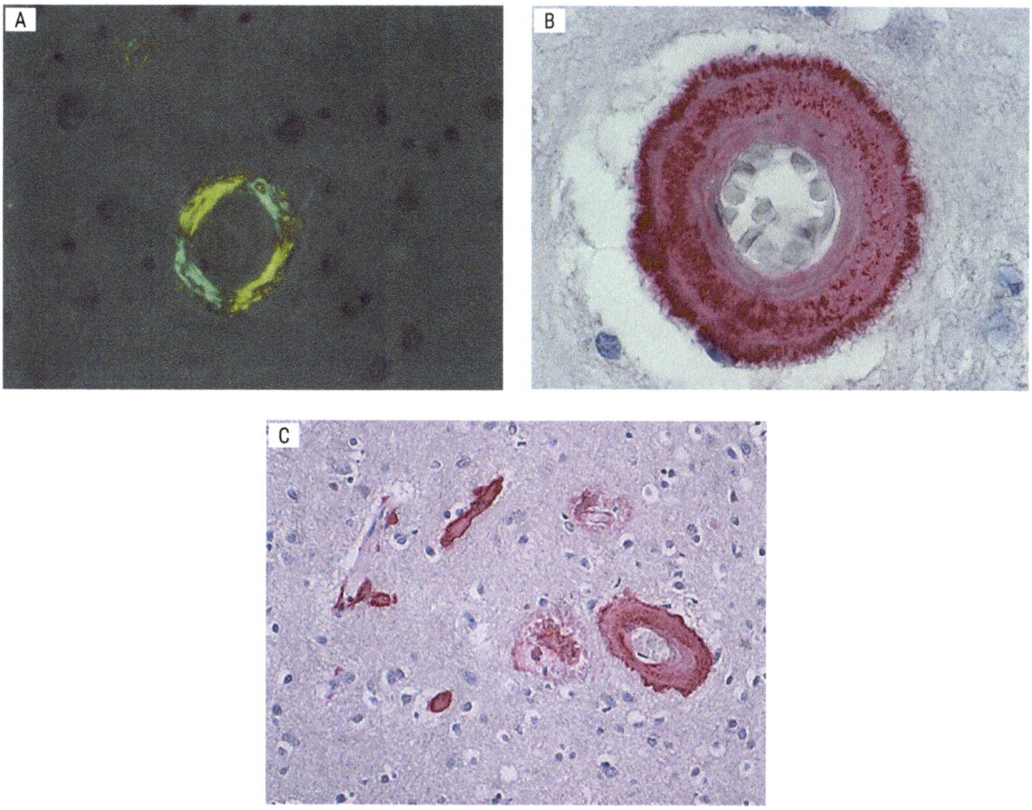

FIGURE 4.16 Cerebral amyloid angiopathy: Apple-green birefringence of the vessel wall under polarized light with Congo red stain (**A**); immunocytochemistry for Aβ shows diffuse infiltration of the arteriolar wall by amyloid (**B, C**). There is also involvement of the capillaries (dysphoric angiopathy), with amyloid appearing to be "leaking" from the capillary wall into brain parenchyma (**C**).

- *APP* codon 692 and 694 mutations appear to cause, respectively, *a rare Flemish form of CAA* (also with frequent intraparenchymal hemorrhage) and *Alzheimer disease with prominent CAA* in a family reported from the US state of Iowa and another family in Ireland.
- An Icelandic form of CAA leading to hemorrhagic stroke, *hereditary cerebral hemorrhage with amyloidosis, Icelandic type* [*HCHWA-I*]), results from mutation in the gene encoding cystatin C/gamma-trace. Hence, this condition is also sometimes described as hereditary cystatin C amyloid angiopathy (HCCAA). This mutation causes cerebral hemorrhages in young and middle-aged adults. Brains from patients with HCHWA-I show extensive deposition of gamma-trace protein within arteriolar walls, associated with degeneration of the affected vessel walls.
- *Familial British and Danish forms of CAA* have also been described and attributed to unique mutations on the *BR12* gene, situated on chromosome 13. These two, and other genetically determined forms of CAA (e.g., *meningovascular amyloidosis associated with transthyretin deposition* and *familial amyloidosis of the Finnish type caused by gelsolin deposition*), are less consistently associated with intraparenchymal hemorrhage than are the Dutch, Flemish, and Icelandic familial variants of CAA.

4.1.2.2.2. Pathology. Cerebral amyloid angiopathy may affect all regions of neocortex and overlying meninges, with minor variations in the distribution of affected arteries in different lobes of the brain. Although the cerebellum and its meninges are occasionally involved by CAA, the microvascular abnormality is almost never found within deep central gray matter, the brainstem, or the spinal cord. The white matter vessels seem mostly unaffected. CAA may be patchy within the cerebral cortex and adjacent leptomeninges; it can be segmental in given small vessels and variable among the cerebral lobes.

The term *cerebral amyloid angiopathy* encompasses amyloid deposition within the walls of small and medium-size venules, arteries, and arterioles (congophilic angiopathy, also called type 2 of Thal) (Fig. 4.16B, C). In dysphoric angiopathy, also called type 1 of Thal, amyloid gives the appearance of "leaking" from the capillary wall into brain parenchyma (Fig. 4.16C). Type 1 is always found when type 2 is present, although sometimes the presence of amyloid renders the accurate identification of the vessel type difficult.

Histologically, there is infiltration of the media and adventitia of small vessels by an acellular amorphous eosinophilic substance, which gives the vessel wall a homogeneous pale appearance, with striking loss of medial smooth muscle cells, often allowing the diagnosis to be made on routine stains. In addition, some affected vessels, particularly pia mater arterioles, have a "double-barrel" appearance (Fig. 4.17A). Amyloid deposition in the arterial wall causes damage of the medial smooth muscle cells. These changes disrupt the vascular architecture and weaken the affected arterial walls. A variety of secondary changes may be found in the affected vessels, including fibrosis; microaneurysm formation; chronic (including granulomatous) (Fig. 4.17B) inflammation; fibrinoid necrosis; thrombosis; and, very rarely, vessel wall calcification.

4.1.2.2.3. Complications of CAA. Clinically, patients with CAA typically present to medical attention due to the onset of a lobar cerebral hemorrhage. Affected individuals are usually elderly. The hemorrhage less commonly occurs as a convexity SAH, or rarely, as cerebellar hemorrhage. The extent of amyloid deposition within vessel walls correlates with the risk of intraparenchymal hemorrhage. CAA causes hemorrhages with highly distinctive clinicopathologic features (Fig. 4.18). When the hemorrhage occurs within the cerebral cortex there may be dissection into the subarachnoid space; when in the subcortical white matter (lobar hemorrhages), rupture into the lateral ventricles may follow. This lobar, and to a lesser extent subarachnoid, localization results from the topography of CAA, a cortical and meningeal vasculopathy. CAA may be detected on neuropathologic examination in neurosurgical specimens of fragments of brain parenchyma evacuated together with a hematoma. Evidence of cerebral bleeding of different ages (months or years) can be seen at postmortem examination affecting different lobes of both cerebral hemispheres. As many as one-third of patients afflicted with CAA-related lobar hemorrhage may also have clinical evidence of hypertensive microangiopathies, and features of associated AS may be seen.

Other clinical manifestations of CAA seen less frequently include SAH *without* an intraparenchymal hemorrhage; CAA with superficial siderosis; CAA-related inflammation with leukoencephalopathy (see Section 4.3.2.3); CAA-related angiitis (amyloid β-related angiitis [ABRA]); granulomatous angiitis (Fig. 4.17B); brain infarct (especially

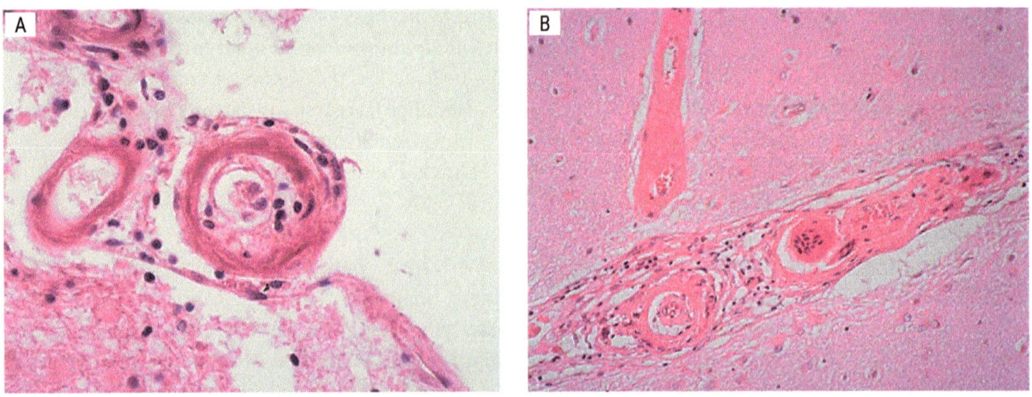

FIGURE 4.17 Cerebral amyloid angiopathy infiltration of the vessel wall by the acellular, amorphous, eosinophilic amyloid substance; note the "double-barrel" appearance of a leptomeningeal arteriole (**A**) and inflammatory granulomatous reaction (**B**) (H&E).

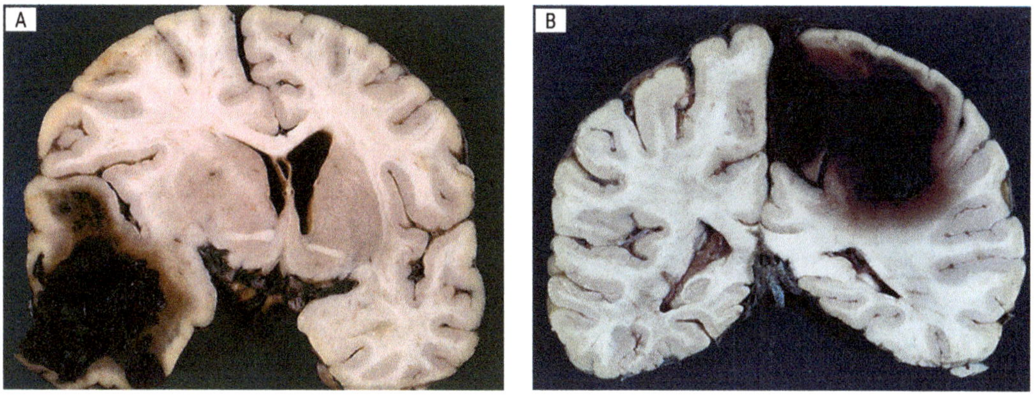

FIGURE 4.18 Intracerebral lobar hemorrhages in patients with CAA involving the temporal lobe (**A**) and the parieto-occipital region (**B**).

microinfarcts); and recurrent transient neurologic symptoms (so-called amyloid spells), possibly due to cortical spreading depression from sites of microinfarct or miliary hemorrhage in the cerebral cortex. When CAA is associated with inflammation in and around the affected vessels, clinical response to anti-inflammatory drugs is sought.

4.1.2.3. VASCULAR MALFORMATIONS

Vascular malformations may be found in the CNS parenchyma, extending to the subarachnoid space overlying dura, or (rarely) both.

4.1.2.3.1. Arteriovenous malformations. AVMs are the most clinically important and most common disorders in this category; these developmental lesions rarely become manifest clinically beyond age 60 years. They include all direct and indirect communications between one or more arteries of the brain or spinal cord parenchyma, and one or more draining veins, without an intervening capillary bed. AVMs have a core of abnormal channels called the nidus. They are variously referred to as arteriovenous varix, varicose aneurysm, aneurysm by anastomosis, pulsating venous aneurysm, and cirsoid aneurysm.

AVMs may cause intraparenchymal hemorrhage, SAH, or both. The lesion usually occurs in the MCA territory, often involving a wedge-shaped area of brain parenchyma and the overlying leptomeninges, but AVMs may be seen anywhere in the CNS, including posterior fossa, and rarely confined to the circle of Willis.

Dural arteriovenous fistulas (DAVFs) are arteriovenous shunts with no nidus. These are acquired lesions that, unlike AVMs, typically present in older age. The arterial feeders are supplied by dural arteries. Rare pial arteriovenous fistulas are fed by pial or cortical arteries. When they occur along the spinal cord, they can give rise to a slowly progressive myelopathy, Foix–Alajouanine disease.

The venous drainage of AVMs and DAVFs may take place in the superficial or the deep draining systems of the brain. The morphologic features of an AVM are characteristic, both grossly and microscopically (Fig. 4.19A). An AVM is recognized histologically as a collection of vascular channels of variable mural thickness and diameter, embedded within abnormal, gliotic, and occasionally malformed brain parenchyma. The CNS parenchyma may show morphologic evidence of old hemorrhage. Thrombosed and recanalized vascular channels are usually present within an AVM. Other associated abnormalities include hyalinized, sometimes calcified (very rarely, ossified) vascular walls or abnormalities in the blood vessels comparable to intimal fibromuscular hyperplasia, as seen in atherosclerotic arteries.

The AVMs become symptomatic following rupture of the vessel wall and bleeding and direct pressure and damage to adjacent brain tissue. Clinical manifestations include partial seizure and focal deficits because of mass effect or "steal" of blood from adjacent structures in the setting of arteriovenous shunting. AVMs are associated with berry aneurysms in 10% of cases. DAVFs commonly affect the spinal cord; true AVMs do so rarely. AVMs and DAVFs are usually treated by surgical excision, radiation therapy, or endovascular embolization therapy.

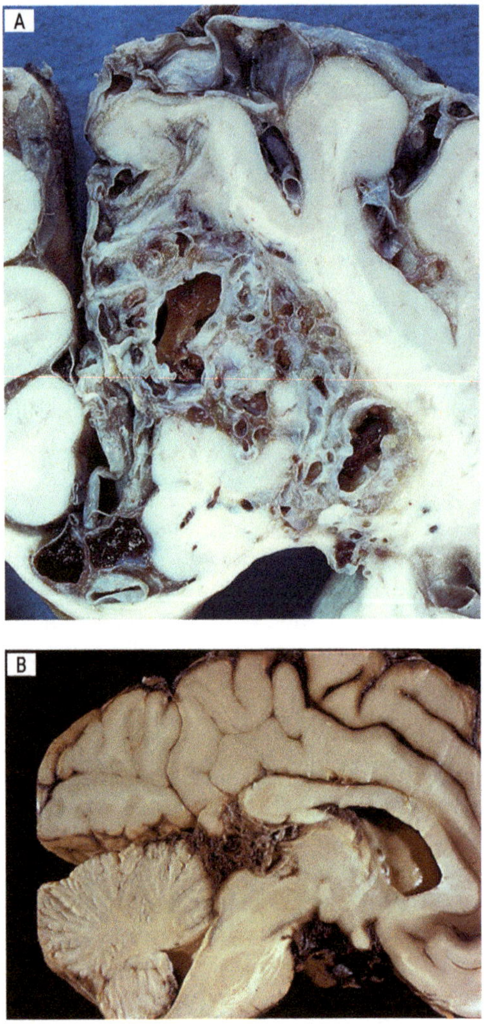

FIGURE 4.19 Vascular malformations: (**A**) medial frontal cerebral arteriovenous malformation; (**B**) vein of Galen aneurysm.

4.1.2.3.2. Developmental venous angiomas. Developmental venous angiomas (DVAs) consist of one or more dilated, often grossly apparent, veins and their smaller tributaries, lacking an obvious arterial component. A single tortuous vein (e.g., in the spinal subarachnoid space) is described as a *varix* (Fig. 4.19B). Component vessels of a DVA are more dilated and have thicker walls than normal veins, and brain parenchyma between the vessels shows negligible reactive changes or old hemorrhage. They are often seen on imaging studies during life and usually found as incidental lesions at autopsy.

4.1.2.3.3. Capillary telangiectasia. Capillary telangiectasias are also common incidental lesions found on imaging studies or at autopsy. On macroscopic examination, both DVAs and capillary telangiectasias appear as small, fairly well-defined hemorrhagic lesions that initially suggest a localized region of petechial hemorrhage. Microscopically, they consist of multiple dilated capillaries without abnormalities (either malformative or hemorrhagic/reactive) of the surrounding brain substance; surrounding glial reactive changes may be seen.

4.1.2.3.4. Cerebral cavernous malformations. Cerebral cavernous malformations (CCMs) appear as closely packed blood vessels of varying wall thickness without intervening CNS parenchyma. The malformation is most often seen in the basis pontis or subcortical white matter; in these locations, the lesion may clinically mimic a primary CNS neoplasms, and patients may present with focal signs from the space-occupying lesion, producing mass effect and/or seizures. Although the lesions do not usually lead to massive hemorrhage, there are almost always surrounding deposits of hemosiderin visible on microscopic examination, suggesting slow or recurrent leakage of blood from component abnormal vessels. Familial syndromes of cavernous malformations have been linked to genes on chromosomes 3q (*CCM3*), 7q (*CCM1*), and 7p (*CCM2*).

4.1.2.4. SYSTEMIC AND MISCELLANEOUS FACTORS

Intracerebral hemorrhages may result from systemic disease and other factors, including thrombocytopenia, iatrogenic coagulopathy, hepatic failure, hemophilia, disseminated intravascular coagulation, and leukemia (Fig. 4.20). The hemorrhages seen in

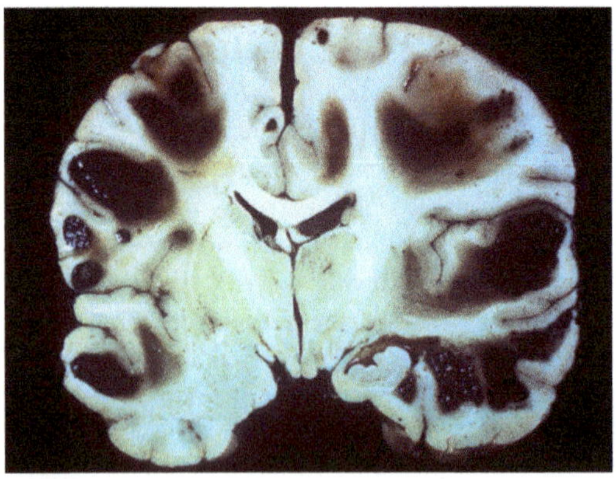

FIGURE 4.20 Multiple lobar hemorrhages in a patient with leukemia.

patients with these diseases may mimic hematomas associated with hypertension or CAA, both in extent and topography.

4.2. ISCHEMIC VASCULAR PATHOLOGY OF ARTERIAL ORIGIN: INFARCTION

The terms *cerebral infarct, cerebral softening,* and *encephalomalacia* are used to denote an area of tissue necrosis localized to a territory of vascular supply. In most cases, an infarct is due to occlusion of a branch of the feeding arterial tree. It may also follow a severe global decrease in blood flow in the absence of arterial occlusion. In venous infarction, the tissue ischemia is due to the occlusion of a large vein (and often its branches) and consequent stasis of blood flow.

4.2.1. General features

Arterial occlusion of sufficient duration produces ischemic necrosis of tissue. The macroscopic and microscopic appearances associated with infarction are manifest by a series of sequential changes that are distinctive regardless of the site of the affected territory within the CNS.

The main types of infarction generally recognized are *anemic,* or *pale, infarcts,* in which the cellular reactions to ischemic necrosis predominate (Fig. 4.21); and *hemorrhagic infarcts,* in which the lesions are associated with hemorrhage. The associated hemorrhages especially involve the cortical ribbon and the basal ganglia (Fig. 4.22).

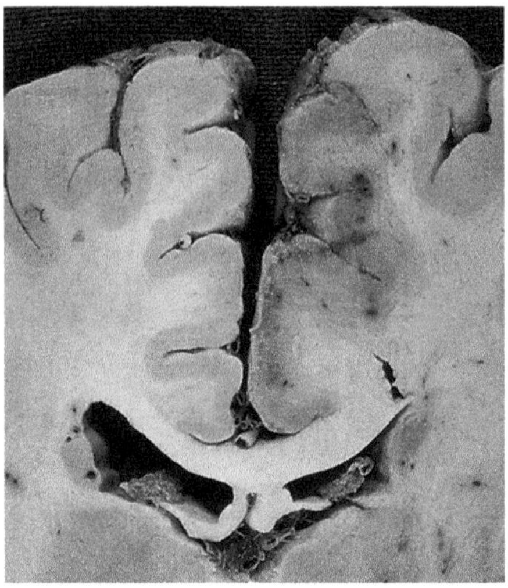

FIGURE 4.21 Recent anemic *or* pale infarct involving the territory of the right anterior cerebral artery.

4.2.1.1. ANEMIC/PALE (BLAND) INFARCTION

On macroscopic examination, the lesions of anemic/pale (bland) infarction are poorly circumscribed early during the evolution of the infarct (Fig. 4.21). In the first 6 hours or so, no visible alteration can be demonstrated with the naked eye, although the neurons are irreversibly damaged. From 8 to 48 hours, the damaged zone becomes discolored, and the demarcation between the white and gray matter is indistinct ("blurred"). Edematous swelling is apparent and is sometimes accompanied by vascular congestion, which is more marked in the cortex. At this stage, the softer consistency of the involved area is the most apparent feature that permits the infarct to be recognized macroscopically after 2 or 3 weeks of formalin fixation. From 2 to 10 days in the course of the evolution of the infarct, the swelling persists, progressively decreasing over time, while the softened tissue becomes more friable, and the boundaries of the infarcted territory become better defined.

Microscopically, after 6–12 hours, the neurons within the infarcted territory demonstrate the features of acute ischemic cell injury; that is, the perikaryal cytoplasm is eosinophilic, the Nissl substance is dispersed, the nucleus is shrunken, and the nucleolus is no longer visible (Fig. 1.2). In the cortex and white matter, the capillary blood vessels show endothelial swelling accompanied by vasogenic and cytotoxic edema and with some extravasation of red blood cells (even in anemic infarction). Simultaneously, glia also manifest ischemic cell damage; somewhat later, myelinated fibers lose their usual tinctorial hue, irrespective of staining technique. Between 24 and 48 hours, there is evidence of a migration of neutrophils, which can be severe and may simulate an acute infectious process (Fig. 4.23). After 48 hours, the leukocytes are replaced by macrophages. These cells, which are laden with breakdown products of cell disintegration, cluster around the swollen capillary blood vessel walls. The macrophage proliferation increases progressively after 5 days, and macrophages may remain in the infarcted tissue for the life of the affected patient.

After 10 days, macroscopically, liquefaction begins, and from the third week onward,

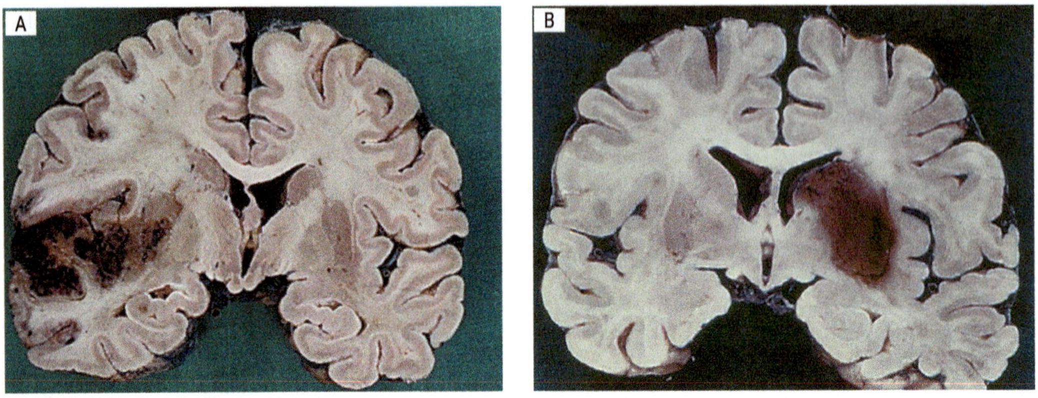

FIGURE 4.22 Hemorrhagic infarcts in middle cerebral artery occlusion. (**A**) The hemorrhages may involve the entire extent of the ischemic region. (**B**) They also occur commonly in the basal ganglia.

the process of cavitation becomes more evident. From that point, yellowish, sunken gray tissue replaces the necrosis. The macrophage proliferation persists, although to a decreasing degree, during the subsequent months, and the number of swollen, reactive astrocytes (gemistocytic) progressively increases. After a few months, the necrotic zone becomes a cystic cavity with ragged outlines, intersected by vascularized connective tissue strands and covered by leptomeninges on its cortical surface (Fig. 4.24). During the phase of scar formation, the residual cystic cavity is surrounded by a glial proliferation, while a few macrophages remain along the persisting connective tissue strands and thin-wall blood vessels that run across the cavity.

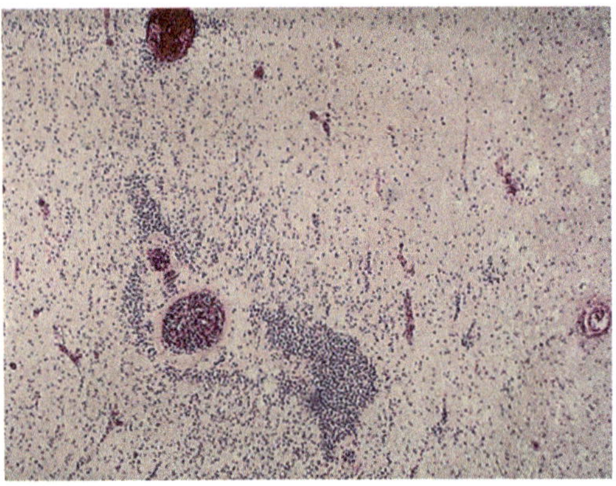

FIGURE 4.23 Microscopic features of cerebral infarcts: perivascular and diffusely infiltrating polymorphonuclear leukocytes at 35 hours after onset of symptoms (H&E).

4.2.1.2. HEMORRHAGIC INFARCTION

Hemorrhagic infarction (Fig. 4.22) is traditionally regarded as distinct from anemic bland infarction, although, as mentioned previously, microscopic evidence of red blood cell extravasation is often found in bland infarcts, especially at the outer border of the lesion. In hemorrhagic infarction, patches or confluent areas of hemorrhage are evident, particularly in the cortex. These hemorrhages may involve the entire extent of the ischemic region (Fig. 4.22A) and, in the cerebral cortex, predominate along boundary zones supplied by leptomeningeal arterial anastomoses; in MCA stem occlusion, the basal ganglia are often involved (Fig. 4.22B). It is generally accepted that an important pathogenetic mechanism of hemorrhagic infarction is tissue reperfusion following endogenous thrombolysis or mobilization of the thrombus. Bleeding then occurs in a capillary bed damaged by the ischemic insult. Indeed, this type of infarction most often follows cerebral embolization, where breakdown of the occluding thrombus and distal migration commonly occur. These processes are enhanced by the concomitant use of antithrombotic or thrombolytic drugs.

4.2.2. Pathophysiology and etiology

Cerebral infarction caused by prolonged ischemia localized to a vascular territory is commonly secondary to arterial occlusion (Fig. 4.25). It may be due to either thrombosis, most often in the setting of atherosclerosis, or embolization (of cardiac origin or via artery-to-artery embolism). When the

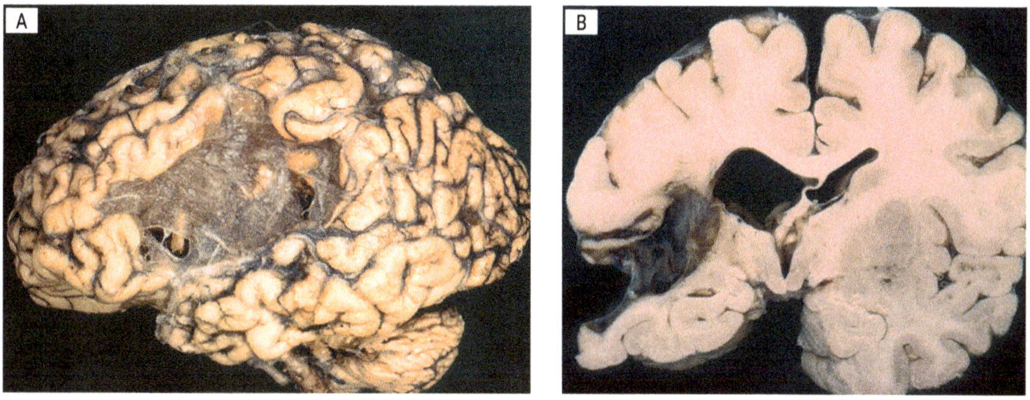

FIGURE 4.24 Old cystic infarct in the territory of the middle cerebral artery: (**A**) left cerebral hemisphere; (**B**) coronal section: note the involvement of a large part of the territory of the middle cerebral artery, sparing the inferior temporal lobe.

neuropathologic examination of cerebral infarcts does not show arterial occlusion, the presumption is that (a) the occluding emboli have undergone secondary lysis, (b) severe and prolonged hypotension involving arteries with extensive or multifocal atheromatous stenosis has resulted in hypoperfusion of tissue, or (c) stenosis has been the result of arterial spasm ("vasospasm"). The appearance and extent of the cerebral infarct depend on several modifying hemodynamic and etiological factors.

4.2.2.1. HEMODYNAMIC FACTORS

4.2.2.1.1. Presence and efficacy of anastomotic pathways of vascular supply. In the course of arterial occlusion, the ischemic cerebral territory is partially re-irrigated by arteries at the base of the brain (circle of Willis and ophthalmic artery) and by superficial corticomeningeal anastomoses (Fig. 4.26A). This potential arterial anastomotic re-irrigation supply explains why, in most cases, the resulting area of cerebral infarct remains smaller

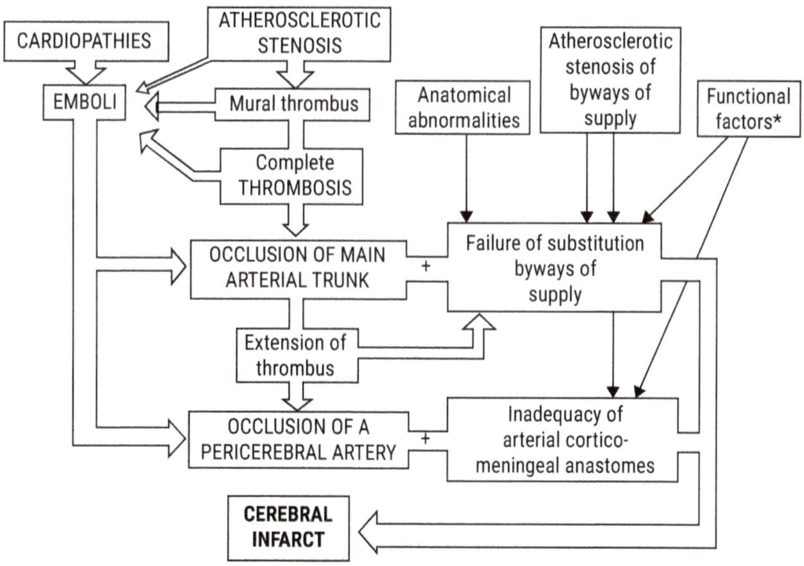

FIGURE 4.25 Etiological and pathophysiological factors determining cerebral infarcts. *Functional factors: decrease in caliber of ischemic arteries, drop in blood pressure, and loss of autoregulation of arterial caliber.

than the vascular territory that is normally supplied by the occluded artery (Fig. 4.26D, E). However, the extent of this collateral reinforcement varies from patient to patient, and anatomical variations from the norm are frequent (Fig. 4.26B). Moreover,

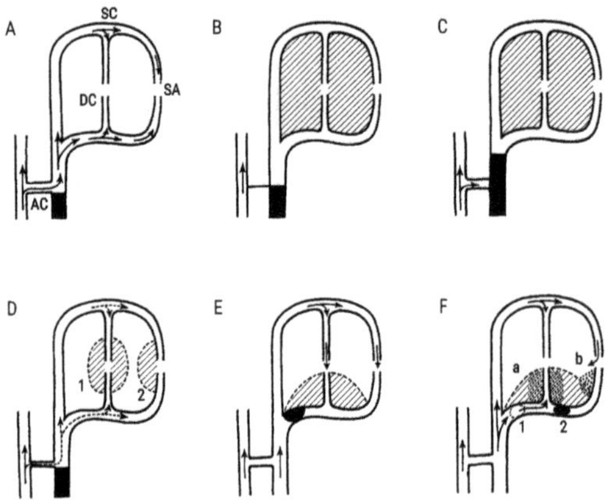

FIGURE 4.26 Respective roles of the anastomotic substitution pathways of circulatory supply and of the type of vascular occlusion in determining the occurrence and extent of cerebral lesions (AC, anastomotic vascular network; DC, deep vascular territory; SA, superficial meningeal anastomoses; SC, superficial arterial circulation). **(A)** Arterial occlusion but with effective and adequate anastomotic substitution network of supply: no infarction. **(B)** Arterial occlusion without anatomically effective anastomotic substitution network of supply (AC): massive infarction of the corresponding vascular territory. **(C)** Arterial occlusion extending beyond the origin of the anastomotic substitution network of supply. No anastomotic substitution by way of vascular supply: massive infarction. **(D)** Occlusion proximal to the anastomotic substitution network of supply. Insufficient anastomotic substitution by way of arterial supply. Anemic infarct of variable extent in the territory (2) distal to the junction of two vascular territories (last field of irrigation or watershed infarct) and in border zone between superficial and deep vascular territories (1). **(E)** Proximal occlusion of one dividing branch; anastomotic substitution by way of vascular supply provided by superficial meningeal anastomoses: limited proximal infarction. **(F)** Embolic occlusion. Mobilization of thrombus from 1 to 2. Sudden occlusion in 1, resulting in total ischemia of both deep and superficial vascular territories and in hemorrhages in the superficial territory when border zones are undergoing reirrigation (b); secondary mobilization of the thrombus in 2, with hemorrhages due to secondary extension of blood into the originally ischemic deep vascular territory (a, hemorrhagic infarct).

these anastomotic pathways may themselves be compromised either by atherosclerotic lesions or because of thrombus propagation leading to a "no-reflow" phenomenon (Fig. 4.26C).

4.2.2.1.2. Site of occlusion. Proximal occlusion of a blood vessel, such as the ICA, may produce only a limited lesion. This is the case when there is sufficient collateral flow from the contralateral arterial network, either via the anterior communicating artery or from the external carotid system via the ophthalmic artery, or from the posterior circulation via the posterior communicating artery. Re-irrigation is generally adequate in the proximal territory, and the lesions will then predominate in the distal regions (last fields of irrigation) or at the "junction" of two vascular territories (*watershed* or *border zone infarct*) (Fig. 4.26D). Should the proximal arterial anastomotic network (i.e., circle of Willis or the ophthalmic artery connection) be anatomically incompetent (Fig. 4.26B) or pathologically completely or partially occluded (Fig. 4.26C), the infarct may then be massive and involve the entire arterial territory. In the case of occlusion involving an end artery distal to these large anastomoses, such as the MCA, collateral flow is dependent on a superficial leptomeningeal anastomotic network, which is often precarious; thus, the infarct, although of variable severity, will usually be extensive (Fig. 4.26E).

4.2.2.1.3. Type of occlusion. In general, thrombosis that leads to gradual occlusion of an artery allows for adaptive mechanisms of collateral flow. The resulting infarct is then usually pale and of relatively limited extent. In contrast, emboli typically produce sudden occlusion, with cessation of flow and inadequate irrigation. Hence, the resulting infarct may be extensive. In addition, migration and secondary fragmentation of the embolus frequently occur. This distal migration of the embolus with sudden reflow of blood into the damaged artery accounts for the hemorrhagic component of the infarct frequently observed in the proximal part of the ischemic territory (Fig. 4.26F).

4.2.2.1.4. Thrombus extension and no reflow. Early neurological deterioration after stroke is usually due to ICH, malignant edema, expansion of the infarct due to failure of collateral flow, or early recurrence of cerebral embolism. Progression of infarction may occur after spontaneous or intravenous thrombolysis due to obstruction of the distal microvasculature (*no reflow phenomenon*). This failure of reperfusion may result from in situ thrombus extension of persistent occlusion, distal emboli beyond the original occlusive site, platelet and inflammatory cell activation within distal vessels, and vasospasm within distal vessels, but conclusive neuropathological studies are lacking. In the modern therapeutic era, infarct size may be affected by the sequelae of endovascular intervention (thrombolytic therapy or thrombectomy).

4.2.2.2. ETIOLOGIC FACTORS

4.2.2.2.1. Atherosclerosis

4.2.2.2.1.1. General features. Atherosclerosis is a principal etiologic factor in the production of many cerebral infarcts. The structural features and development of atherosclerosis in the brain are comparable to those in other organs. In the cerebral circulation, atherosclerosis affects chiefly large intracranial arteries and the cervical carotid arteries in the neck. It predominates at sites of bifurcation (particularly at the level of the carotid sinus), at sites of curvature of the arteries, and at sites where the arteries are anatomically fixed. The distribution of atherosclerosis in the thoraco-cervical arterial tree and in the circle of Willis is illustrated in the classical diagram by Baker and Fisher (Fig. 4.27). The ICAs and the basilar artery are the most heavily involved both at their origins and at their terminations. Atherosclerosis less severely affects the most distal branches of the arterial tree compared to the vessels at the base of the brain.

Increase in the size of the atherosclerotic plaque and focal complications, such as intramural hemorrhage, calcification, and mural thrombosis, lead to increasing arterial stenosis (Fig. 4.28). It is generally believed that stenosis must progress to more than 75% of the original lumen of the artery (or to a residual lumen of <1.5 mm) to cause a clinically significant decrease of blood flow. The evolution of arterial stenosis is variable (Fig. 4.29). The main complication lies in the development of arterial thrombosis secondary to local changes. Thrombosis may occlude the arterial lumen completely; thus, a new event may take place, namely anterograde extension of a so-called stagnation thrombus, usually into the first sizable collateral branch. The thrombus is ultimately replaced by loose-textured connective tissue in which new vessels of variable permeability may develop. In many cases, the mural thrombus can fragment and, in doing so, give rise to arterial emboli (*artery-to-artery emboli*). These emboli are believed

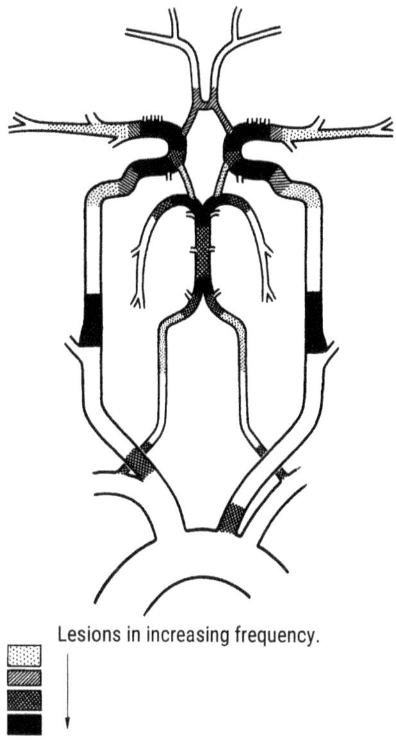

FIGURE 4.27 The frequency and severity of atherosclerotic lesions in the carotid–vertebral cerebral arterial tree.

to account for many small infarcts and *transient ischemic attacks* (TIAs). When the ischemic period is of short duration, there may be no residual infarct (TIA), or permanent infarction may occur when disintegration of the thromboembolism has not been sufficiently rapid.

4.2.2.2.1.2. Atherosclerotic thrombosis. Internal carotid thrombosis develops in a setting of stenosing atheromatous lesions. These lesions are most often observed at the carotid bifurcation or at the level of the carotid sinus. In the setting of complete or near-complete occlusion, a stagnation thrombus is formed. This thrombus usually extends rostrally to the ostium of the first collateral branch, namely the ophthalmic artery; collateral contribution through the external carotid artery may ensure adequate perfusion of the proximal hemispheric territory. The zone of infarction resulting from such low-flow lesions is often limited to the distal portion of the MCA territory and, to a lesser extent, the anterior cerebral territory (i.e., to their border zone). Anterograde extension of the thrombus beyond the ophthalmic artery, as well as beyond the origin of the

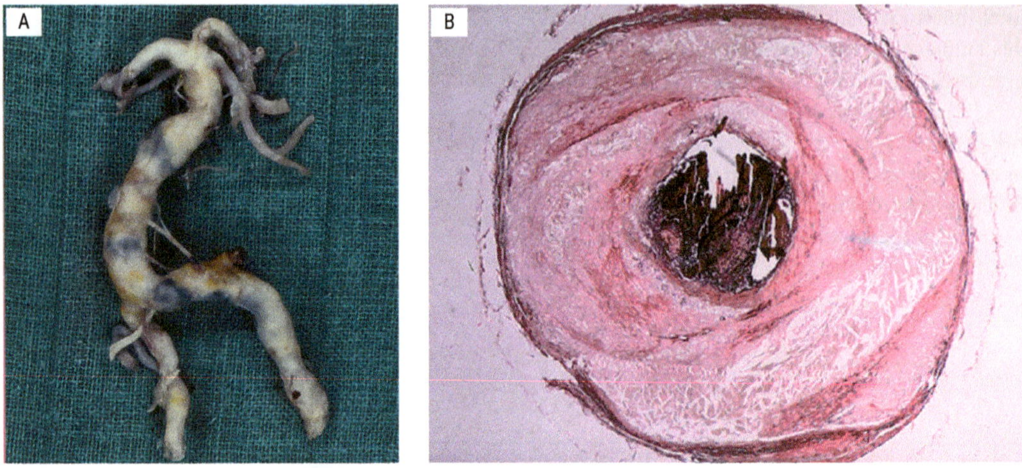

FIGURE 4.28 Stenosing atherosclerotic lesion: (**A**) gross appearance of atherosclerosis of the basilar artery; (**B**) microscopic appearance with narrowing of the arterial lumen by atherosclerotic lesions (H&E).

posterior communicating and the anterior cerebral arteries, may then result in massive infarction. Less often, thrombosis takes place at the level of the carotid syphon (i.e., near the termination of the ICA). Occlusion due to atheromatous lesions in this terminal portion of the artery is usually accompanied by retrograde extension of the thrombus down to the carotid sinus. When the lesion is old and organized, it may be difficult to determine whether thrombosis of the carotid artery originally took place at its distal or proximal end.

Isolated in situ thrombosis of the middle or anterior cerebral artery is much less common than internal carotid thrombosis. It may follow extension of a carotid thrombus beyond the bifurcation of the ICA or progressive occlusion at these sites from intracranial atherosclerosis (or in *moyamoya syndrome*).

Vertebral artery (VA) thrombosis occurs more often at the origin (V1 segment) or the terminal parts (V3 and V4 segments). It is often clinically silent due to the bilateral vertebral supply of the basilar artery. If collateral flow is inadequate, VA occlusion may cause infarction in the territory of the posterior inferior cerebellar artery or the lateral medullary region (Wallenberg syndrome). VA atherosclerotic lesions may also be the source of artery-to-artery embolism to the cerebellum, brainstem, or other structures supplied by branches of the basilar artery.

Basilar artery thrombosis occurs in the setting of atherosclerotic lesions, common at this site, or from ascending extension of VA thrombosis. Infarcts may be limited to the territories of small penetrating arteries supplying the pons or midbrain when the ostia of these arteries are occluded, or it may lead to

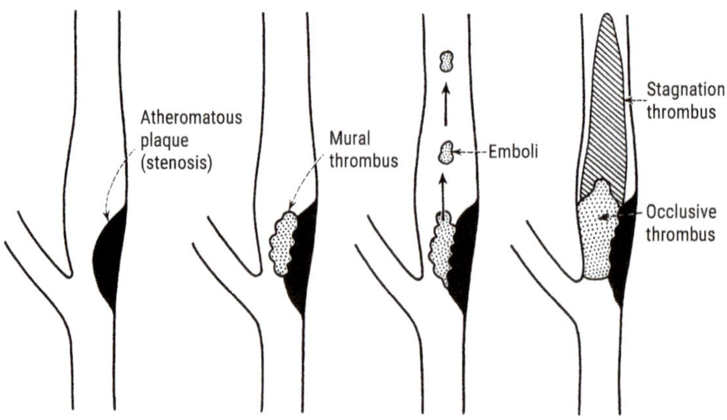

FIGURE 4.29 Evolution of lesions caused by atheromatous carotid stenosis.

extensive and devastating infarction in the pons and midbrain.

Atherosclerotic thrombosis of a posterior cerebral artery (PCA) is seldom an isolated event. It usually occurs as the result of anterograde extension of basilar artery thrombosis. When the PCA is a tributary of the ICA (*fetal PCA*), its occlusion may be secondary to extension from a thrombosed carotid. Thus, these lesions frequently result in massive hemispheric infarction.

Subclavian artery thrombosis may give rise to ischemic lesions in the vertebrobasilar territory via diversion of the arterial flow (*subclavian steal syndrome*).

4.2.2.2.2. Emboli of atherosclerotic origin. For emboli of atherosclerotic origin (Fig. 4.29), artery-to-artery atheroemboli play an important role in the development of cerebral infarcts. They can arise from ulcerated plaques anywhere along the arterial tree or from the aortic arch or from platelet or fibrin thrombi overlying atherosclerotic lesions. The most common sites of origin are the carotid sinus and the vertebral and basilar arteries. The aortic arch is also a source of cerebral emboli that is often overlooked. Platelet emboli frequently detach as small fragments from a thrombus and may cause transient cerebral accidents or occlude terminal arterial branches. Fibrin emboli originate from a mural thrombus or from fragmentation of a stagnation thrombus. They often produce occlusion in the branches of larger arteries (middle, anterior, or posterior cerebral) in a setting of carotid or vertebrobasilar thrombosis. Purely atherosclerotic emboli most often are the result of spontaneous detachment of thrombotic material from ulcerated plaques. Rarely, they may be seen as cholesterol emboli to eye, brain, kidney, feet (blue toes syndrome), and other systemic locations.

4.2.2.2.3. Cardiac-derived emboli. Cardiogenic embolization (Fig. 4.30) may lead to distal arterial occlusion. These can originate from an atrial thrombus with or without atrial fibrillation or from valvular lesions such as mitral stenosis; from a mural thrombus in the course of myocardial infarction; from various forms of endocardial vegetations (e.g., bacterial endocarditis, nonbacterial thrombotic or "marantic" endocarditis) from a cardiac prosthesis; or from other rare lesions, such as flail leaflets, fibroelastomas, and atrial myxomas.

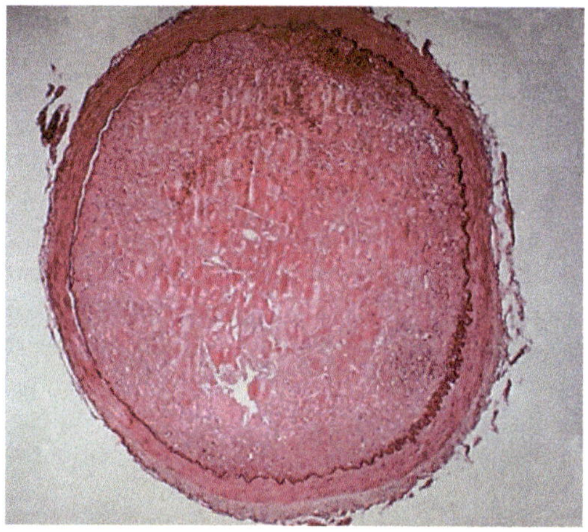

FIGURE 4.30 Arterial embolus (superficial temporal artery). Note the normal appearance of the arterial wall (H&E).

Emboli other than those of cardiac or artery-to-artery origin are less frequent. Fibrocartilaginous and tumoral metastatic emboli have rarely been reported. Also, hydrophilic polymer emboli (foreign body emboli in patients who have undergone vascular procedures using hydrophilic-coated medical devices) may occur after cardiac catheterization, diagnostic or therapeutic cerebral angiography, or orthotopic cadaveric organ transplantation. Last, it should be stressed that often the source of emboli remains unidentified even after careful clinical and postmortem examination. The acronym ESUS (embolic stroke of undetermined sources) is used to refer to these cases.

4.2.2.2.4. Other Causes. Arteritis (or "vasculitis") is a rarer cause of cerebral infarction. Arteritis may be systemic (giant cell arteritis, including temporal arteritis and Takayasu arteritis; polyarteritis nodosa; Churg–Strauss syndrome; and leukocytoclastic vasculitis) or isolated in the CNS (primary CNS vasculitis, granulomatous angiitis of the nervous system). The inflammatory response may be found in small superficial arterioles and, more infrequently, the deep intracerebral or spinal intramedullary vessels. The resulting parenchymatous lesions consist of circumscribed and widely disseminated foci of softening. Syphilitic arteritis, which affects especially the basal arteries, is seen infrequently today. Tuberculous and other bacterial meningitides, as well as meningitis caused by fungal and parasitic organisms (e.g., aspergillosis), can produce occlusive arteritic lesions that may account for cerebral and spinal infarcts (see Chapter 5). Some fungi (e.g., *Aspergillus*) tend to infect blood vessel walls. HIV infection increases the risk of cerebral infarcts for reasons that are not fully understood. In children, otitis media and rhinopharyngitis can occasionally be a cause of internal carotid occlusion, which may result in cerebral infarcts.

Amyloid angiopathy of the cortical blood vessels may cause multiple disseminated cortical and white matter infarcts, in addition to cerebral hemorrhages, as discussed previously (see Section 4.1.2.2). When CNS angiitis is encountered in an elderly subject, amyloid β-related inflammation or angiitis (ABRA) must be considered and treated, as mentioned previously.

Injuries to the neck or in the mouth may give rise to internal carotid occlusion.

Vascular malformations, especially AVMs with aneurysms, are sometimes associated with cerebral infarcts (see Section 4.1.2.3).

Moyamoya disease is a rare chronic, progressive, steno-occlusive disorder believed to be genetic in origin; the gene RING finger protein 213, *RNF213*, has been identified as a susceptibility gene. It occurs at the distal ICAs, typically bilaterally, sometimes extending to the middle and anterior cerebral arteries and to other arteries of the circle of Willis. Abnormal collateral vessels (*moyamoya collaterals, foggy clusters*) adjacent to the stenotic arteries occur at the base of the brain. These moyamoya vessels represent perforators and anastomotic branches. The pia mater may also have reticular conglomerates of small vessels. Children in some Asian populations (Japan, Korea, and Taiwan) are known to be especially affected, as well as adult women in North America in the third and fourth decades of life. The cause of the occlusive vasculopathy is unknown and is probably multifactorial. Associations with sickle cell disease, thyrotoxicosis, trisomy 21, AVMs, and radiation injury have been reported (*secondary* moyamoya or *moyamoya syndrome*). Occluded ICAs and stenotic arteries of the circle of Willis show thicker intima with dense smooth muscle cells and thinning of the media of the MCA compared to controls, with tortuosity and fragmentation of the internal elastic lamina. The distal lenticulostriate arteries show severe medial damage like that seen in hypertensive patients. Fibrin deposits, thrombosis, and formation of microaneurysms have been reported. Moyamoya disease is associated with ischemic and hemorrhagic strokes secondary to progressive stenosis or occlusion compromising flow, thrombosis, or embolization.

4.2.3. Topography

Regardless of the specific cerebral or spinal territory involved by an infarct, the location and extent of the infarct will be determined by the distribution of the occluded artery and the status of compensatory collateral vessels.

4.2.3.1. CEREBRAL INFARCTS

Cerebral infarcts need to be evaluated at postmortem after complete anatomical study of both the carotid and the vertebrobasilar system from the aortic arch up to the cerebral branches (Fig. 4.31). The study must also include a meticulous examination of the heart cavities, heart valves, and myocardium.

4.2.3.1.1. Infarcts in the carotid (anterior) territory. Infarction may involve either the whole or only part of the territories of the branches of the ICA (Figs. 4.32–4.35). A single infarct may be found, but it is important to emphasize the frequency of multiple infarcts. These can vary in size and age.

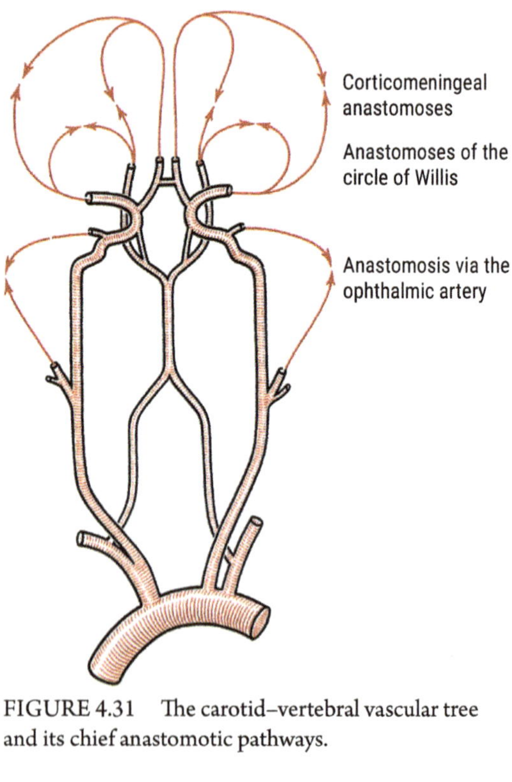

FIGURE 4.31 The carotid–vertebral vascular tree and its chief anastomotic pathways.

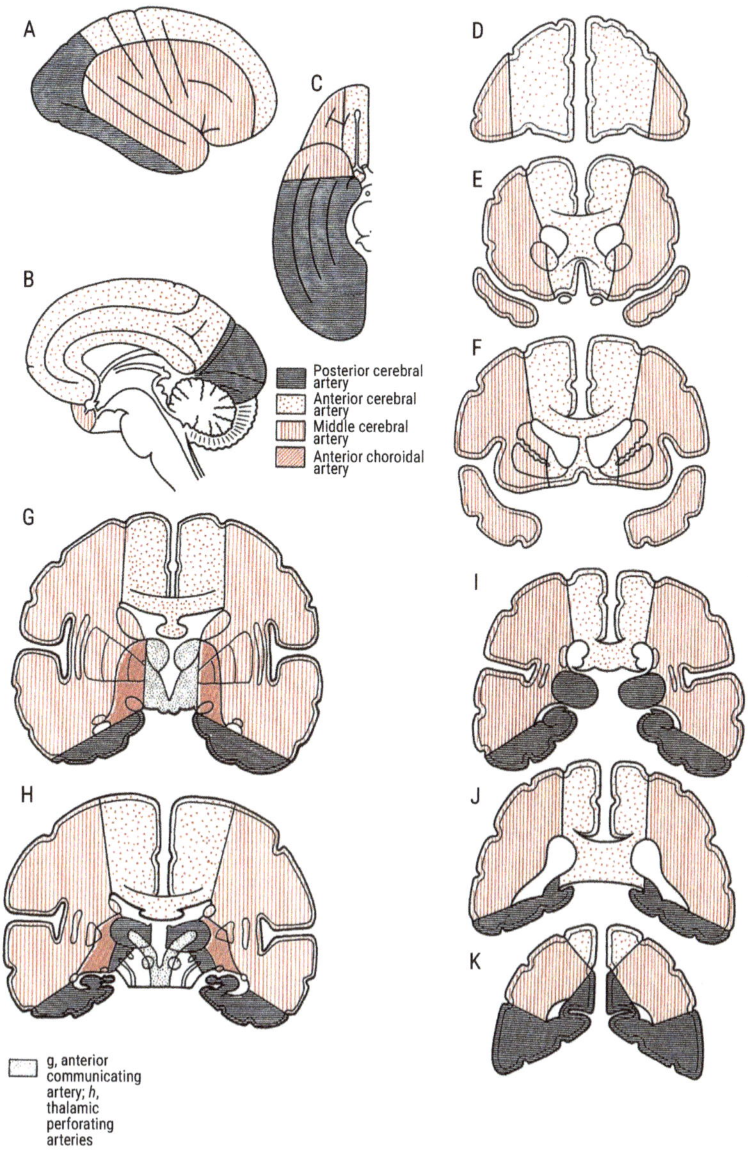

FIGURE 4.32 Cerebral vascular territories: (**A**) lateral surface; (**B**) medial surface; (**C**) basal surface; (**D–K**) coronal slices from frontal poles (**D**), posteriorly to occipital poles (**K**).

- *Infarct in the anterior cerebral artery territory* (Fig. 4.33A–C). This area consists of the superior frontal gyrus, inferior and medial surfaces of the frontal lobe back to the level of the precuneus, genu and body of the corpus callosum, and anterior portion of the basal ganglia supplied by the recurrent artery of Heubner. Because of collateral flow provided by the contralateral anterior cerebral artery via the anterior communicating artery, infarcts in the anterior cerebral territory are less common than those of the middle cerebral territory. Anatomic variations in the circle of Willis (i.e., a single origin of both anterior cerebral arteries) may account for bilateral infarction in some cases (Fig. 4.33B, C). In the case of internal carotid thrombosis, infarction is also associated with involvement of the middle cerebral territory (Fig. 4.35).
- *Infarct in the MCA territory*. This area includes the lateral surface of the frontal and parietal lobes; insula; superior and middle temporal

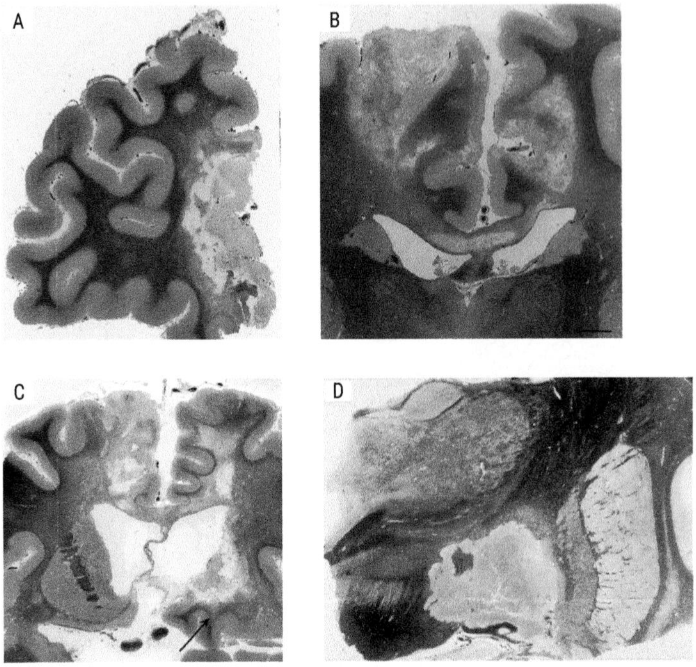

FIGURE 4.33 Principal topographical areas of distribution of infarcts in the internal carotid territory: anterior cerebral artery and anterior choroidal artery (Loyez stain for myelin). (**A**) Infarct in the territory of the anterior cerebral artery involving the cingulate gyrus and inferior rostral gyrus. (**B**) Bilateral infarcts in the territory of the anterior cerebral artery. On the left, infarct involves the cingulate sulcus, the superior frontal gyrus, and the corpus callosum. On the right, there is a circumscribed infarct of the white matter of the superior frontal gyrus and the cingulate sulcus. Note the involvement of the caudate nucleus (within the territory recurrent artery of Heubner). (**C**) Bilateral infarcts in the territory of the anterior cerebral artery. Note an infarct in the corpus callosum. (Figures 4.33A–4.33C from the *Journal of Neuropathology and Experimental Neurology*, 2009, *68*, 113–124, with permission.) (**D**) Right-sided anterior choroidal infarct.

gyri; and deep striatal territory containing the frontopontine, corticobulbar, and corticospinal fibers in the internal capsule. Occlusion of the proximal part of the MCA may result in total middle cerebral infarction (Fig. 4.34C, D) when the superficial collateral arterial circulation is only able to provide little compensatory flow. The occlusion is much more often the result of embolization than of primary intravascular thrombosis. Cerebral infarctions restricted to the superficial branches of the MCA result from occlusions distal to the origin of the perforating branches (i.e., the superior or inferior divisions and their branches) (Fig. 4.34A), whereas occlusion of the ostia of the perforating branches by embolism or atherosclerosis is responsible for deep middle cerebral infarcts (Fig. 4.34B). Such deep territory infarcts may be isolated either when only the ostia of the penetrating vessels are occluded or when leptomeningeal collateral compensation is effective for cortical areas. Most often, infarction involves only part of the vascular territory (e.g., territory of the ascending branches). This sparing may result from occlusion of only the terminal branches, but more often, it results from proximal occlusion of the ICA coupled with adequate re-irrigation of the spared territory through leptomeningeal vascular anastomoses.

- *Infarct in the anterior choroidal artery territory* (Fig. 4.33D). The posterior part of the internal capsule, pallidum, and optic tract are located within this arterial territory, as well as the internal anterior part of the temporal lobes and, at times, part of the base of the mesencephalon. Infarction of this deep area of supply, especially when recent, may be difficult to detect at pathological examination because of the limited extent of the involved territory. Selected infarction of this area, although rather frequent on MRI, is

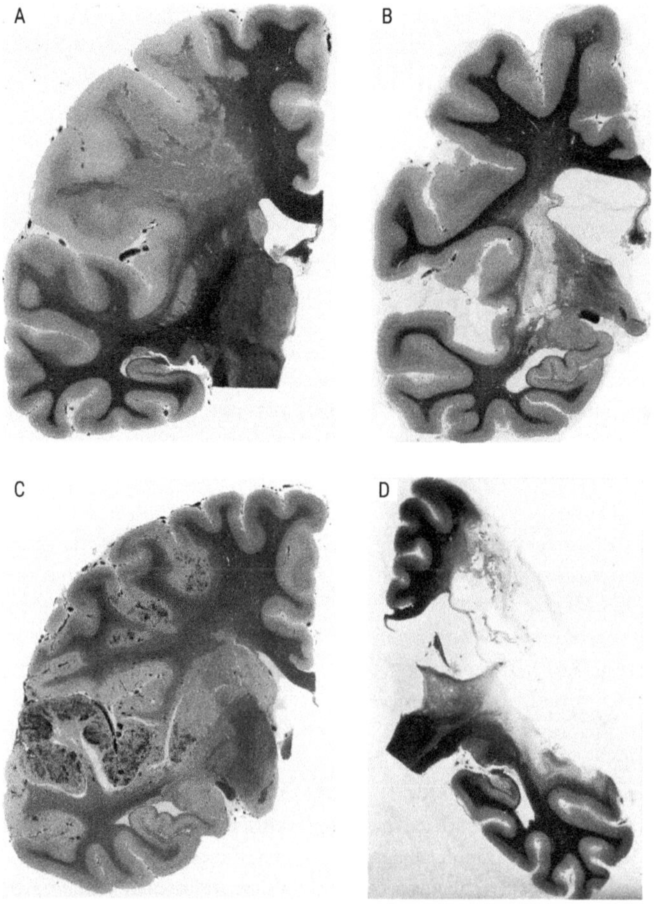

FIGURE 4.34 Principal topographical areas of distribution of infarcts in the internal carotid territory: middle cerebral artery (Loyez stain for myelin). (**A**) The infarct involves the superficial territory of the left middle cerebral artery posteriorly. Note that the entire temporal lobe territory is spared. (**B**) The infarct involves the deep territory of the left middle cerebral artery (putamen, internal capsule, and caudate nucleus) anteriorly. (**C**) A large recent hemorrhagic infarct involves the superficial and deep territories of the middle cerebral artery. (Figures 4.34A–4.34C from the *Journal of Neuropathology and Experimental Neurology*, 2009, *68*, 113–124, with permission.) (**D**) Total right middle cerebral infarct, old with cystic transformation.

seldom seen at autopsy. Isolated embolism to the anterior choroidal artery may occur. In most autopsy cases, however, infarction of the anterior choroidal territory accompanies total infarction of the middle cerebral territory and is therefore part of a massive hemispheric infarct.

- *Massive hemispheric infarct.* A massive hemispheric infarct may involve the entire territory of the ICA vascular supply (Fig. 4.35A, B). It is produced as the result of sudden occlusion of the terminal portion of the ICA, either by an embolus or by extension of an internal carotid thrombus beyond the terminal bifurcation of the artery so that all potential proximal collateral supply is absent. The large extent of the zone of ischemia accounts for the severity of the edematous reaction and for the high frequency of mesial temporal herniation (Fig. 4.35).
- *"Watershed" or border zone infarcts* (Fig. 4.36). These affect mostly the boundaries between the anterior and middle cerebral territories, especially posterior to the interparietal sulcus (Fig. 4.36A). They sometimes occur between the middle or anterior and posterior cerebral territories (Fig. 4.36B). Likewise, watershed infarcts may occur in the centrum semiovale, at the junction of the deep and superficial territories of the MCA. They result from hypoperfusion of the distal arterial territory

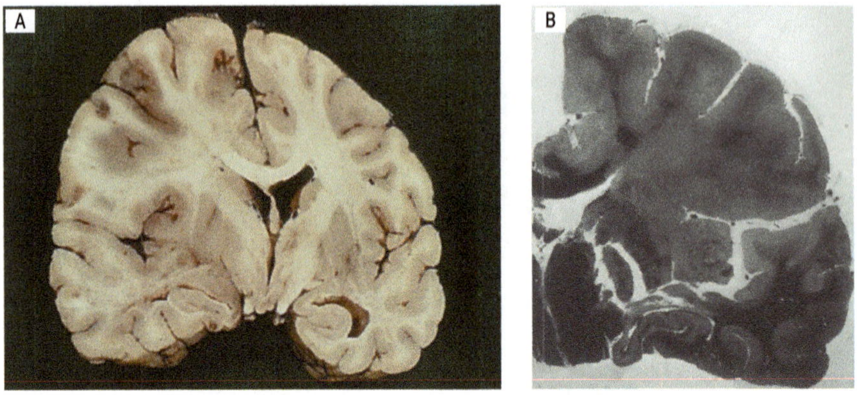

FIGURE 4.35 Recent massive hemispheric infarct. (**A**) Gross appearance, left cerebral hemisphere. (**B**) Infarct involving the entire territories of the right anterior cerebral, middle cerebral, and anterior choroidal arteries. Note right temporal herniation (Loyez stain).

or embolism to the distal artery as a result of internal carotid thrombosis or after prolonged episodes of arterial hypotension.

- *Granular atrophy of the cerebral cortex of arteriopathic origin* (Fig. 4.37). This pathological picture is seen in rare forms of vascular dementia. It is characterized by the presence of small chronic ischemic infarcts forming punched-out foci of cavitated cicatricial softening, or focal glial scars, situated primarily in the cortex. The distribution of the lesions is remarkable; they involve the watershed territories at the junction of the middle and anterior cerebral territories, along the crest of the gyri from the frontal to the occipital pole, along the superior frontal and interparietal sulci, and at the junction of the middle and posterior cerebral artery territories on the inferior surface of the temporal lobes. They may be bilateral. The distribution of the lesions is indicative of chronic watershed ischemia. When bilateral, they may be related either to bilateral ICA thrombosis or to cardiac insufficiency. They may also result from microangiopathy, usually Aβ CAA.

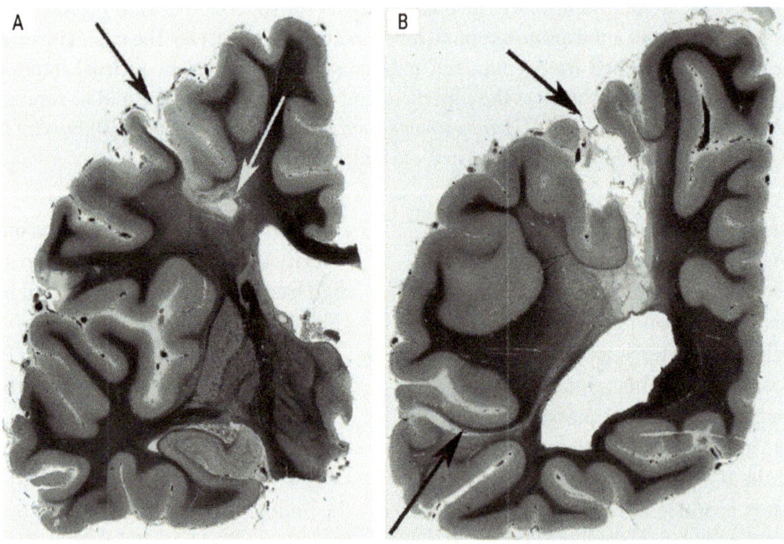

FIGURE 4.36 Infarcts of the junctional ("watershed") territories: (**A**) superficial (*black arrow*) and deep (*light arrow*) junction infarct between the territories of the anterior and middle cerebral arteries; (**B**) superficial and deep junction infarcts (*arrows*) between the superficial territories of the anterior, middle, and posterior cerebral arteries. (Figures 4.36A and 4.36B from the *Journal of Neuropathology and Experimental Neurology*, 2009, *68*, 113–124, with permission.)

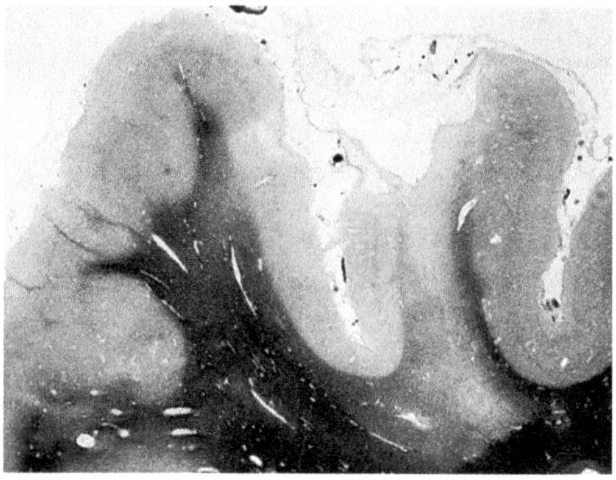

FIGURE 4.37 Granular atrophy; old ischemic lesion involving the watershed territories at the junction of the middle and anterior cerebral territories at the crest of the gyrus along the frontal superior sulcus (Loyez stain for myelin).

4.2.3.1.2. Infarcts of the vertebrobasilar (posterior) territory. Infarcts of the posterior circulation depend on the same general pathophysiological mechanisms as already described; in addition, they have the distinctive anatomic aspects of the posterior circulation and its system of collateral flow. The posterior system consists of a median axis, the basilar artery, formed by the junction of two vertebral arteries originating from the subclavian arteries, which follow a tortuous course through the foramina transversaria terminating in two branches, the PCAs, described by neuroradiologists as the P1 segments of the PCAs. There are considerable variations of this vascular arrangement, especially in the size of the vertebral, posterior communicating, and PCAs. In approximately 15% of patients, the main supply to the PCA is the anterior circulation via a large posterior communicating artery in the setting of an atretic P1 segment (i.e., proximal PCA connecting the basilar tip to the more distal PCA).

Variable anastomotic communications exist with the ICAs, through the posterior communicating arteries, with branches of the external carotid and subclavian arteries, and between the vertebral arteries themselves through the spinal perimedullary arterial network. Finally, there are lateral anastomotic rings formed between the cerebellar arteries.

These special anatomic features account for the frequent bilaterality and asymmetry of the ischemic lesions and for their multifocal distribution along the brainstem axis and cerebellum.

- *Infarcts of the PCA territory* (Fig. 4.38). These are often bilateral, producing necrosis of the inferomedial surface of the occipital lobe; of the cuneus; and especially of the calcarine

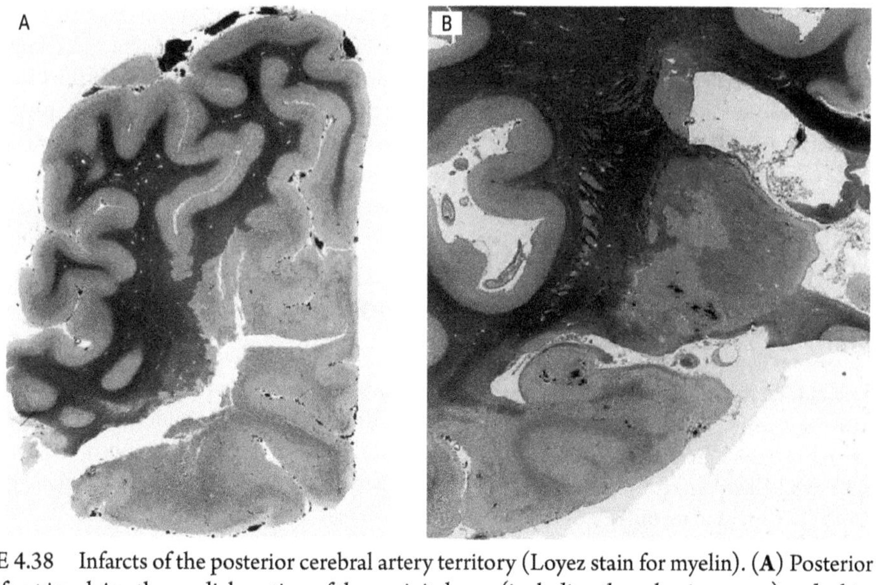

FIGURE 4.38 Infarcts of the posterior cerebral artery territory (Loyez stain for myelin). (**A**) Posterior cerebral artery infarct involving the medial portion of the occipital gray (including the calcarine gyrus) and white matter, including the striate area and optic radiations. (**B**) Recent infarct of the thalamo-geniculate territory. Note involvement of Ammon horn. (Figures 4.38A and 4.38B from the *Journal of Neuropathology and Experimental Neurology*, 2009, *68*, 113–124, with permission.)

cortex as well as the inferomedial temporal lobe, including part of Ammon's horn. These infarcts follow occlusion of the PCA beyond its junction with the posterior communicating artery (the P2 segment of this artery). Such an occlusion is generally embolic in origin, secondary to underlying vertebrobasilar thrombosis/embolism or cardioembolism. The most frequent infarcts of the deep territory of the PCA affect either the thalamogeniculate territory (i.e., the ventrolateral thalamus and the pulvinar), in case of occlusion of the P1 segment, or the paramedian thalamic territory (i.e., the intralaminar nuclei). These infarcts often affect both thalamic and mesencephalic territories of the PCA (thalamomesencephalic infarct). In some patients, the two paramedian thalamic penetrators arise from a single trunk (artery of Percheron), in which case a bilateral butterfly-shaped lesion develops and is associated with variable involvement of the mesencephalon. PCA territory infarcts may also result from severe compression of this artery in transtentorial herniation.

- *Infarcts of the brainstem* (Fig. 4.39). These infarcts may be secondary to atherosclerotic thrombosis of the vertebral or basilar artery; to small arterial disease of the penetrating arteries; or to cardiac embolism, most commonly to the top of the basilar artery. The general pattern of arterial supply is that of a relatively constant and simple arterial intraparenchymal network supplied by a variable and complex extraparenchymal network. This explains why these lesions often defy classification. They fall roughly into the following types:

  Localized lesions corresponding to necrosis in a particular vascular territory: Either paramedian branches of the basilar artery (midline infarct of the midbrain tegmentum with or without associated thalamic infarcts from involvement of paramedian thalamic [thalamoperforating] arteries); paramedian pontine penetrators (paramedian infarct of the pontine tegmentum and massive softening); short circumferential branches of the basilar arteries (infarct of the middle cerebellar peduncle); medullary penetrators (paramedian medullary or lateral medullary infarction causing *Wallenberg syndrome*) due to occlusion of three or four branches from the V4 segment of the VA or, at times, from the posterior and inferior cerebellar artery [PICA]) (Fig. 4.39F).

  Multiple and diffuse lesions. These may involve many vascular territories and sometimes consist of lesions of different ages. They may also form relatively localized lesions that extend beyond the usual topographical limits of irrigation.

- *Cerebellar infarcts* (Fig. 4.40). Cerebellar infarction is three to five times more frequent than cerebellar hemorrhage. The lesions frequently appear as infarcts in the territory of distribution of the occluded long circumferential branches originating from the vertebral and basilar arteries (Fig. 4.40A). These may involve (a) the territory of the superior cerebellar artery (SCA), which comprises the superior portion of the cerebellum down to the dentate nucleus and the posterolateral portion of the upper pontine tegmentum (Fig. 4.40B); (b) the territory of PICA on the ventral surface of the hemisphere and at times the ipsilateral posterolateral part of the medulla; and(c) the anterior inferior cerebellar artery, which usually supplies the flocculus, the middle cerebellar peduncle, and the inferior lateral territory of the pons (Fig. 4.40C). Cerebellar infarcts are mainly due to emboli. The infarcts can be of considerable size and may often be associated with multiple other foci of infarction in the brainstem. Large cerebellar infarcts behave as space-occupying masses that can cause compression of the fourth ventricle and obstructive hydrocephalus and cerebellar herniation with brainstem compression. Border zone infarcts, situated at the boundaries between the territories of distribution of the cerebellar arteries, are not uncommon at autopsy and are frequent on MRI scans, even in asymptomatic patients.

4.2.3.2. SPINAL INTRAMEDULLARY INFARCTS

Spinal intramedullary infarcts are much less common than cerebral infarcts. Because it is usually difficult to carry out a complete and satisfactory anatomical study of the blood supply of the spinal cord, these infarcts may raise complex problems of pathophysiological interpretation.

- *Arterial organization of the spinal cord* (Figs. 4.41 and 4.42). The general pattern is that of a relatively constant and simple arterial intramedullary network associated with a highly

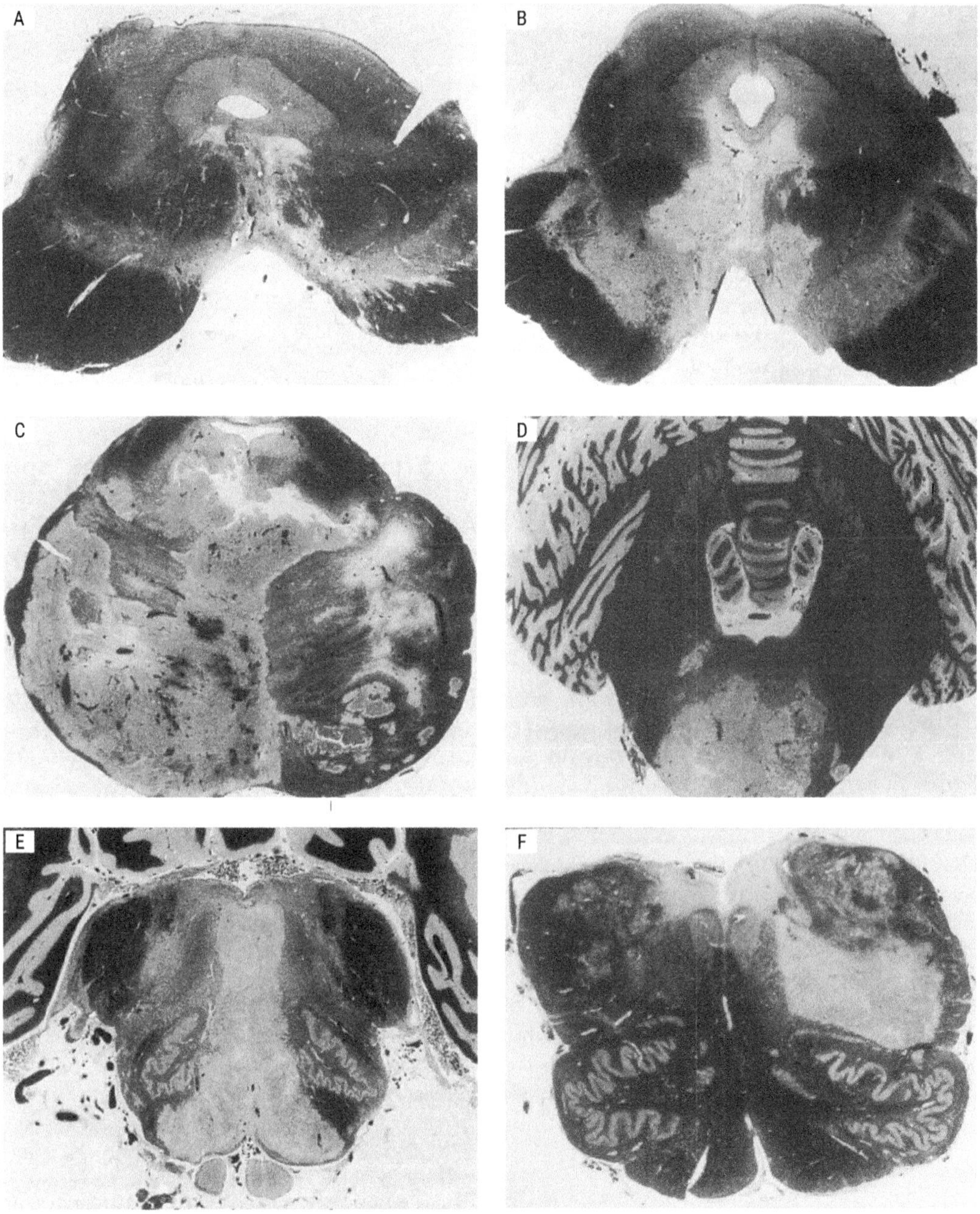

FIGURE 4.39 Infarcts of the brainstem (Loyez stain for myelin): (**A**) midbrain infarct; (**B**) massive infarct of the midbrain tegmentum; (**C**) massive upper pontine infarct with paramedian predominance on the left; (**D**) massive infarct of the basis pontis; (**E**) central medullary infarct; (**F**) lateral medullary infarct (causing Wallenberg syndrome).

variable and complex extramedullary network. The intramedullary network depends on one major anterior spinal artery, which extends downward along the ventral aspect of the spinal cord and ensures the supply of the anterior two-thirds of the cord (therefore including most of the gray matter in the anterior horns and the corticospinal tracts in the lateral cord), through the sulco-commissural arteries. Two posterior spinal arteries irrigate the dorsal three-fourths

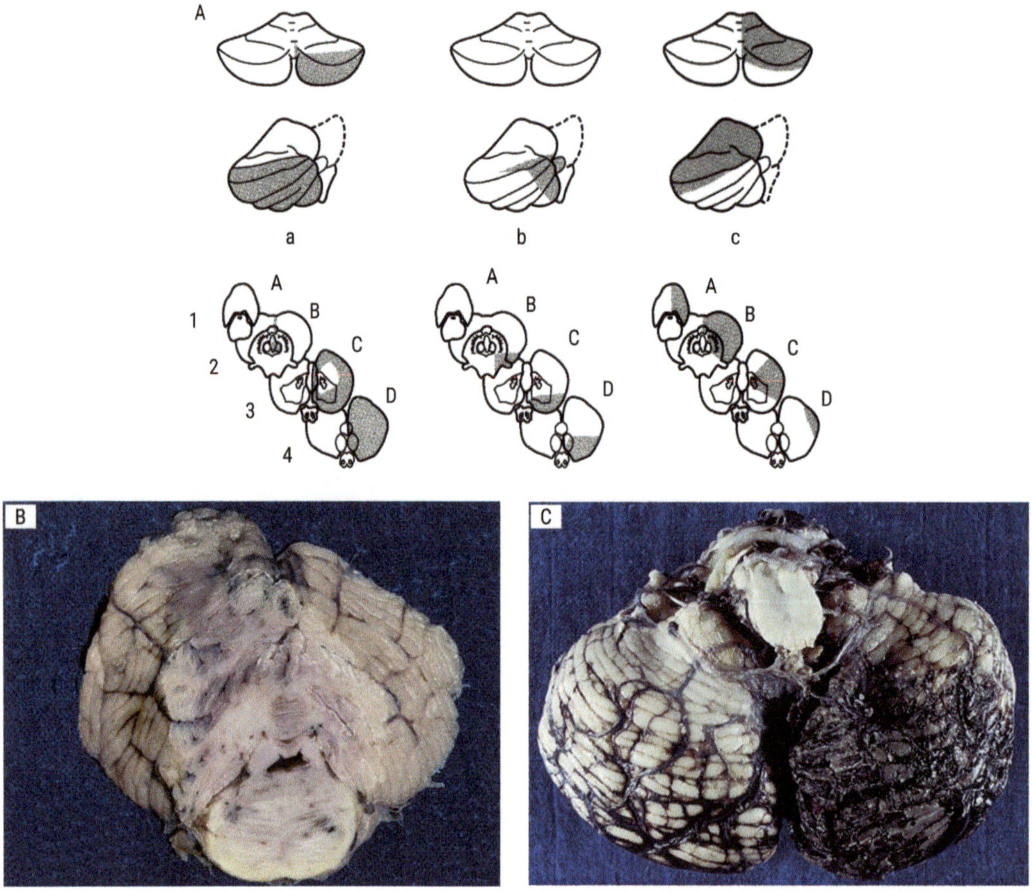

FIGURE 4.40 Cerebellar infarcts: (**A**) Diagram showing the full extent of cerebellar infarcts. From top to bottom: Posterior view; lateral view; and transverse sections through the superior cerebellum and pons (A), middle cerebellum and lower pons (B), middle cerebellum and rostral medulla (C), and inferior cerebellum and medulla (D). (**a**) Posterior inferior cerebellar artery territory; (**b**) anterior inferior cerebellar artery territory; and (**c**) superior cerebellar artery territory. (Modified from Amarenco, P., & Hauw, J. J. (1989). Anatomie des artères cérébelleuses. *Revue Neurologique (Paris)*, *145*, 267–276, with permission. See also Amarenco, P., Hauw, J. J., & Caplan, L. R. (1993). Cerebellar infarction. In R. Lechtenberg (Ed.), *Handbook of cerebellar diseases* (pp. 251–290). Marcel Dekker.) (**B**) Right-side recent pale infarct of the vascular territory of the superior cerebellar artery (on left). (**C**) Left-side hemorrhagic infarct of the posterior inferior cerebellar artery (on the right).

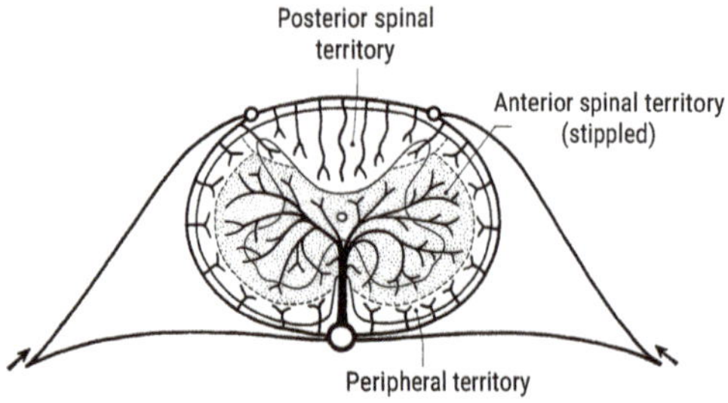

FIGURE 4.41 Transverse arterial territories of the spinal cord.

of the posterior columns. A perimedullary anastomotic network gives off a few branches to the periphery of the cord. The extramedullary network, which is highly complex and variable, depends on the presence of radicular arteries. The following territories are recognized:

- A superior, or cervicothoracic, territory corresponding to the cervical and upper two or three thoracic segments and supplied by arterial twigs originating from the vertebral arteries or from branches of the subclavian arteries.

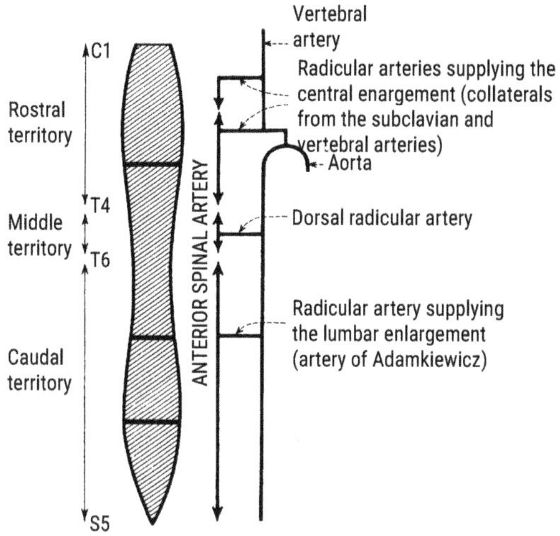

FIGURE 4.42 The three principal longitudinal arterial territories of the spinal cord.

- An intermediary, or middle thoracic, territory extending from T4 to T8 with a blood supply derived from the vertebral arteries via the anterior spinal artery.
- An inferior, or thoracolumbar, territory whose abundant vascularization is supplied by a single lumbar artery (i.e., the *artery of the lumbar enlargement* or *artery of Adamkiewicz*). This artery is situated on the left and most frequently accompanies one of the lower thoracic or upper lumbar nerve roots and is sometimes reinforced by an upper or a lower branch.

- *Topographical features* (Figs. 4.43–4.45)
  - *Massive infarction* (Fig. 4.43A) of the spinal cord usually occurs in the middle thoracic zone, which is a vulnerable border zone between the vertebral and Adamkiewicz supply to the anterior spinal artery. It is usually the result of sudden total ischemia when re-irrigation of the middle thoracic segments by the abundant cervical and lumbar networks is inadequate. The infarct extends over several segments and is often lengthened into a proximal and a caudal fusiform pencil of centromedullary softening, which is situated in the ventral part of the posterior columns at the boundary between the anterior and posterior spinal territories (Fig. 4.43B, C). In rare instance, a severe hypoxic or hypotensive episode may result in anoxic neuronal change among anterior horn cells, with sparing of myelin ("hypoxic myelinopathy"), usually affecting the lumber spinal cord.
  - *Anterior spinal artery infarction* involves a greater or lesser portion of the anterior spinal territory, especially the ventral horns (Fig. 4.44). It is the most frequent type of infarct in the spinal cord. It may be found in the cervical region but is more often in the lumbar region because of the special vulnerability of this territory, which depends on a single artery without potential collateral supply from an invariably slender middle thoracic arterial network.
  - *Infarcts of the posterior spinal territory* (Fig. 4.45) are much rarer.
- *Microscopic features.* The microscopic lesions are identical to those of cerebral infarcts; that is, they consist of an initial edematous stage and of secondary processes of liquefaction and tissue resorption through the mobilization of macrophages. Axonal spheroids may be prominent in long tracts.
- *Chief etiological factors.* Atherosclerosis with arterial thrombosis within an aneurysm of the aorta or dissection of the aorta involving either the feeding vessels or the aorta itself plays an important role. The pathological changes usually result from obstruction of the orifices of the intercostal and lumbar arteries. This may occur in the setting of aortic aneurysm, and supplying arteries may be injured in the course of surgical repair of a thoracic or abdominal aortic aneurysm (AAA).

Except for cholesterol emboli originating from ulcerated aortic atheromatous plaques, arterial embolism can seldom be demonstrated to be an etiological factor. Cartilaginous embolism following relatively minor trauma to the spine has been recorded as a mechanism of spinal cord infarction.

Thoracic surgery and aortography may be special etiological factors in vascular disorders of the spinal cord. Spontaneous dissecting aneurysm of the aorta may cause occlusion of the spinal radicular arteries, including the artery of Adamkiewicz. As noted previously, spinal cord supply arising from the descending aorta may be injured in the course of AAA repair.

4.3. PATHOLOGY OF SMALL ARTERIES

We have referred to small artery disease as underlying hypertensive intracranial hemorrhage and acute ischemic stroke. This section addresses the

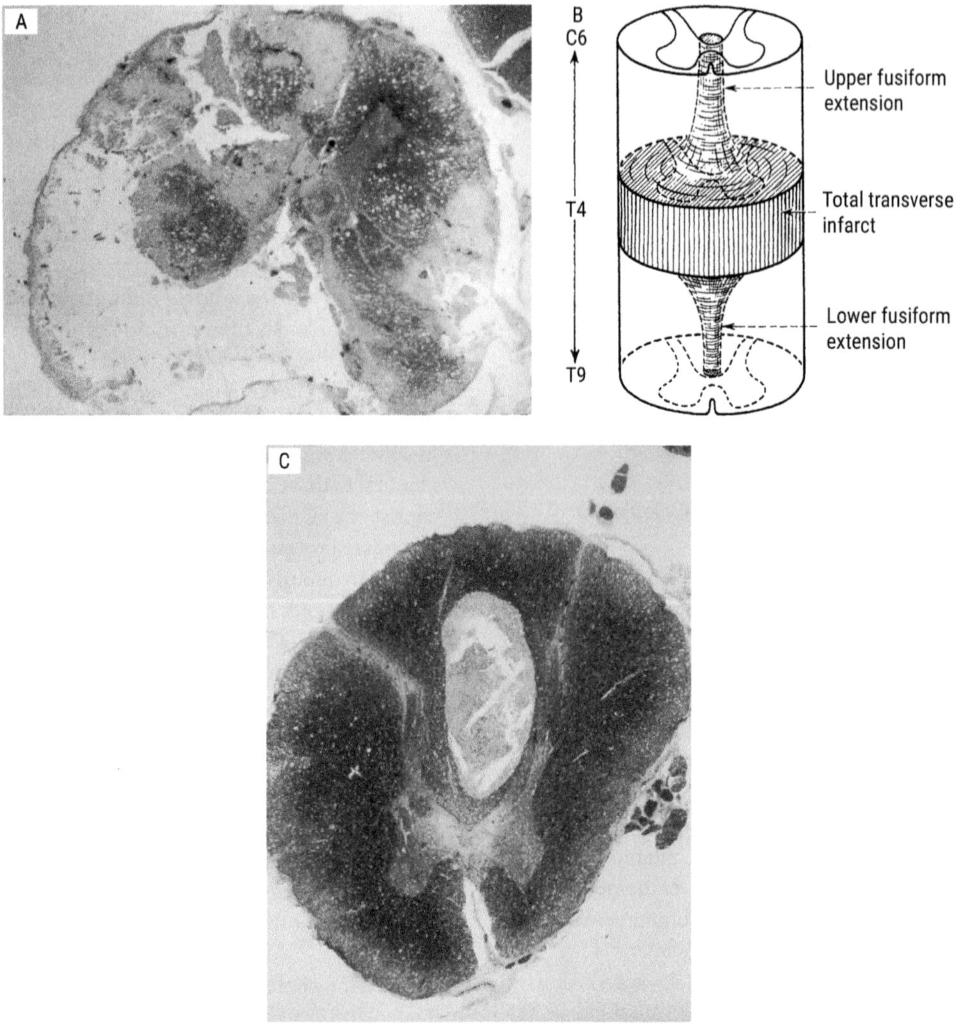

FIGURE 4.43 Transverse infarcts of the spinal cord: (**A**) maximal transverse extent of the infarct (Loyez stain for myelin); (**B**) diagram of the fusiform shape of the infarct; (**C**) upper fusiform extent of the infarct in transverse section (Loyez stain for myelin).

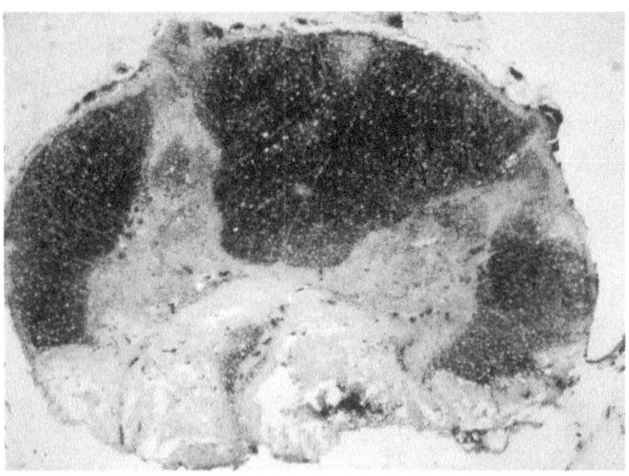

FIGURE 4.44 Focal infarct of the spinal cord (Loyez stain for myelin). Anterior spinal artery.

pathology of small arterial lesions. The improved imaging resolution introduced by MRI has allowed identification of small lacunar lesions, microbleeds, and leukoencephalopathy during life and has increased considerably the interest in the pathology and pathogenesis of these lesions. In addition to underlying ischemic strokes and hemorrhages, microvascular disease is a frequent feature of vascular dementia and may be an aggravating factor in degenerative dementia (see Chapter 8). The term "microvascular disease" encompasses all forms of microangiopathy.

These so-called small arteries are perforating arteries with diameters from 40 to 400 μm that

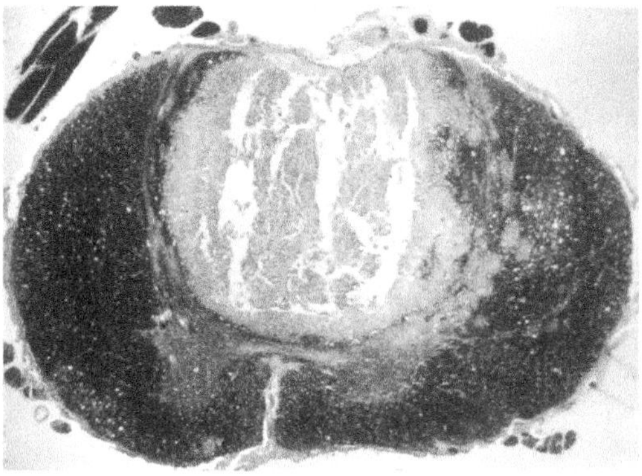

FIGURE 4.45 Focal infarct of the spinal cord (Loyez stain for myelin). Posterior spinal artery infarct.

emerge from the leptomeningeal arteries, enter the brain parenchyma from the surface of the brain, and extend a variable depth into the parenchyma. Among small arteries, one may distinguish the deep perforators at the base of the brain supplying the basal ganglia, thalamus, and adjacent white matter, in addition to the brainstem, from the superficial perforators originating from the pial branches of the anterior, middle, and PCAs, over the surface of the brain. Short superficial perforators supply the cortex, and longer ones—the medullary arteries—nourish the deep white matter. The perforators are end arteries with very limited collateral connection with neighboring blood vessels until they divide into capillaries.

4.3.1. Diseases of small arteries

Diseases of small arteries include hypertensive arteriosclerotic cerebrovascular disease (see Section 4.1.2.1); CAA (see Section 4.1.2.2); and hereditary small vessel diseases distinct from CAA, particularly cerebral autosomal dominant arteriopathy with subcortical infarcts and leukoencephalopathy (CADASIL) and its autosomal recessive counterpart (CARASIL).

4.3.1.1. CEREBRAL AUTOSOMAL DOMINANT ARTERIOPATHY WITH SUBCORTICAL INFARCTS AND LEUKOENCEPHALOPATHY

A hereditary disease of the brain vessels, CADASIL is caused by a mutation of the *NOTCH3* gene on chromosome 19. It is characterized by deposition of pathognomonic granular osmiophilic material seen by electron microscopy in the media and adventitia of the wall of small arteries (Fig. 4.46D, E), including dermal arteries (where the deposit can easily be identified on skin biopsy), since the arteriopathy is generalized. The extracellular domain cleaved from the Notch-3 protein accumulates outside the degenerating vascular smooth muscle cells in response to ligand binding and can be identified by immunohistochemistry. Its topography is different from that of granular deposits (Fig. 4.46). This accumulation is associated with degeneration of vascular smooth muscle cells, progressive wall thickening and fibrosis, and luminal narrowing of small and medium-size penetrating arteries. Multiple small infarcts in the white matter or deep gray matter are frequent. The cerebral cortex is usually less affected, and ICHs are uncommon.

Other hereditary cerebral and retinal vascular diseases have been described. The relevant gene and gene mutations have been identified in many of these. Some diseases, such as CADASIL, are autosomal dominant. Other autosomal dominant diseases include *retinal vasculopathy with cerebral leukodystrophy* (RVCL) resulting from mutations of the *TREX1* gene (and previously described as cerebroretinal vasculopathy), *cerebral small vessel disease related to* COL4 *mutations, hereditary extensive vascular leukoencephalopathy* (HEVL) mapping to chromosome 20q13, *Swedish hereditary multi-infarct dementia,* and *pontine autosomal dominant microangiopathy and leukoencephalopathy* (PADMAL) with mutations upregulating *COL4A* expression. Others are autosomal recessive. These include CARASIL as well as *leukoencephalopathy calcifications and cysts* (LCC) due to mutations in *SNORD118*.

Except for CADASIL, which remains the prototypic hereditary disease of cerebral small vessels, neuropathological postmortem studies of these disorders are either lacking or limited to single-case reports or small series. In most cases, there is variable association of lacunar infarcts, microhemorrhages, and vascular leukoencephalopathy, the shared markers of cerebral small vessel disease. Distinctive vascular changes may be observed in some of these conditions. In the case of CADASIL, or LCC, the findings are very specific, even diagnostic. In other cases (e.g., RVCL or HEVL), the morphologic changes may be suggestive of a diagnosis that then requires genetic confirmation. In some of these conditions, there is systemic vascular involvement that will be demonstrable in skin, muscle, nerve, or renal biopsy.

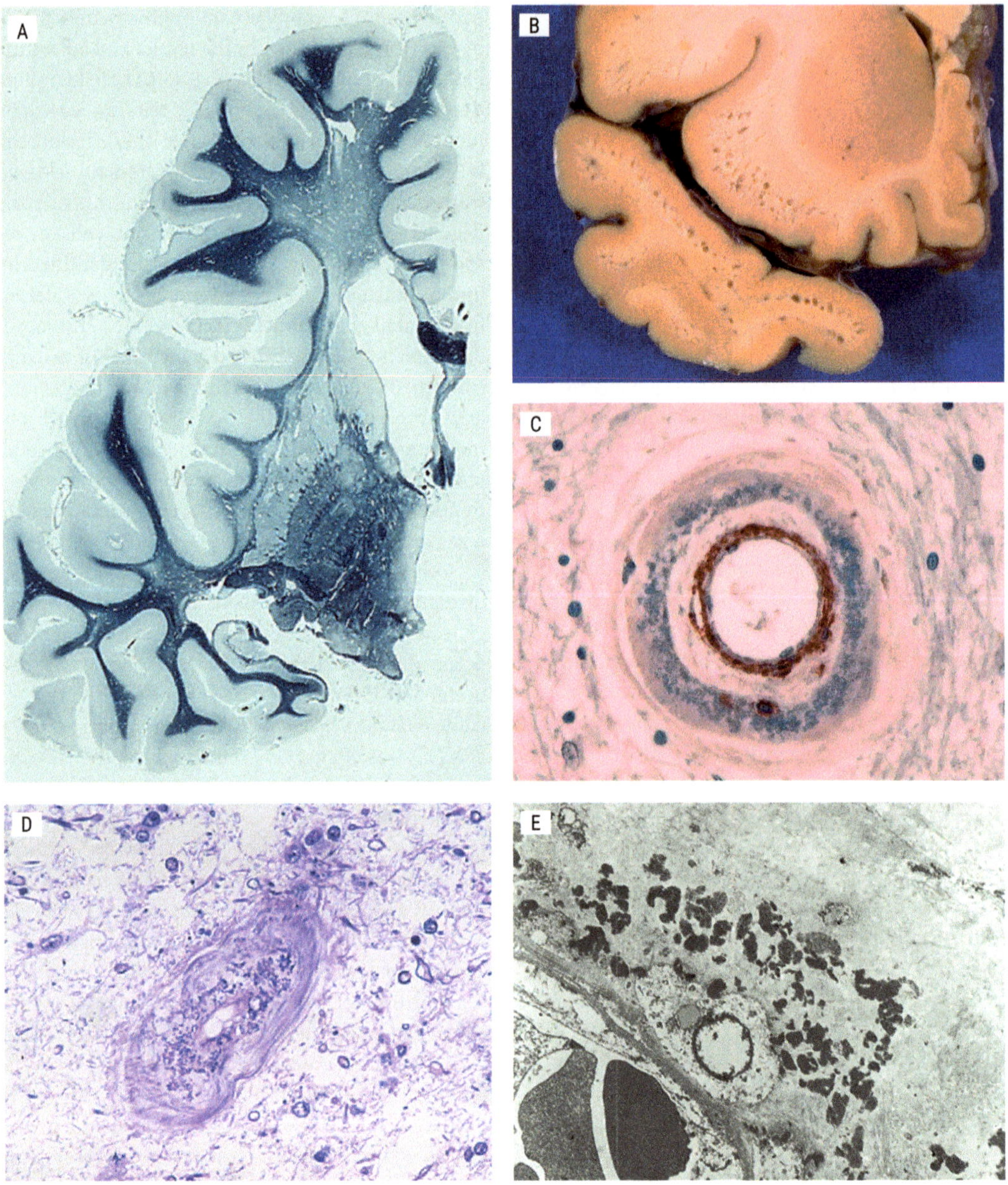

FIGURE 4.46 CADASIL: (**A**) Overview of subcortical infarcts and leukoencephalopathy (whole mount; Woelcke stain). (**B**) Gross appearance of status cribrosus at the cortico–subcortical junction in the anterior temporal and frontal lobes. (**C**) White matter arteriole, immunostaining of the extracellular domain of Notch 3. Note positive deposit around the lumen and the vascular smooth muscle cells. It is clearly different from the unstained granular deposit deeper in the arteriolar wall. (**D**) Granular osmiophilic material in arterial walls on semithin section and (**E**) on ultrastructural examination.

4.3.1.2. SMALL VESSEL INVOLVEMENT IN SYSTEMIC CONDITIONS

Small vessel involvement has been described in rare, chronic, systemic conditions that may present clinically with comparable vascular complications, with leukoencephalopathy as a frequent and characteristic feature. These conditions include *mitochondrial encephalopathy, lactic acidosis, and stroke-like episodes* (MELAS), in which infarcts are usually cortical (see Chapter 10), and merosin-negative congenital muscular dystrophies (see Chapter 12).

4.3.1.3. ACUTE INFLAMMATION OF SMALL VESSELS: CNS VASCULITIS

Inflammatory diseases of the CNS blood vessels can occur in a wide range of disorders with multiple causes. Certain pathological features are common to all, namely intramural inflammation and necrotic changes within the vascular wall. These disorders may be further subdivided into infectious vasculitides, due to direct infection ofblood vessels by microorganisms, and noninfectious CNS vasculitides, resulting from immune-mediated injury.

4.3.1.3.1. Infectious vasculitides. Infectious vasculitides, caused by direct infection of blood vessels by microorganisms, have been described with viral infections (HIV, varicella zoster virus, Epstein–Barr virus, and herpes simplex virus), cytomegalovirus, bacterial infections (tuberculosis, syphilis, mycoplasma, and rickettsiae), mycoses, aspergilloses, and parasitoses (see Chapter 5).

4.3.1.3.2. Noninfectious CNS vasculitides. The noninfectious vasculitides are caused by immune-mediated injury. These disorders are difficult to diagnose and treat because of the wide range of clinical manifestations, role of symptom progression/evolution, and variable response to drug therapy. They are also a challenge for the pathologist because their etiology and pathogenesis are often not established, and the histopathological features are variable and nonspecific. A system of classification of CNS vasculitides to direct treatments and anticipate prognosis has been an ever-evolving goal.

Vasculitis of the CNS may be divided into two categories—*primary* and *secondary*:

- *Primary angiitis of the CNS (PACNS)* is defined as vasculitis occurring predominantly in the CNS in the absence of systemic inflammatory diseases, infections, neoplasms, or exposure to drugs. It was once considered a uniformly progressive and fatal disease. However, patient prognosis has improved with immunosuppressive therapy. Clinical, laboratory, and imaging data are not sufficiently specific to ascertain the diagnosis, although some angiographic features are suggestive of angiitis in a subset of patients, and a biopsy is usually sought to guide diagnosis and management. Yet, the establishment of a firm pathologic diagnosis can be problematic because the lesions are focal, and brain biopsy has a suboptimal sensitivity; a negative biopsy does not necessarily rule out the diagnosis. Sampling the leptomeninges and cortex and targeting radiologically/angiographically abnormal areas increase the diagnostic yield. In the absence of focal lesions, the temporal tip of the nondominant hemisphere is the preferred biopsy site. The changes on biopsy involve the small and medium vessels of the brain and spinal cord, arterioles, and venules. Rarely, the vasculitis may be confined to the spinal cord. The abnormalities are focal and segmental in distribution. Histologically, granulomatous changes are the most characteristic (hence the other name *granulomatous angiitis of the nervous system*, GANS) and consist of infiltration of the vessel walls by histiocytes, giant cells, and mononuclear cells (Fig. 4.47). Necrotizing, lymphocytic, or mixed lesions are also frequent. Acute lesions often coexist with more chronic healing or healed lesions. A special feature is the SICRET syndrome or Susac's syndrome, which is

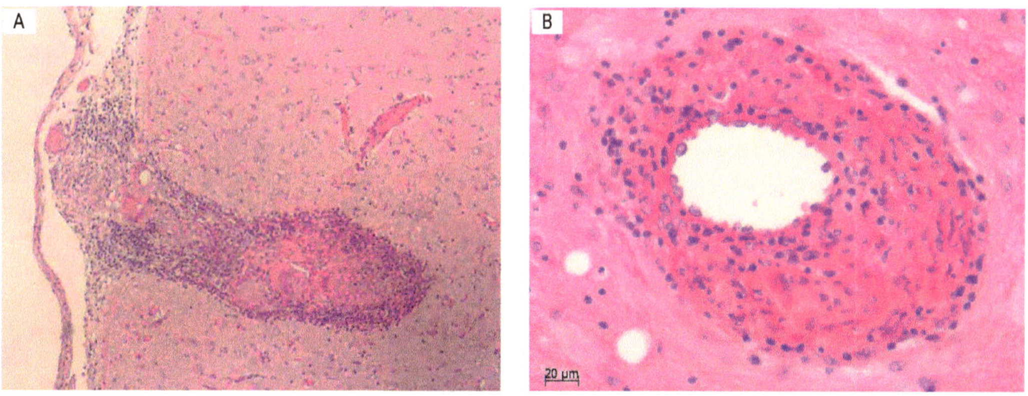

FIGURE 4.47 Primary angiitis of the CNS: infiltration of the vessel walls by histiocytes, giant cells, and mononuclear cells involving a leptomeningeal and a perforating artery (**A**) and an intraparenchymal artery (**B**).

- characterized by small infarcts of cochlear, retinal, and encephalic tissues in the young.
- *Secondary inflammation of CNS blood vessels* may occur as a manifestation of various systemic diseases, malignancy-related vasculitis, and drug-induced vasculitis. In CNS vasculitis associated with systemic diseases (*polyarteritis nodosa, granulomatosis with polyangiitis, and Churg–Strauss syndrome*; also, *Sjögren–Larsson syndromes* and *neuro-Behçet disease* when involving venules in particular, and rarely *systemic lupus erythematosus*), involvement of the CNS is a serious complication in the course of the disease. The characteristic features of CNS vasculitis in these disorders are not clearly established and are not specific in the relatively few neuropathological studies, mostly postmortem. In evaluating a brain biopsy for possible vasculitis, it is valuable to know if the patient has serologic evidence of an autoimmune or connective tissue disorder.

Vasculitides of the nervous system may occur in patients with neoplasia. These cases have most commonly shown involvement of the peripheral nervous system (see Chapter 13). CNS vasculitis has been described in patients with Hodgkin disease. In most cases, the typical histopathologic appearance is that of granulomatous angiitis. The neurological symptoms may precede the diagnosis of the underlying neoplasm, and brain biopsy may be necessary to establish a definite diagnosis.

Drug allergies may cause leukocytoclastic vasculitis, which may affect peripheral nerves and the CNS. The neuropathologic features of other forms of drug-induced vasculitis are not well established. Cases of biopsy-proven cerebral vasculitis in cocaine abusers have been reported. Necrotizing angiitis affecting cerebral arteries and arterioles has been described in autopsy studies of drug addicts who used multiple amphetamine drugs. The etiology of these vasculitides is unclear. The association between polyarteritis nodosa and hepatitis B and C may be one explanation for necrotizing vasculitis in drug abusers.

4.3.2. Cerebrovascular complications of diseases of small arteries

Three common cerebrovascular disorders are specifically associated with diseases of small arteries: nontraumatic intraparenchymal hemorrhage, lacunes, and arteriopathic leukoencephalopathies.

4.3.2.1. CEREBRAL MICROBLEEDS

Apart from large intraparenchymal hemorrhages (see Section 4.1.2), which are mainly associated with hypertensive cerebrovascular disease (see Section 4.1.2.1) and CAA (see Section 4.1.2.2), the frequent occurrence of small, often asymptomatic "microdeposits of hemosiderin" has been discovered by sensitive MRI techniques. This discovery has introduced the concept of CMBs as small, well-demarcated, hypointense, rounded lesions seen on MRI sequences sensitive to magnetic susceptibility. Studies suggest that CMBs are an imaging marker for small vessel pathology. These lesions have a high prevalence (approximately 5%) and are observed more frequently with increasing age. They have been observed mostly in patients with primary ICH and in a few patients with ischemic cerebrovascular disease. The neuropathologic correlate of these imaging studies is still being analyzed. The first studies have shown that "microbleeds" seen by MRI usually correspond pathologically to microscopic hemorrhagic foci of different ages (usually clusters of hemosiderin-laden macrophages), such as cortical miliary hemorrhages observed in CAA (see Section 4.1.2.2.3). They also may correspond to calcium or iron deposits, vascular malformations, or cross sections of pial blood vessels.

4.3.2.2. LACUNES

Lacunes (Fig. 4.48) are small cavitary lesions in the brain that are less than 15–20 mm in diameter. They are mostly associated with hypertensive cerebral microvascular (arteriosclerotic) disease (see Section 4.1.2.1) but can also be seen in small vessel disease of other types (e.g., CADASIL). It has been proposed they be subdivided into three types.

4.3.2.2.1. Lacunar infarcts (or microinfarcts) (type 1). The small cavities of lacunar infarcts (microinfarcts; type 1) are the result of remote, small, deep cerebral infarcts due to occlusion of small penetrating arteries (200–800 μm in diameter). These irregular, ragged cavities have all the characteristics of ischemic necrosis. They contain small amounts of parenchymatous debris, lipid-filled macrophages (Fig. 4.48B), and occasionally macrophages filled with hemosiderin. Like all infarcts, most lacunar infarcts are laced with small-caliber vessels and are surrounded by reactive changes. Lacunar infarcts may be solitary or

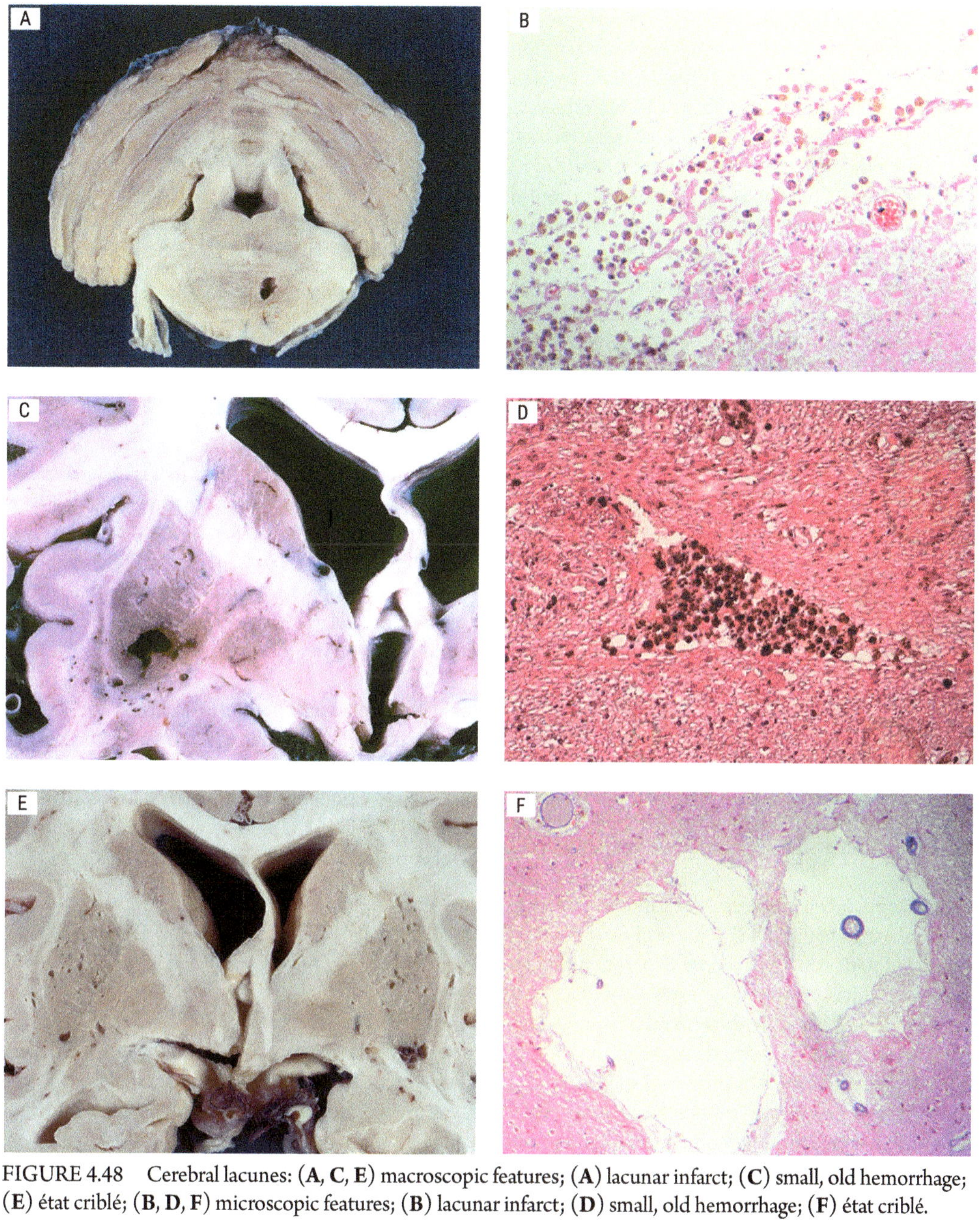

FIGURE 4.48 Cerebral lacunes: (**A**, **C**, **E**) macroscopic features; (**A**) lacunar infarct; (**C**) small, old hemorrhage; (**E**) état criblé; (**B**, **D**, **F**) microscopic features; (**B**) lacunar infarct; (**D**) small, old hemorrhage; (**F**) état criblé.

multiple; they involve preferentially the basal ganglia, the pons (Fig. 4.48A), and the internal capsule. They are associated with increasing age, arterial hypertension, and diabetes mellitus. In most cases, they result from a segmental process of AS of the penetrating arteries linked to arterial hypertension. They may also be related to atherosclerosis involving arterial trunks when a plaque occludes the ostium of the artery. Artery-to-artery emboli or emboli of cardiac origin may infrequently cause infarcts indistinguishable from lacunar infarcts due to small vessel disease. However, the pattern in this case is more a single lacunar infarct, whereas in hypertensive small vessel disease there are multiple accompanying older lacunar infarcts, with leukoaraoisis, microdeposits of hemosiderin, and dilatation of perivascular spaces.

4.3.2.2.2. Small old hemorrhages (type 2). There are cavitated destructive lesions resulting from small, old hemorrhages (type 2). Their outline is usually more regular than that of lacunar infarcts (Fig. 4.48C). Their wall is the site of ocher-yellow pigmentation due to the abundance of hemosiderin-laden macrophages (Fig. 4.48D), which are found also inside the cavity. Small, old hemorrhages are usually solitary and located in the basal ganglia, commonly associated with hypertension or, in the hemispheric white matter or cortex, commonly associated with CAA. They are considered to be due to the rupture of a microaneurysm, but necrosis and amyloid degeneration of the vessel wall have also been implicated. Indeed, necrosis within an affected vessel wall may contribute to microaneurysm formation.

4.3.2.2.3. État criblé (status cribrosus) (type 3). Status cribrosus (état criblé; type 3) results from dilation of the perivascular spaces. The cavities are rounded with a smooth outline. They always contain one or two cross sections of an artery with an open lumen (Fig. 4.48F). The cavity is lined by simple flattened cells, which are the normal lining cells that form the outer walls of the Virchow–Robin spaces and correspond to the invaginated pial covering surrounding the blood vessels. The cerebral parenchyma that surrounds them is usually devoid of gliosis.

No single mechanism can explain état criblé. In the basal ganglia (Fig. 4.48E), the lesions are usually associated with AS. They can be experimentally induced in models of arterial hypertension. État criblé can also be associated with cerebral atrophy, whatever the cause, and is more frequent in the elderly. It is also a feature of CADASIL, and specific to this disease is the dilation of the perivascular spaces at the cortico–subcortical junction, particularly in the temporal lobe (Fig. 4.46B). État criblé is often seen in association with lacunar infarcts and/or small old hemorrhages.

Although often asymptomatic, both lacunar infarcts and small hemorrhages, when clinically significant, often present with one of the characteristic syndromes of lacunar stroke. The features depend on the location of the lesion and include ataxic hemiparesis (most commonly basis pontis or posterior limb of the internal capsule), pure motor hemiparesis (most typically posterior limb of the internal capsule), dysarthria and clumsy hand syndrome (classically the genu of the internal capsule, but often other locations, such as the basis pontis), and pure unilateral sensory syndrome (classically lateral thalamus). A diffuse progressive neurological deficit may be seen when there are many lacunes; the most classical clinical consequences are a pseudobulbar syndrome and vascular dementia.

4.3.2.3. ARTERIOPATHIC LEUKOENCEPHALOPATHIES

The diffuse white matter lesions of arteriopathic leukoencephalopathies are seen in certain forms of vascular dementia. The changes consist of diffuse myelin pallor of the white matter, with sparing of the subcortical U fibers, the corpus callosum, and the internal capsule (Fig. 4.49A, B). On microscopic examination, ill-defined, incomplete myelin destruction, spongiosis, swollen oligodendrocytes (Fig. 4.49C), dilation of the perivascular spaces, and reactive astrocytosis with perivascular reinforcement are seen. In arteriopathic subcortical encephalopathy (Binswanger disease), numerous lacunes are present in the white matter and basal ganglia (Fig. 4.49A), and the arterioles of these regions are the site of severe advanced arteriolosclerosis (Fig. 4.49D). This is typically seen in patients with long-standing hypertension. In CADASIL, subcortical infarcts or lacunes are frequent in the white matter and basal ganglia (Fig. 4.46A), as they are in CARASIL and cerebroretinal vasculopathies.

4.4. VASCULAR PATHOLOGY OF VENOUS ORIGIN

In the past, the study of cerebral venous lesions was closely linked to that of the pathology of infectious diseases in the brain because cerebral phlebitis was most often secondary to infectious lesions. With the widespread and early use of antibiotics, cerebral venous thrombosis due to sinus and cerebral infections has become rare. Cerebral venous sinus thrombosis and cortical vein thrombosis are now most commonly seen in the setting of disturbances of coagulation. Venous occlusion leads to circulatory stasis, diapedesis of red blood cells, and hemorrhages proximal to the site of vascular occlusion. A venous infarct is the final outcome of this process. In contrast to arterial hemorrhagic infarcts, which predominate in the cortex, hemorrhages in venous infarction involve simultaneously the leptomeninges, the cortex, and the subcortical white matter. In superior sagittal sinus thrombosis (Fig. 4.50), hemorrhagic lesions

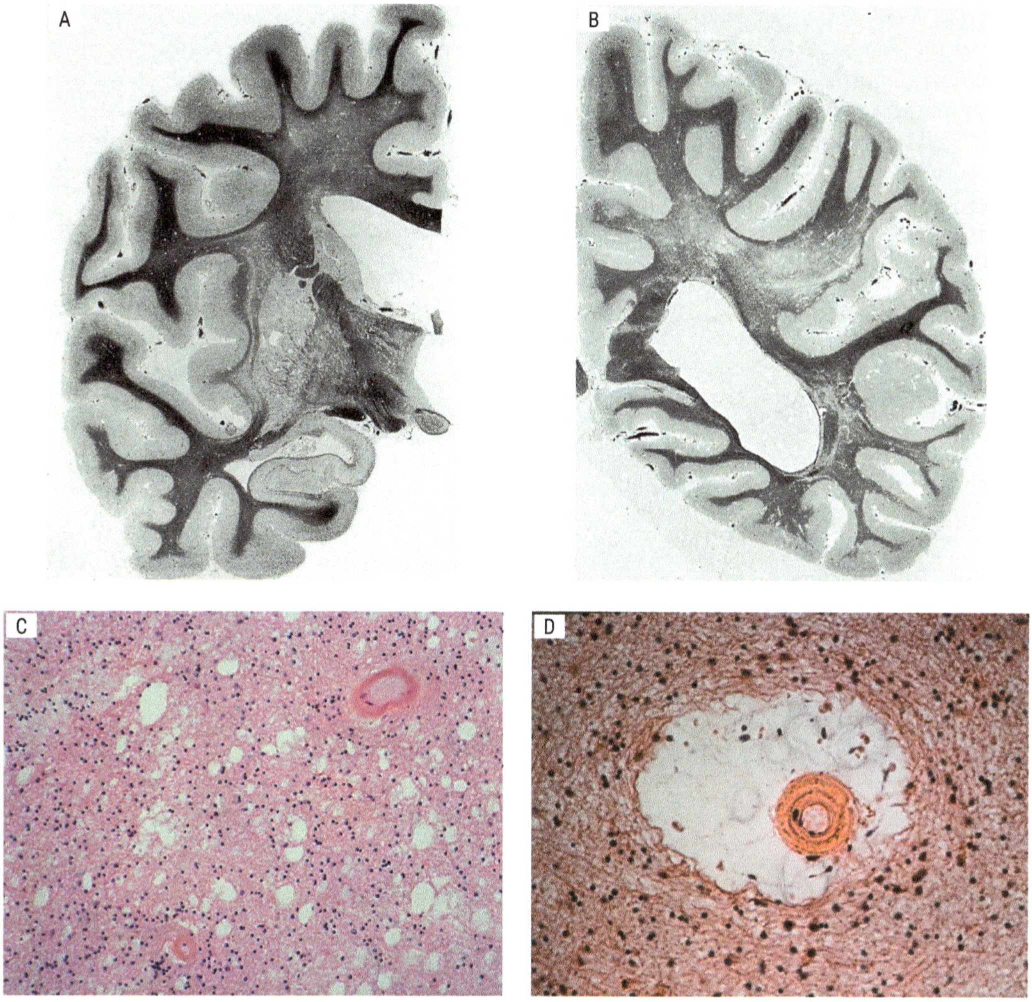

FIGURE 4.49 Arteriopathic subcortical encephalopathy (Binswanger). (**A, B**) Macroscopic appearance on Loyez stain for myelin. Note the presence of myelin pallor of the white matter and lacunar infarcts in the basal ganglia (**A**) and in the posterior white matter (**B**). (**C, D**) Microscopic features (H&E). Edema and glial swelling (**C**), dilation of perivascular space, and arteriolar hyalinosis (**D**).

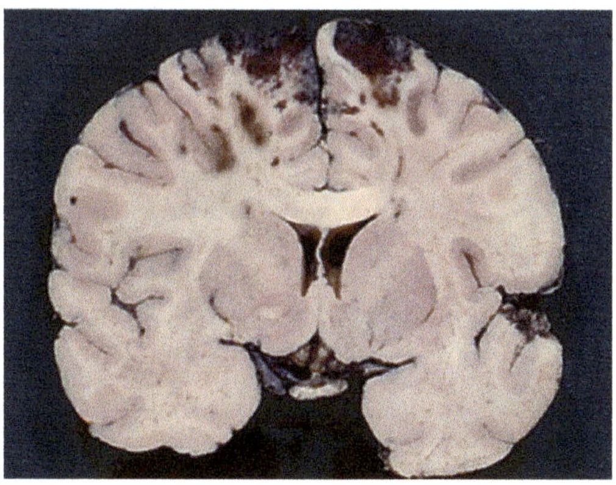

FIGURE 4.50 Bilateral venous infarction resulting from thrombosis of the superior sagittal sinus.

may symmetrically affect the hemispheric white matter bilaterally and predominate in the centrum semiovale. In thrombosis of the vein of Galen, the lesions involve the periventricular regions and the thalamic areas. In superficial phlebitis, lesions are often seen in the hemispheric gray matter and the underlying white matter.

4.5. MULTIPLE PATHOLOGIC PROCESSES

Patients (especially the elderly) often exhibit combinations of disease processes that frequently affect the CNS. These may be either of vascular origin (hemorrhages and infarctions or other disorders; see Section 4.1) or, more frequently, of vascular origin associated with other pathologies, such as neurodegenerative diseases. For example, Alzheimer disease patients have a high incidence of severe cerebral amyloid angiopathy and microinfarcts: The same proteins (Aβ) are involved in some amyloid angiopathies and Alzheimer disease. This leads to the concept of "mixed dementia." In addition, the coexistence of cerebral vascular lesions, whatever the origin, and degenerative lesions in a patient leads to a more rapidly progressive manifestation of the symptoms of dementia.

5

Infections of the Central Nervous System

FABRICE CHRÉTIEN, ISAAC H. SOLOMON, LEILA CHIMELLI, AND LEROY R. SHARER

A WIDE range of pathogenic infectious organisms—bacteria, fungi, parasites, viruses, and prions—may affect the central nervous system (CNS). Organisms can be classified as pathogenic or opportunistic. Infections by the former group cause diseases in every individual; those by the latter group affect patients with a compromised immune system. Infectious agents enter the CNS in multiple ways: through the blood; by retrograde spread via peripheral nerves; through congenital defects in the neuraxis, such as meningomyelocele; or by direct invasion, often in the postoperative setting. The hematogenous route is most common, either by direct spread or via host cells.

The brain and spinal cord are relatively well protected from infective agents by the skull and vertebral column, by the meninges, and by the blood–brain barrier. However, once a pathogen enters the CNS, host defense mechanisms are suboptimal to control its replication and pathogenicity. In addition, immunodeficiency conditions in the host are becoming increasingly frequent. This may account for the continuing high mortality and morbidity rates from infections of the CNS, despite the advances in diagnosis and treatment that have been made in recent years.

5.1. BACTERIAL INFECTIONS

Depending on virulence/pathogenicity determinants, bacteria can induce (a) purulent lesions with recruitment and lysis of polymorphs; (b) cellular inflammatory reactions with influx of mononuclear leukocytes; or (c) inflammatory edema due to toxins and other inflammatory substances released by bacterial secretions or lysis, in the absence of bacterial replication. Precise identification of an organism is difficult on morphologic grounds alone, thereby requiring additional diagnostic methods, including cultures and molecular techniques (e.g., 16S rRNA sequencing) for diagnosis and optimal antibiotic treatment based on susceptibility data.

5.1.1. Pyogenic infections

Bone, dura mater, arachnoid, and pia mater delimit four compartments and tend to prevent the spread of infection from one compartment to another. Infections can arise in each of the four compartments: epidural, subdural, subarachnoid, and intraparenchymal.

5.1.1.1. EPIDURAL ABSCESSES

Infection of the epidural space is relatively rare. It more commonly occurs in the epidural space along the vertebral canal compared to the intracranial epidural space. Spread is frequently from osteomyelitis secondary to frontal or mastoid sinusitis, trauma, or surgery or may complicate epidural analgesia. Spinal epidural abscesses can extend over several vertebral levels. Intracranial epidural abscesses are biconvex and circumscribed by the skull and the displaced dura.

5.1.1.2. SUBDURAL ABSCESSES OR EMPYEMA

Infection of the subdural space most often extends from an adjacent sinusitis, otitis, or osteomyelitis. Infection associated with purulent leptomeningitis is the main cause of subdural empyema in infants. Subdural infection tends to spread over the convexity of one cerebral hemisphere but is ordinarily contained from crossing the midline by the falx cerebri. In most cases, the empyema is situated above the tentorium, occasionally adjacent to the falx cerebri. Empyema occurs less commonly in the posterior fossa and rarely involves the spinal canal.

5.1.1.3. ACUTE BACTERIAL MENINGITIS

Purulent infection of the leptomeningeal spaces is the most frequent pyogenic infection of the CNS. Most cases of pyogenic meningitis are secondary to hematogenous dissemination of bacteria. Meningitis may also complicate trauma, surgery, or developmental malformations. Various bacterial species–gram positive or gram negative, aerobic or anaerobic—can cause acute bacterial meningitis. Some species are more often found in children older than 1 year and in adults in whom infection results from either otitis or a primary respiratory infection (sinusitis, rhinopharyngitis, or pneumonia). Three major agents—pneumococcus (*Streptococcus pneumoniae*), meningococcus (*Neisseria meningitidis*), and *Haemophilus influenzae*—each account for one-third of the recorded cases. Other species, such as *Streptococcus agalactiae, Escherichia coli, Citrobacter koseri,* and *Listeria monocytogenes,* are most frequently isolated in affected young children or newborns, and the infection can be transmitted from mother to infant.

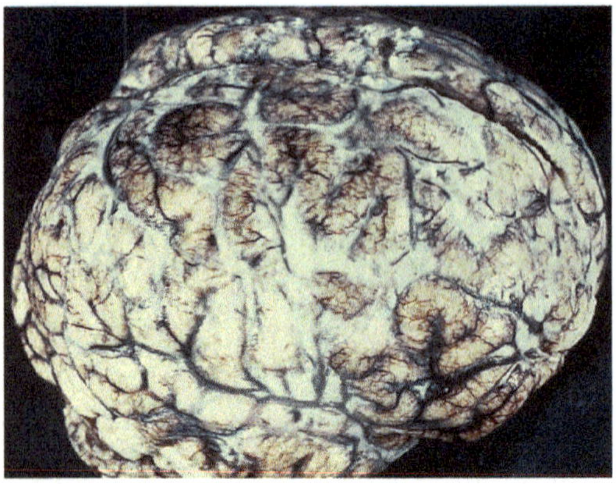

FIGURE 5.1 Macroscopic appearance of purulent leptomeningitis.

The purulent exudate may be recognized macroscopically in the leptomeninges (Fig. 5.1). Microscopically, large numbers of polymorphonuclear leukocytes invade the leptomeningeal (Fig. 5.2) and Virchow–Robin spaces. Bacteria, highlighted by Gram, Warthin–Starry, or Steiner stains, may be seen either free or within neutrophils. Over time, in the absence of early resolution, such as by appropriate antibiotic therapy, the polymorphonuclear leukocytes degenerate and disappear to be replaced by a fibrinous exudate containing lymphocytes, plasma cells, histiocytes, and macrophages. After persistent infection over the course of weeks, the exudate organizes into fibrous connective tissue.

All the CNS structures in contact with the cerebrospinal fluid (CSF) are involved in the infectious process. Thus, (a) there is a polymorphic

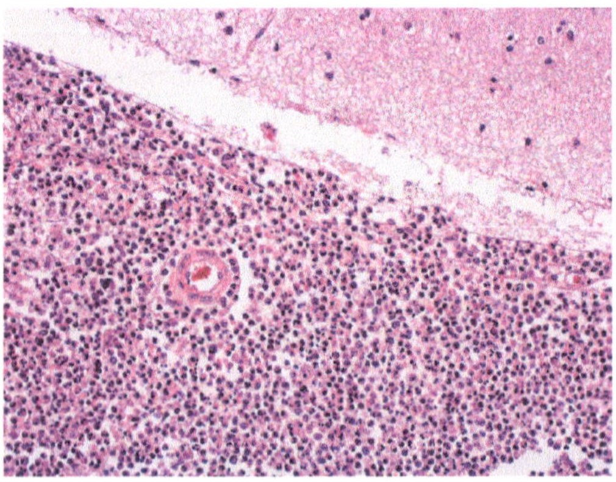

FIGURE 5.2 Microscopic appearance of purulent leptomeningitis (hematoxylin and eosin [H&E]).

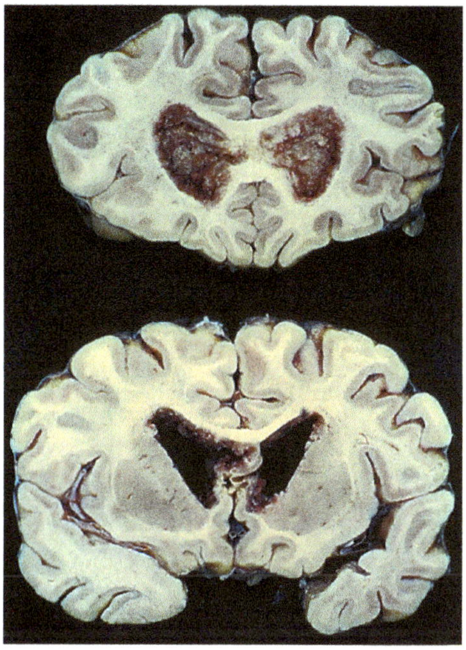

FIGURE 5.3 Purulent ventriculitis.

inflammatory cellular infiltrate in the walls of the leptomeningeal blood vessels, mainly the veins, that may undergo thrombosis and cause cerebral venous infarcts; (b) there is cellular infiltration of the cranial nerves and spinal roots, sometimes with degeneration of the myelinated fibers; and (c) there is invasion of the ventricular walls with consequent purulent ventriculitis (Fig. 5.3). The process may also spread to the subpial and subependymal neural parenchyma. Cerebral abscesses secondary to purulent meningitis are not unusual in infants and newborns. The production of a fibrinocellular exudate and its subsequent fibrous organization may obstruct the outflow of the CSF and result in the development of hydrocephalus or, sometimes, pyocephalus.

Listeria monocytogenes infections deserve separate mention because of the frequency with which microabscesses ("*Listeria* nodules"), localized particularly in the brainstem, are associated with this type of purulent meningitis.

5.1.1.4. BRAIN ABSCESSES

Brain abscess is the second most common purulent infection of the CNS after bacterial meningitis and is the most frequent space-occupying infection. Neuroimaging has been very useful in reaching a diagnosis of brain abscess, resulting in a decrease of the mortality rate. It has also become possible to treat cases with antibiotics alone.

As in leptomeningitis, the source of infection that leads to brain abscesses may be local or blood-borne. Post-traumatic abscesses occur at the site of craniocerebral wounds or neurosurgery. Abscesses of hematogenous origin tend to occur at the junction between the gray and white matter (Fig. 5.4) and are often multiple. They are secondary to septic emboli from bacterial endocarditis or chronic suppurative intrathoracic infection. Paradoxical cerebral septic emboli may occur in congenital cyanotic heart disease. Abscesses resulting from direct spread from an adjacent suppurative focus are usually situated in the temporal lobe (Fig. 5.5A) or in the cerebellum following otitis media or mastoiditis or in the frontal lobe following sinusitis.

The initial stage of *focal cerebritis* (Days 1–3 after inoculation) appears macroscopically as an ill-defined region of hyperemia surrounded by edema. Microscopically, it is characterized by early parenchymal necrosis with vascular congestion, petechial hemorrhage, microthrombosis, perivascular fibrinous exudate, and infiltration by polymorphs. Surrounding edema is an invariable finding and contributes to the mass effect of the abscess. *Late cerebritis* (Days 4–9) is characterized by a necrotic purulent center resulting from the confluence of adjacent foci of necrosis. The pus is surrounded by a narrow, irregular layer of inflammatory granulation tissue infiltrated by

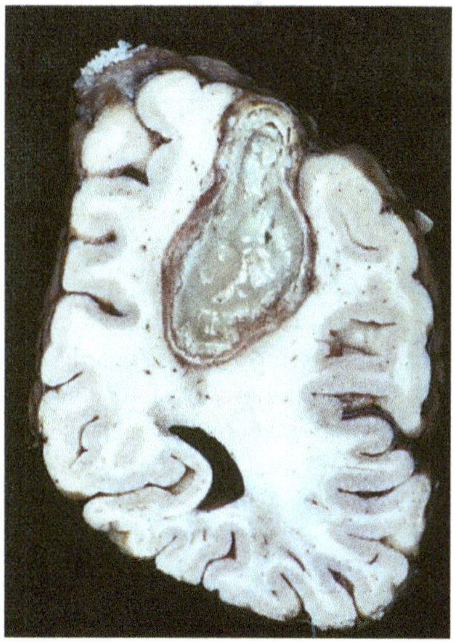

FIGURE 5.4 Parietal lobe abscess with central necrosis and a peripheral capsule with granulation tissue.

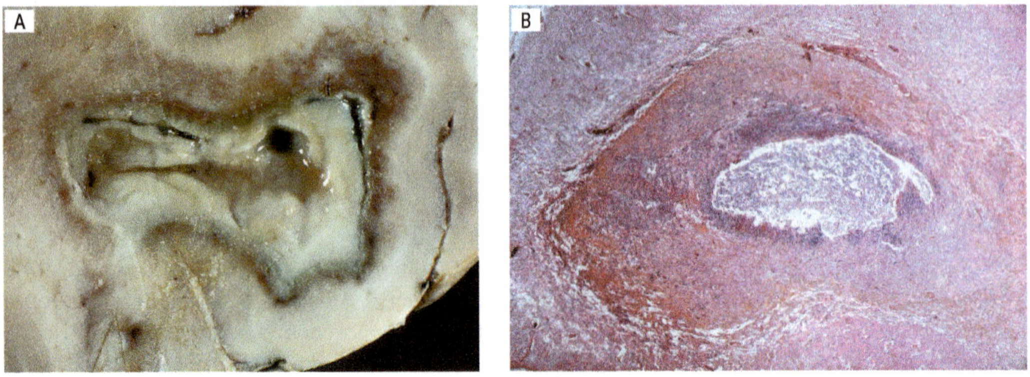

FIGURE 5.5 Temporal lobe abscess with purulent necrosis in the center and surrounding granulation tissue: (**A**) macroscopic appearance; (**B**) microscopic appearance (H&E).

neutrophils, lymphocytes, and some macrophages. The perivascular spaces in the vicinity become cuffed with polymorphs and lymphocytes.

The *early abscess capsule* develops over Days 10–13 and is made up of granulation tissue, which includes lymphocytes, plasma cells, monocytes and macrophages, numerous newly formed blood vessels, and scattered fibroblasts. The developing capsule is at first poorly defined; it is thickest on its cortical surface and often very thin or even deficient on its ventricular surface. For this reason, abscesses tend to expand inward and rupture into the ventricular system, resulting in ventriculitis. As time evolves (Day 14 and later), *the capsule becomes firmer* and can be stripped easily from the surrounding edematous white matter. Microscopically, more fibroblasts invade the tissue so that a well-encapsulated abscess consists of five layers: a necrotic center invaded by macrophages; granulation tissue with proliferating fibroblasts and capillaries, and long, radially oriented blood vessels; a zone of lymphocytes and plasma cells in granulation tissue; dense fibrous tissue with embedded astrocytes; and a surrounding edematous area of gliosis (Fig. 5.5B). Fibrosis is an unusual phenomenon within the CNS, with brain abscess being a notable exception.

The two major and most serious complications of brain abscesses are raised intracranial pressure with the risk of cerebral herniation and rupture of the abscess into a ventricle, resulting in ventricular empyema.

5.1.1.5. SEPTIC EMBOLISM

Apart from cerebral abscesses, a septic embolus, whenever of sufficient size, may cause cerebral infarction that can become infected by extension from the embolus. Implantation of a septic embolus in a cerebral artery may result in a mycotic aneurysm due to local infection and weakening of the arterial wall. Despite the name, mycotic aneurysms are due to pyogenic bacteria rather than fungi (see Chapter 4). A mycotic aneurysm may rupture, causing either hemorrhage into the brain or subarachnoid space or, less frequently, meningitis.

5.1.1.6. SUPPURATIVE INTRACRANIAL PHLEBITIS

Septic intracranial thrombophlebitis most frequently follows infection of paranasal sinuses, middle ear, mastoid, face, or oropharynx. The infection spreads centrally along the emissary veins. Septic thrombophlebitis may also occur in association with epidural abscess, subdural empyema, or meningitis. Septic intracranial phlebitis may cause hemorrhagic infarction. In addition, local suppuration may produce venous hemorrhage, venous necrosis, epidural abscess, subdural empyema, meningitis, and brain abscess.

5.1.2. Tuberculosis

5.1.2.1. TUBERCULOUS EPIDURAL OR SUBDURAL ABSCESSES

Epidural tuberculous abscess is a recognized complication of tuberculosis of the spine (Pott disease), involving either the vertebral bodies or the intervertebral disks. Subdural tuberculous abscess is also a frequent co-occurrence.

5.1.2.2. TUBERCULOUS MENINGITIS

Tuberculous meningitis is the most common form of tuberculosis of the CNS. In most cases, the disease complicates the initial hematogenous dissemination that follows primary infection; it may also follow late reactivation of latent infection elsewhere in the body. Tuberculous meningitis may be associated with miliary tuberculosis.

Unlike purulent meningitis, which spreads over the cerebral convexities, in tuberculous meningitis, the meninges at the base of the brain are the site most often involved (Fig. 5.6). There may be some gray-green opacity of the meninges over the cerebral convexities, but a much thicker exudate fills the basal cisterns, covering the basis pontis and extending into the Sylvian fissures and cisterna magna. The spinal cord may also be enveloped by exudate. Tubercles are not easily found in the exudate, but they can sometimes be seen along the banks of the Sylvian fissure and near veins over the convexities.

Microscopically, the inflammatory infiltrate involves the leptomeninges and the subpial regions, as well as the ependyma and subependymal parenchyma. It is mostly composed of lymphocytes, mononuclear cells, and epithelioid nodules, with Langhans and other giant cells, and tubercles. Tubercles consist of a central area of caseous necrosis surrounded by an epithelioid macrophage reaction with a peripheral ring of lymphocytes (Fig. 5.7). Acid-fast bacilli, highlighted by Ziehl–Neelsen, Fite–Faraco, or anti-mycobacteria immunohistochemical stains, may be either abundant or scanty.

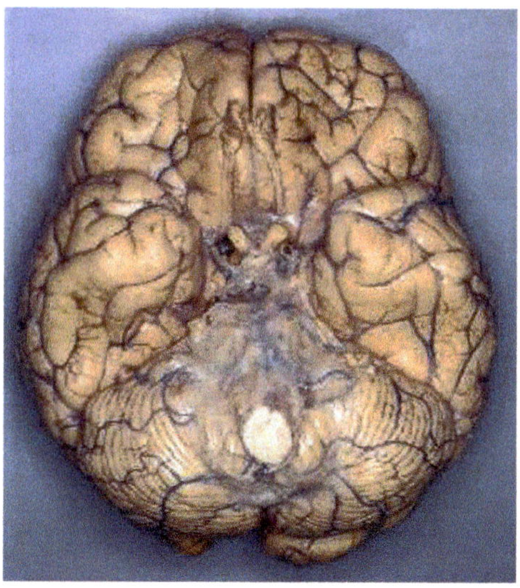

FIGURE 5.6 Tuberculous meningitis: thick exudate involving the basal meninges.

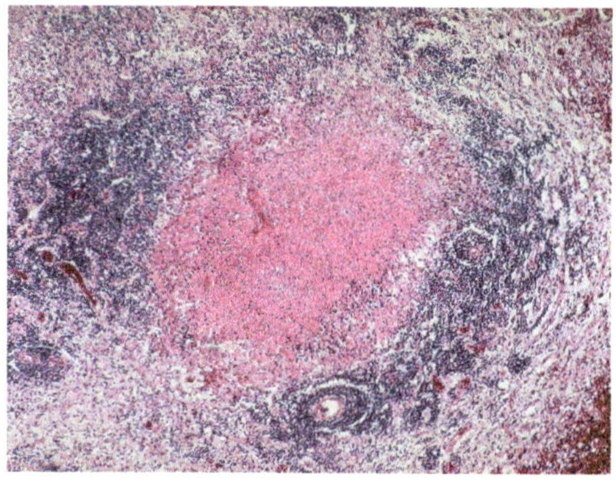

FIGURE 5.7 Tuberculous meningitis: tubercles consisting of a central area of caseous necrosis surrounded by an epithelioid macrophage reaction with a peripheral ring of lymphocytes and multinucleated giant cells (H&E).

Arterial lesions of reactive endarteritis obliterans (Fig. 5.8A) are constant and are frequently responsible for ischemic parenchymal lesions, particularly within the basal ganglia due to involvement of lenticulostriate penetrating blood vessels (Fig. 5.8B).

In treated patients who die several weeks after onset of the illness, the exudate is more fibrous. It is especially thick over the base (Fig. 5.9A) of the brain and in the cisterna ambiens, where the reactive changes in the meninges may cause obstruction of the flow of CSF and lead to hydrocephalus (Fig. 5.9B).

5.1.2.3. TUBERCULOMA OF BRAIN AND SPINAL CORD

The formation of a mass lesion, tuberculoma, was formerly a relatively common occurrence in patients with intracranial tuberculosis and remains a serious problem in some areas of the world. These may be single mass lesions but are more often multiple (Fig. 5.10A). The more commonly affected sites include the cerebellum, the pontine tegmentum, and the paracentral lobule. Tuberculoma has occasionally been described in the spinal cord. The lesions are spherical or multilobular with a caseous center, necrotic but firm and of a semi-liquid white macroscopic appearance, surrounded by a granulomatous reaction that includes giant cells, lymphocytes, and fibrosis to a variable extent (Fig. 5.10B). Surrounding brain edema is less prominent than what is found around cerebral abscesses.

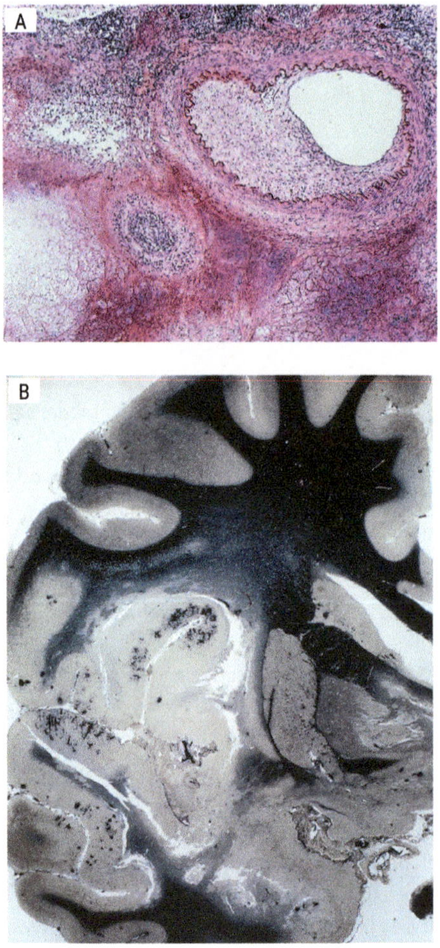

FIGURE 5.8 Tuberculous meningitis: (**A**) marked vascular changes forming endarteritis obliterans (H&E); (**B**) arterial lesions causing extensive cerebral infarction (Loyez stain).

Tuberculoma, particularly when in supratentorial locations, may spontaneously become cystic, fibrous, or calcified; bacilli may be difficult to detect, and inflammatory exudates can be scant. Rupture into the subarachnoid space may occur.

5.1.2.4. TUBERCULOUS ABSCESS

True tuberculous abscesses of the brain, as opposed to tuberculomas, are composed of a necrotic center containing pus in which *Mycobacterium tuberculosis* bacilli are abundant. These lesions are surrounded by a fibrous capsule like that in pyogenic abscesses, without the characteristic granulomatous reaction. Tuberculous abscesses of the CNS are usually multiple. In true abscesses, the absence of a granulomatous epithelioid reaction suggests the failure of immune mechanisms. Tuberculous abscesses have more recently been seen in patients with AIDS.

5.1.3. Atypical mycobacteriosis

Nontuberculous mycobacteria ("atypical mycobacteria"), which are saprophytic organisms, have recently become more common than tuberculous infections in North America. The *Mycobacterium avium* complex (MAC), including *M. avium, M. intracellulare,* and *M. chimaera,* is now recognized as one of the more common causes of opportunistic infection (OI) in patients with AIDS, in whom it produces disseminated systemic infection. However, in most cases of generalized MAC infection, involvement of the CNS is asymptomatic. Neuropathological examination only reveals diffuse perivascular

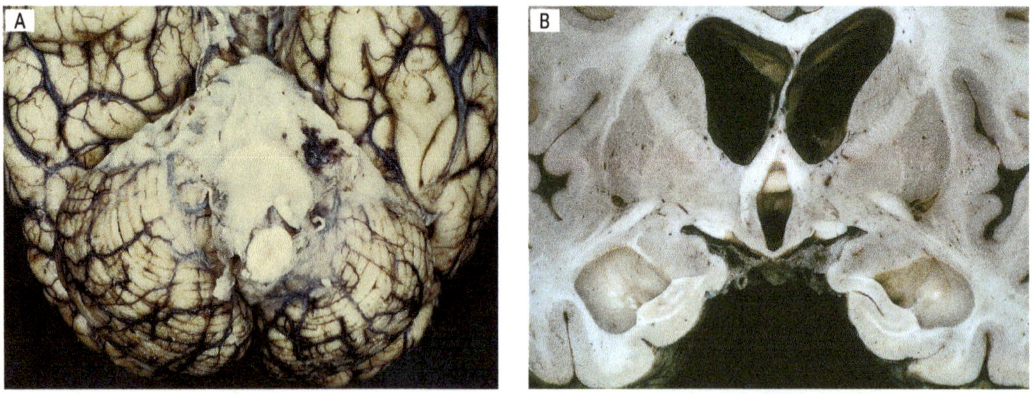

FIGURE 5.9 Chronic tuberculous meningitis: (**A**) massive fibrous infiltration of the basal meninges; (**B**) basal obstruction of CSF pathways with ventricular dilation.

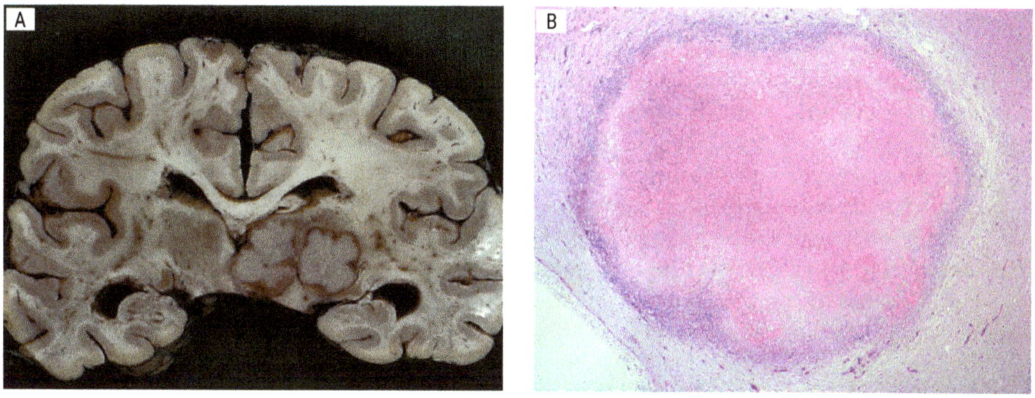

FIGURE 5.10 Tuberculoma: (**A**) macroscopic appearance of multiple tuberculomas in the thalamus; (**B**) microscopic appearance showing a caseous center surrounded by a granulomatous reaction (H&E).

macrophages containing clusters of acid-fast and periodic acid–Schiff (PAS)–positive mycobacteria. Symptomatic infection of the CNS due to MAC, *M. fortuitum*, and *M. genavense* and brain abscesses due to *M. kansasii and M. haemophilum* have been recorded in rare case reports in patients with AIDS.

5.1.4. Whipple disease

Whipple disease is a multisystem disorder often involving the intestine, caused by a gram-positive actinomycete, *Tropheryma whippelii*. Involvement of the CNS is uncommon and is usually associated with systemic disease. In rare instances, Whipple disease may be confined to the brain.

At neuropathological examination, small lesions are disseminated throughout the entire CNS but are especially abundant in the cortex, with a tendency to localize in the subpial regions, the basal ganglia, the hypothalamic nuclei, the periaqueductal gray matter, the nuclei of the brainstem, and the dentate nuclei of the cerebellum. The lesions may become confluent to form more extensive foci.

The microscopic picture consists of meningeal and parenchymal lymphocytes and multinucleated cells (Fig. 5.11A). The macrophages with lipid-filled cytoplasm contain tiny sickle-shaped inclusions that are PAS positive (Fig. 5.11B), gram negative, and methenamine silver positive. The bacteria also occur extracellularly in the tissue. By electron microscopy, lamellar, partially degraded bacterial cell walls and better-preserved bacilli are present in macrophages, astrocytes, and pericytes.

5.1.5. Actinomycosis

Actinomyces are small, anaerobic, gram-positive organisms whose appearance as thin, branching

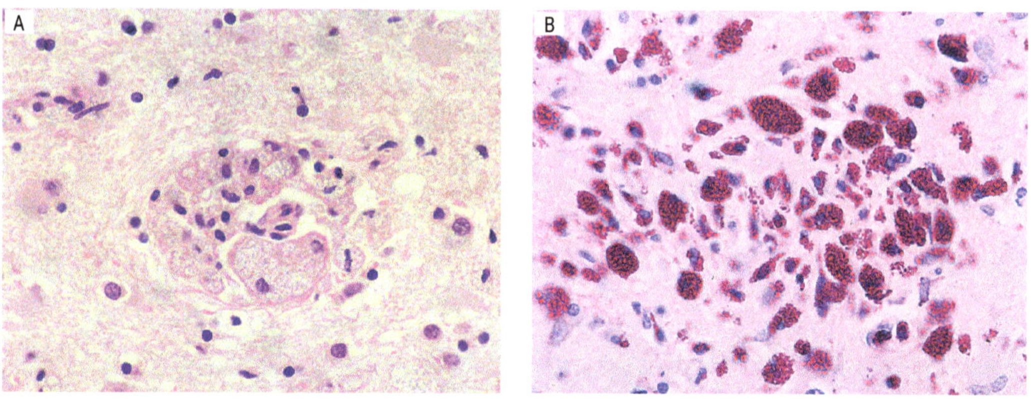

FIGURE 5.11 Whipple disease: (**A**) perivascular accumulation of lipid-laden macrophages surrounded by reactive astrocytosis (H&E); (**B**) foamy macrophages containing PAS-positive inclusions in the cytoplasm (PAS).

filaments has long led to their inclusion (with *Nocardia*) among fungi. Actinomyces have a worldwide distribution but occur predominantly in patients living in rural areas. Most infections in humans are produced by *Actinomyces israelii* and *A. bovis* and are acquired from organisms situated in the oral cavity or in the large intestine; they invade the tissues through a breach in the mucosa. Bone (mainly the mandible) is the most often affected site. Lesions of the CNS are rare and are usually secondary to a focus elsewhere in the body, spreading to the nervous system either by direct extension or via the bloodstream. Multilocular abscesses are formed, with a central necrotic inflammatory exudate containing polymorphs, necrotic debris, and colonies of branching organisms forming "sulfur granules" (naked eye appearance of the bright yellow lesion), surrounded by granulation tissue.

5.1.6. Nocardiosis

Nocardia asteroides is a ubiquitous aerobic organism that can be pathogenic, particularly in immunosuppressed patients. The nervous system is usually invaded through the hematogenous route from a primary pulmonary lesion. In the brain, *Nocardia* produces abscesses or meningitis. Microscopically, the abscesses have fibrous walls and polymorphs (Fig. 5.12A). The organism appears as thin, branching filaments, about 1 μm in diameter. They cannot be recognized in routinely stained preparations but can be identified using a modified Grocott methenamine silver stain (Fig. 5.12B) or Gram stain, where they are gram positive, and can be distinguished from *Actinomyces* by weak acid-fast staining with modified acid-fast stains. *Nocardia* is one of the more common causes of bacterial brain abscess in patients with AIDS, in whom brain abscesses are not especially common.

5.1.7. Neurosyphilis

Involvement of the CNS is a sequel of primary luetic disease that either has been undetected or has been inadequately treated. Although invasion of the leptomeninges during secondary syphilis is relatively common, symptomatic neurosyphilis occurs predominantly at the tertiary stage of the disease. Classically, neurosyphilis may be separated into meningovascular (inflammatory) syndromes occurring within a few years of the primary infection and parenchymatous (degenerative) syndromes, which have a latency of decades. However, considerable overlap of these syndromes is regularly observed.

5.1.7.1. MENINGOVASCULAR NEUROSYPHILIS

Meningovascular neurosyphilis is due to a combination of chronic meningitis, multifocal arteritis, and gummatous, necrotic lesions.

- Chronic meningitis composed of lymphocytes and plasma cells often leads to fibrous organization and obstruction of the CSF flow with consequent hydrocephalus. Extension of

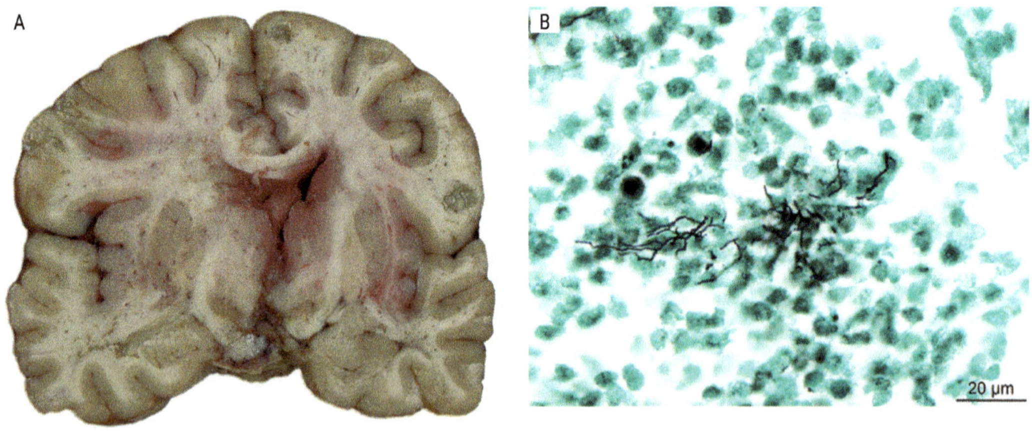

FIGURE 5.12 Cerebral nocardiosis: (**A**) macroscopic appearance of multiple abscesses at the gray–white matter junction; (**B**) filamentous bacteria (Gomori Grocott).

the inflammatory process into cranial and spinal nerves and periarteritis may cause optic atrophy or cranial nerve palsies.

- The vascular component of meningovascular syphilis, "Heubner arteritis," consists of an infiltration of the arterial wall by lymphocytes and plasma cells associated with intimal proliferation (*endarteritis obliterans*). This arteritis involves large and medium-sized blood vessels and may cause ischemic lesions in the brain or spinal cord.
- Cerebral gumma is now rarely seen in Europe and North America. Lesions may occur in the meninges and can involve the cerebral convexity, or they may be found in the midbrain, hypothalamus, and spinal cord. They are usually adherent to both the dura mater and the brain and consist of round, red-tan-gray lesions that are focally firm and rubbery, with a central area of necrosis (Fig. 5.13). Microscopically, they consist of central gummatous necrosis with ghost-like outlines of dead cells. This is surrounded by a granulomatous reaction, including epithelioid cells and fibroblasts with scattered multinucleated giant cells. Spirochetes, highlighted by Warthin–Starry or *Treponema pallidum* immunohistochemistry, are rarely demonstrable because the gumma represents a hyperimmune form of tissue necrosis.

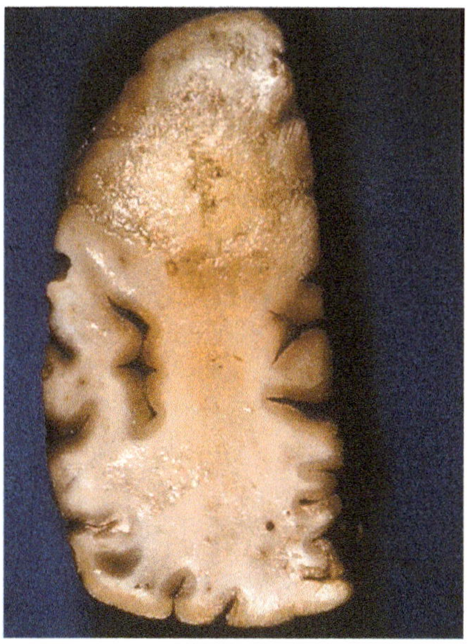

FIGURE 5.13 Cerebral gumma in a patient with AIDS. (Courtesy of the late Dr. Marius Valsamis.)

5.1.7.2. PARENCHYMATOUS NEUROSYPHILIS

Parenchymatous neurosyphilis takes two forms: paretic dementia (general paralysis of the insane [GPI]) and tabes dorsalis. Both forms may coexist as "tabo-paresis."

Reports of the older literature of patients dying after many years of *GPI dementia* described characteristic macroscopic changes in the brain; it was shrunken, firm, and covered by a thick and opaque pia–arachnoid. These lesions were most marked frontally, gradually decreasing in intensity posteriorly. The ventricles were enlarged, and the ependyma showed diffuse granular ependymitis. GPI is now rare. In the healed stages of the disease, the brain is usually grossly normal except perhaps for ependymal granulations.

On microscopic examination, there is meningeal thickening and striking involvement of the cerebral cortex, which is atrophic with loss of the normal laminar pattern. There is multifocal neuronal loss and reactive changes at various stages of development with proliferation of reactive astrocytes and rod-shaped microglia. This pattern of involvement gives a low power image of "bush-fire" or "windswept" cellular aggregates in the isocortex. Perivascular cuffing by lymphocytes and plasma cells is found in the cortex and leptomeninges. Specific silver impregnation stains may occasionally demonstrate spirochetes.

- *Tabes dorsalis* consists of degeneration of the posterior columns (Fig. 5.14) and dorsal roots and ganglia. It is apparently the result of

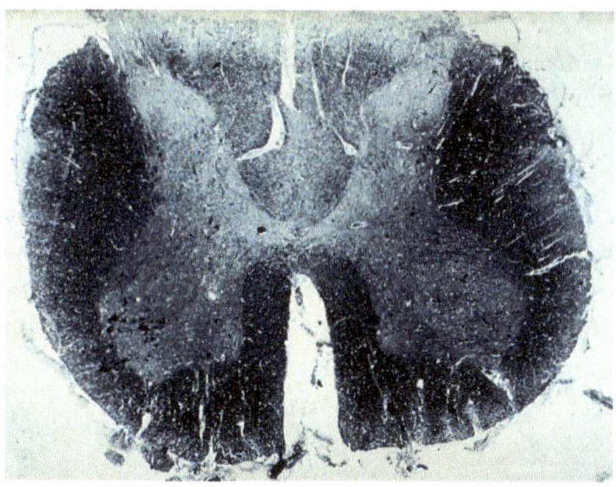

FIGURE 5.14 Tabes dorsalis: horizontal section of the lumbar cord showing degeneration of the posterior columns (Loyez stain).

inflammatory meningovascular lesions localized to the subarachnoid portion of the dorsal nerve roots. Spinal cord involvement is secondary to dorsal root/dorsal root ganglion lesions. It is characterized by Wallerian degeneration of the dorsal columns. Unlike in GPI, no inflammatory reaction is demonstrable in the cord parenchyma, and *T. pallidum* is absent in the dorsal columns.

5.1.7.3. SYPHILIS AND HIV INFECTION

Neurosyphilis is not uncommon in patients with AIDS. Co-infection with HIV may modify the clinical spectrum of syphilis. Patients with HIV infection are likely to progress rapidly to symptomatic neurosyphilis and to show an accelerated disease course. Treatment failure is also more frequent. The most common manifestations of symptomatic neurosyphilis in HIV-infected patients are syphilitic meningitis and meningovascular syphilis. General paresis, syphilitic meningomyelitis, syphilitic polyradiculopathy, and cerebral gummas have been recorded in case reports.

5.1.8. Borreliosis

Borreliosis is due to an infection by a spirochete of the *Borrelia* group, which is transmitted to a human by insect bites from ticks or lice. Examples include relapsing fever and Lyme disease. The latter is a multisystem disorder due to the spirochete *Borrelia burgdorferi*. Lyme disease affects the skin, cardiovascular system, joints, and central and peripheral nervous systems. Neurological signs usually develop several weeks after an *Ixodes scapularis* (blacklegged tick, deer tick) bite, which may cause *erythema chronicum migrans*, and culminate in lymphocytic meningitis, where the exudate is rich in plasma cells. Involvement of the spinal or cranial nerve roots is frequent. Encephalomyelitic complications are much rarer. Tertiary neurological complications occurring years after initial infection include the manifestations of axonal neuropathies and smoldering encephalopathy. The pathogenesis of CNS lesions is unclear; an immunopathological process rather than a direct effect of bacterial invasion has been speculated.

5.1.9. Brucellosis

Brucellosis, or Malta fever, is a zoonosis transmitted to humans by raw dairy products or by direct contact with animal products (e.g., the placenta). The disease is endemic in cattle-breeding countries. Leptomeningeal involvement is common in the septicemic phase of the disease. Either spontaneously or after inadequate treatment, the disease may give rise to subacute neurological manifestations, either infectious or hyperergic. The different clinical forms of neurobrucellosis correspond to the underlying neuropathologic substrate, including meningoencephalitis, meningomyelitis, and meningomyelitis–radiculitis, with frequent involvement of the cranial nerves, particularly the acoustic nerve.

5.1.10. Sarcoidosis

Sarcoidosis is a granulomatous multisystem disorder of unknown etiology. The lung is predominantly affected; skeletal muscle or peripheral nerve involvement is not uncommon; CNS involvement occurs in approximately 5% of cases.

The lesions may affect any part of the CNS but preferentially involve the base of the brain, especially the suprasellar and hypothalamic regions, the optic nerves and chiasm, the basal ganglia, and the posterior fossa. Hydrocephalus may result from thickening of the basal meninges or aqueductal obstruction by a periventricular parenchymal lesion.

The sarcoid granulomas consist of a central mass of epithelioid cells and multinucleated giant cells (MGCs) surrounded by lymphocytes, monocytes, and fibroblasts (Fig. 5.15A). The granulomatous changes involve predominantly the leptomeninges; they are often perivascular and may extend to the underlying parenchyma along the Virchow–Robin spaces. Cerebral vasculitis may give rise to vascular occlusion and brain infarction. Within the brain, granulomas may be confined to the perivascular spaces (Fig. 5.15B). Parenchymal lesions may also involve the periventricular areas, particularly around the third ventricle, and the choroid plexus; they are often surrounded by marked astrocytic proliferation. Coalescence of granulomas may form larger meningeal or parenchymatous masses, simulating neoplasms.

5.1.11. Chronic pachymeningitis

In rare instances, there can be a chronic inflammatory condition of the cerebral dura, which causes thickening of the dura, with a mixed inflammatory cell infiltrate consisting of plasma cells, lymphocytes, and occasional eosinophils. The inflammation often

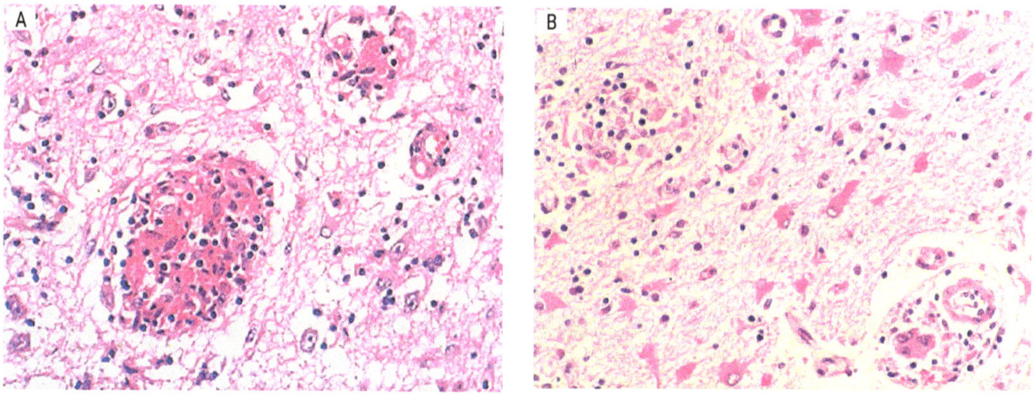

FIGURE 5.15 Sarcoidosis: (**A**) intraparenchymal epithelioid granulomas (H&E); (**B**) perivascular granuloma, including lymphocytes, monocytes, and multinucleated cells; note marked reactive astrocytosis (H&E).

has a storiform or whorled appearance, and germinal centers can also be seen. Cultures of this inflammatory lesion are negative, and microorganisms cannot be demonstrated within them with special staining techniques. These lesions of the dura resemble similar inflammation of the orbit and, in some instances, are referred to as inflammatory pseudotumors. Some patients with this disorder may have elevated serum levels of immunoglobulin (Ig) G4, and a diagnostic feature is the presence of 30 or more IgG4-positive plasma cells per high-power field on immunohistochemistry. This disorder is thought to be part of the spectrum of IgG4-related disease.

5.1.12. Toxin-induced neurological disease

In addition to direct invasion of the CNS, bacteria can cause neurological damage indirectly by producing neurotoxic substances. Several neurotoxins have been identified in specific bacterial infections (diphtheria, tetanus, and botulism). In other instances (shigellosis, *Bordetella pertussis* infection, melioidosis, and legionellosis), the possibility of toxin-induced CNS involvement has been postulated because of the clinical features and persistent negative CSF cultures. Although the encephalopathy may be lethal, there are few well-decanted neuropathological descriptions.

5.2. MYCOSES AND PARASITIC INFECTIONS

Fungi, protozoa, and metazoa may affect the CNS. These infections used to be uncommon in neuropathological practice in industrialized countries, restricted to certain geographical areas or affecting small groups. However, the epidemiology has changed due to multiple factors, including increased intercontinental travel, relaxation of health control measures, and the AIDS epidemic. Also, the incidence of some OIs (particularly mycoses and toxoplasmosis) has increased in the past few decades due to the increase in the number of immunocompromised patients.

5.2.1. Mycotic infections

Although fungal infections of the CNS are usually secondary to a primary focus elsewhere in the body (respiratory system, gastrointestinal tract) or to a direct extension from the sinuses or bone, in some instances these infections may arise and be confined only in the CNS. The morphologic form of the organisms on histologic tissue sections may be that of yeasts or hyphae, which can be best appreciated on Grocott–Gomori's methenamine silver (GMS) and periodic acid–Schiff with diastase (PAS-D). Identification of yeast forms is mostly based on size, budding mode (broad or narrow based), and the presence of a capsule or pseudo-hyphae. Identification of hyphae is based on pigmentation (hyaline vs. dematiaceous), size (thickness and homogeneity), and the presence of branching and septa. Different fungal species may display similar morphological features; precise identification of the organism is difficult on morphologic grounds alone. Additional diagnostic methods are required for species identification (immunohistochemistry, in situ hybridization, molecular techniques including internal transcribed spacer and 28S ribosomal RNA gene sequencing, and culture).

The characteristics of the organism may in some cases determine the type and extent of the lesions: meningitis in infections by the smallest fungi; extensive infarcts following occlusion of blood vessels by the largest fungi; and multiple small infarcts in case of infection by organisms of intermediate size, with infection of the ischemic lesions in turn causing abscesses and granulomas.

The classical distinction of fungi into pathogenic and opportunistic organisms is not absolute. The most important fungal infections that may affect the CNS are summarized in Table 5.1 and Figs. 5.16, 5.17.

5.2.2. Protozoal infections

The principal protozoa responsible for human infections are listed in Box 5.1.

5.2.2.1. AMOEBIASIS

In humans, cerebral lesions are caused by *Entamoeba histolytica* and free-living amoebae. Cysts and trophozoites are visible on H&E stains and may also be highlighted by GMS and PAS-D stains.

- Although rare, *E. histolytica* is responsible for hematogenous brain abscesses that are usually associated with hepatic or pulmonary involvement.
- Free-living organisms may produce primary meningoencephalitis (by *Naegleria fowleri*) and a granulomatous encephalitis (*Acanthamoeba* and *Leptomyxid*).
- Primary amoebic meningoencephalitis due to *N. fowleri* is usually contracted during the summer by healthy young people swimming in infected water. Parasites reach the CNS through the nasal mucosa and the olfactory epithelium. Affected individuals develop an encephalitis with hemorrhagic necrosis, identifiable parasites, and basal leptomeningitis. Virtually all cases are fatal.
- Patients with granulomatous amoebic encephalitis present with brain swelling with moderate meningitis and confluent areas of hemorrhagic necrosis. On microscopic examination, there is chronic vasculitis with the presence of parasites and a variable granulomatous reaction (Fig. 5.18).

5.2.2.2. CEREBRAL MALARIA

Responsible for 800,000 deaths a year in Africa alone, cerebral malaria is prevalent in at least 100 countries. There is marked clinical heterogeneity between cases, probably reflecting host susceptibility. *Plasmodium falciparum* is still the most important pathogen causing morbidity and mortality, but there are reports from Borneo that emerging *Plasmodium knowlesi* may be as lethal, albeit on a much smaller scale.

Macroscopically, the brain is swollen with dusky leptomeninges, and on section it appears pale or slate gray. Microscopically, the most common feature is sequestration of parasitized blood cells within cerebral microvessels, which also contain dark malarial pigment (Fig. 5.19A). Petechial hemorrhages of various types are also frequent. Focal necrosis within the white matter is followed by a macrophage/microglial reaction (Dürck's granuloma) (Fig. 5.19B).

5.2.2.3. TOXOPLASMOSIS

Feline species, particularly the domestic cat, are the definitive host of the protozoan *Toxoplasma gondii*. Toxoplasmosis in humans can manifest as congenital toxoplasmosis or as acquired/primary toxoplasmosis in adults.

Congenital toxoplasmosis is secondary to transplacental infection. In these cases, there are diffuse necrotic and inflammatory lesions of the cortex and white matter that are accompanied by calcifications, especially in periventricular regions.

In immunocompetent adults, CNS involvement is uncommon, usually minimal, and most often asymptomatic. In contrast, in immunocompromised patients (HIV, post-transplantation, and congenital immunodeficiencies), toxoplasmosis is often fatal. Cerebral toxoplasmosis is one of the most frequent CNS complications of AIDS and represents the main infectious cause of focal and space-occupying cerebral lesions in these patients. Typically, the disease develops as multiple abscesses involving predominantly the cerebral hemispheres, particularly the basal ganglia and the cortico–subcortical junction (Fig. 5.20A). The lesions contain central, eosinophilic, and acellular pseudo-ischemic necrosis surrounded by a cellular inflammatory reaction, usually with neutrophils. Parasites are seen either within pseudocysts (bradyzoites) (Fig. 5.20D) or as free forms (tachyzoites) (Fig. 5.20C). The combination of encysted bradyzoites and

Table 5.1 Principal Fungal Infections Affecting the Central Nervous System

MYCOSIS	ORGANISM	TYPE OF ACTION	GEOGRAPHIC DISTRIBUTION	NEUROPATHOLOGY
Aspergillosis	*Aspergillus*: *flavus*, *fumigatus*, *niger*	Predominantly opportunist	Ubiquitous	Usually secondary to foci in lungs, nasopharynx, and gastrointestinal tract. Abscesses and granulomas; vascular involvement, with extensive hemorrhage. Acute angle branching and narrow, septate hyphae.
Blastomycosis	*Blastomyces dermatitidis*	Predominantly pathogenic, mainly in agricultural workers	North America, Africa	Primary focus in lungs. Meningeal lesions, epidural lesions. Pachymeningitis, purulent or granulomatous meningitis (mimicking tuberculosis). Central, basophilic body with wall; single bud.
Candidiasis	*Candida albicans* other species	Opportunistic, mainly in premature infants, immunosuppressed and diabetic patients	Ubiquitous	Saprophyte in digestive and genital mucosae. Abscesses or granulomas; vascular involvement. Sometimes meningitis. Chains of elongated cylindrical pseudo-hyphae (and hyphae for *Candida albicans*). Gram-positive yeast.
Phaeohyphomycosis: heterogeneous group of organisms that appear pigmented microscopically or in cultures (dematiaceous)	*Alternaria*, *Cladophialophora*, *Curvularia*, *Exophialia*, *Fonsecaea*, *Madurella*, *Phialophora*, *Rhinocladiella*	In both immunocompetent and immunocompromised patients	Ubiquitous	Primary focus usually in the skin. Meningitis, abscesses, or diffuse encephalitis. Mainly hyphae, less often spores. Pigmented and stain positive with Fontana–Masson.
Coccidioidomycosis	*Coccidioides immitis*, *Coccidioides posadasii*	Predominantly pathogenic, can be opportunistic	South America, Mexico, southwestern United States	Primary foci in lungs. Basal meningitis with nodules; vasculitis. Spherules and endospores. Hyphae.

(*continued*)

Table 5.1 Continued

MYCOSIS	ORGANISM	TYPE OF ACTION	GEOGRAPHIC DISTRIBUTION	NEUROPATHOLOGY
Cryptococcosis (Fig. 5.17)	*Cryptococcus neoformans, Cryptococcus gattii*	Predominantly opportunistic	Ubiquitous, but predominates in southern United States and Australia	Usually secondary to a focus in the lungs. Meningitis with occasional tubercles. Amount of inflammation depends on degree of immunosuppression. Yeast (positive with Fontana–Masson) with capsule (positive with Mucicarmine).
Histoplasmosis	*Histoplasma capsulatum*	Pathogenic; but for CNS infections, it tends to be opportunistic	Ubiquitous, but common in the United States	Secondary to pulmonary infection. Meningitis with vasculitis. Granulomas are rare. Small ovoid budding bodies, intracellular.
Paracoccidioidomycosis	*Paracoccidioides brasiliensis*	Predominantly pathogenic	Brazil	Primary focus in the lungs. Space-occupying lesions; meningitis. Multiple budding.
Scedosporiosis	*Scedosporium/Pseudallescheria* species complex	Opportunistic (immunodeficiency, diabetes)	Ubiquitous	Associated with disorders of the respiratory system. Meningitis and abscesses; vasculitis. Sometimes granulomas. Septate hyphae and chlamydospores.
Mucormycosis	*Rhizopus, Mucor, Lichtheimia*	Opportunistic, mainly diabetic patients, but also drug users, patients on antibiotics and corticosteroids	Ubiquitous	Secondary to focus in skin, nasal mucosa, or lungs. Necrosis and polymorphs with giant cells. Vasculitis with hemorrhage. Broad branching, pauciseptate hyphae.

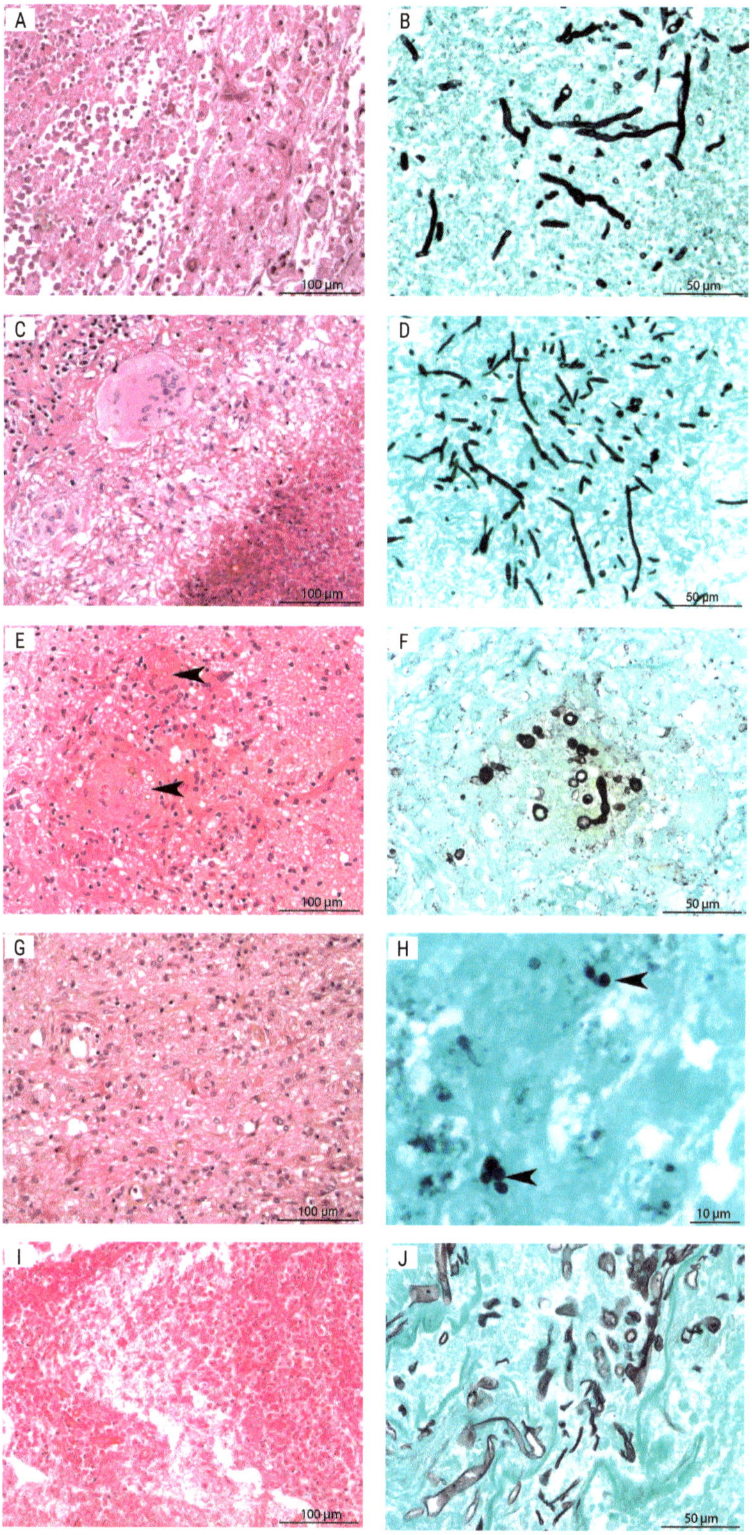

FIGURE 5.16 Histopathological profile of principal fungal infections affecting the central nervous system: (**A**, **B**) aspergillosis; (**C**, **D**) candidiasis; (**E**, **F**) phaehyphomycosis; (**G**, **H**) histoplasmosis; (**I**, **J**) mucormycosis (left panels **A**, **C**, **E**, **G**, **I**: H&E; right panels **B**, **D**, **F**, **H**, **J**: Gomori Grocott).

Box 5.1 Principal Protozoa Responsible for Human Infections

1. Amoebiasis
   a. *Entamoeba histolytica*: cerebral amoebic abscesses
   b. Primary amoebic encephalitis
      i. Primary amoebic meningoencephalitis (*Naegleria fowleri*)
      ii. Granulomatous amoebic encephalitis (*Acanthamoeba* spp. and *Leptomyxid*)
      iii. *Acanthamoeba* keratitis
2. Cerebral malaria (*Plasmodium falciparum* infection)
3. Toxoplasmosis (*Toxoplasma gondii* infection)
4. Trypanosomiasis
   a. African trypanosomiasis (*Trypanosoma brucei* spp.)
   b. South American trypanosomiasis (*Trypanosoma cruzi*)

free tachyzoites is characteristic of *T. gondii* infection. The identity of organisms can be confirmed by immunohistochemistry using an antibody to *T. gondii*. Associated hemorrhages are frequent. The abscesses can evolve during the illness and in the course of treatment, and they appear at postmortem as (a) necrotizing abscesses (Fig. 5.20A), (b) organizing abscesses (Fig. 5.20B), or (c) chronic "treated" lesions with a central cystic space. Rarely, in patients with AIDS, diffuse "septicemic" encephalitic forms may occur with dissemination of microglial nodules, in some cases containing encysted bradyzoites or tachyzoites.

An algorithm has been proposed for patients with AIDS and a space-occupying lesion that directs treatment for toxoplasmosis with antibiotics for a 10-day to 2-week period. If lesions persist, brain biopsy is advised because primary brain lymphoma can clinically/radiologically mimic cerebral toxoplasmosis. This algorithm is not applied to children with AIDS, particularly in developed countries, because these patients are less often exposed to

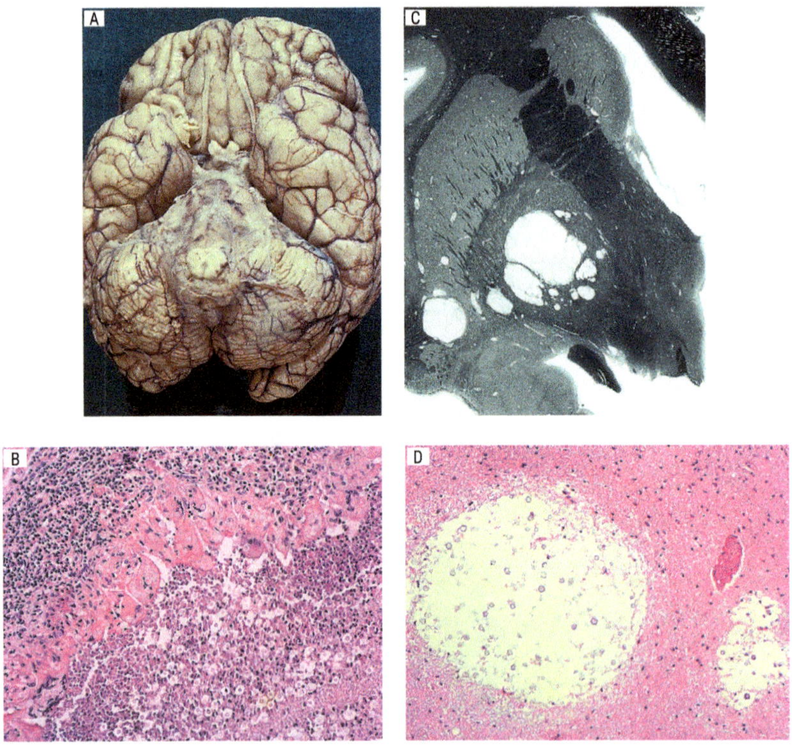

FIGURE 5.17 Cryptococcosis: (**A**) cryptococcal meningitis, macroscopic appearance: chronic meningitis involving the basal leptomeninges; (**B**) cryptococcal meningitis in an immunocompetent patient, marked lymphocytic and giant cell inflammation (H&E); (**C**) parenchymal cryptococcal cysts in a patient with AIDS (Loyez stain); (**D**) dilation of the perivascular space forming a cystic cavity filled with cryptococci; note the absence of inflammation or astrocytic reaction in the surrounding parenchyma (H&E).

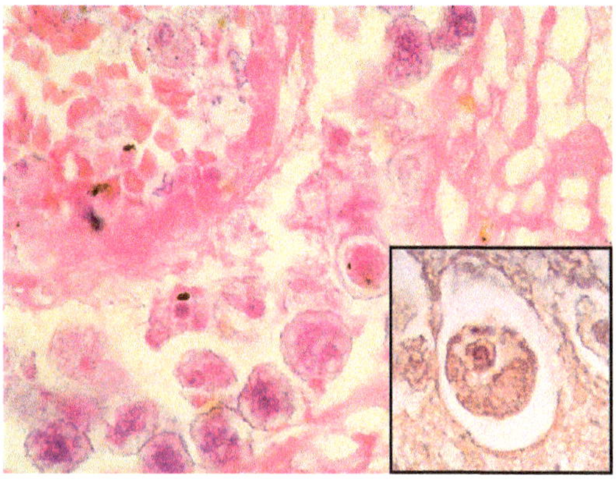

FIGURE 5.18 Amoebiasis, granulomatous encephalitis: chronic vasculitis with the presence of parasites (H&E).

T. gondii and are probably more likely to have primary brain lymphoma.

5.2.2.4. TRYPANOSOMIASIS

African trypanosomiasis is caused by *Trypanosoma brucei* subspecies transmitted to humans by the tsetse fly. The disease is characterized neuropathologically by meningoencephalitis. There is perivascular inflammation with microglial nodules. Mott cells, characteristic of this form, are plasma cells with prominent eosinophilic cytoplasmic Russell bodies. Parasites are not usually seen in brain tissue.

South American trypanosomiasis (Chagas disease) remains a health problem in many areas of Central and South America, where it affects up to 18 million individuals. The agent, *Trypanosoma cruzi*, is responsible for both an acute and a chronic form of the disease. The former can be asymptomatic or present as a mild meningoencephalitis with microglial nodules in the brain, sometimes containing parasites. The chronic form includes a "chagasic" encephalopathy with neuronal loss and focal inflammatory changes and, more commonly, a peripheral autonomic and occasionally somatosensory neuropathy with ganglion cell loss. In patients with AIDS, *T. cruzi* infection may cause multifocal necrotizing encephalitis, in which abundant amastigote parasites are present, particularly within glial cells and neurons (Fig. 5.21).

5.2.3. Metazoal infections

The major helminthic infections of the CNS are listed in Box 5.2.

5.2.3.1. CYSTICERCOSIS

Cysticercosis is the most common parasitic infection of the CNS and is endemic in all countries, particularly in Latin America. It is caused by the larval stage of the pig tapeworm *Taenia solium*. The disease occurs between 2 months and 30 years after initial infection. The number of cysts in the CNS varies from one to several hundred (Fig. 5.22A). The cysts have uniform structure; they contain a single scolex with four suckers and a double row of hooklets (Fig. 5.22B). The cyst wall consists of three layers: (a) outer or cuticular, (b) middle cellular with a pseudo-epithelial appearance, and (c) inner reticular or fibrillary (Fig. 5.22C). Dying organisms elicit an inflammatory reaction, including eosinophils. A granulomatous reaction with fibrosis and calcification occurs when the organism

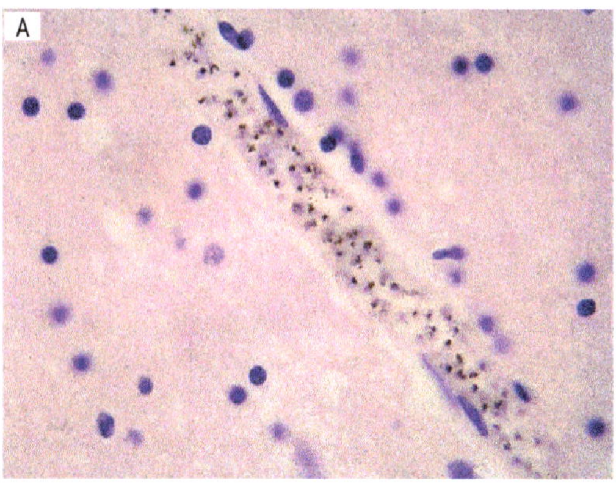

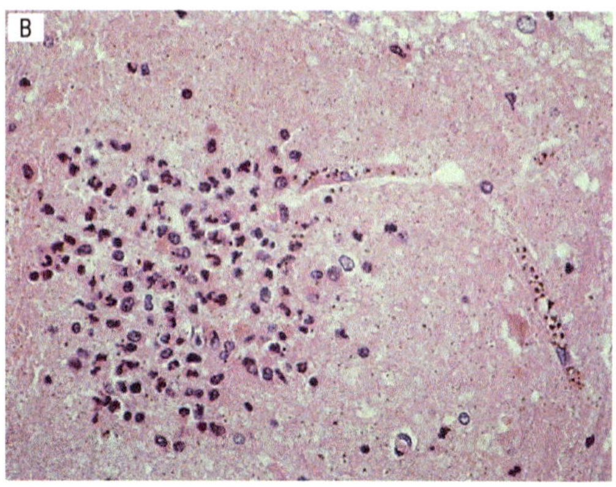

FIGURE 5.19 Cerebral malaria: (**A**) sequestration of parasitized blood cells within cerebral microvessels, which also contain dark malarial pigment (H&E); (**B**) Dürck's granuloma (H&E).

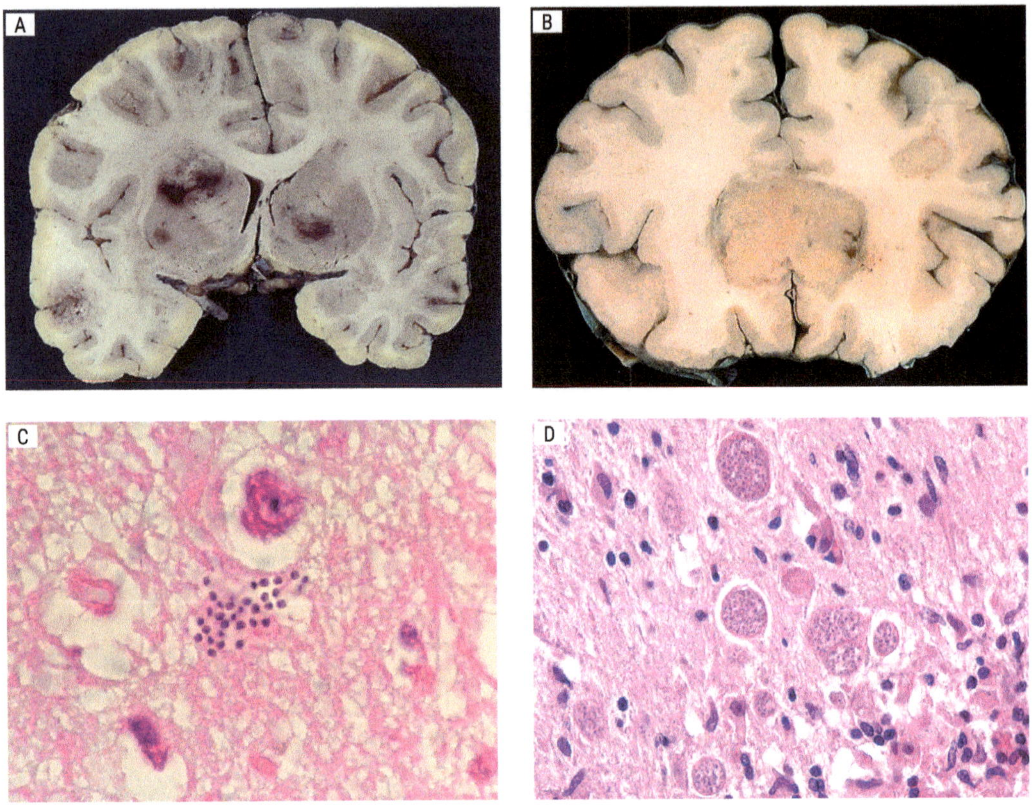

FIGURE 5.20 Toxoplasmosis: (**A**) multiple necrotizing abscesses, some of which are hemorrhagic involving the basal ganglia and the cortico–subcortical junction; (**B**) organizing abscesses with central necrosis and hyperemic border in the genu of corpus callosum and in the white matter of the right frontal lobe; (**C**) free tachyzoites at the periphery of a necrotic lesion (H&E); (**D**) numerous pseudocysts (bradyzoites) around a necrotic lesion (H&E).

dies. Racemose cysticercosis is an aberrant form that lacks a scolex and can develop into a large multiloculated mass.

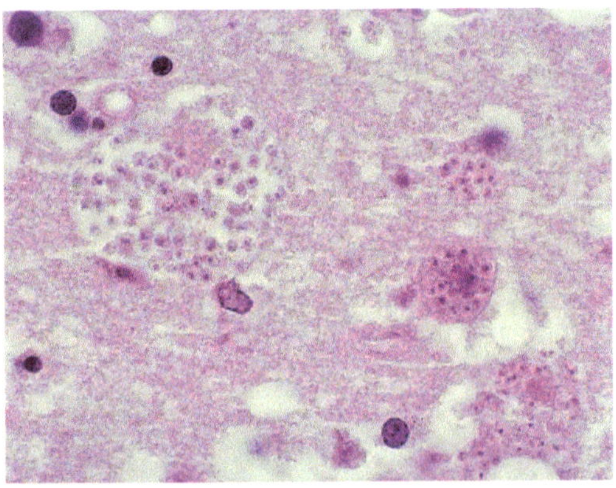

FIGURE 5.21 Trypanosomiasis: Abundant amastigote parasites are present within glial cells in a case of multifocal necrotizing encephalitis (H&E).

5.2.3.2. HYDATIDOSIS

Hydatid cyst is endemic in the Mediterranean regions and the Middle East, as well as in Latin America. Dogs and other canids are the definitive hosts. Cysts in the brain are usually solitary and unilocular, and their wall consists of two layers: (a) the outer, laminated, cuticular layer; and (b) the inner germinal layer (Fig. 5.23), within which are multiple proto-scolices.

5.2.3.3. SCHISTOSOMIASIS

Schistosomiasis is caused by flukes of the genus *Schistosoma*, which have humans and other mammals as definitive hosts. The infection is endemic in South America, the Middle East, Asia, and Africa. CNS lesions involve predominantly the spinal cord. Macroscopic changes are uncommon. Histological examination reveals three principal tissue reactions:

Box 5.2 Major Helminthic Infections of the CNS

1. Cestodes
   a. Neurocysticercosis (*Taenia solium*)
   b. Hydatid cyst (*Echinococcus granulosus*)
   c. Coenuriasis (*Taenia multiceps*)
   d. Sparganosis (*Spirometra*)
2. Trematodes
   a. Paragonimiasis (*Paragonimus westermani*)
   b. Schistosomiasis (*Schistosoma mansoni, japonicum, haematobium, mekongi*)
   c. Other trematode infections
3. Nematodes
   a. Eosinophilic meningoencephalitis
      i. *Angiostrongylus cantonensis*
      ii. *Gnathostoma spinigerum*
   b. Toxocariasis (visceral larva migrans)
      Other forms of larva migrans
      Trichinella spiralis
   c. Human filariases
      i. Loa-loa
      ii. *Dracunculus medinensis*
      iii. *Onchocerca volvulus*
   d. Nematodes and immunosuppression
      i. *Strongyloides stercoralis*

(a) necrotic–exudative with variable number of eggs and with the area surrounded by eosinophils, lymphocytes, plasma cells, and macrophages; (b) a productive stage in which eggs have lost the embryo; and (c) a late stage with a granulomatous reaction and giant cells (Fig. 5.24).

5.2.3.4. EOSINOPHILIC MENINGITIS

Eosinophilic meningitis is due to infection by *Angiostrongylus cantonensis* or *Gnathostoma spinigerum*. Larvae may be demonstrated in the brain or meninges and show a predominantly eosinophilic infiltrate.

5.2.3.5. TOXOCARIASIS

Toxocara canis is a common agent and important canine zoonosis that occurs worldwide. It may occasionally affect humans, particularly children. Death of the parasite in the brain is followed by a nonencapsulated granulomatous reaction consisting of lymphocytes, eosinophils, plasma cells, fibroblasts, and epithelioid and giant cells.

5.2.3.6. TRICHINOSIS

The trichinosis infection exists in North and South America, but outbreaks have been reported also in Europe, including Mediterranean countries. Involvement of striated muscle is the main complication (see Fig. 12.26). Involvement of the CNS is uncommon. Macroscopic features may be manifest as a nonpurulent meningitis, mild edema, and occasional small hemorrhages. Histological findings include granulomatous nodules, predominating in the white matter and consisting of lymphocytes; microglia; and histiocytes. Larvae are only rarely identified in nodules, suggesting an immune-mediated pathogenesis of the lesions.

5.2.3.7. SARCOCYSTOSIS

Sarcocystosis is a zoonotic infection due to *Sarcocystis nesbitti*, a protozoon whose natural life cycle is still uncertain but likely involves snakes (definitive host) and monkey and other mammals (intermediate hosts). Human infection is accidental and probably linked to ingestion of water contaminated by sporocysts excreted in snake feces. Symptomatic cases have been reported from Malaysia and other areas of Southeast Asia. Clinical manifestation of sarcocystosis includes headache, relapsing fever, myalgia, and muscle swelling. Muscle biopsies have shown small cysts within muscle fibers, with very mild or occasionally moderate surrounding inflammation. Each cyst comprises a thin cyst wall with numerous bradyzoites within.

5.2.3.8. STRONGYLOIDES STERCORALIS INFECTION

Strongyloides stercoralis infection is known to occur in the presence of severe immunosuppression, during which larval infection can affect every organ. In these circumstances, larvae can be seen in the subarachnoid spaces, and microinfarcts may be produced by obstruction of capillaries by the parasite.

5.3. VIRAL INFECTIONS

The lesions of the CNS induced by viral infections may result from various mechanisms. Some

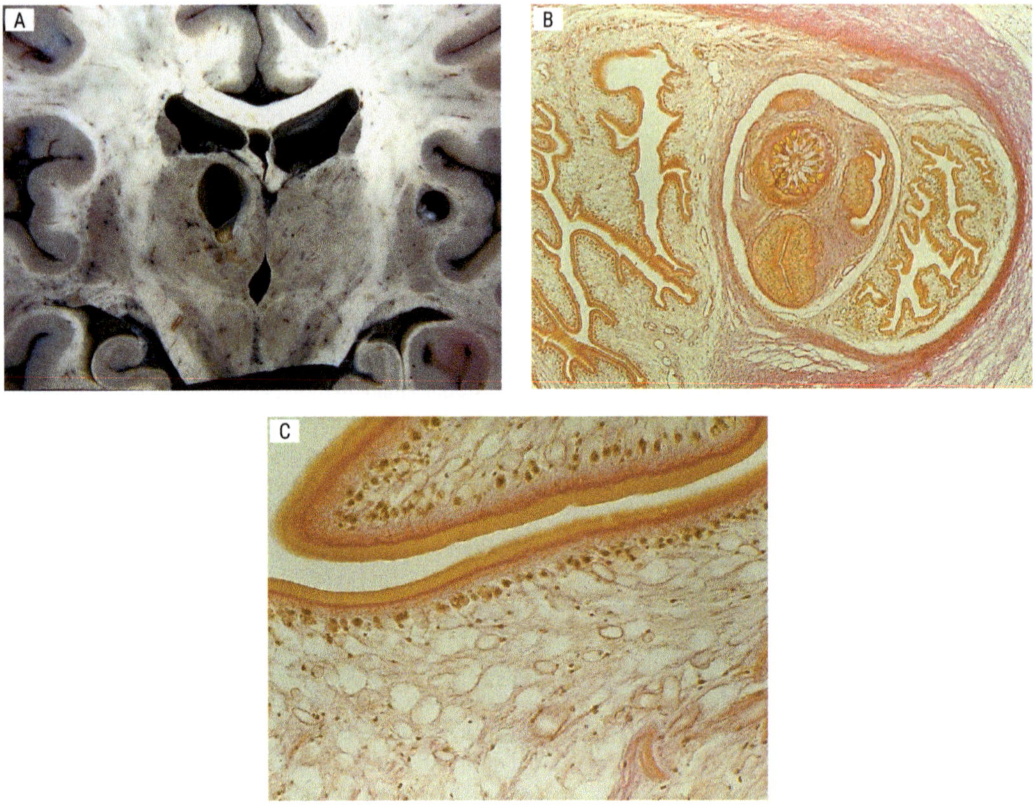

FIGURE 5.22 Cysticercosis: (**A**) macroscopic appearance: two cystic cavities containing a parasite are present in the thalamus and insular cortex; (**B**) microscopic appearance of the scolex with suckers and a double row of hooklets; (**C**) higher magnification showing the three layers of the cyst walls (H&E).

are nonspecific and are due to immunoallergic reactions that are secondary to the viral infection; they involve the leptomeninges and especially the white matter (leukoencephalitides). Other, more specific, lesions are directly caused by the infection of the CNS by the virus. They involve mainly, but not exclusively, the gray matter (polioencephalitides).

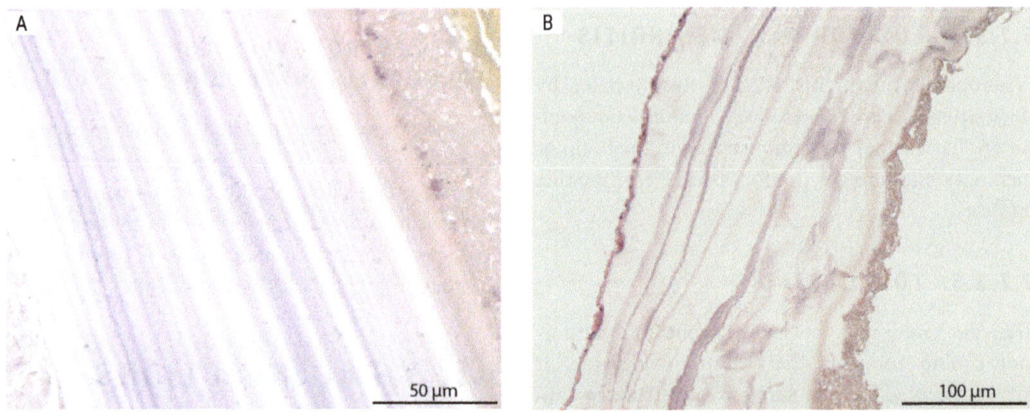

FIGURE 5.23 Wall of hydatid cyst: (**A**) outer laminated cuticular layer and (**B**) inner germinal layer (H&E).

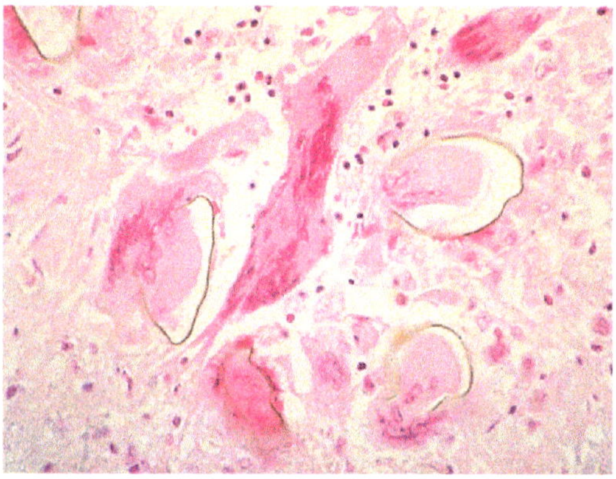

FIGURE 5.24 Schistosomiasis: eggs within a granulomatous reaction with multinucleated giant cells (H&E).

Most viral encephalitides run an acute course. However, special immunological phenomena may modify the course of the disease and result in the development of a latent infection, notably as in herpes, or a persistent infection, as in subacute sclerosing panencephalitis (SSPE), which is presumably caused by a defective measles virus. In AIDS, infection by the retrovirus HIV causes both immunodeficiency and subacute encephalitis. CNS viral infections are increasingly diagnosed by molecular testing of CSF and occasionally brain tissue (targeted panels or unbiased metagenomic sequencing).

5.3.1. Nonspecific CNS involvement in viral infections

5.3.1.1. ACUTE VIRAL LYMPHOCYTIC MENINGITIS OR ASEPTIC MENINGITIS

The term *aseptic* applies when culture of the CSF fails to grow bacteria or fungi; in these cases, viruses may be either isolated or detected by polymerase chain reaction (PCR). Acute viral lymphocytic meningitis or *aseptic* meningitis occurs in several types of viral infections, mainly enteroviruses (echovirus, coxsackieviruses, and enterovirus 71), but also mumps virus, herpes simplex virus 2 (HSV-2), arboviruses, lymphocytic choriomeningitis virus, measles, parainfluenza, and adenoviruses.

Microscopically, aseptic meningitis is characterized by vascular congestion and scanty infiltrate of lymphocytes in the leptomeninges, in the perivascular spaces surrounding some of the superficial cortical blood vessels, and in the choroid plexus.

5.3.1.2. ACUTE DISSEMINATED ENCEPHALOMYELITIS, ACUTE DISSEMINATED LEUKOENCEPHALITIS, OR ACUTE POSTINFECTIOUS/POSTVACCINIAL PERIVENOUS ENCEPHALITIS

Postinfectious encephalitis (see Chapter 7) (acute disseminated encephalomyelitis [ADEM], acute disseminated leukoencephalitis, or acute postinfectious/postvaccinial perivenous encephalitis) may complicate a variety of systemic viral diseases, including measles, mumps, chickenpox, rubella, influenza, severe acute respiratory syndrome coronavirus 2 (SARS-CoV-2), and infectious mononucleosis caused by Epstein–Barr virus (EBV). Reports in the literature have documented the disease following smallpox or rabies vaccination. The microscopic findings closely resemble those of experimental allergic encephalomyelitis produced by injecting experimental animals with myelin proteins and adjuvant. The pathogenesis of the lesions is believed to be due to a T-cell–mediated hypersensitivity reaction. Clinically, ADEM manifests a few days to 3 weeks after the causative viral infection or vaccination.

Microscopic examination shows infiltrates of lymphocytes, plasma cells, and macrophages around the venules of the neural parenchyma. These involve mainly the white matter, where they are associated with perivenous foci of demyelination (Fig. 5.25A, B) with relative sparing of the axons (see Chapter 7). There may also be small perivascular hemorrhages. Arteries are relatively free of inflammation, but there are often inflammatory cells in the leptomeninges.

5.3.1.3. ACUTE HEMORRHAGIC LEUKOENCEPHALOPATHY OF HURST

Acute hemorrhagic leukoencephalopathy of Hurst (AHLE; Weston–Hurst syndrome) is a fulminant, usually fatal, disorder, regarded by some as a hyperacute form of ADEM. It is characterized by the presence of numerous scattered hemorrhagic foci, which are more prominent in the cerebral (Fig. 5.26) and cerebellar white matter and in the pons. Microscopically, many small blood vessels undergo fibrinoid necrosis and are surrounded by a variable zone of necrotic tissue and a larger zone of hemorrhage (ring- or ball-shaped perivascular hemorrhages). Still recognizable vessels are veins or venules, and they may be surrounded by fibrin and

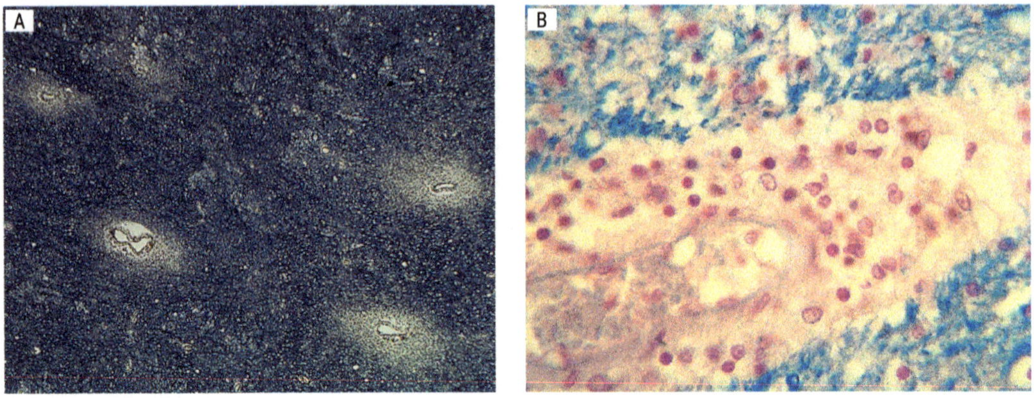

FIGURE 5.25 ADEM: (**A**) perivenous foci of demyelination in the white matter (Loyez stain); (**B**) higher magnification showing perivenous inflammatory infiltrates (Klüver–Barrera stain).

an inflammatory infiltrate, including neutrophils and mononuclear cells. There is demyelination, but many areas also show axonal fragmentation.

5.3.2. Viral encephalitis and encephalomyelitis

Viral encephalitis—in the strict meaning of the term—is due to infection of the brain by a virus. However, quite often, viral infection also involves the meninges (meningoencephalitis) or the spinal cord (encephalomyelitis, meningoencephalomyelitis) as well as the nerve roots (meningoencephalomyelor adiculitis).

Nervous system involvement is ordinarily secondary to infection elsewhere in the body. In fact, most viral infections of the CNS are rare complications of common systemic viral diseases. The portal of entry that has been directly exposed to infection may be the skin (through direct contact or by an animal or insect bite), the airways (after inhalation), or the alimentary tract (after ingestion). The virus may spread to the CNS directly along the olfactory or peripheral nerves or by the hematogenous route in the course of viremia. This is followed by obligatory intracellular viral replication in one or more of the cell types in the CNS—neurons, glial cells, or macrophages/microglial cells, depending on cell tropism. Some viruses have a rather restricted or narrow cell tropism in the CNS; for example, JC virus infects oligodendroglial cells in progressive multifocal leukoencephalitis (PML), and poliomyelitis viruses infect lower motor neurons. Other viruses have wide cell tropism, infecting most of the cells in the CNS, including endothelial cells, which is the case for many of the herpes viruses. Cell tropism is largely determined by cell receptors that allow entry of virus into the cell.

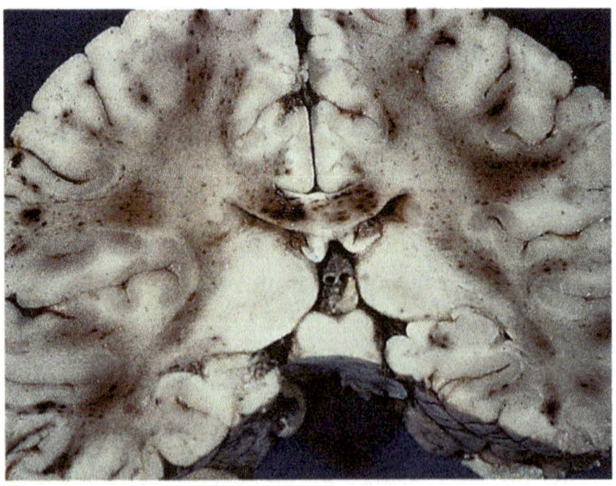

FIGURE 5.26 Acute hemorrhagic leukoencephalopathy, macroscopic appearance.

Whatever the causative virus, the basic neuropathological picture of viral encephalitis includes the following:

- Involvement of the neuronal cell body, resulting in death of the cell and engulfment by macrophages (neuronophagia) (Fig. 5.27A).
- Perivascular cuffing of inflammatory cells, mainly lymphocytes, macrophages, and sometimes plasma cells (Fig. 5.27B).
- Microglial proliferation with the formation of microglial nodules and the appearance of rod cells (Fig. 5.27C).
- In some cases, intranuclear or intracytoplasmic inclusion bodies are indicative of the presence of virus in neurons and glia.

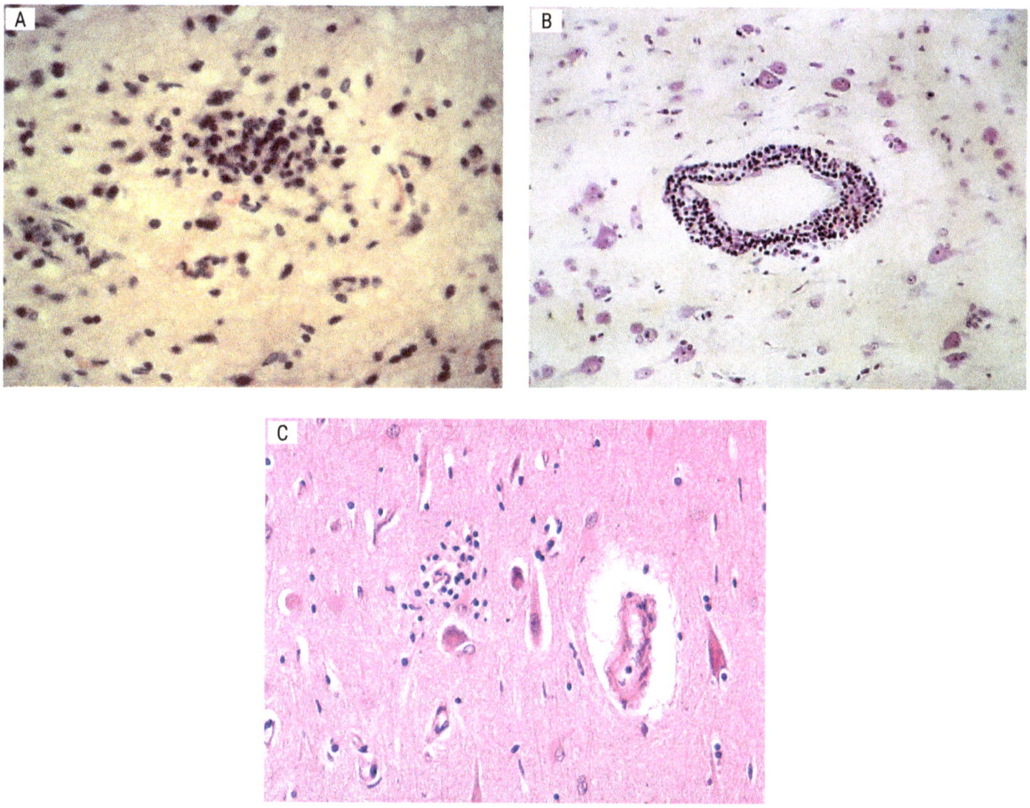

FIGURE 5.27 Microscopic features of encephalitis: (**A**) neuronophagia (Nissl stain); (**B**) lymphocytic perivascular cuffing (Nissl stain); (**C**) proliferation of rod-shaped microglia (H&E).

According to the type of the offending virus, one may separate encephalitis due to RNA viruses (enterovirus, arbovirus [orthobunyavirus, alphavirus, and flavivirus], rabies, paramyxovirus, rubivirus, and retrovirus), encephalitis due to DNA viruses (herpes viruses, adenoviruses, and polyomaviruses), and encephalitis suspected of being due to as yet unidentified viruses (encephalitis lethargica, Behçet's uveomeningoencephalitis, and chronic localized encephalitis of Rasmussen).

5.3.2.1. ENCEPHALITIDES DUE TO RNA VIRUSES

5.3.2.1.1. Poliomyelitis. Poliomyelitis is due to infection of the CNS by a poliovirus, a small RNA virus of the genus *Enterovirus*. The most frequent form of the disease, "acute anterior poliomyelitis," is characterized by lytic infection of the motor neurons. The lesions selectively involve the motor neurons of the anterior horns and the cranial nerve nuclei but may extend to the frontal gyri, the hypothalamus, the reticular formation, and the posterior horns of the spinal cord. As a result of viral infection and lysis of the neurons, the tissue reaction that ensues is neuronophagia and microglial nodules with microglial/macrophage cell proliferation. Inflammation in the leptomeninges and affected gray matter is intense (Fig. 5.28A, B). There is edema and vascular congestion, which may be associated with perivascular hemorrhages and, occasionally, focal necrosis.

Following resolution of the acute phase, the residual lesions consist of atrophy of the anterior horns with neuronal loss and astrocytic gliosis. There is atrophy and fibrosis of the anterior nerve roots, which appear thin and grayish on macroscopic examination. The skeletal muscles innervated by the affected motor nerve cells show denervation atrophy. Following a prolonged latent period after recovery from poliomyelitis, often decades later, weakness, fatigue, and muscle atrophy may develop, a condition known as post-polio syndrome. The syndrome is treated symptomatically and is not life-threatening.

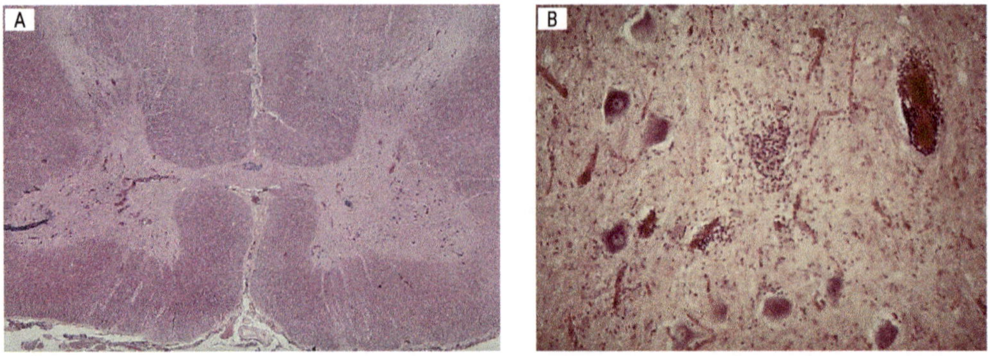

FIGURE 5.28 Poliomyelitis: (**A**) transverse section of the cervical spinal cord showing inflammation in the anterior horns; (**B**) higher magnification showing neuronophagia, microglial proliferation, and perivascular cuffing of lymphocytes (H&E).

The introduction of vaccines for poliomyelitis viruses has resulted in a sharp decline in the incidence of poliomyelitis. However, outbreaks of paralytic infection by wild-type poliovirus still occur in developing countries. In vaccinated populations, poliomyelitis is usually caused either by the rare reversion to neurovirulence of attenuated vaccine-related strains of poliovirus or by other groups of enteroviruses, especially group A coxsackieviruses and enterovirus 71. The latter, a cause of hand, foot, and mouth disease, has also been responsible for fulminant fatal brainstem encephalitis in children. There is increasing evidence that neurotropic enteroviruses, including poliovirus, could invade the CNS by retrograde axonal transmission in motor nerves.

5.3.2.1.2. Arbovirus (arthropod-borne virus) encephalitides. The arbovirus (arthropod-borne virus) encephalitides, predominantly belonging to the *Alphavirus*, *Flavivirus*, and *Orthobunyavirus* genera, are transmitted by insects and have a distinct geographical distribution, often indicated by the name of the virus.

The best-known forms of the mosquito-borne encephalitides include St. Louis encephalitis, and the Eastern, Western, and Venezuelan equine encephalitides in America; Japanese encephalitis in South and East Asia; Murray Valley encephalitis in Australia; and West Nile fever, primarily in Africa but also in Europe, Asia, and America. In all of these forms, the typical lesions of encephalitis are widely distributed throughout the neuraxis.

In Japanese encephalitis, which is the most important of the arboviral encephalitides in terms of global incidence, morbidity, and mortality, the inflammation tends to be particularly severe in the thalamus, substantia nigra, pons, medulla, and spinal cord and is occasionally necrotizing (Fig. 5.29A, B).

Chikungunya and Zika arbovirus infections have rapidly expanded throughout the world in recent years, with large-scale outbreaks and with CNS involvement. Chikungunya virus is a re-emerging alphavirus. Severe forms of the disease include rare fatal cases with CNS affecting both adults and neonates. Zika virus, a member of the genus *Flavivirus*, Flaviviridae family, is transmitted by a mosquito bite; also, more recently, vertical and sexual transmission have been described. After the outbreak of Zika viral infections in the Americas and Caribbean nations in 2015–2016, the World Health Organization announced that Zika virus infection during pregnancy can be a cause of congenital brain abnormalities (congenital Zika syndrome) and also that Zika virus is a trigger of Guillain–Barré syndrome. The most relevant neuropathological findings in fetuses and neonates infected with Zika virus early in gestation (due to viral tropism for proliferating cells in the germinal matrix) are microcephaly with ex vacuo ventriculomegaly or large head circumference associated with obstructive hydrocephalus due to severe midbrain and aqueduct distortion. Brain damage includes various degrees of parenchymal hypoplasia involving neurons and glial cells, calcifications, various disturbances of neuronal migration, reactive gliosis, microglial hyperplasia, and occasional perivascular cuffs of lymphocytes. Hypoplastic lesions secondary to injury of descending pathways include small basis pontis, pyramids, and spinal corticospinal tracts. Cerebellar hypoplasia is also common. Severe motor neuron loss in the anterior horn of the spinal

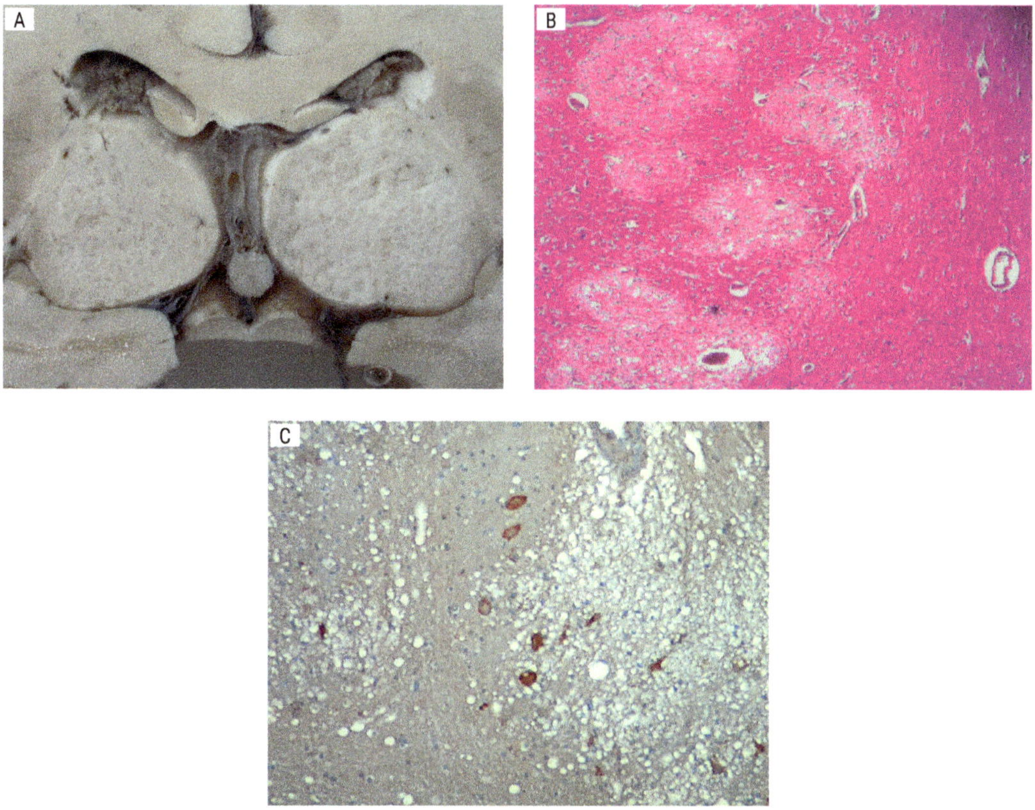

FIGURE 5.29 Japanese encephalitis: (**A**) macroscopic appearance of necrotic lesions in the thalamus (courtesy of Pr. S. K. Shankar and Dr. A. Mahadevan); (**B**) necrolytic lesions in the neuronal areas (H&E); (**C**) viral antigens in neurons around edematous/necrolytic areas (viral immunohistochemistry [IHC]).

cord is responsible for fetal akinesia and consequent arthrogryposis. There seem to be only very rare well-documented cases of dengue affecting the CNS.

Tick-borne encephalitides, which include Russian spring–summer encephalitis, Central European encephalitis, and Powassan encephalitis, are characterized by meningoencephalitic lesions and by involvement of the lower cranial nerves and spinal cord anterior horn cells, especially at cervical levels. In these encephalitides, inclusions are not detectable by light microscopy, but organisms have been observed ultrastructurally. In many cases, the virus can be demonstrated immunohistochemically (Fig 5.29C).

5.3.2.1.3. Rabies. Rabies is caused by a rhabdovirus that is transmitted to humans by the bite of a rabid animal. The animal reservoir includes foxes, skunks, coyotes, jackals, and bats. However, dogs remain the main source of human infection. The disease may present as "furious" rabies or "dumb" (paralytic) rabies. Post-exposure immunoglobulin therapy is effective in prevention after a bite, but once symptomatic, the disease is almost always fatal.

On neuropathological examination, rabies is characterized by the presence of diagnostic cytoplasmic inclusions in neurons called Negri bodies (Fig. 5.30A, B). These are mainly found in the pyramidal neurons of the hippocampus and in Purkinje cells. Accompanying lesions include leptomeningeal and perivascular inflammation, microglial nodules (Babès nodules), and microglial proliferation. The severity and distribution of these lesions are variable, but there may be disparity between the abundance of virus and the paucity of inflammation.

5.3.2.1.4. Measles encephalitides. Measles virus, a member of the family paramyxoviridae like parainfluenza and mumps, is known to cause two rare forms of encephalitis: SSPE and immunosuppressive measles encephalitis. In addition,

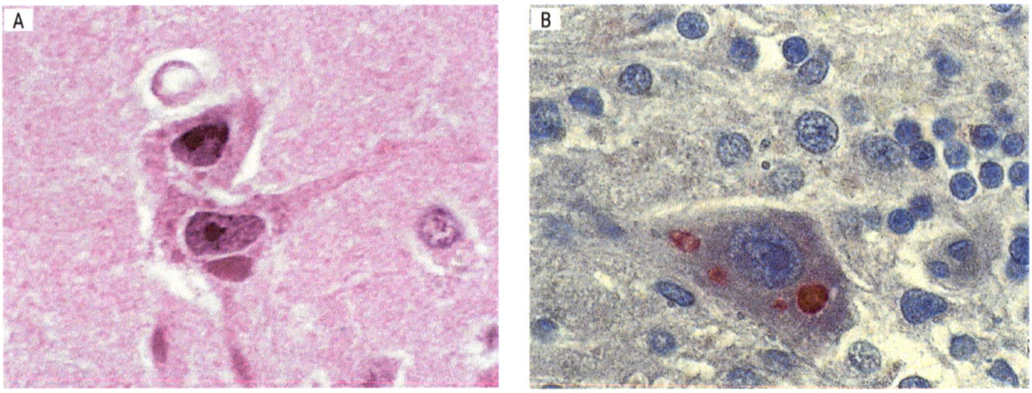

FIGURE 5.30 Rabies: (**A**) Negri bodies in a pyramidal neuron of the hippocampus (H&E); (**B**) rabies viral antigen detection in Negri bodies in a Purkinje (rabies IHC; red chromogen).

it may induce postinfectious encephalitis (see Section 5.3.1.2).

Subacute sclerosing panencephalitis occurs in children several years after an episode of measles. About half of the patients are known to have had measles before age 2 years. The lesions involve both the gray and the white matter. In the gray matter, the cortex is predominantly affected, but involvement of the basal ganglia, mainly the thalamus, is frequent, and occasionally there may be extension to the brainstem. Microscopic examination shows the features of subacute encephalitis. There is neuronal loss, occasional neuronophagia, and astrocytic and microglial reaction. Inclusion bodies may be found in neuronal and glial nuclei (Fig. 5.31A). In the white matter, there is thinning and demyelination with severe gliosis (Fig. 5.31B). Inflammatory cells may be very scanty, as may inclusion bodies, which may be better detected immunohistochemically. There are leptomeningeal, perivascular, and parenchymal (gray and the white matter) inflammatory infiltrates. In late cases, there may be extensive neuronal loss with atrophy of the cortex and basal ganglia; neurofibrillary degeneration of the Alzheimer type has been reported.

Although measles virus has been demonstrated to be the causative agent by electron microscopy (Fig. 5.32), in tissue culture and by immunological and virological assays, the pathogenesis of this type of prolonged viral infection remains uncertain. A viral mutation resulting in defective M protein expression enabling the virus to elude the host immune response has been postulated.

Measles inclusion body encephalitis (immunosuppressive measles encephalitis) develops within months of the initial systemic infection in patients with impaired cell-mediated immunity. In patients

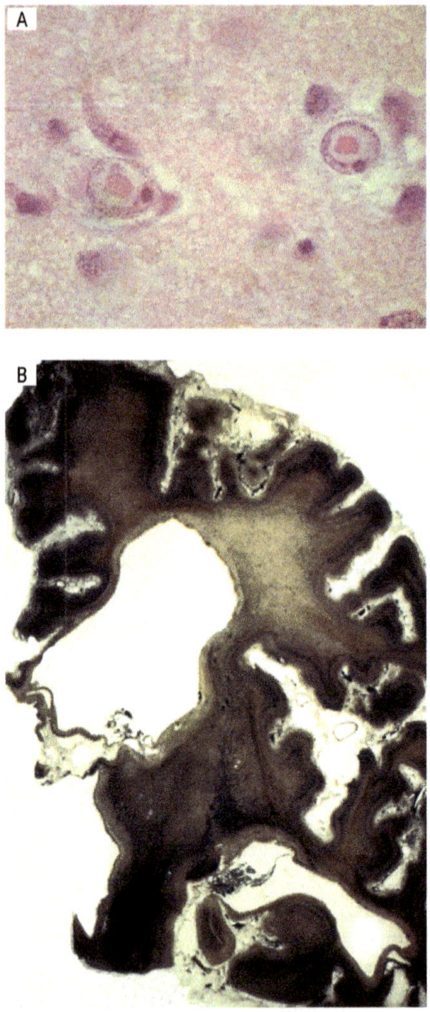

FIGURE 5.31 Subacute sclerosing panencephalitis: (**A**) intranuclear inclusion bodies in neurons (H&E); (**B**) massive demyelination of the white matter and severe cortical atrophy (Loyez stain).

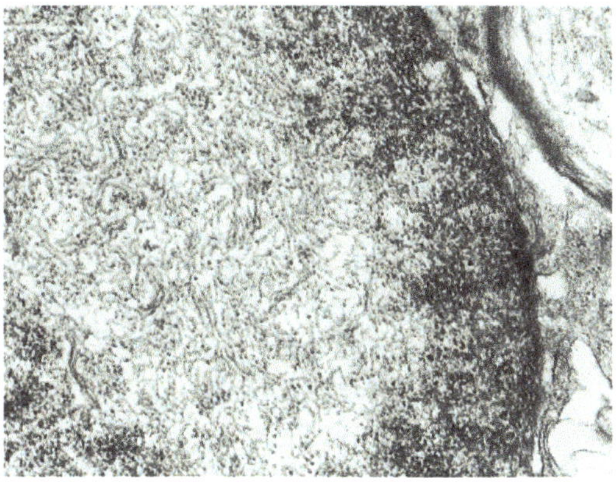

FIGURE 5.32 Electron micrograph showing intranuclear tubular formations characteristic of measles myxovirus in a case of subacute sclerosing panencephalitis.

with AIDS, similar changes have also been reported to occur after measles vaccination.

The brain may be normal or may show extensive zones of necrosis of gray and white matter. Clinically, there may be *epilepsia partialis continua*, but the diagnosis can be made only on microscopic examination. The lesions may be focal or widespread throughout the brain; involvement of the spinal cord has been found in children with AIDS. The diagnostic feature is the presence of eosinophilic inclusion bodies that are readily seen on routine stain (Fig. 5.33) but can also be demonstrated by immunohistochemistry and electron microscopy. These are mostly intranuclear and involve predominantly neurons and, to a lesser extent, astrocytes and oligodendrocytes. Occasionally, MGCs containing virus may be found. There may be accompanying inflammatory infiltrates and reactive astrocytes and microglia, but these may be very scanty, even absent, and the presence of inclusions may thus be missed.

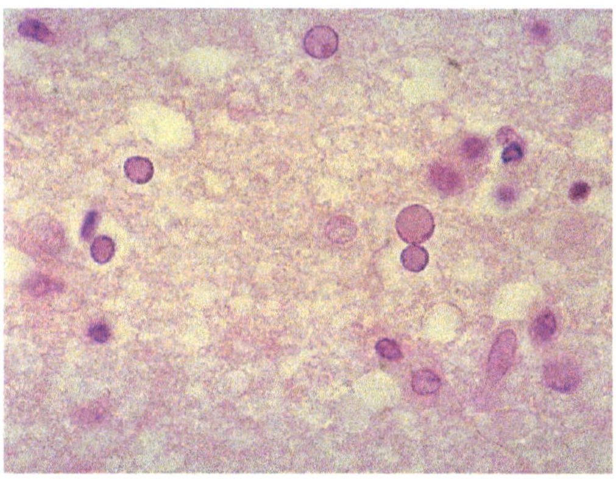

FIGURE 5.33 Measles inclusion body encephalitis: presence of numerous eosinophilic intranuclear inclusion bodies (H&E).

5.3.2.1.5. Henipavirus encephalitis. Henipavirus is a new genus of RNA viruses belonging to the Paramyxoviridae family that was first recognized to cause severe human encephalitis in the 1990s. The genus includes the two closely related, fruit bat–originated viruses, Hendra virus and Nipah virus. Important intermediate hosts for transmission to humans are horses, pigs, and possibly other domestic animals. Both viruses appear to cause similar acute and relapsing henipavirus encephalitides.

Acute henipavirus encephalitis is characterized by disseminated small vessel vasculopathy and parenchymal pathology, mainly in the CNS, but these features are also found in many extra-CNS organs, including lung and kidney. Vasculopathy consists of true vasculitis with intramural necrosis, inflammation, and endothelial ulceration (Fig 5.34A). Vascular occlusion by vasculitis-induced thrombosis or thromboembolism is readily observed, and there may be perivascular hemorrhages. Occasionally, MGCs or syncytia arising from the endothelial surface can be found (Fig. 5.34B). Viral inclusions, antigens, RNA, and nucleocapsids can be detected in vascular endothelium, MGCs, and smooth muscle.

Parenchymal pathology of acute encephalitis comprises discrete necrotic or more subtle vacuolar, plaque-like lesions often found adjacent to blood vessels involved by vasculopathy (Fig. 5.34C). These lesions are characterized by necrosis, edema, inflammation, neuronal loss, and often viral inclusions; antigens (Fig. 5.34D) and RNA can be demonstrated in surviving or adjacent neurons and more rarely in glial cells. Hence, necrotic plaques are probably caused by a dual pathogenic mechanism of microinfarction and neuronal infection. In some cases, focal neuronophagia, microglial nodule formation, clusters of foamy macrophages, perivascular cuffing, and meningitis can be found.

In contrast to acute henipavirus encephalitis, where there is systemic involvement, the pathology of relapsing henipavirus encephalitis is confined to the CNS, and vasculopathy is absent throughout. In affected neuronal areas and adjacent white matter, extensive confluent parenchymal necrosis, edema, and inflammation are observed. Reactive gliosis and prominent vascular proliferation in areas of severe

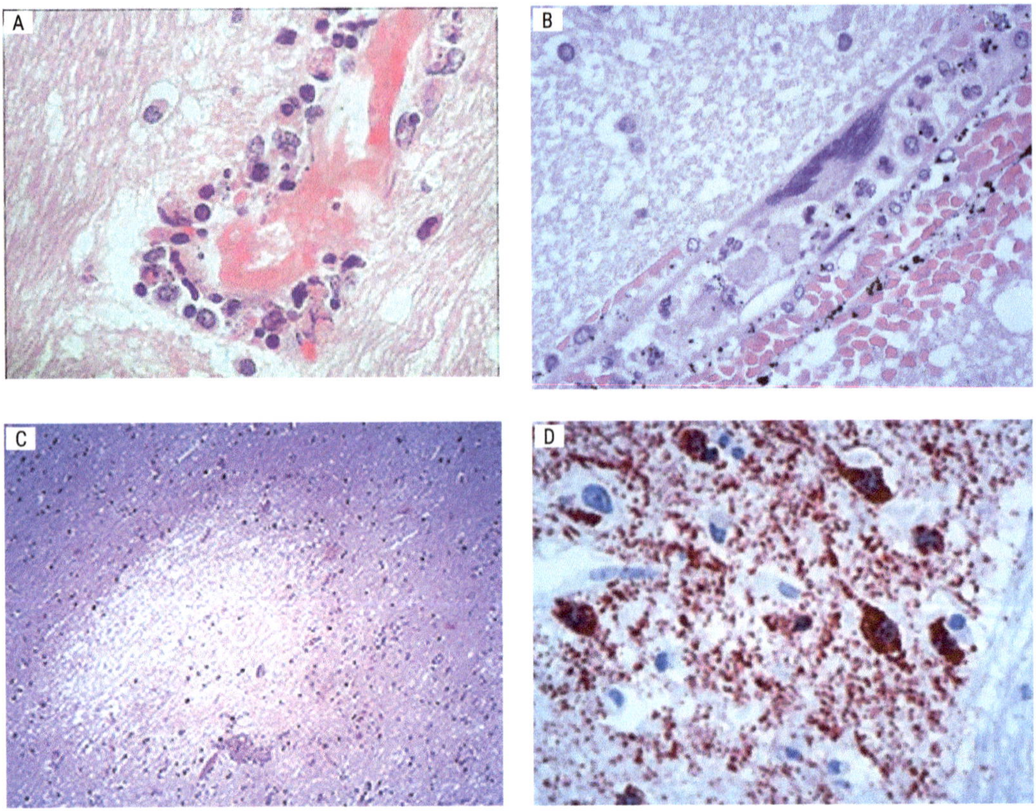

FIGURE 5.34 Acute Nipah encephalitis: (**A**) vasculopathy consisting of vasculitis and thrombo-occlusion of vessel (H&E); (**B**) multinucleated syncytia arising from the endothelial surface (H&E); (**C**) necrotic plaque with adjacent thrombotic vessel (H&E); (**D**) viral antigens in neurons (viral IHC).

neuronal loss are also seen. Severe meningitis may be found in many areas. Like in acute henipavirus encephalitis, viral inclusions, antigens, and RNA can be demonstrated in neurons and glial cells.

5.3.2.1.6. Progressive rubella panencephalitis. Progressive rubella panencephalitis is a very rare, delayed complication of congenital or childhood rubella infection. At neuropathological examination, there is widespread neuronal loss with gliosis and leptomeningeal and perivascular inflammation containing lymphocytes and macrophages, and there also is vasculitis with fibrinoid necrosis and mineral deposition. There is extensive myelin destruction with relative sparing of axons. Inclusion bodies are not found, and rubella virus is not detected by either electron microscopy or molecular techniques. The lesions may result from vasculitis produced by immune complex deposition.

5.3.2.1.7. Infection by HIV-1. HIV-1 is a retrovirus of the lentivirus subfamily, properly classified as an immunodeficiency virus, a subgroup of lentiviruses that also includes HIV-2 as well as the closely related simian immunodeficiency virus. HIV-1 infects cells that carry on their surface the CD4 antigen, which is present on both $CD4^+$ helper T lymphocytes and monocytes/macrophages, with the chemokine receptor CCR5 serving as an important coreceptor for HIV-1 on monocyte/macrophage cells. On the one hand, infection of $CD4^+$ lymphocytes leads to their destruction and cell-mediated immunodeficiency (AIDS). On the other hand, HIV-1 can invade the CNS via infected macrophages, which represent a major cell type capable of supporting viral replication and thus potentially serving both as a reservoir for the virus and as an agent for its dissemination. Viral particles can also freely cross the blood–brain barrier, gaining entry into the CNS parenchyma.

The CNS neurological complications of HIV infection are frequent and result from various mechanisms. Apart from lesions directly related to infection of the CNS by the virus, OIs and lymphomas may occur as a result of the immunodeficiency syndrome; HIV-associated systemic disorders may also cause neuropathological changes. They include cerebrovascular disease (marantic [noninfectious] endocarditis, thrombocytopenia, coagulopathy, and cerebral atherosclerosis), metabolic and nutritional abnormalities (hypoxia, vitamin deficiencies causing Wernicke encephalopathy and, possibly, vacuolar myelopathy, as well as electrolyte disturbances responsible for central pontine myelinolysis), liver failure causing hepatic encephalopathy, or increased levels of circulating pro-inflammatory cytokines likely to be responsible for multifocal necrotizing leukoencephalopathy. Finally, neurological complications of treatment, particularly those involving the peripheral nervous system, are increasingly frequent.

HIV-induced CNS lesions are defined as original and specific changes that had never been observed before the AIDS epidemic and are found only in HIV-infected individuals, without evidence of another cause. They include HIV encephalitis resulting from direct infection of the CNS by the virus, HIV leukoencephalopathy, and diffuse poliodystrophy, which may be variably associated.

- *HIV encephalitis* due to productive infection of the CNS by the virus is the most characteristic. It includes marked astrocytic and microglial activation with frequent MGCs (Fig. 5.35A) and abundant viral load demonstrated by either immunocytochemistry (Fig. 5.35B) or in situ hybridization. MGCs have been proposed as the hallmark of HIV encephalitis. These cells are of macrophage lineage, contain HIV in their cytoplasm, and result from the fusing capacity of the virus. Thus, their presence provides evidence of productive HIV infection and of a cytopathic effect of the virus. The lesions consist of multiple disseminated foci that may affect any part of the CNS but are more frequently found in the deep white matter and basal ganglia.
- *Involvement of the white matter, HIV leukoencephalopathy*, is also a prominent feature of HIV-specific neuropathology (Fig. 5.36). It is often but not invariably associated with HIV encephalitis. It is characterized both by diffuse myelin pallor, without true demyelination, involving predominantly the deep white matter and usually sparing of the U fibers, and by widespread axonal damage. The white matter pallor is thought to be secondary to alterations in the blood–brain barrier.
- *Involvement of the gray matter, diffuse poliodystrophy*, is characterized by diffuse reactive astrocytosis and microglial activation in the cerebral gray matter. It is associated with neuronal loss resulting, at least partly, from an apoptotic process and, when severe, may cause macroscopic cortical atrophy.

None of these HIV-induced CNS lesions can be precisely correlated with the specific progressive cognitive/motor syndrome termed *HIV-associated neurocognitive disorder* (HAND), suggesting that HAND more likely reflects a specific neuronal dysfunction resulting from the combined effects of several neurotoxic factors, including those produced by

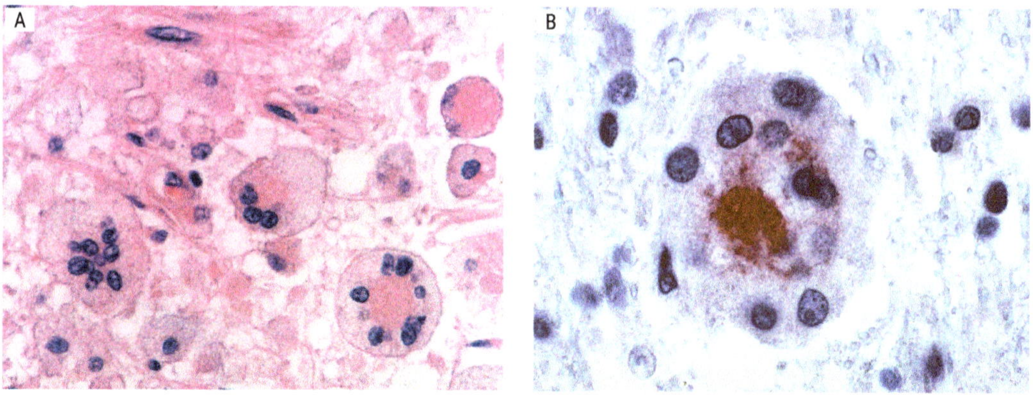

FIGURE 5.35 HIV encephalitis: (**A**) presence of abundant multinucleated giant cells (H&E); (**B**) immunocytochemistry with anti-HIV p24 antibody demonstrates the presence of HIV antigen in the cytoplasm of a multinucleated giant cell (HIV IHC).

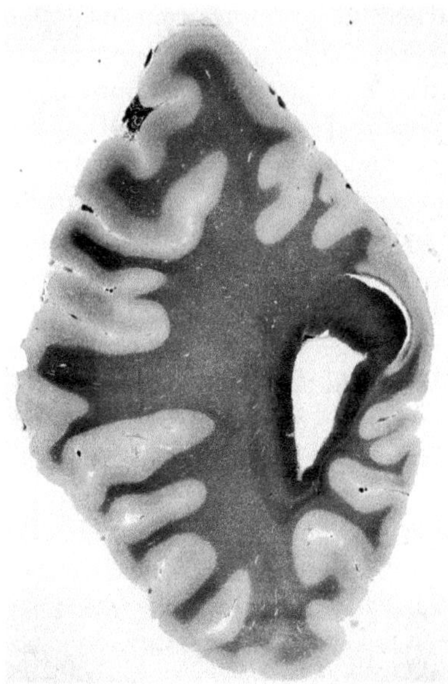

FIGURE 5.36 HIV leukoencephalopathy with diffuse myelin pallor sparing subcortical fibers (Loyez stain).

HIV itself, substances produced by activated glial and microglial cells, as well as antiretroviral drugs, some of which may be reversible.

5.3.2.1.8. Human T-cell leukemia/lymphotropic virus 1–associated myelopathy. Human T-cell leukemia/lymphotropic virus 1 (HTLV-1), an oncogenic retrovirus (oncovirus) that can cause T-cell leukemia, was the first human retrovirus to be identified. It is endemic in the Caribbean, the southern United States, South America, parts of Africa, and Japan. In rare cases, it may cause myelopathy, HTLV-1–associated myelopathy (HAM), characterized by progressive spastic paraparesis with sphincter and sensory disturbances.

In long-standing cases of HAM, there may be macroscopic meningeal thickening, spinal cord atrophy, and degeneration of the lateral columns. Microscopic examination shows myelin loss and some axonal degeneration in the long tracts of the spinal cord, particularly in the lateral columns. There is fibrosis and lymphocytic infiltration of the leptomeninges and astrocytosis and mononuclear inflammation in the spinal cord, more marked in the lower thoracic region.

5.3.2.1.9. Severe acute respiratory syndrome coronavirus 2/coronavirus disease 2019/COVID-19. SARS-CoV-2, the coronavirus responsible the global pandemic beginning in late 2019, has been associated with numerous neurological symptoms in the acute and subacute/postinfectious setting, including anosmia/ageusia, headache, and fatigue. Most notably, encephalopathy, commonly referred to as "brain fog," occurs in a large proportion of individuals in the post-acute setting and is of unclear etiology. Minimal evidence exists to support significant viral entry or replication within the CNS, either hematogenous or through olfactory nerve axonal transport, and indirect mechanisms are favored, including a systemic inflammatory response and damage to endothelial cells in cerebral blood vessels. Postmortem gross and histological findings are nonspecific but most commonly show infarcts (ranging in size from microinfarcts to large vessel), hypoxic–ischemic injury, and microglial predominant inflammation with minimal lymphocytes. Co-infections, particularly rhino-orbital-cerebral mucormycosis, have been reported. Rare demyelinating features have been described consistent with ADEM/AHLE. Multisystem inflammatory syndrome in children includes brain involvement, although neuropathological reports are limited.

5.3.2.2. ENCEPHALITIDES DUE TO DNA VIRUSES

The encephalitides due to DNA viruses include encephalitis due to herpes viruses and polyomaviruses. The main herpes viruses causing CNS infection in humans include herpes simplex virus type 1 (HSV-1) and HSV-2 (human herpes virus types 1 and 2, or HHV1 and HHV2, respectively); varicella zoster virus (VZV or HHV3); and cytomegalovirus (CMV or HHV5). The main human infection caused by polyomaviruses is PML due to infection by the JC virus.

5.3.2.2.1. Herpes simplex virus encephalitis. Herpes simplex virus is the most common cause of sporadic acute encephalitis. Most cases are due to infection by HSV-1, but in immunosuppressed individuals and neonates, HSV-2 may also cause encephalitis. Following a primary infection (oropharyngeal for HSV-1, genital for HSV-2), HSV establishes a latent infection in the sensory ganglia, with periodic reactivation of the virus leading to recurrent lesions at mucocutaneous junctions, at or near the site of primary infection. The mechanism of HSV-1 entry into the CNS to cause encephalitis is debated. Possibilities include (a) spread along olfactory nerve fibers either during primary nasopharyngeal infection or after reactivation of a latent virus in the olfactory bulbs; (b) reactivation of a latent virus in the trigeminal ganglia and axonal spread into the brain; and (c) reactivation of a previously established latent infection in the CNS, mainly in the temporal lobes.

In patients who die at the acute stage of the disease, gross examination has shown generalized swelling and bilateral asymmetric necrotic and hemorrhagic lesions involving predominantly the temporal lobes and the limbic regions (Fig. 5.37A) (insulae, cingulate gyri, and posterior orbital frontal cortex). On microscopic examination, the earliest lesions consist of meningeal, perivascular, and scanty parenchymal inflammation with scattered cells (neurons and glial cells) containing intranuclear inclusion bodies. The presence of HSV may be identified by immunohistochemistry or electron microscopy (Fig. 5.37D). At a more advanced stage, the lesions are more characteristic and include foci of hemorrhage and necrosis, with parenchymal infiltration by lymphocytes and macrophages (Fig. 5.37B). Changes more characteristic of meningoencephalitis (mononuclear inflammation of the leptomeninges, perivascular cuffing, neuronophagia, and diffuse microglial hyperplasia) are also present. Nuclear inclusions (Fig. 5.37C) are usually sparse, and the virus is more easily identified by immunohistochemistry. Early diagnosis is essential so that treatment with antiviral therapy, usually acyclovir, can be initiated promptly to achieve a good therapeutic response. The untreated case fatality rate is very high, approaching 80%, with a significant reduction of mortality in people who are treated. Reactivation of encephalitis after therapy has been reported.

In long-term survivors of untreated or unsuccessfully treated herpes encephalitis, the affected

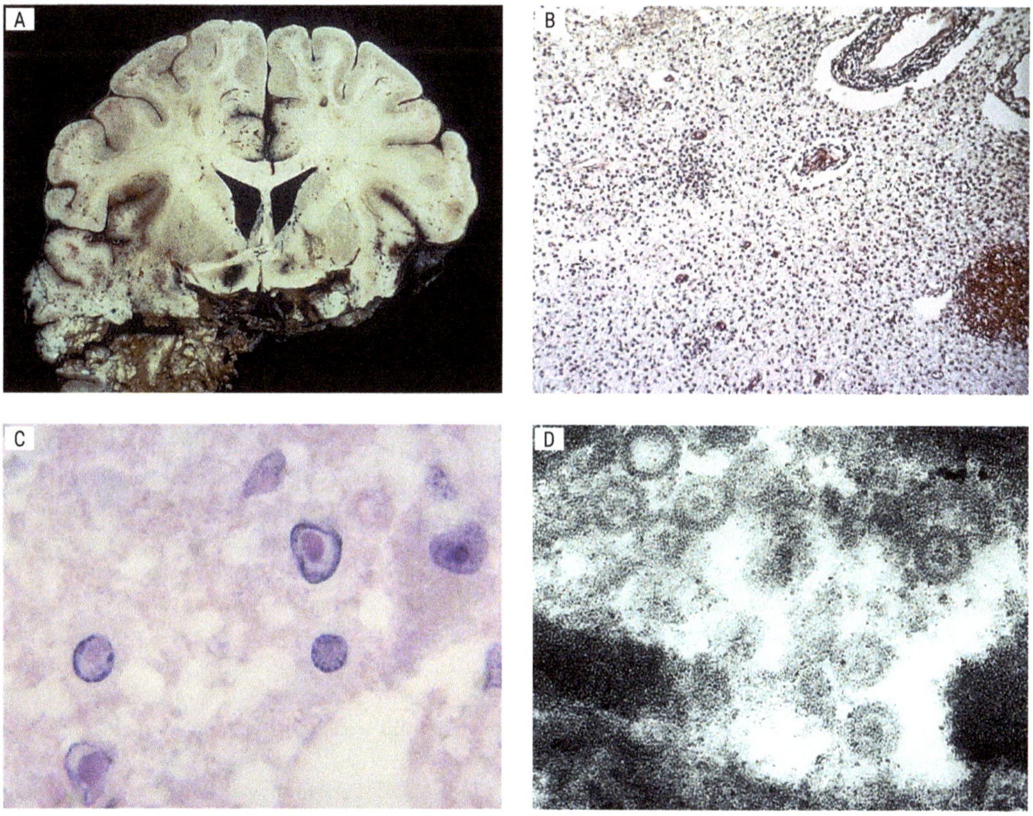

FIGURE 5.37 Herpes virus encephalitis: (**A**) necrosis of the left temporal lobe (the right temporal lobe was surgically excised); (**B**) microscopic appearance: necrosis with parenchymal infiltration by macrophages; note the presence of hemorrhage and perivascular cuffing by lymphocytes (H&E); (**C**) characteristic Cowdry type A intranuclear inclusion bodies (H&E); (**D**) electron micrograph showing typical "target-like" intranuclear viral particles (electron microscopy).

parts of the brain are shrunken and cavitated with yellow-brown discoloration. The entire parenchyma is replaced by cavitated glial scar tissue. Occasional clusters of lymphocytes are still seen in the leptomeninges and brain parenchyma. The virus is no longer demonstrable by culture, immunohistochemistry, or electron microscopy, but viral DNA may be identified by PCR.

Neonatal HSV encephalitis differs from the adult disease in that it is usually due to HSV-2 (acquired from a mother who has genital HSV-2 infection) by passage through the infected birth canal, causing a more generalized encephalitis without any predilection for any part of the brain. It also presents as necrotizing encephalitis. Nuclear inclusions, viral antigen, and DNA are usually demonstrable in abundance.

5.3.2.2.2. Varicella zoster virus infection. Primary infection by VZV causes chickenpox. Latent infection is subsequently established in the dorsal root or trigeminal ganglia. Reactivation of latent virus usually manifests as shingles, with a vesicular rash typically in the distribution of dermatome.

The pathological changes in zoster infection are usually limited to the dorsal root ganglia or to the ganglia of a sensory cranial nerve and the nerve root, but changes may extend to the corresponding metameric segment of the spinal cord, where there can be intense lymphocytic inflammation that may be associated with vasculitis and necrosis. Arteritis of large arteries may cause extensive infarction of brain tissue.

In immunocompromised patients, particularly those with AIDS, several patterns of VZV encephalitis and myeloradiculitis have been described, including multifocal lesions predominantly involving the white matter, likely to be due to hematogenous spread of the virus; ventriculitis secondary to ventricular spread; encephalitis involving the visual system or the brainstem; and myeloradiculitis resulting from spread from ophthalmic, trigeminal, or dorsal root zoster. In all cases, inflammatory necrotizing lesions are associated with vasculitis. Intranuclear inclusion bodies are present, and the virus may be identified by immunohistochemistry or in situ hybridization. In addition, granulomatous, necrotizing, or noninflammatory (endarteritis obliterans) lesions involving small or large intracranial vessels may cause infarcts or hemorrhages.

5.3.2.2.3. Cytomegalovirus infection. Early fetal infection by CMV may result in necrotizing encephalitis or ventriculoencephalitis. Residual lesions in children surviving the acute neonatal illness include microcephaly, microgyria, porencephalic cysts, hydrocephalus, and periventricular calcifications.

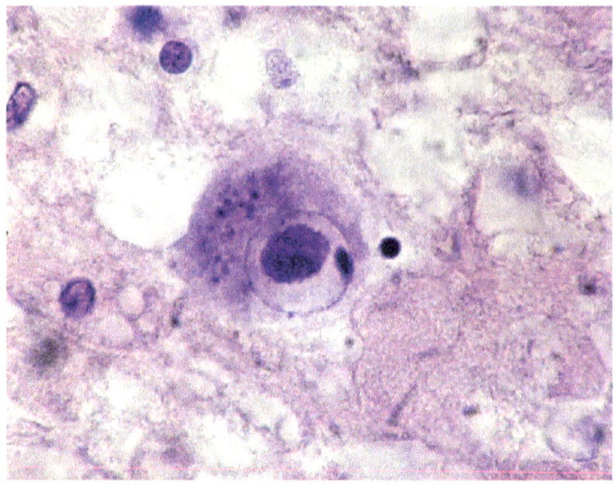

FIGURE 5.38 Cytomegalic cell in a case of CMV encephalitis in a patient with AIDS (Nissl stain).

In immune-compromised adults, CMV may cause an OI. Diffuse, nonnecrotic encephalitic lesions consisting of disseminated microglial nodules, some of which contain characteristic cytomegalic cells (Fig. 5.38), have been described, especially in transplant recipients. In patients with AIDS, in addition to microglial nodule encephalitis, other lesions have been observed, including necrotizing ventriculoencephalitis, ependymitis, necrotizing encephalitis with large cystic foci of encephalomalacia, and acute meningomyeloradiculitis, the latter usually with numerous neutrophils. Cytomegalic cells containing intranuclear and intracytoplasmic inclusion bodies are numerous and involve many types of cells (neurons, glial cells, endothelial cells, and macrophages). The virus may be identified by immunohistochemistry, in situ hybridization, or electron microscopy, but these are usually not necessary for the diagnosis because the appearance of the infected cells on routine stains is so characteristic. Indeed, CMV is one of the few viral infections that can be accurately diagnosed by light microscopy because of the unique appearance of the cytomegalic cells with dark intranuclear inclusions.

5.3.2.2.4. Progressive multifocal leukoencephalitis. The disease PML is due to infection by JC virus. This is an OI occurring most often in patients with immunodeficiency, particularly AIDS. The virus infects specifically oligodendrocytes, causing a demyelinating disease. The lesions are usually bilateral and asymmetrical. They involve predominantly the subcortical hemispheric white matter, especially in the parieto-occipital regions, but the cerebellum, brainstem, and even the spinal cord may be affected. They develop as punctate foci that subsequently coalesce to form larger confluent demyelinating areas (Fig. 5.39A). On microscopic examination of the lesions, there are lipid-laden macrophages and only scanty perivascular lymphocytes. The presence of giant astrocytes with bizarre hyperchromatic nuclei (Fig. 5.39B) and oligodendrocytes with enlarged nuclei containing viral inclusions (Fig. 5.39C) is a striking and very characteristic feature of PML. The virus may be identified in oligodendrocytes by immunocytochemistry, in situ hybridization, or electron microscopy.

Since the AIDS epidemic, there has been a considerable increase in the incidence of PML. The disorder is relatively frequent in patients with AIDS, in whom the lesions may be particularly severe, with sometimes necrotic, very extensive damage involving particularly the cerebellum (Fig. 5.39D). Viral inclusions are abundant and may be found in cells other than oligodendrocytes, including neurons.

5.3.2.3. ENCEPHALITIS OF UNCERTAIN ORIGIN

5.3.2.3.1. Encephalitis lethargica (epidemic encephalitis of von Economo). The supposed viral disease called encephalitis lethargica (epidemic encephalitis of von Economo) was rampant from 1916 to 1930, but attempts, with the limited techniques then available, to implicate a virus, as well as efforts to relate the encephalitis with the contemporaneous pandemic of influenza, were unsuccessful. The disorder was characterized by preferential involvement of the midbrain and basal ganglia. In many cases, a postencephalitic parkinsonism developed.

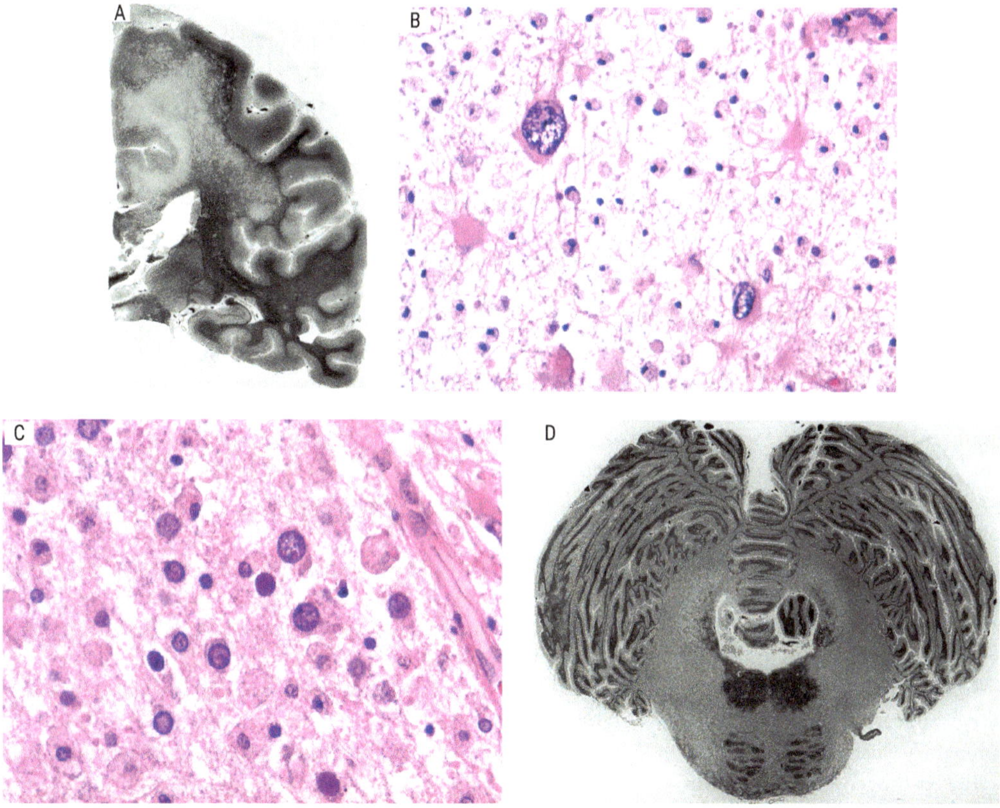

FIGURE 5.39 Progressive multifocal leukoencephalitis: (**A**) confluent demyelination in the subcortical white matter of the parietal lobe (whole mount, Loyez stain); (**B**) presence of giant "bizarre" astrocytes in a demyelinated area (H&E); (**C**) presence of abnormal oligodendrocytes with enlarged nuclei containing viral inclusions (H&E); (**D**) extensive demyelination of the cerebellum and pons in a patient with AIDS (Loyez stain).

5.3.2.3.2. Behçet's uveomeningoencephalitis. Uveomeningoencephalitides is present as inflammatory encephalitis, meningitis, and uveal lesions involving the choroid, ciliary body, and iris. The etiology is uncertain. Behçet's disease is a rare disorder that most commonly presents as recurrent ulceration of the mouth and genitalia accompanied by uveitis or iridocyclitis. An encephalitic syndrome may occur occasionally, consisting of multifocal necrotizing lesions that involve predominantly the thalamus, hypothalamus, and midbrain. The inflammatory changes are often necrotic and sometimes hemorrhagic. Vasculitis is considered to be the underlying lesion, but cerebral blood vessel changes are nonspecific. Attempts to demonstrate a virus as the cause of Behçet's disease have failed.

5.3.2.3.3. Chronic localized encephalitis of Rasmussen. The rare, devastating disorder called chronic localized encephalitis of Rasmussen is characterized by progressive, unilateral, neurological deficit with sudden onset of seizures, usually in childhood, which are refractory to treatment. Seizures are of partial complex type, and they become generalized and associated with hemiplegia, hemianopia, and intellectual deterioration.

Macroscopic changes vary from case to case and are predominantly unilateral. They consist of cerebral atrophy, which may be patchy, and dusky discoloration of the cortex (Fig. 5.40A). Histological examination confirms the largely unilateral distribution of the lesions, although bilateral involvement also occurs. Lesions are more diffuse and severe than can be assumed from macroscopic observation and have a concentric distribution. They are necrotic and destructive in the center, whereas at the periphery they have all the features of active encephalitis. Microscopic findings include thickening of the leptomeninges with mild lymphocytic infiltration and accompanying intraparenchymal cuffing of the vessels by lymphocytes and macrophages (Fig. 5.40B). Microglial nodules and neuronophagia are ubiquitous (Fig. 5.40C–E), and the former are seen also in the white matter. In older lesions, there may be thinning of the cortex with loss of neurons and spongiosis, severe glial reaction, and less intense inflammatory clusters.

The pathogenesis of Rasmussen encephalitis (RS) is unknown. The possibility of an infectious etiology has been raised by some studies, which have shown similarities between RS and the epilepsy seen in Kozhevnikov encephalitis, a tick-borne viral encephalitis with intractable seizures seen almost exclusively in Russia. The presence of an infectious ipsilateral uveitis and chorioiditis are also consistent with this hypothesis. Other supporting data include the demonstration by in situ hybridization of EBV and CMV reported in some studies, although not confirmed by others.

Autoimmune mechanisms of injury, including immune complex deposits and vasculitis, have also been postulated. Antibodies to GluR3 have been identified in RS, but they have also been identified in other cases of focal seizures. More recently, direct T-cell–mediated cytotoxicity against the neurons has been demonstrated.

The observation of cortical dysplasia, tuberous sclerosis, cavernous angioma, and tumors in patients with RS has raised the possibility that these lesions may be instrumental in inducing seizures, altering the blood–brain barrier, which could in turn trigger a viral or autoimmune disorder.

5.4. RICKETTSIOSIS

Some forms of rickettsial infection (murine/endemic typhus due to *Rickettsia prowazeki*, exanthematic/epidemic typhus due to *Rickettsia typhi*, and Rocky Mountain spotted fever due to *Rickettsia rickettsii*) may cause encephalitis characterized histologically by perivascular mononuclear cuffing and microglial nodules that preferentially involve the gray matter of the cerebral hemispheres and the brainstem. The agents, which are obligatory intracellular microorganisms that have the staining properties of gram-negative bacilli, may be demonstrated in the cytoplasm of endothelial cells.

5.5. OPPORTUNISTIC INFECTIONS

By definition, an OI is an infection that takes the opportunity of a deficiency in the immune response of the host to develop. It may be either a primary infection or a reactivation of a latent infection. OIs are due to saprophytic organisms, which do not cause diseases in immunocompetent individuals and differ from primary pathogens by several characteristics (Table 5.2). However, included in this group of infections are common pathogens such as tuberculosis, syphilis, measles, or VZV, where the disease may take the course of an OI in patients with impaired immunity. One may also extend the concept

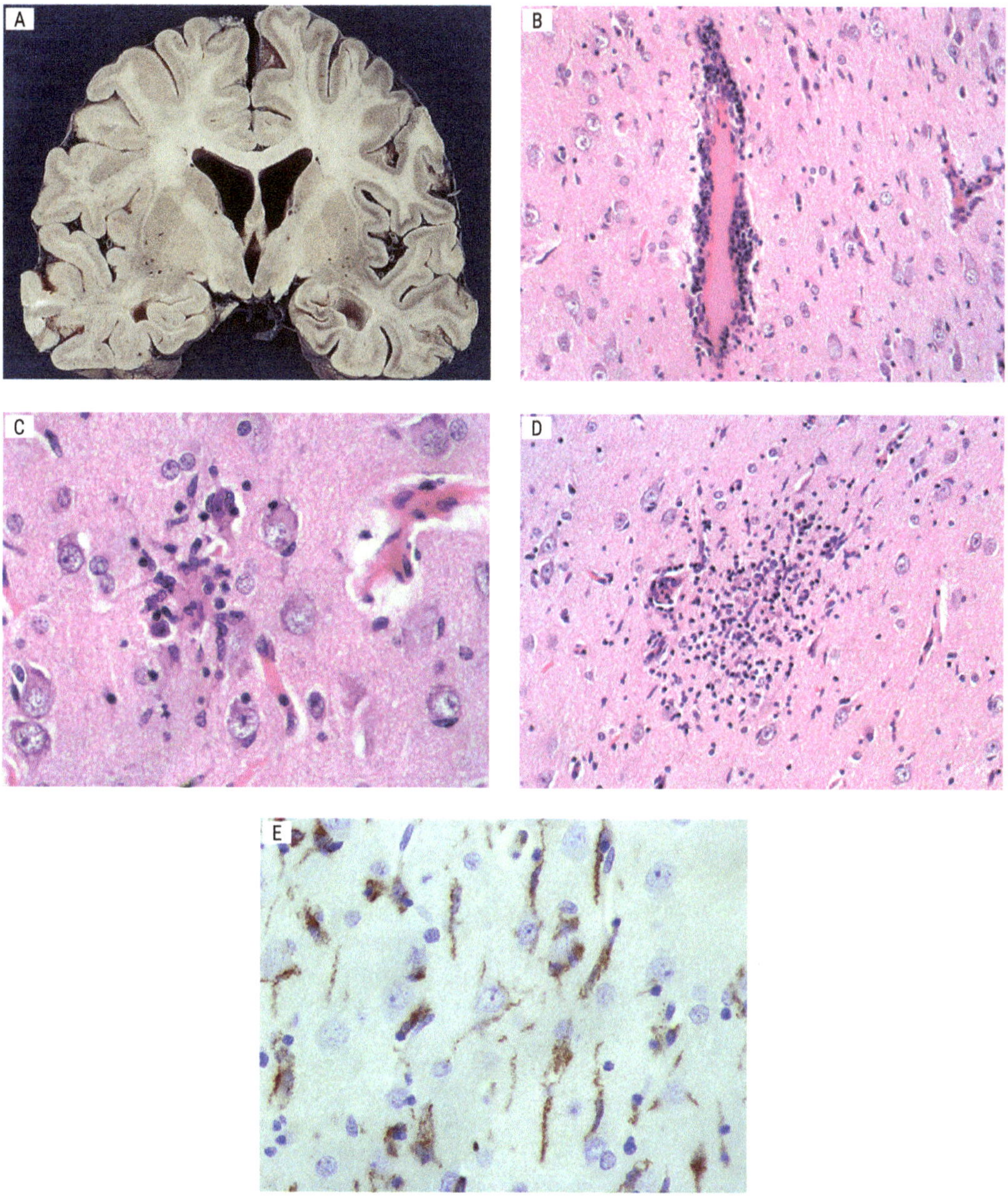

FIGURE 5.40 Rasmussen encephalitis: (**A**) gross appearance with unilateral darkened atrophic cortex; (**B**) intraparenchymal perivascular cuffing by lymphocytes and macrophages (H&E); (**C**) nodule of neuronophagia (H&E); (**D**) microglial nodule (H&E); (**E**) proliferation of rod cell microglia (CD68 IHC).

of OIs to some neoplasms related to a specific viral infection that develops only in immunocompromised individuals; these include Kaposi sarcoma of patients with AIDS, related to infection by HHV type 8 (also known as Kaposi sarcoma–associated virus); and primary brain lymphoma related to infection by EBV (or HHV type 4), occurring in patients with AIDS and organ transplant recipients. There is only one report of Kaposi sarcoma metastatic to the CNS.

In addition to the rare congenital and idiopathic immunodeficiency disorders, there has been a dramatically increasing number of patients with acquired immunodeficiencies in the past 20 years. This public health problem is partly due to the steadily increasing age of the general population, as well as

Table 5.2 Differential Characteristics of Primary and Opportunistic Pathogens

PRIMARY PATHOGENS	OPPORTUNISTIC PATHOGENS
Induce specific diseases in immunocompetent hosts with identified reservoirs and routes of infection	Induce atypical infections in immunocompromised patients Present in wide environmental reservoirs, in commensal (endogenous) flora, or latent in host
Interacts with specific cellular or humoral target molecules	Lack defined cellular or humoral host receptors
Share specific virulence/pathogenicity determinants	May express potentially virulent and pathogenic molecules (constitutive or inducible) once they have colonized the host
Can be transmitted from host to host and induce the same disease (potential for epidemics)	Are acquired from the environment, from food sources, or from the endogenous flora, and, for nosocomial infections, are communicable to susceptible contacts
Clonal origin with limited genetic variability	Genetic diversity and plasticity, which hamper indirect diagnosis and specific immunotherapies and vaccines
Induce specific immune responses, allowing for specific immunological diagnoses and vaccines	High frequency of genetic variations and rearrangements, allowing acquired resistance to antimicrobial agents

a growing number and longer survival of patients with debilitating diseases, such as diabetes, alcoholism, and lymphoid neoplasms. Patients who have received immunosuppressive drugs for rheumatic and neoplastic diseases and for organ transplantation are also at risk. The occurrence of the AIDS epidemic has represented a major cause of acquired immunodeficiency.

Different types of immunodeficiency may be associated with specific OIs, as described in the following sections.

5.5.1. Opportunistic infections of the CNS in patients with granulocytic disorders

Severe depletion of granulocytes is usually the consequence of decreased or absent production in the bone marrow. This may occur in myeloid leukemia or more often in the course of treatment with cytotoxic drugs. More rarely, severe granulocytopenia may result from peripheral sequestration as in hypersplenism or as an idiosyncratic reaction to medication. In people who develop severe granulocytopenia, the most common OIs are mycoses, particularly those due to *Aspergillus* species and *Candida* species and to certain bacterial infections, particularly *Pseudomonas aeruginosa*, *L. monocytogenes*, and *N. asteroides*.

5.5.2. Opportunistic infections of the CNS in patients with combined granulocytic and lymphocytic disorders

Immunodeficiency resulting from both granulocytic and lymphocytic impairment is the rule in transplant recipients. It may also occur in patients with lymphoid neoplasms (Hodgkin diseases or lymphoid leukemia); with other malignancies treated with chemotherapy; or on prolonged, high-dose corticosteroid therapy.

In addition to mycoses (aspergillosis, cryptococcosis) and bacterial infections (listeriosis, nocardiosis), other cerebral OIs may occur, including toxoplasmosis, PML, and CMV infection. Primary malignant non-Hodgkin lymphomas of the brain, related to EBV infection, may also be seen. It is of historical interest that primary brain lymphomas were first recognized as an opportunistic event in patients who had undergone renal transplantation.

5.5.3. Opportunistic infections of the CNS in patients with lymphocytic disorders, particularly in AIDS

Prior to the introduction of highly active combination antiretroviral therapy (cART) or combination therapy including an HIV protease inhibitor, OIs secondary to the depletion in CD4+ T cells causing the cell-mediated immunodeficiency syndrome characteristic of AIDS were a frequent complication of the disease. OIs usually occurred during the late stages, in full-blown AIDS, in people with depletion of CD4 cells and with high viral loads; they included multiple parasitic (*Toxoplasma*), fungal (cryptococcal), bacterial (mycobacterial), and viral (CMV, PML) infections, as well as primary brain lymphomas. Unlike the situation with granulocytopenia, these patients, by and large, did not have frequent infections due to *Aspergillus* sp. Although bacterial infections were rare, note that a brain abscess in a patient with AIDS who did not have bacterial endocarditis was more likely to be due to *Nocardia* species than to any other agent.

The occurrence of many OIs in immunosuppressed patients, particularly in those with AIDS, has modified the clinical presentation of these complications in these patients and has consequently made diagnosis difficult for the following reasons: (a) An increased range of organisms may be involved; (b) a particular patient may have successive or simultaneous infections by different agents; (c) there can be involvement of several organs at the same time, as well as an increased incidence of neurological disease; and (d) there is generally a reduced inflammatory reaction.

The occurrence of OIs of the CNS in patients with AIDS varies with the geographical location where the patient has lived, with the age of the patient, and with therapy both for OIs and for HIV infection.

- With regard to geographic location, several points can be made. Cerebral toxoplasmosis is more frequent in France and Germany than it is in either the United States or the United Kingdom. In addition, this CNS complication has been reported in patients from sub-Saharan Africa, South America, and India. CNS histoplasmosis, blastomycosis, and coccidioidomycosis are much more frequent in America than in Europe. Acute or reactivated cerebral trypanosomiasis causing devastating necrotic lesions occurs only in South America. *Mycobacterium tuberculosis* infection of the CNS is especially common in patients with AIDS living in developing countries that have a high incidence of tuberculosis, particularly in Africa.
- Children up to age 13 years in general have a lower incidence of CNS OIs than do adults, a phenomenon that is particularly manifest in AIDS, probably because children have had less time than adults to be exposed to common opportunist pathogens. This is especially true for toxoplasmosis, which is a much less common cause of CNS mass lesion than is primary brain lymphoma in children with AIDS in the United States. For this reason, it is recommended that children with AIDS who have a mass lesion in the CNS be biopsied at presentation rather than after a trial of anti-*Toxoplasma* therapy (see Section 5.2.2.3). Cryptococcal meningitis and PML are also rare in children with AIDS. The most common opportunistic pathogen in this age group, even in young children, continues to be CMV. In addition, children with AIDS are also at risk for developing bacterial meningitis, including that caused by *S. pneumoniae*, as well as disseminated candidiasis, which often involves the CNS.
- Introduction of cART has dramatically modified the course and prognosis of HIV disease.

In the developed world, where cART is readily available and where there have been progressive improvements in the management of OIs in general, the incidence of CNS OIs has declined dramatically from the 1980s, and epidemiological studies have shown that AIDS-defining events are no longer the major causes of death in HIV-infected patients. The benefit is mainly due to a decrease of HIV viral load and a restored, functional immune system.

However, in addition to those related to drug toxicity, new types of complications have occurred. On the one hand, "burned out" forms of treatable infections in which no inflammation and no infectious agent can be detected have become more frequent. "Scar lesions" have been found with increasing frequency in clinically and biologically cured patients who died from other causes. In other instances, despite efficient treatment, the disease continued to progress clinically and often radiologically. This pattern was particularly prevalent in patients with severe, multifocal toxoplasmosis, PML, or HIV encephalitis (HIVE) when treatment had been administered too late in the course of the disease, after irreversible cerebral destruction had occurred with secondary progressive Wallerian degeneration.

On the other hand, *new inflammatory lesions related to the restoration of the immune system* have appeared. An "immune reconstitution inflammatory syndrome" (IRIS), was identified with four diagnostic criteria: (a) patients with AIDS; (b) those efficiently treated by cART; (c) patients with presenting symptoms consistent with an infectious/inflammatory condition that appeared while the patient was on antiretroviral therapy; and (d) those with symptoms that could not be explained by a newly acquired infection, the expected course of a previously recognized infection, or side effects of therapy. In the CNS, IRIS caused paradoxical exacerbation of tuberculosis and cryptococcal infection, as well as exacerbation of CMV retinitis.

In some patients with PML or HIVE, onset or worsening of neurological signs following cART institution was associated with contrast enhancement on magnetic resonance imaging, suggestive of an unusually intense inflammation with impairment of the blood–brain barrier. Neuropathological studies have confirmed intense inflammation, with an influx of $CD8^+$ lymphocytes variably associated with an acute worsening of the underlying infection (HIV or JC virus) and a nonspecific immunopathologic reaction of the ADEM or MS type. In most cases, IRIS is correlated with prolonged survival, interpreted as a marker of both improved immune status and outcome; however, in rare instances, IRIS has coincided with clinical and radiological aggravation and death.

Also, people with undiagnosed or unsuspected HIV infection are still at risk of presenting with a CNS OI, as are HIV-infected individuals who are not compliant with their antiretroviral and prophylactic therapy. In addition, this complication of AIDS can be seen in people who develop HIV mutations resistant to antiretroviral agents. Finally, and of great importance, CNS OIs in AIDS also continue to be a major problem in developing countries, where effective treatment and prevention are often not available.

5.5.4. Opportunistic infections of the CNS in patients on B-cell–depleting antibodies

Increased use of rituximab and other B-cell–depleting monoclonal antibodies for treatment of autoimmune disease and hematologic malignancy has resulted in infectious side effects. Hepatitis B and JC virus can reactivate, and arboviruses including West Nile, tick-borne encephalitis, Eastern equine encephalitis, Cache Valley, Jamestown Canyon, and Powassan viruses have all been reported to have neuroinvasive disease in patients on rituximab. Blood and CSF serological testing is frequently negative in these cases, requiring molecular testing, immunohistochemistry, or in situ hybridization to confirm a diagnosis.

6

Human Prion Diseases

MARKUS GLATZEL AND STÉPHANE HAIK

6.1. INTRODUCTION

Prion diseases, also known as transmissible spongiform encephalopathies, are rare fatal neurodegenerative disorders with a specific biologic mechanism. Human prion diseases are distinct from other neurodegenerative disorders in that they occur in sporadic (idiopathic), genetic (inherited), or acquired (transmissible) forms (Table 6.1). These diseases are characterized pathologically by varying combinations of spongiform change (vacuolation of the gray matter due to distention and swelling of neuronal cell processes); neuronal loss; reactive gliosis (involving microglia and astrocytes); and accumulation of the disease-associated form of the prion protein in the brain, sometimes in the form of amyloid plaques. Prion diseases also occur in other mammals, with implications for spread to humans, the best example of which is bovine spongiform encephalopathy (BSE).

Table 6.1 Classification of Human Prion Diseases

Idiopathic	Sporadic Creutzfeldt–Jakob disease
	Sporadic fatal insomnia
	Variably protease-sensitive prionopathy
Genetic	Familial Creutzfeldt–Jakob disease
	Gerstmann–Sträussler–Scheinker disease and variants
	Prion disease with cerebral amyloid angiopathy
	Prion diseases associated with octapeptide repeat region insertional mutations (variable phenotype)
	Fatal familial insomnia
Acquired	From human: Kuru
	Iatrogenic: Creutzfeldt–Jakob disease
	From bovine: Variant Creutzfeldt–Jakob disease

6.2. BIOLOGY OF PRIONS

6.2.1. The transmissible agent

The transmissible agent in prion diseases consists of pathological prion proteins (PrP^{Sc} or PrP^{res}, see below). These are misfolded and pathologically aggregated forms of the cellular form of the prion protein (PrP^{C}) that can induce a conformational change in other prion proteins toward pathological prion protein forms. This mechanism of disease initiation was discovered while attempting to identify the agent responsible for scrapie (a transmissible disease affecting sheep and goats). It was found that the agent did not contain RNA or DNA, thus the term "prion" for proteinaceous infectious particles was proposed by Prusiner in 1982. The prion hypothesis stated that the prion has a molecular weight of 27–30 kDa, is partially resistant to proteolytic cleavage, and co-purifies with infectivity in extracts of scrapie-infected brain. It was subsequently demonstrated that this protein was an abnormal conformer of the cellular, physiological form PrP^{C}, where "C" stands for cellular, and was termed PrP^{Sc}, where "Sc" stands for the scrapie form of the protein. The sequence is encoded by the prion protein gene (*PRNP*), located on the short arm of chromosome 20 in humans, and the protein is mainly expressed in the mammalian brain.

6.2.2. The normal prion protein

The normal prion protein PrP^{C} is a 253-residue peptide that is translated from a single exon within the *PRNP*. The peptide undergoes a series of post-translational modifications, including cleavage of a signal peptide, addition of up to two N-linked oligosaccharide chains (at residues 181 and 197), and attachment of a glycosylphosphatidylinositol anchor. The protein contains five octapeptide repeats from codons 51–91. Four putative α-helices in PrP^{C} are located between codons 109 and 122, 129 and 140, 178 and 191, and 202 and 218.

Most PrP^{C} is membrane-associated and has a short half-life, but approximately 10% of total PrP^{C} is subject to ectodomain shedding by the protease ADAM10, which leads to the release of almost full-length soluble shed PrP^{C} into the extracellular matrix. As with other proteins, it is sensitive to proteolytic digestion in standard in vitro conditions (commonly assessed using the bacterial enzyme proteinase K). PrP^{C} is a multifunctional protein with roles in axonal guidance, synaptic function, and control of circadian rhythms. PrP^{C} can act as a copper-binding protein, and it has roles in oxidative cell stress and signal transduction. Several *PRNP* polymorphisms have been identified, of which the most significant is M129V because it affects susceptibility to prion diseases (Table 6.2).

Table 6.2 Prion Protein Genotypes in the Normal Population and in Prion Diseases

	PRION PROTEIN GENE CODON 129 POLYMORPHISMS (%)		
	MM	MV	VV
Normal population	44	45	11
Sporadic CJD	60	21	19
Variant CJD	>99	<1	—

CJD, Creutzfeldt–Jakob disease; M, methionine; V, valine.
Source: Data from https://www.cjd.ed.ac.uk.

6.2.3. The abnormal prion protein

PrP^{Sc} has an identical amino acid sequence and the same molecular weight as PrP^{C}, but it has a much longer half-life and is partially resistant to proteolytic digestion (Fig. 6.1). Structural studies have indicated that PrP^{Sc} has a predominant β-pleated sheet structure, with a relative loss of the α-helix regions that are present in PrP^{C}. This conformer, PrP^{Sc}, is resistant to proteolytic degradation, and it aggregates and accumulates within the central nervous system (CNS), sometimes as amyloid fibrils. The accumulation of PrP^{Sc} results in the degeneration of neurons and spongiform changes within the brain, eventually leading to rapidly progressing neurologic symptoms and death.

The mechanisms and cellular sites of the conversion of PrP^{C} into PrP^{Sc} are not fully understood. Conversion of PrP^{C} to PrP^{Sc} can be achieved in cell-free systems, including in vitro amplification systems such as the protein misfolding cyclical amplification (PMCA) reaction and the real-time quaking-induced conversion (RT-QuIC). In PMCA, small amounts of seeding-active PrP^{Sc} are incubated with a comparatively larger amount of PrP^{C} and other components present in the cell (lipids, RNA, etc.) to generate growing aggregates of PrP^{Sc} using

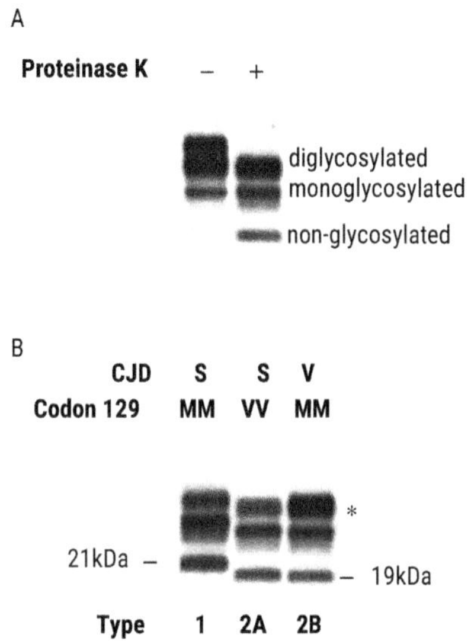

FIGURE 6.1 Western blot analysis. (**A**) Western blot of prion protein (PrP) in variant CJD brain tissue with (+) or without (–) prior digestion with proteinase K. Proteinase K results in complete degradation of PrP^{C} (top band, seen on left) and in N-terminal truncation of PrP^{Sc}. Normal brain shows no bands remaining after proteinase K digestion (not shown). The protease-resistant PrP (PrP^{res}) occurs in di-, mono-, and nonglycosylated forms. (**B**) Western blot analysis of protease-resistant prion protein (PrP^{res}) in sporadic (S) and variant (V) CJD brain. Nonglycosylated PrP^{res} occurs as either a 21-kDa band (termed type 1) or a more extensively truncated 19-kDa band (termed type 2). Variant CJD exhibits a characteristic predominance of the diglycosylated band (*), and this protein is termed type 2B to distinguish it from the type 2A isotype seen in sporadic CJD, where the diglycosylated form does not predominate. The cases shown were homozygous for methionine (MM) or valine (VV) at codon 129 of the *PRNP* gene. (Courtesy of Dr. Mark W. Head and Ms. Helen Yull.)

ultrasound treatments. Thus, minute amounts of PrP^{Sc} can be detected and prion infectivity can be amplified. RT-QuIC also detects the seeding activity of PrP^{Sc} in material under investigation. Here, small amounts of seeding-active PrP^{Sc} are incubated with a relatively larger amount of PrP^{C}, and through cycles of shaking, minute amounts of PrP^{Sc} are amplified, allowing detection of these. There are no indications that the thus-generated products are infectious.

The mechanisms of neurotoxicity of PrP^{Sc} are not fully understood, although a range of possibilities exist, from a direct toxic effect on neurons to indirect toxicity mediated by microglia and possibly astrocytes. No pathologic changes occur outside the CNS in prion diseases, although in some diseases, PrP^{Sc} can be found in the peripheral nervous system, in lymphoid tissues such as the spleen and tonsil, and in skeletal muscle (see variant CJD Section 6.3.3.3).

6.2.4. Diagnostic methods for detecting PrP^{Sc}

The resistance of PrP^{Sc} to protease digestion forms the basis for its biochemical detection in tissue, which lies at the heart of confirming the diagnosis of prion diseases. When tissue homogenates are examined by Western blot analysis with antibodies to PrP, samples containing PrP^{Sc} will show immunoreactivity even after treatment with proteinase K, whereas PrP^{C} is completely digested. Although resistant to complete digestion, PrP^{Sc} is partially cleaved; there are two common sites of cleavage, resulting in fragments of protease-resistant PrP (PrP^{res}) of different lengths. The size of the immunoreactive PrP^{res} fragment, along with the pattern of glycosylation, is used to define PrP^{Sc} isotypes (Fig. 6.1). Experimental animals inoculated with a prion strain associated with a particular isotype of PrP^{Sc} will typically propagate the same isotype, which is maintained on subsequent passage in the same experimental model and is associated with a stable clinicopathologic phenotype. The term *molecular strain typing* has been used to describe the biochemical characterization of individual PrP^{Sc} isoforms and their associated disease phenotypes. The classification proposed by Parchi et al. in 1999 that distinguishes two principal types of PrP^{Sc} isoforms (Fig. 6.1) is used to describe the PrP^{Sc} isoforms by most laboratories worldwide. This classification identifies relationships between the predominant PrP^{Sc} isotypes and disease phenotypes to be examined.

In fluids, Real-Time Quaking-induced Conversion (RT-QuIC), which uses recombinant PrP^{C} as the conversion substrate during repeated cycles of incubation and high-speed agitation, is a very effective technique for the diagnosis of sCJD in the CSF that shows high sensitivity and outstanding specificity. CSF RT-QuIC documented robustness and interlaboratory replicability led to its inclusion in the international criteria for sCJD diagnosis in 2017. Less effective is PMCA (protein misfolding cyclic amplification), which works best with PrP^{C} from normal brain homogenate as the substrate during repeated cycles of incubation and sonication. It has been shown to detect PrP^{Sc} in the urine, CSF and plasma of patients with symptomatic variant CJD (vCJD) with high sensitivity and specificity, but its use in detecting sCJD has proven to be more challenging.

6.3. THE HUMAN PRION DISEASES

6.3.1. Sporadic prion diseases

6.3.1.1. SPORADIC CREUTZFELDT–JAKOB DISEASE

Sporadic Creutzfeldt–Jakob disease (sCJD) is the most commonly diagnosed human prion disease, occurring with a relatively uniform incidence of approximately 1 or 2 individuals per 1 million per year in countries with a functioning surveillance system. Although a wide range of ages at onset has been reported, most cases of sCJD occur in the seventh decade of life, with males and females affected equally. The disease usually presents as a rapidly progressive dementia accompanied by other neurological abnormalities, among which ataxia, myoclonus, visual abnormalities, pyramidal, and extrapyramidal signs are common. The duration of the clinical illness of sCJD is typically four to seven months, but both shorter and in some cases markedly longer clinical courses have been observed.

Use of a combination of diagnostic tests can assist in identifying cases of sCJD. These include the electroencephalogram (EEG), which shows a characteristic abnormality (periodic sharp wave complexes with a biphasic or triphasic morphology) in approximately 65% of patients, although not at all phases of the illness. Elevated levels of the chaperone protein 14-3-3 in the cerebrospinal fluid (CSF) can also be found, although this is also true in other clinical settings. More recently, the detection of PrP^{Sc} in the CSF in sCJD by RT-QuIC (see Section 6.2.3) has shown a high sensitivity and specificity for sCJD and is now employed in clinical diagnosis. Brain imaging studies can also assist in making the diagnosis of sCJD, with restricted diffusion and hyperintensity on fluid-attenuated inversion recovery (FLAIR) sequences evident in anatomically involved regions such as cerebral cortex and striatum. These imaging changes typically progress along with clinical signs and symptoms during the disease. These investigations have allowed diagnostic criteria for sCJD and other prion diseases to be established; a definite diagnosis of a human prion disease requires progressive neurological syndrome and a neuropathological or biochemical confirmation for the presence of PrP^{Sc}.

The etiology of sCJD is unknown. It has been suggested that this disease might occur as a consequence of a random event that results in the spontaneous conversion of PrP^{Sc} within the brain. Case–control studies have failed to identify any consistent predisposing factors in terms of occupation or diet; a past history of surgery (not specifically neurosurgery) or blood transfusion has been reported to be significantly higher in patients with sCJD than in controls in some case–control studies, possibly due to biases in study design. Analysis of the *PRNP* has shown that most patients with sCJD are methionine homozygotes at codon 129, in contrast to the normal population (Table 6.2). This finding has been reproduced consistently in many countries, but the significance of this genetic predisposing factor remains uncertain.

Clinical and pathologic heterogeneity occur in sCJD, and a wide range of eponyms has been applied to some of these clinical subgroups (e.g., Heidenhain variant with a short clinical history and cortical blindness as a prominent feature; Brownell–Oppenheimer variant with prominent cerebellar ataxia). Recent studies on large cohorts of patients with sCJD have identified an association between the clinicopathologic phenotype, the *PRNP* codon 129 genotype (MM, MV, or VV [M, methionine; V, valine]) (Table 6.2), and the PrP^{Sc} isotype (type 1 or type 2) on Western blot analysis (Fig. 6.1). These allow for six combinations (MM1, MM2, MV1, MV2, VV1, and VV2) that appear to be associated with certain neuropathologic and clinical features (Fig. 6.2; Table 6.3). There is some overlap between these groups; for example, the MM1 and MV1 subgroups share neuropathologic and clinical features and are therefore combined into a single subgroup, MM/MV1, which is the most common sCJD subgroup. In contrast, the MM2 subgroup is heterogeneous in its neuropathologic and clinical features and is therefore subdivided into the MM2 cortical (MM2C) and MM2 thalamic (MM2T) subgroups. The MM2T subgroup corresponds to a phenotype closely resembling the genetic prion disease fatal familial insomnia (FFI) and is now referred to as sporadic fatal insomnia.

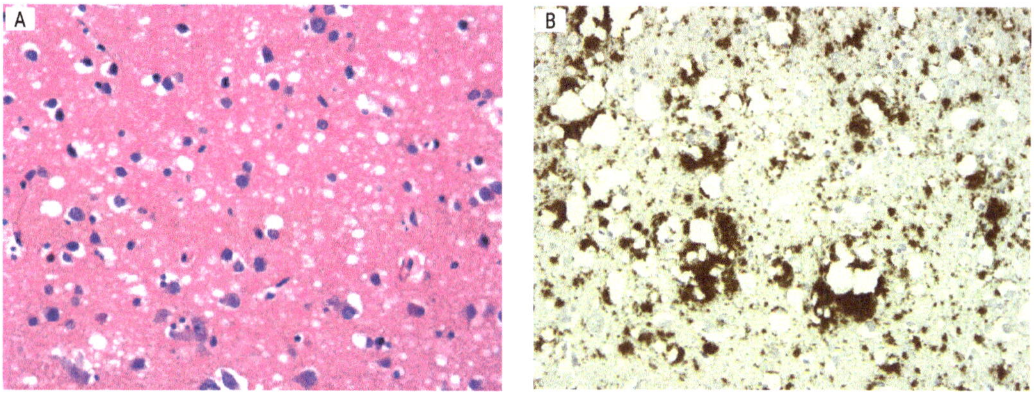

FIGURE 6.2 Sporadic CJD. (**A**) Spongiform change in the cerebral cortex in sporadic CJD MM1 consists of multiple small vacuoles in the gray matter that occasionally join to form larger cyst-like spaces (hematoxylin and eosin [H&E]). (**B**) Immunostaining for PrP shows accumulation of PrP in amorphous deposits around areas of spongiform change.

6.3.1.2. VARIABLY PROTEASE-SENSITIVE PRIONOPATHY

In 2008, a novel form of prion disease now known as variably protease-sensitive prionopathy (VPSPr) was defined. More than 40 patients have been identified worldwide. It differs in clinical features from sCJD, with features including psychiatric symptoms; language deficits (including aphasia); cognitive impairment; and motor signs, including parkinsonism. The disease duration is longer than in sCJD. All three *PRNP* codon 129 genotypes are affected. Interestingly, the *PRNP* codon 129 MM genotype is rare.

Spongiform change is present, particularly in the neocortical and subcortical regions of the cerebrum, and spongiform change and microplaques are present in the cerebellar cortex (Fig. 6.3). The most

Table 6.3 Summary of Genotypes and Phenotypes of Sporadic Human Prion Diseases

CLINICAL DISEASE	*PRNP* MUTATION	*PRNP* CODON 129	PRP^{SC} ISOTYPE	PROPOSED PRP-IMMUNOHISTOCHEMISTRY CORRELATE
Sporadic CJD (myoclonic, Heidenhain variants)	None	MM, MV	Type 1A	Synaptic and coarse granular staining in cerebral cortex and cerebellum
Sporadic CJD (Brownell–Oppenheimer variant)	None	VV	Type 2A	Plaque-like, focal, and perineuronal staining with severe cerebellar involvement
Sporadic CJD (Kuru-plaque variant)	None	MV	Type 2A	Kuru-type amyloid plaques in the cerebellum
Sporadic CJD (sporadic fatal insomnia)	None	MM	Type 2A	Staining faint and variable, similar to that in fatal familial insomnia
Sporadic CJD (cortical variant)	None	MM	Type 2A	Cortical perivacuolar staining
Sporadic CJD	None	VV	Type 1A	Faint synaptic cortical staining
Variant CJD	None	MM	Type 2B	Florid and cluster plaques in cerebral cortex and cerebellum

CJD, Creutzfeldt–Jakob disease; M, methionine; V, valine.

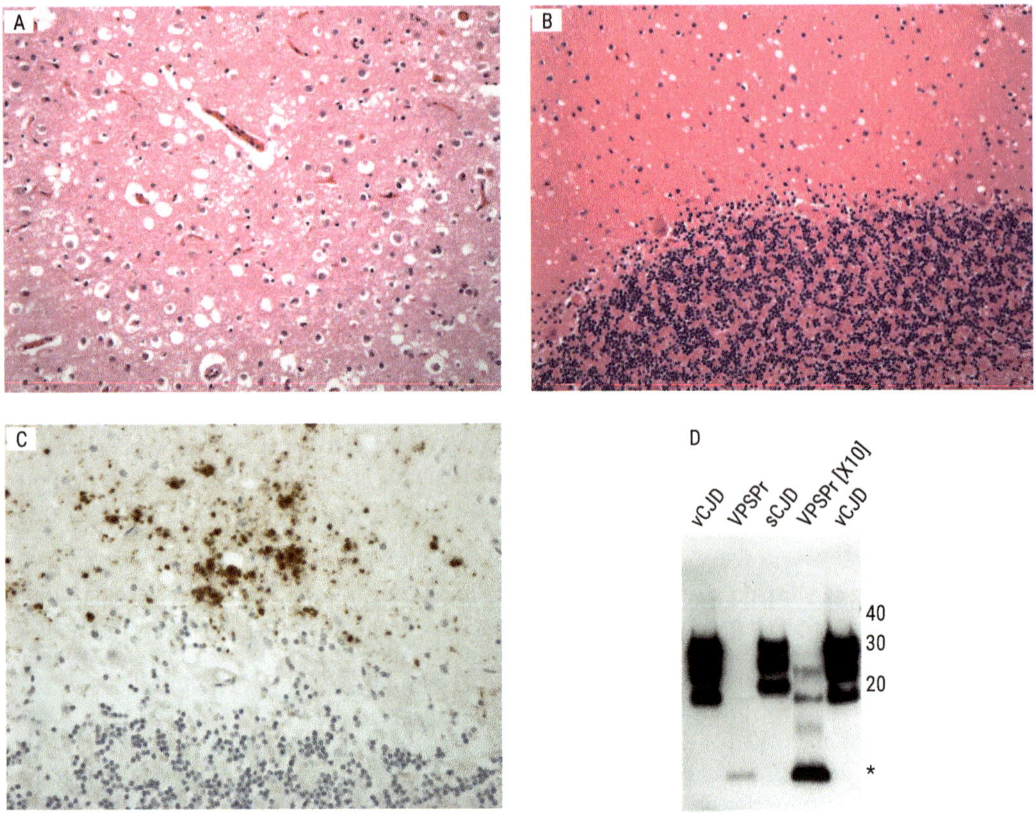

FIGURE 6.3 Variably protease-sensitive prionopathy (VPSPr). (**A**) VPSPr shows spongiform change in the frontal cortex (H&E); (**B**) focal fine vacuolation in the cerebellar cortex (H&E); (**C**) microplaques in the cerebellar cortex (PrP immunohistochemistry [IHC]). (**D**) Western blot analysis of protease-resistant PrP in VPSPr compared to that of variant Creutzfeldt–Jakob disease (vCJD) and sporadic Creutzfeldt–Jakob disease (sCJD) shows a faint ladder of higher molecular weight bands in addition to the prominent approximately 8-kDa band (*) that characterizes VPSPr.

striking feature of VPSPr is the banding pattern of the disease-associated prion protein in the brain on Western blot examination (Fig. 6.3). This shows a ladder-like electrophoretic profile with five major bands, in which the 7- to 8-kDa band may predominate. This appearance is in marked contrast to other human prion diseases.

The full characterization of this novel disorder is still underway; the results of experimental transmission studies indicated that VPSPr differs from sCJD in its transmission properties, thus indicating that it may derive from a different human prion strain. However, its potential for human-to-human transmission remains unclear.

6.3.2. Genetic prion diseases

Genetic prion diseases occur as autosomal dominant disorders with high penetrance and include a wide range of clinicopathologic phenotypes, which are categorized as familial CJD (fCJD), Gerstmann–Sträussler–Scheinker (GSS) disease, FFI, and a range of other variable phenotypes. The first genetic abnormality to be identified in a familial prion disease was the *PRNP* P102L mutation in GSS in 1989. Since then, more than 40 different *PRNP* mutations, including missense, deletion, insertion, and amber mutations, have been identified. The insertional mutations are in the octapeptide repeat region. In addition to mutations, the polymorphic codon 129 on both the mutant and non mutated alleles of *PRNP* can strongly influence disease phenotype: The amino acid at codon 129 on the same allele as the disease-causing mutation can influence the clinical and pathologic features of the disease, whereas the amino acid at codon 129 on the other allele predominantly influences age of onset and disease duration. For this reason, it has been proposed that mutations which cause familial forms are to be identified with both the details of the mutation and the codon 129 context.

6.3.2.1. FAMILIAL CREUTZFELDT-JAKOB DISEASE

In fCJD, the range of clinical and pathologic phenotypes resembles those observed for sCJD. Some cases, initially suspected to be sCJD because of the apparent absence of a positive family history, have subsequently been found to be associated with a *PRNP* mutation. The most common *PRNP* haplotypes to be associated with fCJD are E200K-129M and D178N-129V (Table 6.4). Phenotypic variability occurs within affected families in terms of both the clinical and pathologic features of the disease.

6.3.2.2. GERSTMANN-STRÄUSSLER-SCHEINKER DISEASE

Gerstmann–Sträussler–Scheinker disease is a progressive cerebellar syndrome, accompanied by pyramidal signs and progressive cognitive decline, which may result in dementia. The histological feature in GSS is the presence of multicentric PrP-amyloid plaques in the cerebral and cerebellar cortex, while spongiform change may or may not be present (Fig. 6.4). Several point mutations resulting in a similar clinicopathologic phenotype have been described (Table 6.4). The F198S and Q217R mutations are associated with neocortical neurofibrillary tangles (similar to those found in Alzheimer disease), in addition to widespread multicentric and unicentric PrP-amyloid plaques.

6.3.2.3. PRION DISEASE WITH CEREBRAL AMYLOID ANGIOPATHY

While PrP-amyloid deposits in the parenchyma in some forms of prion disease, selective vascular wall accumulation of this material can be seen in the rare setting of stop mutations in *PRNP* (Y145stop, Y226stop). In these cases, the clinical course is usually a relatively prolonged progressive cognitive decline leading to dementia, whereas the common histological feature is the vascular and perivascular amyloid deposits, minimal spongiform change, and neurofibrillary tangle accumulation in neurons near the affected vessels. Interestingly, this pattern of disease does not always result from truncation mutations in PrP, as another missense mutation (Q227stop) gives rise to a pattern more in keeping with GSS, again with abundant neurofibrillary tangles.

Table 6.4 Most Common Haplotypes and Phenotypes of Familial Human Prion Diseases

CLINICAL DISEASE	*PRNP* HAPLOTYPE	PRP^{SC} ISOTYPE	HISTOLOGICAL CORRELATES
Gerstmann–Sträussler–Scheinker disease	P102L-129M	Type 1B and 8 kDa	Spongiform change, synaptic PrP, amyloid plaques
		8 kDa only	PrP-amyloid plaques, no spongiform change
	P105L-129V A117V-129V H187R-129V	8 kDa	Multicentric amyloid plaques, no spongiform change
	F198S-129V Q217R-129V	8 kDa	Multicentric amyloid plaques, no spongiform change and neurofibrillary tangles
Fatal familial insomnia	D178N-129M	Type 2B	Thalamic atrophy, inferior olivary gliosis
Familial Creutzfeldt–Jakob disease	D178N-129V	Type 1B	Cortical spongiform degeneration
	E200K-129M	Type 1B	Diffuse PrP staining
	E200K-129V	Type 2B	Diffuse PrP staining in cortex, focal deposits in the cerebellum or plaque-like deposits in the cerebellum

M, methionine; V, valine.

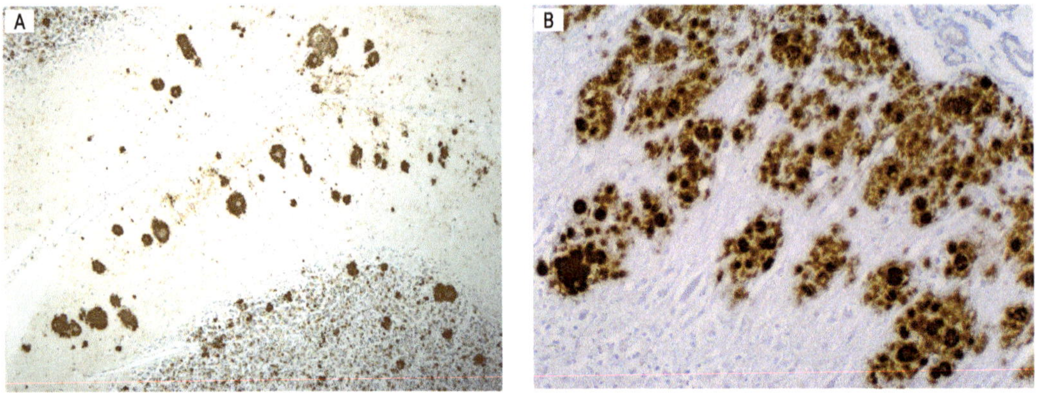

FIGURE 6.4 Gerstmann–Sträussler–Scheinker disease: (**A, B**) multicentric PrP plaques in the cerebellar molecular layer; smaller plaques are present in the granular layer (PrP IHC).

A novel clinicopathologic phenotype of genetic human prion disease has recently been reported, characterized by diarrhea, autonomic neuropathy, and systemic PrP amyloidosis. A previously unreported *PRNP* Y163X truncation mutation was found in affected family members.

6.3.2.4. PRION DISEASES ASSOCIATED WITH OCTAPEPTIDE REPEAT REGION INSERTIONAL MUTATIONS (VARIABLE PHENOTYPES)

In patients with insertional mutations in the octapeptide repeat region of the *PRNP*, the clinical manifestations are highly variable both in terms of disease duration and in the disease phenotype. In general, patients with up to four additional copies of the octapeptide repeats have a clinical phenotype similar to sCJD, with rapidly progressive dementia and characteristic EEG abnormalities. In patients with a larger number of extra repeats, the clinical phenotype is more variable, often with progressive ataxia and other movement disorders. Histologically, these cases often show unusual linear PrP deposits in the molecular layer of the cerebellum (Fig. 6.5); however, the other neuropathologic features are somewhat more variable.

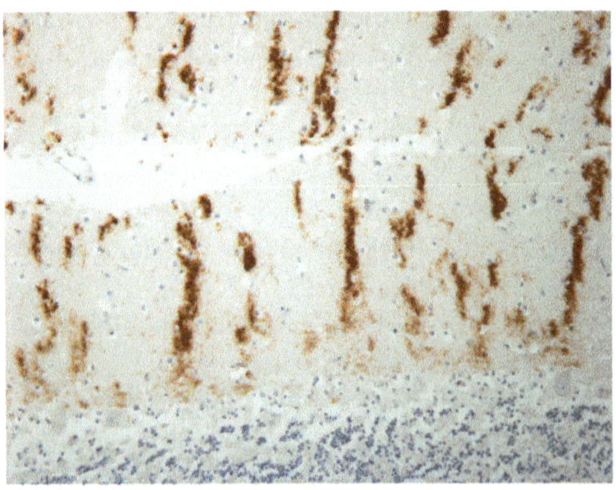

FIGURE 6.5 Prion disease with octapeptide repeat region insertional mutations. Linear deposits of PrP in the molecular layer of the cerebellum (PrP IHC).

6.3.2.5. FATAL FAMILIAL INSOMNIA

Fatal familial insomnia is a disorder characterized by sleep disturbance, dysautonomia, and motor signs, with cognitive abnormalities, which are often relatively mild but tend to increase with the duration of the disease. The neuropathology of FFI is characterized by severe neuronal loss and gliosis in the anterior thalamic nuclei (Fig. 6.6) and in the hypothalamus, in the absence of spongiform change and PrP^{Sc} deposition. Neuronal loss and gliosis are also evident in the inferior olivary nuclei (Fig. 6.6) and to a lesser, but variable, extent in the cerebral and cerebellar cortex. Spongiform changes can be remarkably difficult to detect in this disorder but are usually apparent on careful study of the cerebellar cortex. In some cases, tissue blots obtained from sections of paraffin-embedded tissue may help identify PrP^{Sc} deposition, particularly in the entorhinal cortex (Fig. 6.6).

The discovery that FFI is caused by a mutation in *PRNP* highlights the impact of codon 129 on disease phenotype (Table 6.4). The identified mutation, shared across FFI kindreds, is D178N, which had already been demonstrated to cause fCJD. It was recognized that D178N-129M results in FFI,

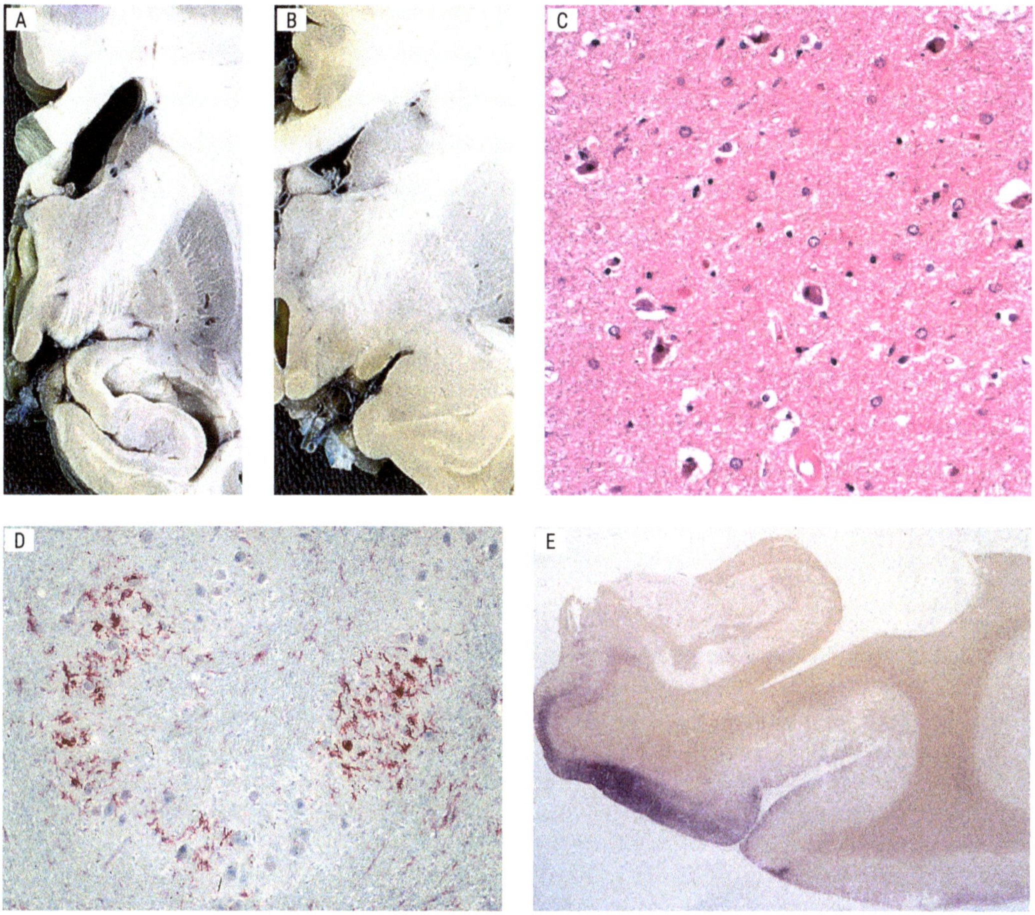

FIGURE 6.6 Fatal familial insomnia. Coronal section of the right thalamus through the mammillary bodies showing atrophy of the anterior and medial nuclei in an FFI case (**A**) compared to a normal control (**B**). (Courtesy of Professor Danielle Seilhean.) (**C**) Microscopic appearance of the medial thalamus with neuronal loss and gliosis (note the absence of spongiosis; H&E). (**D**) Immunohistochemistry for glial fibrillary acidic protein (GFAP) showing neuronal loss and gliosis in the medullary olive (GFAP IHC). (**E**) Paraffin-embedded tissue immunoblotting shows PrP deposition in the entorhinal cortex. (Courtesy of Professor Francesco Scaravilli.)

whereas D178N-129V results in fCJD. Phenotypic variability has been described within FFI, usually under the influence of the codon 129 genotype on the nonmutated allele.

6.3.3. Acquired prion diseases

There are several types of acquired prion diseases: kuru, iatrogenic CJD, and variant CJD.

6.3.3.1. KURU

Kuru was described as an endemic disease among the Fore tribe of Papua New Guinea in the 1950s. The disease was characterized by progressive ataxia and tremor with marked emotional instability, but rapidly progressive dementia was not a common feature. The disease was associated with ritualistic cannibalism, and since this practice has been discouraged, the incidence of disease has declined significantly. The disease is now extinct, and some of the last symptomatic patients sustained incubation periods of approximately 40 years.

The pathology of kuru is similar to that of sCJD VV2 and MV2 subsets, with amyloid plaques, so-called kuru plaques, present in the cerebellum, particularly in the granular cell layer (Fig. 6.7), and spongiform change noted in the cerebellum, basal ganglia, and thalamus, with a variable distribution in the cerebral cortex. Immunohistochemistry for PrP not only has highlighted the presence of the amyloid deposits in the cerebellum (Fig. 6.7) but also has

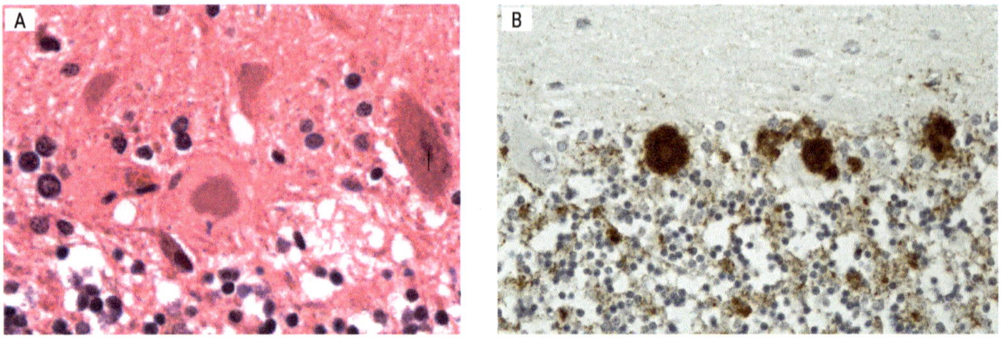

FIGURE 6.7 Kuru. (**A**) Kuru plaque in the molecular layer of the cerebellum (H&E). (**B**) Kuru plaques are well identified on PrP immunostaining in the granular layer of the cerebellum.

demonstrated diffuse deposits, which are not identifiable on routine stains.

6.3.3.2. IATROGENIC CJD

In 1974, the occurrence of iatrogenic CJD (iCJD) was reported in a recipient of a corneal transplant. Since then, more than 500 cases of human transmission of CJD have been identified; the majority of these have been recipients of autopsy-derived human pituitary hormones (mostly growth hormone) or human dura mater grafts. A summary of the routes of transmission of iCJD is given in Table 6.5. There is a relationship between the route of infection and incubation times, with a central route of infection having the shortest incubation times, whereas the peripheral route of infection (particularly in growth hormone recipients) has a longer incubation period.

The clinical features of iCJD are variable; some patients (particularly those with a "central" route of transmission) have features resembling those of sCJD, whereas others (including the human pituitary hormone recipients) often present with a progressive cerebellar ataxia and other focal neurological symptoms, as well as dementia occurring only later in the illness.

Histologically, iCJD is similar to sCJD, although the cerebellar pathology in the pituitary hormone recipients tends to be more severe than in sCJD (Fig. 6.8). In general, iCJD has developed more frequently in the setting of homozygosity at codon 129. There is an intriguing observation that cases from the United Kingdom are more commonly 129VV, whereas those from France are more commonly 129MM; this may reflect differences in the strains of the contaminating prion agents.

Recent studies of iCJD in human growth hormone and human dura mater graft recipients have found evidence of increased Aβ deposition in the brain, both as diffuse and neuritic plaques and as cerebral amyloid angiopathy. Because low levels of Aβ

Table 6.5 Routes of Iatrogenic Transmission of Creutzfeldt–Jakob Disease

SOURCE OF INFECTION	NO. OF REPORTED CASES	INCUBATION PERIOD (YEARS)
Neurosurgical instruments	4	1.4–2.2
Intracerebral electrodes	2	1.3–1.7
Dura mater graft	244	1.3–30
Corneal graft	2	1.5–30
Human growth hormone	242	5–42
Human gonadotrophin	4	12–16
Blood transfusion (vCJD)	3	6.5–8.3

vCJD, variant Creutzfeldt–Jakob disease.

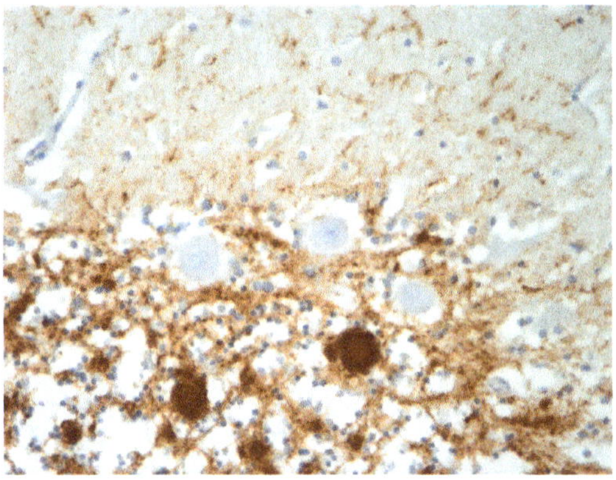

FIGURE 6.8 Iatrogenic CJD. Iatrogenic CJD in a growth hormone recipient: The cerebellum contains small kuru-type plaques as well as more diffuse PrP deposits (PrP IHC).

can be present in both the pituitary gland and dura mater, these findings raise the possibility that iatrogenic amyloid seeding of Aβ has occurred in the brains of these patients by a prion-like mechanism.

6.3.3.3. VARIANT CJD

In 1996, a novel form of prion disease with unusual clinical, biological, and pathologic features was identified by the National CJD Surveillance Unit in the United Kingdom. A causative relationship with the epidemic of BSE in cattle seemed likely. Since then, more than 200 patients with this disease, subsequently known as variant CJD (vCJD), have been identified worldwide.

Clinically, there is a relatively young age at onset (mean: 27 years; range: 12–74 years). The lengthy duration of illness (13 months) and clinical presentation are also characteristic. The latter includes psychiatric or sensory manifestations at onset, followed by severe progressive ataxia, extrapyramidal and pyramidal signs, and progressive dementia that in some cases is severe. The EEG is abnormal and may occasionally exhibit the characteristic abnormalities seen in sCJD. Cranial magnetic resonance imaging (MRI) scans show a symmetrical area of hyperintensity on FLAIR sequences in the posterior thalamus (the "pulvinar sign") (Fig. 6.9), which is highly characteristic and has been incorporated into the clinical diagnostic criteria for vCJD. Analysis of CSF 14-3-3 levels has not proven useful in making the diagnosis of vCJD, but detection of elevated CSF phosphorylated tau can contribute to establishing such a diagnosis.

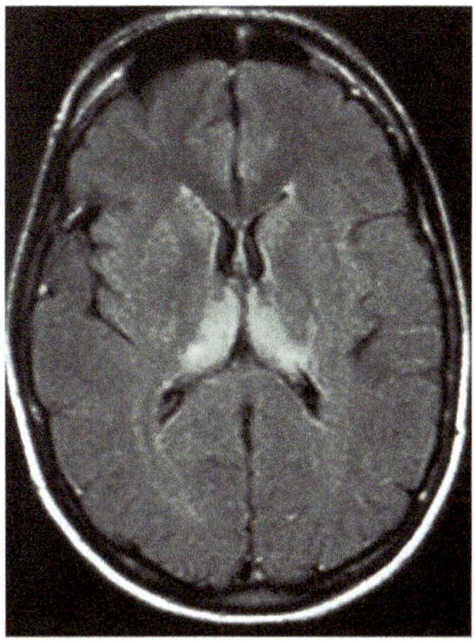

FIGURE 6.9 Variant CJD, brain imaging. Axial MRI FLAIR image at the level of the basal ganglia showing bilateral hyperintensity of the pulvinar and dorsomedial thalamic nuclei in variant CJD.

Pathologically, vCJD differs from other forms of human prion disease by the presence of large numbers of "florid" plaques with a widespread distribution in the cerebral cortex (Fig. 6.10) and in the cerebellum. These lesions comprise a central eosinophilic amyloid core with radiating bundles of amyloid fibrils, surrounded by spongiform change. Apart from the florid plaques, other characteristic neuropathologic features of vCJD include extensive PrP^{Sc} accumulation as both small cluster plaques and diffuse deposits (Fig. 6.10), with spongiform change most marked in the caudate nucleus and putamen. In the thalamus, there is extensive neuronal loss and gliosis in the posterior nuclei, corresponding to the abnormalities on MRI.

Western blot analysis of the brain in vCJD shows a characteristic PrP^{Sc} isotype, with a predominant diglycosylated band and an unglycosylated band that migrates around 21 kDa (Fig. 6.1). This glycosylation pattern is similar to that on Western blots for PrP^{Sc} in cattle with BSE and in other species (e.g., cats) that have been infected with BSE.

At the time of the original description, it was suggested that the most likely hypothesis for the emergence of vCJD is exposure of the human population to the BSE agent. A number of independent investigations have demonstrated that the structural characteristics of the transmissible agent in vCJD are quite similar to those for BSE but share no similarities with those of sCJD. On this basis, it is assumed that most human cases of vCJD result from exposure to BSE through the food chain (i.e., by the consumption of contaminated meat products). There is also evidence from a case–control study to suggest that consumption of certain meat products is higher in patients with vCJD than in controls.

Because the most likely route of exposure to BSE in humans is the oral route, studies have been performed on tissues outside the CNS in order to investigate the peripheral pathogenesis of this disease. PrP^{Sc} is detectable in follicular dendritic cells within germinal centers in lymphoid tissues, including the tonsil (Fig. 6.10), lymph nodes, spleen, thymus, and gut-associated lymphoid tissues in the appendix and small intestine. Experimental transmission studies have confirmed the presence of transmissibility from the spleen and tonsil

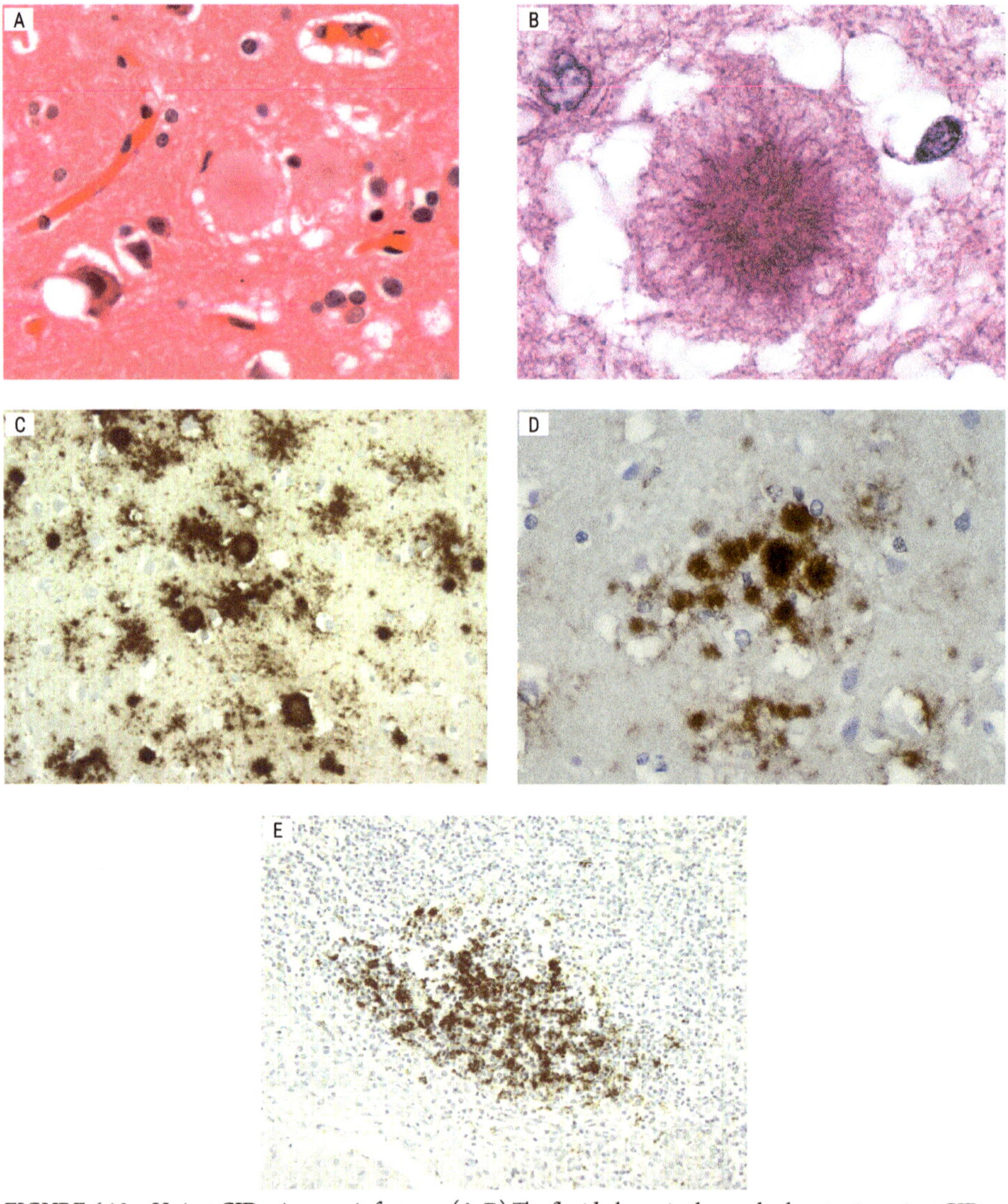

FIGURE 6.10 Variant CJD microscopic features. (**A, B**) The florid plaque in the cerebral cortex in variant CJD comprises a dense core with paler outer layer of amyloid fibrils, surrounded by spongiform change (H&E). (**C, D**) Florid plaques, as well as multiple smaller plaques and diffuse PrP deposits (PrP IHC). (**E**) PrP accumulation in the palatine tonsil in variant CJD within follicular dendritic cells and macrophages in a germinal center (PrP IHC).

of individuals with vCJD; however, the level of infectivity is two or three times lower than that in the brain.

At the time of writing, 233 cases of vCJD had been reported worldwide, of which 178 occurred in the United Kingdom. Until 2016, all patients with definite vCJD were homozygous for methionine at codon 129 in the *PRNP*. However, a case of definite vCJD was recently reported in a *PRNP* codon 129 MV patient, raising the possibility of future cases in this genotype, which is the most common codon 129 polymorphism in Caucasians (Table 6.2). In the United Kingdom, vCJD infection has been transmitted on four occasions by blood transfusion from asymptomatic donors who subsequently died from vCJD. Three of the four recipients were 129MM and later died from vCJD, but the fourth recipient was a heterozygote (129MV). This recipient died from other causes but with no evidence of a neurological disorder; at autopsy, PrP^{Sc} was detected in the spleen and lymph nodes, although not in the brain and spinal cord. Subsequent experimental transmission from the spleen showed a typical incubation period, neuropathology, and PrP^{Sc} isotype for vCJD. The number of new vCJD cases worldwide is declining, and the number of future vCJD cases is uncertain. Although there is evidence of asymptomatic vCJD infection and there are novel techniques to detect PrP^{Sc}, not only in CNS and non-CNS tissues but also in urine or blood of patients with vCJD, there have been no new cases of vCJD since 2020. Thus epidemiological models estimate low numbers of future vCJD cases.

6.4. PRACTICAL CONSIDERATIONS FOR THE INVESTIGATION OF HUMAN PRION DISEASES

A definite diagnosis of a human prion disease requires neuropathologic or biochemical confirmation. The autopsy should be performed according to World Health Organization guidelines to minimize the potential risks of accidental exposure to prion infectivity and to reduce contamination of the mortuary environment. Both fixed and frozen brain tissue should be retained for further investigations. Sampling of non-CNS tissues (particularly lymphoid tissues) may also be of diagnostic value, especially in cases of suspected vCJD. Extensive sampling of the brain for microscopy is essential because the distribution of pathology is highly variable, even between cases of the same form of prion disease. All regions of the cerebral cortex should be examined, along with the hippocampus, basal ganglia, thalamus, brainstem, and cerebellum. Formalin-fixed tissue blocks can be decontaminated by incubation in 96% formic acid for 1 hour. Subsequent washing and renewed formalin fixation and processing allow embedding of decontaminated tissue in paraffin.

7

Multiple Sclerosis and Related Inflammatory Demyelinating Diseases

HANS LASSMAN AND DANIELLE SEILHEAN

INFLAMMATORY DEMYELINATING diseases are defined by the selective destruction of myelin sheaths and oligodendrocytes, which arises in a background of acute or chronic inflammation. There is a spectrum of inflammatory demyelinating diseases that includes multiple sclerosis (MS), acute disseminated encephalomyelitis (ADEM), concentric sclerosis (Baló disease), and neuromyelitis optica (NMO). These diseases have a diverse pathogenesis but share some morphologic features and molecular pathways of tissue injury. Within typical demyelinating lesions, myelin sheaths are lost, whereas axons are relatively preserved; they appear naked and are surrounded by reactive glial tissue. However, as demonstrated even in the earliest descriptions of the pathology of MS, axons are affected and variably reduced in all lesions. Rather than only demyelination, neuroaxonal degeneration is a major correlate of irreversible functional deficits in affected patients. Slower impulse conduction also occurs in demyelinated axons. Demyelination and oligodendrocyte loss can, at least in part, be repaired by remyelination due to recruitment and differentiation of oligodendrocyte progenitor cells. In contrast, spontaneous regeneration of axons or neurons does not occur in the affected central nervous system (CNS). There is evidence that inflammation drives the formation of lesions in inflammatory demyelinating diseases, but the cause of the chronic inflammation, whether of primary autoimmune nature or as a reaction to a chronic infectious or another injurious process, is still unresolved.

7.1. MULTIPLE SCLEROSIS

The clinical spectrum of MS is highly variable. It is determined by the location of lesions within the CNS and the stage of evolution of the disease. The symptoms most commonly start with episodes of neurologic deficits that may resolve, but they are followed by phases of relapses (relapsing/remitting MS [RRMS]). After approximately 10 years of disease duration, this pattern evolves to a phase of less episodic and uninterrupted progression (secondary progressive MS [SPMS]). In a minority of patients, the relapsing stage of the disease is absent, and the patients show uninterrupted progression from the onset (primary progressive MS [PPMS]). Acute MS (Marburg type) is a fulminant, usually monophasic, disease that leads to death of the patient within 1 year after onset.

There are several features of the clinical picture that are particularly important for interpretation of the pathology and understanding the pathogenesis of the disease. In RRMS, clinical disease is largely characterized by new lesions in the white matter that show contrast enhancement on magnetic resonance imaging (MRI) (i.e., reflect inflammation and blood–brain barrier damage). In this stage, anti-inflammatory and immunosuppressive treatments are most effective. Clinically, the progressive stage of the disease mainly occurs later in life; the onset of disease in PPMS generally occurs at the same age as when disease in other patients switches from RRMS to SPMS. In the progressive stage, clinical deterioration does not correlate as well with new white matter lesions, and enhancing lesions on MRI are rare or absent. The speed of progression of the disease is surprisingly uniform and is poorly correlated to the number, or the clinical severity, of previous relapses. Most important, the efficacy of anti-inflammatory or immunosuppressive treatments is minimal or absent at this stage of the disease. Thus, from a clinical standpoint, MS seems to start as an inflammatory disease that gives rise to white matter lesions and subsequently may evolve into a neurodegenerative disease as the disease progresses. This is the current understanding of the disease.

7.1.1. The pathology of multiple sclerosis

The pathology of MS is defined by the triad of inflammation, demyelination, and glial scar formation.

7.1.1.1. INFLAMMATION

Inflammation can be present in all stages of MS. Inflammatory infiltrates are present around small veins and venules within active white matter lesions. Parenchymal infiltration by inflammatory cells is generally associated with active demyelination or neurodegeneration in discrete lesions known as plaques and, to a variable extent, in the more normal-appearing white and gray matter. Inflammatory infiltrates mainly consist of T cells, of which $CD8^+$ cells outnumber $CD4^+$ ones. $CD8^+$ T cells show dominant clonal expansion, suggesting the expansion of this particular cell type through local recognition of their cognate antigen(s). The phenotype of these T cells suggests that they are tissue-resident memory cells. The B lymphocytes are also components of the infiltrates and contribute to less than 50% of the total lymphocyte population. The B cells and plasma cells are mainly present in the leptomeninges and perivascular Virchow–Robin spaces, whereas their infiltration into the parenchyma is less common. Inflammation in the brain of patients with MS is accompanied by additional recruitment of monocytes and macrophages and even more abundantly by pro-inflammatory activation of the local microglia population. Active demyelination and tissue injury are invariably associated with the presence of activated microglia and macrophages.

At the sites of inflammation, and in particular within active lesions, molecules that are involved in induction, propagation, and control of the inflammatory process are expressed. They include class I and class II major histocompatibility complex molecules (necessary for antigen presentation for T cells); adhesion molecules; chemokines and their receptors (which are important for recruitment and migration of inflammatory cells); cytokines (which are involved in propagation or termination of the inflammatory process); Fc receptors and complement (involved in antibody-mediated cell injury); and molecules involved in macrophage toxicity (e.g., cytotoxic cytokines, proteases, and enzymes responsible for the production of reactive oxygen and nitric oxide species).

Inflammation is most extensive in active lesions at early stages of MS (acute and RRMS) but is invariably also present in patients at the progressive stage of the disease when there is ongoing active demyelination and neurodegeneration. In newly developing lesions in the early stages of the disease, inflammation is associated with increased permeability of the blood–brain barrier, which is associated with the migration of newly recruited inflammatory cells from the blood into the CNS. With increased disease duration, part of the inflammatory response becomes trapped or compartmentalized within the brain and spinal cord. The compartmentalized inflammatory response is composed of tissue resident T cells and B cells/plasma cells. The latter are the source of intrathecally produced immunoglobulins, detected in the cerebrospinal fluid as oligoclonal bands of immunoglobulin. During phases of active progression, tissue resident T and B cells show signs of focally or temporally restricted activation and proliferation. In the very late stages of the disease, inflammation may subside to levels observed in age-matched controls. In these patients, no active demyelination is seen, and active neurodegeneration is similar to that seen in age-matched controls. However, when the threshold of functional compensation has been passed due to the accumulated brain damage, clinical disease may progress due to age-related neurodegeneration.

7.1.1.2. DEMYELINATED LESIONS IN THE WHITE MATTER

Focal demyelinated plaques in the white matter are the hallmark of MS pathology. They occur at any sites of the brain and spinal cord but are more frequently located in certain sites that include the periventricular areas of the cerebral hemispheres, subcortical cerebral white matter, the optic nerves, the optic chiasm, the optic tracts, the periventricular regions of the brainstem, the cerebellum, and the spinal cord (Figs. 7.1 and 7.2). In the spinal cord, the lesions generally show a triangular, fan-shaped appearance with the tip of the triangle pointing toward the central gray matter. There is no predilection of plaque localization for specific neuroanatomical tracts, functional systems, neuronal populations using a particular neurotransmitter, or vascular territories. However, areas with a high density of venules and veins are more likely to be affected, and a topographical relationship between plaques and draining veins was demonstrated in the earliest descriptions of the disease.

On gross examination of the CNS, the plaques become more visible after a brief exposure to room air; they are localized predominantly in the white matter but may also extend into gray matter. Their outline is rounded but of variable shape, and they are sharply demarcated from surrounding normal brain tissue (Fig. 7.3). Recent lesions tend to be pink or yellowish and are less sharply defined, whereas older lesions tend to have sharp borders and are grayish or translucent and firm. On microscopic examination, plaques are characterized by loss of myelin in discrete, well-circumscribed areas; this results in a punched-out appearance when sections are stained for myelin (e.g., Heidenhain–Woelcke, Loyez, or Luxol fast blue stains) (Figs. 7.1, 7.2, and 7.4). Methods to demonstrate axons, including silver impregnation or immunohistochemistry for neurofilaments, show a network of variably reduced, but relatively preserved, axons in the plaque, with some axonal swellings or "spheroids" that indicate acute axon injury. Overall axonal density can be reduced by 60% on average within chronic lesions compared to the surrounding white matter. Also, in a given case, the extent of axonal loss is variable from one lesion to another (Fig. 7.5).

Reactive glial cells (astrocytes and microglia) are intimately involved in the pathology of MS lesions. Perivascular cells and parenchymal microglia show evidence of immune activation, and astrocytes show marked hypertrophy and proliferation. Astrogliosis is maximal at the edge of the plaque. Toward the center of the plaque, gliosis tends to become more fibrillary and, in older lesions, forms a dense glial scar consisting of expanded and thickened arborization of astrocytic processes (Fig. 7.6). When gliosis is abundant and particularly active, some large astrocytes have fragmented nuclei. These are known as Creutzfeldt–Peters cells (Fig. 7.6D); they may occur in any condition with long-standing gliosis and should not be confused with malignant glial cells.

Actively demyelinating MS lesions (Fig. 7.7) are seen as both classical active plaques and slowly expanding lesions. Classical active plaques are mainly seen in acute and RRMS. They transform from initial to inactive or remyelinated stages within weeks. In early stages, they are characterized by marked inflammation and damage to the blood–brain barrier. The lesions are heavily infiltrated with macrophages, which contain early myelin degradation products that have staining properties similar to those of normal myelin (e.g., appearing as blue granules in sections stained with Luxol fast blue). Macrophages are either dispersed throughout the whole lesion (as is seen in acute plaques) (Fig. 7.7B) or concentrated at the margin in chronic active plaques (Fig. 7.4). The outer rim of chronic active plaques varies in thickness and contains large numbers of oligodendrocyte progenitor cells or newly differentiated remyelinating oligodendrocytes; myelin sheaths in these areas are in the initial stage of dissolution and are associated with activated microglia. These peripheral regions are the advancing edge of demyelination and tissue injury. Macrophages remaining in the center of the plaques, which have ingested and degraded myelin (Fig. 7.7D), express low levels of pro-inflammatory activation markers (e.g., inducible nitric oxide synthase or NADPH [reduced nicotinamide adenine dinucleotide phosphate]

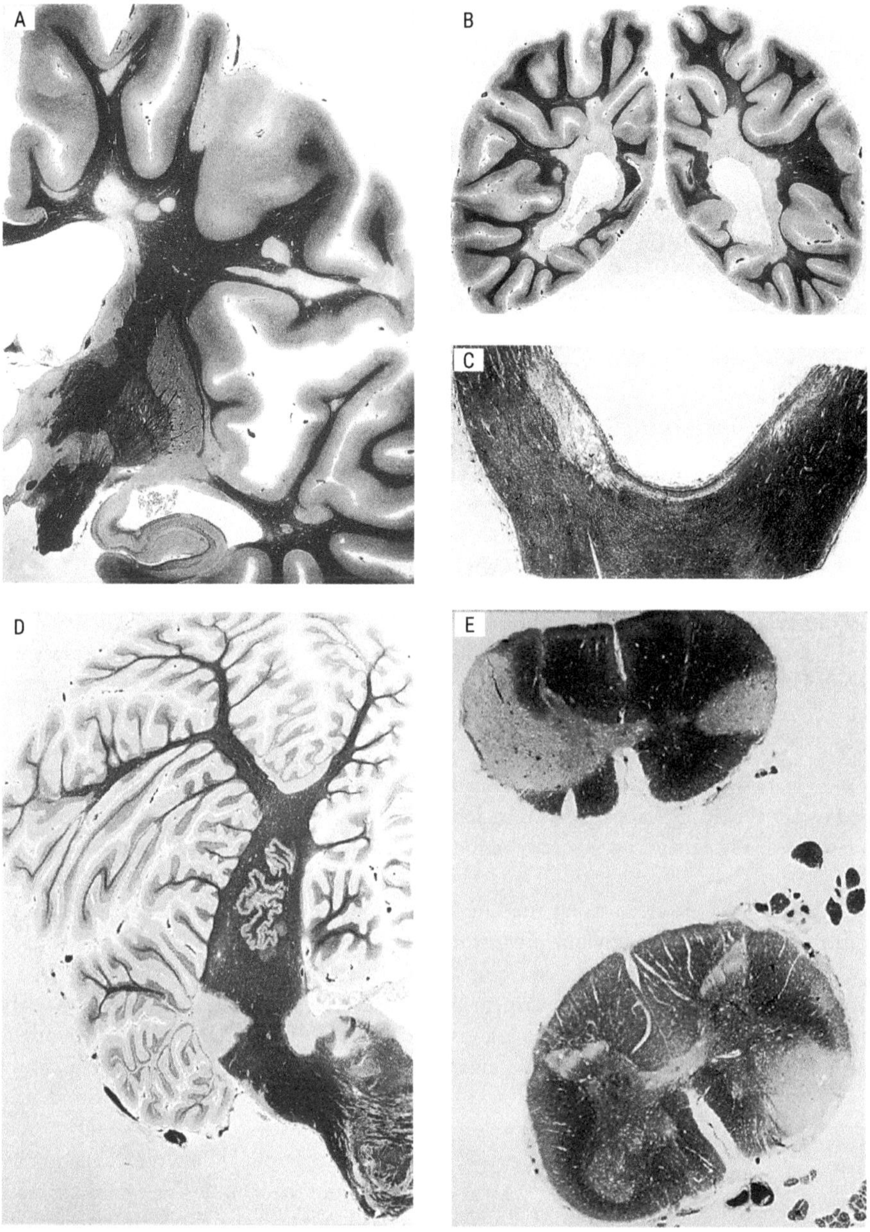

FIGURE 7.1 Principal topographical features of MS lesions (Loyez stain for myelin): (**A**) right cerebral hemisphere with multiple plaques disseminated in the white matter; (**B**) parieto-occipital region of cerebral hemispheres with confluent periventricular distribution of plaques; (**C**) demyelination in the optic chiasm; (**D**) left hemicerebellum and pons with plaques in the anterior aspect of the fourth ventricle and in the cerebellar peduncle; (**E**) plaques involving the spinal cord at the thoracic (upper) and lumbar (lower) levels; although a plaque is present in the right cerebrospinal tract at the thoracic level, there is no degeneration at the lumbar level, demonstrating the absence of Wallerian degeneration.

oxidases) and change their polarization toward an anti-inflammatory or neuroprotective phenotype.

In contrast, slowly expanding lesions are abundant in patients with late relapsing or progressive disease (PPMS, SPMS). These lesions are centered on an inactive demyelinated lesion core with profound fibrillary gliosis (Fig. 7.8) and are surrounded by a small rim of activated microglia, few macrophages with early myelin debris, and a variable extent of acute axonal injury. Some of these lesions contain

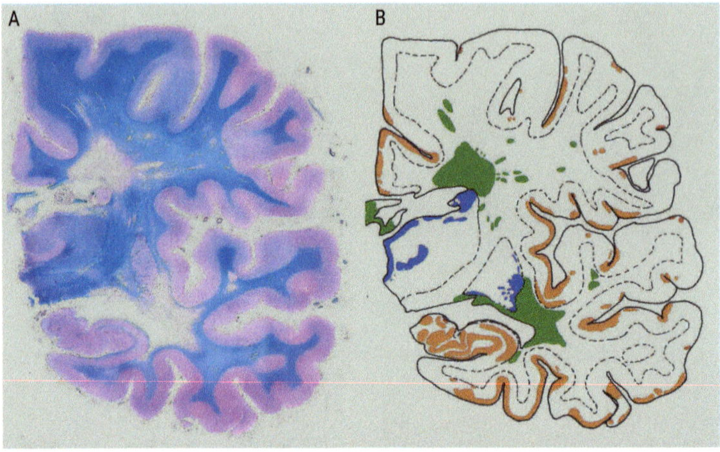

FIGURE 7.2 Distribution of demyelinated lesions in MS (secondary progressive MS). Focal white matter lesions are the hallmark of MS pathology. They are easily demonstrated in fresh brain slices and on sections stained for myelin. (**A**) Hemispheric brain section with multiple plaques (Luxol fast blue). The lesions tend to accumulate in the periventricular white matter, whereas smaller lesions are seen in the depth of the white matter and subcortical area. (**B**) Detailed lesion map that includes white matter and gray matter lesions. In addition to the white matter lesions (*green*), cortical lesions (*orange*) are present as cortico–subcortical lesions, as small intracortical lesions, and, most abundantly, as band-like subpial lesions. In addition, lesions are present in deep gray matter nuclei (*blue*). Subpial cortical lesions are predominantly found in invaginations of the brain surface (sulci, insular cortex, cingulate cortex, and hippocampus).

microglia cells loaded with iron, and their fate can be followed by serial MRI. Serial MRI has revealed that such lesions slowly expand over a time period of years (Fig. 7.9).

Axonal injury is best detected using immunohistochemistry to demonstrate amyloid precursor protein (APP) in axonal swellings and end bulbs. Perivascular inflammatory infiltrates and dispersed T cells are also present in slowly expanding lesions but are not associated with any increase of vascular permeability for serum proteins. In inactive lesions (Fig. 7.8), demyelinated areas are sharply demarcated from the surrounding normal-appearing white matter. They may contain some foci of inflammatory infiltrates and acutely injured axons, but they lack the rim of activated microglia and ongoing demyelination at the outer limit of the lesion.

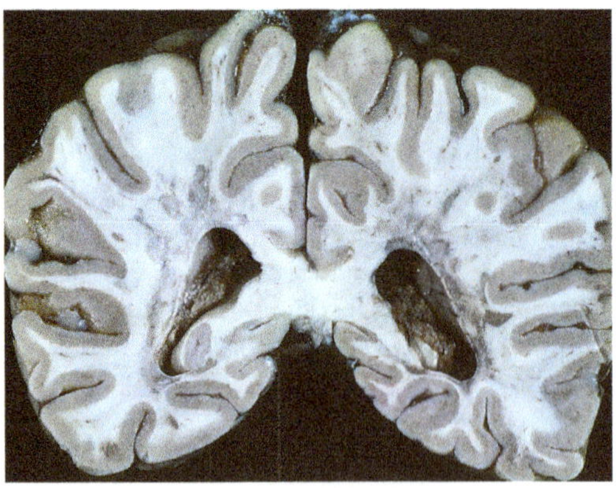

FIGURE 7.3 Gross appearance of MS. Coronal section of the parieto-occipital region at the level of the splenium of the corpus callosum; note the periventricular distribution of many plaques.

Remyelination in MS lesions is variable; when it does occur, the thickness of the individual myelin sheaths never regains its original, normal diameter. Remyelination may be restricted to the outer margins of the lesion (Fig. 7.4A, D) or may be present throughout. When remyelination is present throughout the plaque, the lesions are referred to as a "shadow plaques"; these are sharply demarcated areas of myelin pallor due to widespread reduction in the thickness of the individual myelin sheaths, formed around one or more central veins with similar shape and location as other MS inactive plaques. Although the extent of remyelination in most patients with MS is limited, rarely it can be quite considerable. Remyelination is more pronounced in lesions within the cortex and the subcortical white matter than in periventricular areas. Thus, the extent of repair may be related to the individual (genetic) predisposition of the patients and to focal differences in tissue susceptibility, such as perfusion and oxygen tension in different brain regions.

Initial stages of remyelination with recruitment of oligodendrocytes from the progenitor cell pool and appearance of thin remyelinated fibers are frequently seen in active lesions in early stages of MS. However, newly formed myelin in patients with MS appears to be unstable because new active demyelination occurs more frequently in previously remyelinated areas than in the normal-appearing white matter. In addition, remyelination is sparse or absent in slowly expanding lesions of patients with progressive MS. These observations may explain the low degree of remyelination in the brain of patients with primary or secondary progressive disease.

7.1.1.3. MULTIPLE SCLEROSIS LESIONS IN CEREBRAL CORTEX AND DEEP GRAY MATTER

Since the initial recognition of MS as a distinct pathologic entity, it has been regarded as a disease primarily affecting the white matter. However, with the introduction of more sensitive tools for the immunohistochemical analysis of myelin proteins, it has now become clear that extensive demyelination also can occur in the gray matter, particularly in the cerebral cortex (Figs. 7.2 and 7.10). Cortical demyelination is scant in the early stages but increases with disease duration, reaching its peak in progressive MS. Three different types of cortical lesions have been described: cortico–subcortical, intracortical perivascular, and band-like subpial lesions. Subpial lesions are the most abundant in patients with progressive MS. They affect the outer cortical layers and can span over several cortical gyri and sulci (Fig. 7.2). They are preferentially located within invaginations of the brain surface, such as cortical sulci; insular, cingulate, or temporal cortex, including the hippocampus; and cerebellar cortex. Because active subpial cortical demyelination occurs at sites of meningeal inflammation, the location of the lesions in the infoldings of the brain surface may be due to preferential persistence of inflammation at sites of low flow of the cerebrospinal fluid. Subpial cortical lesions are unique for MS and are not seen in any other inflammatory, infectious, or degenerative disease of the CNS. Like white matter plaques, cortical plaques show primary demyelination with relative sparing of axons and neurons. When they arise in early stages of MS, inflammation is prominent in active lesions even within the cortical parenchyma. However, in progressive MS, inflammatory cells are sparse in the perivascular spaces and the

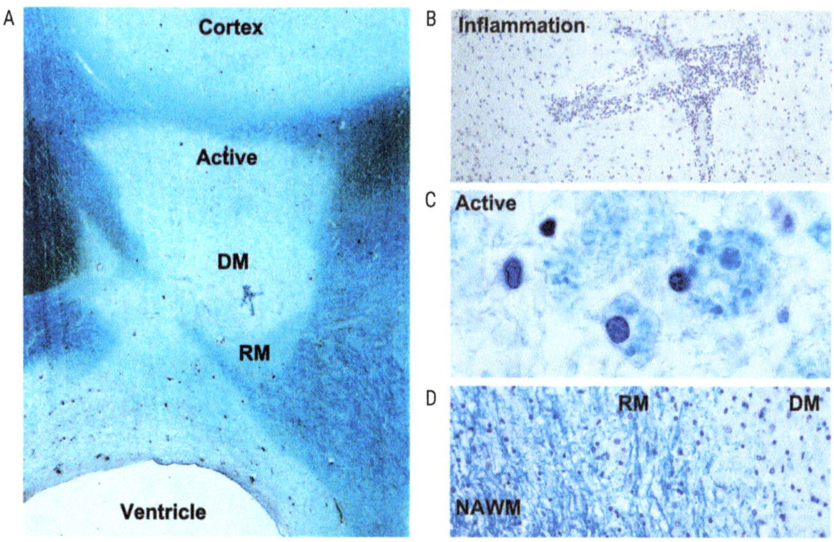

FIGURE 7.4 Structural features of white matter lesions. (**A**) Periventricular lesion in continuity with a large white matter plaque. The central portion of the white matter plaque shows demyelination (DM); a small region of remyelination (RM; shadow plaque) and a broad zone of recent activity (Active) are at the periphery of the plaque. (**B**) Severe perivascular inflammation is seen in the center of the plaque (hematoxylin and eosin [H&E]). (**C**) The active zone of the lesion contains numerous macrophages with early (Luxol fast blue [LFB] positive) myelin degradation products (LFB). (**D**) The zone of remyelination (RM) contains myelin sheaths, which are thinner compared to those in the normal-appearing white matter (NAWM).

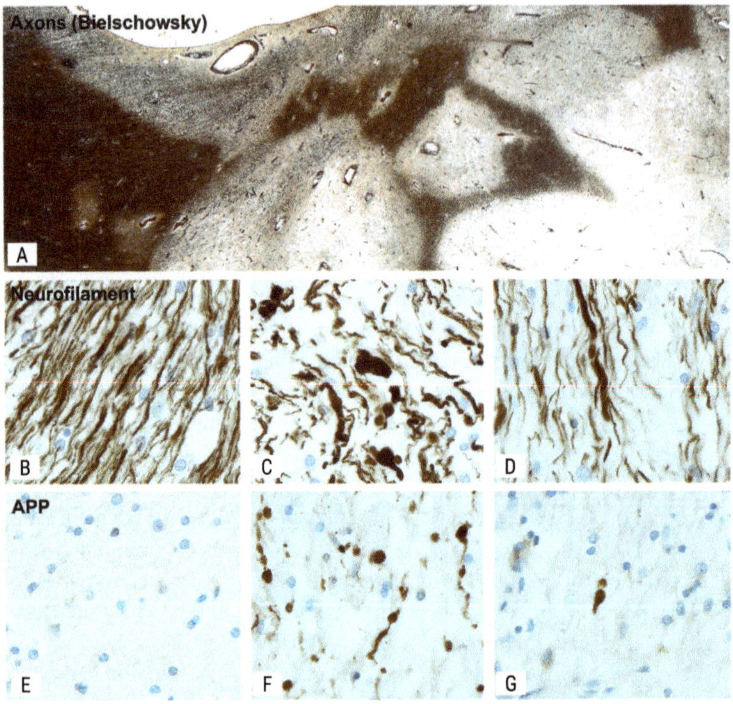

FIGURE 7.5 Axonal pathology in MS lesions. (**A**) Low magnification of the periventricular white matter that contains numerous demyelinated plaques. The different staining intensity in the Bielschowsky silver impregnation reflects the extent of axonal loss in the lesions. (**B–D**) Sections stained for phosphorylated neurofilament show the relative difference in axon density between normal-appearing white matter (**B**), active plaques (**C**), and inactive plaque center (**D**). (**E–G**) Immunocytochemistry for amyloid precursor protein (APP) highlights injured axons with impaired fast axonal transport. This is rarely seen or absent in the normal white matter (**E**); it is pronounced in active lesions (**F**), where there are also concomitant axon spheroids well demonstrated with neurofilament stains (**C**). In the center of the inactive plaque, a single dystrophic axon is seen (**G**).

cortical parenchyma, and blood–brain barrier leakage is minimal or absent. Active subpial cortical lesions are associated with inflammation in the adjacent leptomeninges, either as diffuse meningeal infiltrates or as lymphocyte aggregates, which may show features of secondary B cell follicles.

A B C D

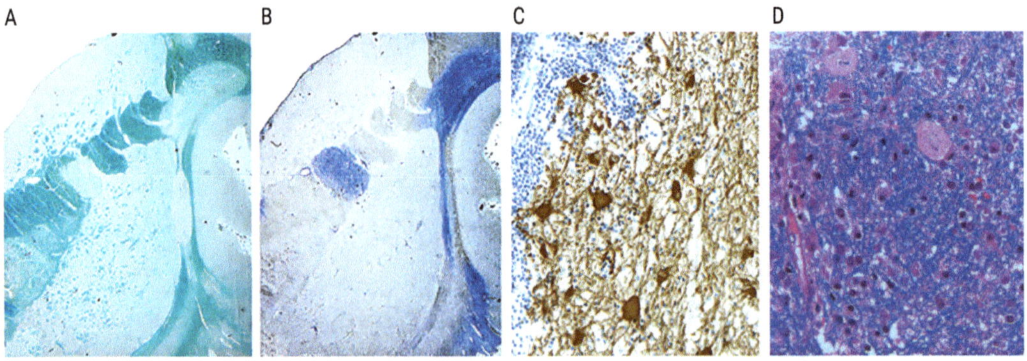

FIGURE 7.6 Astrocytic gliosis in MS lesions. (**A**) Several chronic focal white matter lesions are present in the internal and external capsule (LFB). (**B**) Fibrillary gliosis demonstrated with a Holzer stain, showing intense blue staining in the plaques (Holzer). (**C**) Extensive gliosis with enlarged astrocytic cell bodies showing abundant glial fibrillary acidic protein (GFAP immunohistochemistry [IHC]). This occurs on the background of severe inflammation and active demyelination. (**D**) Creutzfeldt–Peters cells with fragmented nuclei (H&E, LFB).

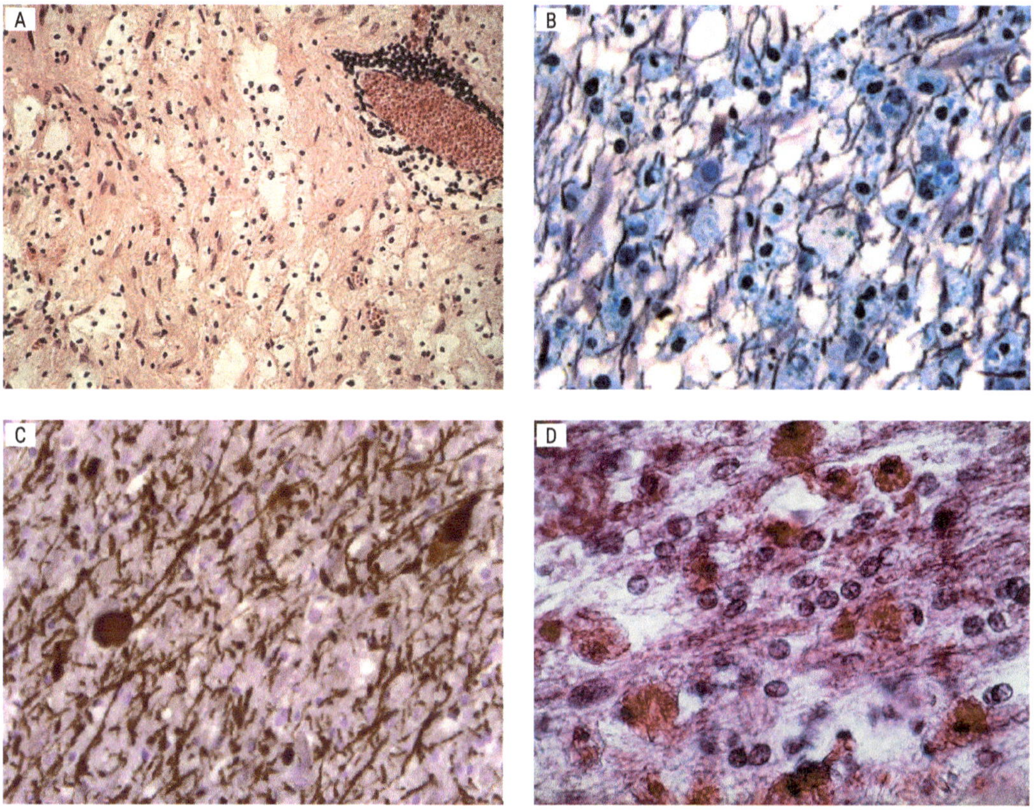

FIGURE 7.7 Microscopic features of MS in active lesions. (**A**) Perivascular lymphocytic infiltrate associated with macrophage infiltration and reactive astrocytosis (H&E). (**B**) Active plaque with diffuse infiltration by macrophages containing myelin debris and relative preservation of axons (Bodian silver for axons, LFB). (**C**) The same plaque as (**B**) showing axonal swellings (neurofilament IHC). (**D**) Active MS plaque showing the sudanophilic (orthochromatic) breakdown of myelin. Macrophages containing myelin degradation products (neutral lipids) are strongly stained (oil red O).

Demyelination in the cortex occurs at sites of microglial activation, which in chronic active lesions demarcate them from the surrounding normal-appearing gray matter.

Demyelinated plaques are also present in the deep gray matter, such as the hypothalamus, thalamus, and the basal ganglia (Fig. 7.2). In contrast to cortical lesions, deep gray matter lesions are already prominent in early stages of the disease, such as acute MS or RRMS. In addition, deep gray matter in MS is affected by profound diffuse neuronal loss, associated with oxidative injury and microglia activation.

7.1.1.4. PATHOLOGY OF THE NORMAL-APPEARING WHITE AND GRAY MATTER

Although focal demyelinated plaques are the hallmark of MS pathology, there are profound diffuse alterations in the normal-appearing white and gray matter. They consist of perivascular and less conspicuous parenchymal inflammatory infiltrates, microglial nodules, diffuse rarefaction of myelin and axons, and diffuse astrogliosis. As a consequence, this gives rise to severe white and gray matter atrophy with expansion of cerebrospinal fluid spaces. These diffuse brain and spinal cord changes can be explained, in part, by Wallerian degeneration following axonal transection within demyelinated plaques. However, diffuse white matter atrophy does not correlate with number, distribution, and extent of damage of focal white matter plaques and correlates only in part with the extent of cortical demyelination. It therefore appears that diffuse white and gray matter changes occur in part independently from focal demyelination in the white and gray matter.

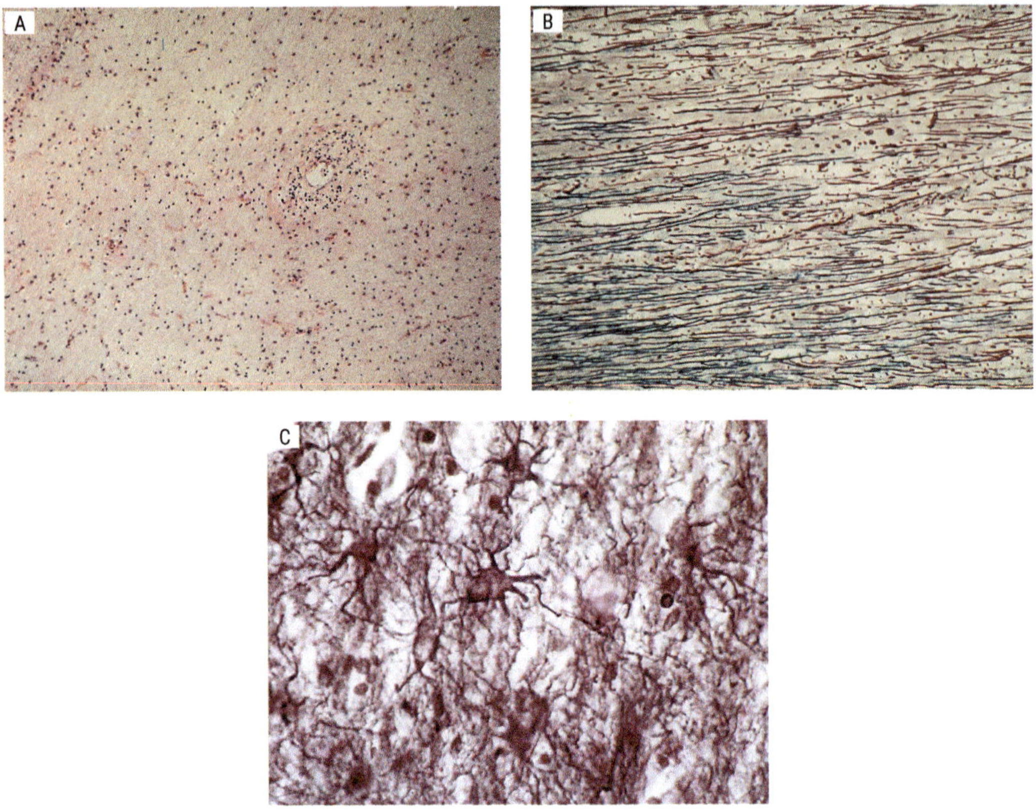

FIGURE 7.8 Microscopic features of MS in inactive lesions. (**A**) Gliosis with Rosenthal fibers and absence of inflammation. Note rare remaining perivascular macrophages (H&E). (**B**) The periphery of an old plaque shows myelin–axonal dissociation with relative preservation of axons. Note the normal staining of myelin on the left (Bodian silver, LFB). (**C**) Metallic impregnation preparation shows fibrillary gliosis in the center of an old plaque, but no axons.

7.1.1.5. PATHOLOGICAL DIFFERENCES BETWEEN RELAPSING REMITTING AND PROGRESSIVE MULTIPLE SCLEROSIS

There is no single pathological feature that distinguishes early relapsing MS from PPMS or SPMS, but the relative frequency of different types of lesions varies with disease duration. In RRMS, newly formed active demyelinating lesions in the white matter are frequent; they occur on the background of new waves of inflammatory cells, entering the brain and spinal cord from the peripheral immune system through a damaged blood-brain barrier. Such lesions are also seen in PPMS and SPMS, although their incidence is rare at this disease stage. In the progressive stage of the disease, inflammation is in part trapped behind a closed or repaired blood–brain barrier, and this process is associated with slow expansion of preexisting white matter lesions (Fig. 7.9), with a gradual increase in number and size of cortical lesions (Fig. 7.10) and with diffuse damage of the normal-appearing white and gray matter. This slow and gradual tissue damage, resulting in progressive atrophy of the brain and spinal cord, is the substrate of progressive tissue injury in the MS brain. It starts already in the initial stages of the disease process and accumulates with disease duration, reaching a peak during the late stages of relapsing disease and early progressive disease. Thus, these changes are also the pathological substrate of "clinically silent" progression, which can now be monitored in patients with advanced MRI techniques and the detection of increased levels of neurofilament light in the serum or cerebrospinal fluid.

A key issue related to clinicopathological correlation in MS is the existence of a functional threshold, which determines the clinical manifestation of damage in the CNS. On average, clinical disease is only seen when more than 50% of axons

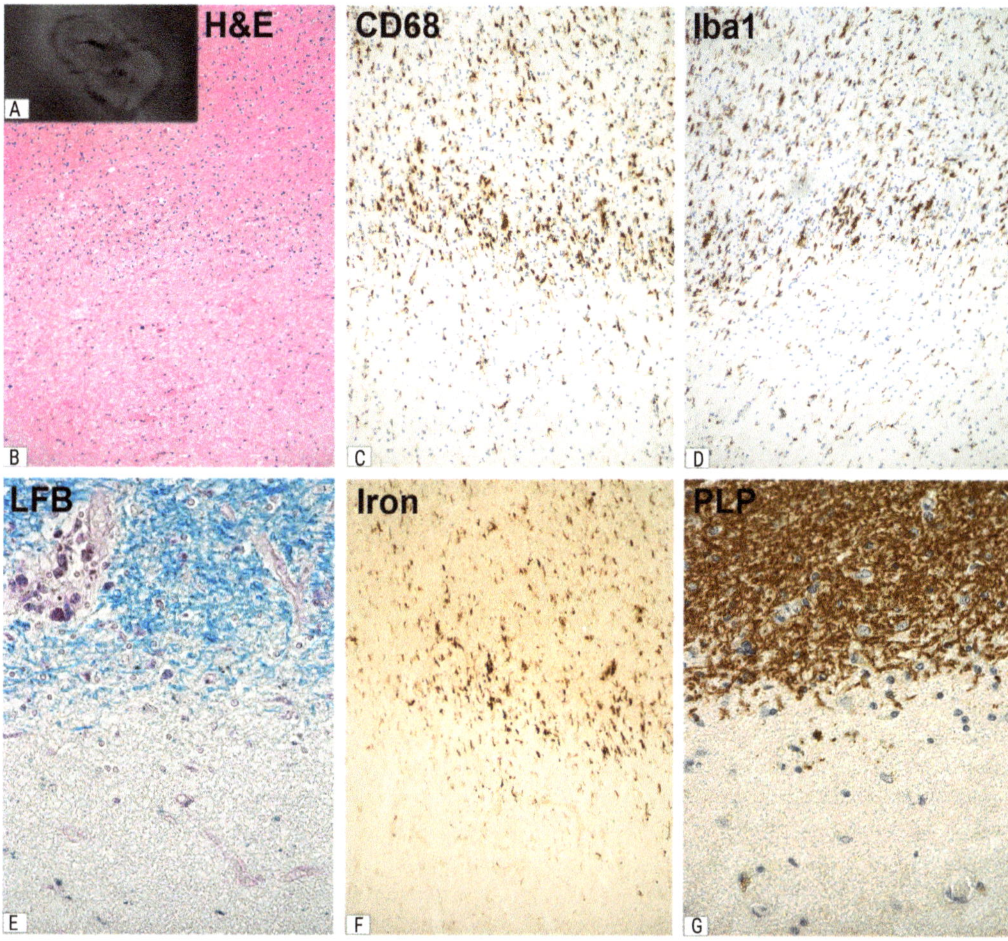

FIGURE 7.9 Pathology of slowly expanding lesions in the white matter. (**A**) White matter lesion depicted on MRI by susceptibility weighted imaging together with a fluid attenuated inversion recovery FLAIR sequence. The dark rim marks the lesion border, defined by a zone of activated microglia containing iron. In the center of the lesion are two large veins, seen in iron-sensitive imaging modalities (central vein sign of a typical MS lesion). (**B**) Edge of a slowly expanding plaque shows the increased cell density at the lesion edge and the reduced cell density in the lesion center (lower part of the figure) (H&E). (**C, D**) The edge of the lesion contains a rim of activated CD68$^+$ microglia (CD68 IHC), also highlighted by the pan-microglia marker Iba1 (Iba1 IHC). (**E**) Myelin is lost within the lesion; at the edge, few microglia/macrophages contain LFB+ early myelin degradation products; perivascular inflammation with macrophages is seen in adjacent vessels (H&E, LFB). (**F**) Diaminobenzidine-enhanced Turnbull blue staining reveals high iron content in the microglia at the lesion's edge, which is depicted as an iron signal in MRI (**A**). (**G**) There is complete demyelination in the lesion (lower portion of image) and the presence of early myelin degradation products in macrophages at the edge (PLP IHC).

in a clinically relevant tract are lost in the brain or spinal cord. This, together with the potential location of lesions in clinically silent areas, explains why the majority of new lesions in MS patients are clinically silent despite the presence of focal plaques with inflammation, demyelination, and axonal loss. Similarly, progressive focal or diffuse brain damage becomes clinically apparent only when its extent surpasses the level of functional compensation, and this is in the majority of patients only the case after several years of disease duration.

7.1.2. Etiology and pathogenesis of multiple sclerosis

There is little doubt that inflammation drives the disease process in genetically susceptible patients, but

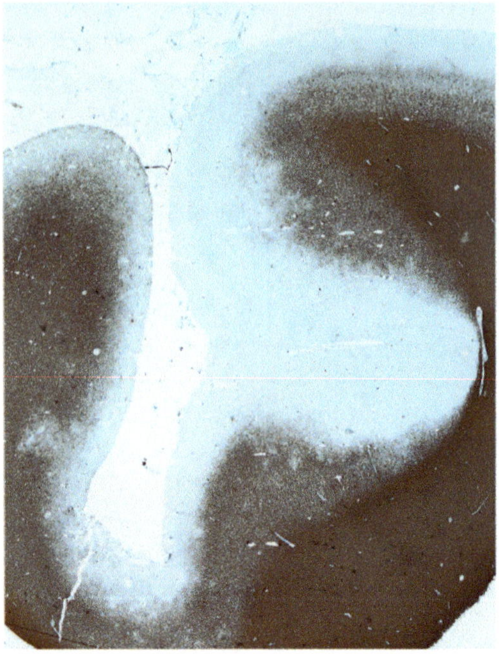

FIGURE 7.10 Cortical lesions in the MS brain. Cortical lesions are not easily seen in sections stained with conventional myelin stains, but they are clearly visible on immunocytochemistry for major myelin proteins. In this section, there is widespread subpial demyelination and smaller perivascular intracortical lesions.

it is entirely unclear what induces and propagates the inflammatory process. Most researchers in the field favor the autoimmune hypothesis. This view is supported by the fact that a disease model with similarities in clinical presentation, pathology, and immunology (i.e., experimental autoimmune encephalomyelitis [EAE]) can be induced in experimental animals sensitized with brain or myelin antigens. However, recent data indicate that EAE may be more relevant for other demyelinating diseases, such as acute disseminated encephalomyelitis, neuromyelitis optica, or myelin oligodendrocyte glycoprotein (MOG) antibody-associated disease.

An alternative view is that chronic inflammation is driven by infection(s), particularly by infection with Epstein–Barr virus. This view has received profound support by a very large epidemiological study, providing compelling evidence for primary EBV infection during adolescence as an essential trigger for the disease. It remains to be clarified whether this EBV infection drives the disease process and chronic inflammation through the presence of the virus within the CNS, by the induction of autoimmunity via molecular mimicry, or through the induction of a chronically dysregulated B lymphocyte response. Chronic inflammation induces a complex cascade of immune mechanisms, which may evoke different mechanisms of tissue injury involving cytotoxic T cells, autoantibodies, and products of activated macrophages and microglia. In addition, the genetic makeup of the tissue in which an immune response occurs may determine its susceptibility to immune-mediated damage. The variable involvement of these different mechanisms provides an explanation of inter-individual differences of clinical disease, pathology, and immunological findings in patients.

Regarding the mechanisms of tissue injury, results from gene expression and neuropathological analysis suggest a dominant role of oxidative injury and mitochondrial damage and dysfunction. The production of reactive oxygen species mainly occurs in microglia and recruited macrophages, which are in part activated by inflammation and in part as a consequence of previous brain tissue damage. Oxidative injury drives mitochondrial dysfunction and induces mutations and deletions of mitochondrial DNA, resulting in further amplification of oxidative injury and a state of energy deficiency (virtual or histotoxic hypoxia). In addition, the human brain accumulates iron (mainly in oligodendrocytes) with aging. In active lesions, the release of iron from intracellular stores into an environment of oxidative damage may give rise to the formation of highly toxic hydroxyl radicals that are able to propagate further oxidative injury.

The central role of mitochondrial dysfunction and energy deficiency in the brain of patients with MS is supported by the observation that focal lesions and diffuse neurodegeneration are concentrated in areas of low arterial perfusion and oxygen tension. Similar mechanisms of oxidative stress and mitochondrial injury, involved in normal brain aging, appear to synergize with MS-related pathogenetic mechanisms in driving neurodegeneration in the progressive stage of MS. Considering the characteristic features of progressive MS, it is not surprising that current anti-inflammatory or immunomodulatory treatments are largely ineffective at this stage, despite the key role played by inflammation during the course of the disease.

7.2. ACUTE MULTIPLE SCLEROSIS

The designation *Marburg type* has been given to MS that follows a rapidly progressive, relapsing or monophasic course and is usually fatal in a few months, always within 1 year of onset. This form of the disease is most often seen in children and young adults but has also been described in older patients.

Neuropathological examination shows multiple plaques whose edges may be poorly defined, making them difficult to see macroscopically. All the plaques are active, hypercellular with prominent perivascular lymphocytic cuffing, numerous foamy macrophages, and scattered reactive astrocytes. Edema may be present in the surrounding white matter, with mass effect in occasional cases. Necrotic changes may be found, and in cases with a more prolonged course, they may result in cavitary lesions (Fig. 7.11). Some of these cases have now been reclassified as ADEM, neuromyelitis optica spectrum disorder, or MOG antibody-associated disease (see Section 7.4). In addition, a similar clinical disease with large focal inflammatory demyelinated lesions can also be present in patients with graft versus host disease, in patients treated with drugs interfering with signaling of the tumor necrosis factor-alpha, or in patients with primary CNS lymphomas with sentinel lesions. Thus, a diagnosis of acute MS has to exclude these other possibilities.

In the so-called Schilder type of MS, which is mostly encountered in children and preferentially runs a progressive course, the lesions are characterized by extensive, acute plaques with clear-cut borders, often asymmetrical and sparing the subcortical white matter (Fig. 7.12). Axonal lesions may be prominent, and Wallerian degeneration is frequent. Some of the cases originally described by Schilder included not only various forms of MS but also the hereditary adrenoleukodystrophy and perhaps other diseases as well. "Transitional sclerosis" has also been described wherein extensive hemispheric lesions may be associated with typical disseminated plaques.

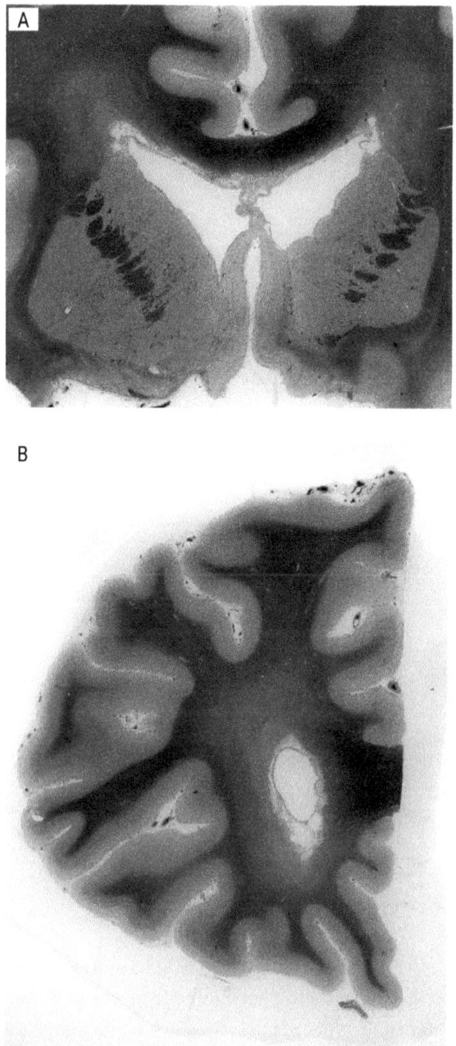

FIGURE 7.11 Cavitating multiple sclerosis. Periventricular plaques with sharp borders on the inferior aspect of corpus callosum (**A**) and around the right frontal horn of the lateral ventricle (**B**).

7.3. BALÓ CONCENTRIC SCLEROSIS

Baló concentric sclerosis is a rare variant of inflammatory demyelinating diseases. The clinical course is generally subacute, very severe, and often fatal, resulting in profound neurological deterioration within months after disease onset. It is characterized by the alternation of demyelinated foci with zones in which the myelin is preserved, thereby resulting in a concentric or irregular pattern of demyelination (Fig. 7.13). The demyelinating lesions have all the histologic features of acute plaques, and axonal injury is often prominent. Rare cavitating forms have been reported. Baló disease is generally regarded as a variant of MS because single layers of concentric demyelination are seen within acute plaques of acute and early chronic MS and large concentric lesions may occur in parallel with MS typical

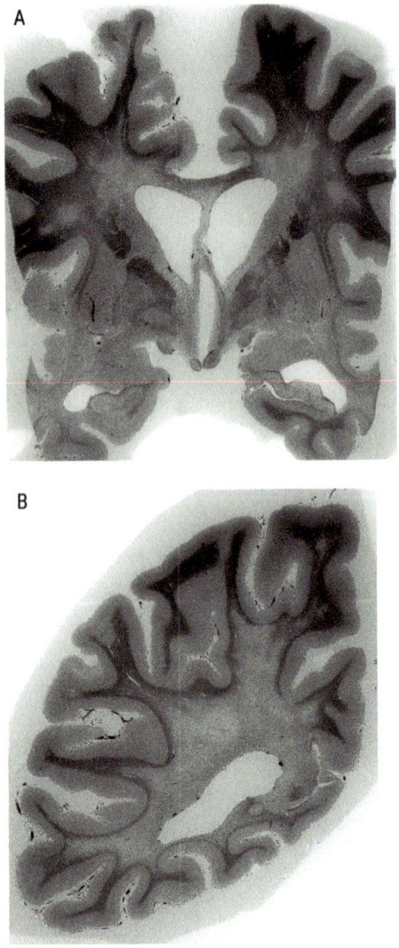

FIGURE 7.12 Schilder-type MS. Extensive hemispheric demyelination emanating from the periventricular zone. Note the presence of smaller plaques at a distance from the large lesions.

lesions at other locations in the same patient. The mechanisms of tissue injury in these lesions are not fully understood, but it seems likely that demyelination, as in other MS lesions, occurs through oxidative damage and mitochondrial injury (as discussed previously), and the preserved concentric rings of myelinated tissue may be protected by hypoxic tissue preconditioning.

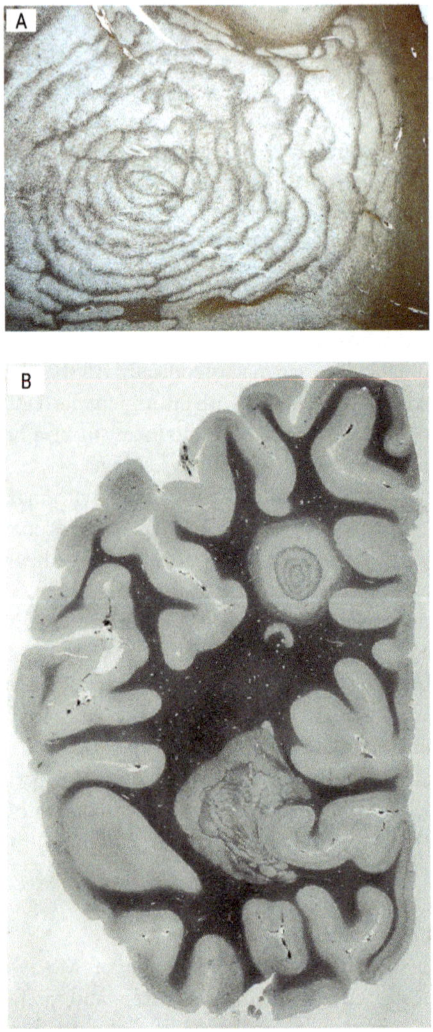

FIGURE 7.13 Concentric sclerosis of Baló type. The lesions of Baló disease are characterized by alternating rings of myelinated and demyelinated white matter. (**A**) A 5-cm-diameter lesion located in the frontal white matter is identified by rings of preservation of myelin proteins. Smaller lesions with some concentric layering of myelinated and demyelinated tissue are sometimes also seen in patients with typical MS with severe active disease (myelin protein IHC). (**B**) Two lesions in the occipital white matter, one periventricular and one with a characteristic concentric pattern (Loyez stain).

7.4. ACUTE DISSEMINATED ENCEPHALOMYELITIS

The disease discussed in this section has several different names, including ADEM, acute disseminated leukoencephalitis, and acute postinfectious/postvaccinal perivenous encephalitis. A particularly severe variant is acute hemorrhagic leukoencephalopathy of Hurst (see Chapter 5). In contrast to typical MS, this is in general a monophasic illness that may occur spontaneously or may follow an infection (e.g., measles) or a vaccination. It affects children more frequently than adults. In patients who survive, there

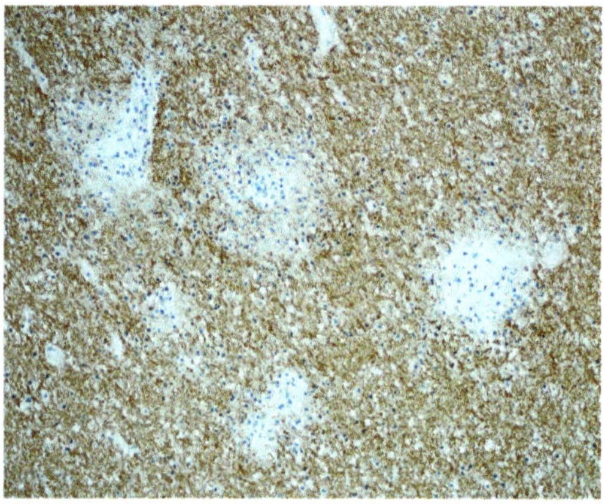

FIGURE 7.14 Acute disseminated (postinfectious) encephalomyelitis (ADEM). Lesions in the cerebellar white matter of a patient with postinfectious measles encephalomyelitis. On immunostaining for myelin proteins, there is marked perivascular inflammation with some perivascular demyelination. Unlike in MS, large confluent plaques of demyelination are absent.

is usually rapid recovery, often without neurological sequelae. The CNS lesions are characterized by small, perivenous, inflammatory infiltrates, centering sleeves of demyelination, without confluent MS-like plaques (Fig 7.14). The disorder is thought to be an autoimmune-mediated complication of a non-CNS infection, and its pathogenesis seems mainly to be driven by T lymphocytes. In some patients, particularly in the rare cases with a relapsing clinical course, circulating demyelinating antibodies, such as against MOG, are present. Such patients may suffer from a different disease, possibly best defined as MOG autoimmune syndrome.

7.5. NEUROMYELITIS OPTICA SPECTRUM DISORDERS

Neuromyelitis optica has long been regarded as a subtype of MS, also termed opticospinal MS or Devic Disease, but recently has been considered as a separate disease. In the majority of patients with NMO, there are autoantibodies against the astrocytic water channel, aquaporin 4 (AQP4), that can be detected in the serum. The presence of these antibodies has an extremely high specificity (100%) and a very high sensitivity (>90%); they have been shown to be pathogenic after transfer into experimental animals.

The pathology of NMO is in some respects different from that seen in MS. Lesions mainly target the spinal cord and the optic system and also can be demonstrated as thin sleeves of tissue injury around the third and fourth ventricles. Very characteristic is their location in the dorsal medulla oblongata, close to the area postrema, and when present in this location they are clinically reflected by severe hiccups. In the spinal cord, the central gray matter is more severely affected than the white matter, and the lesions are extensive along the length of the cord, spanning over several segments (Fig. 7.15). In some patients, very large, ill-defined lesions are seen in the forebrain white matter. When lesions do not show the full spectrum of classical NMO or when they are present

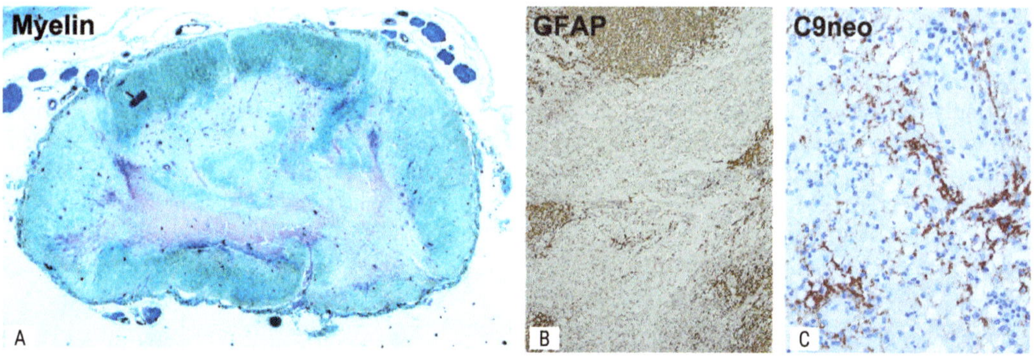

FIGURE 7.15 Neuromyelitis optica (NMO). (**A**) NMO lesions of the spinal cord are mainly located in the center, extensively involving the gray matter, but leaving the subpial white matter largely unaffected. These lesions typically extend longitudinally, spanning several segments of the spinal cord (LFB). (**B**) In NMO lesions, there is extensive destruction of tissue, including glia with areas devoid of GFAP reactivity (GFAP IHC). (**C**) The inflammatory infiltrates in active NMO lesions contain numerous polymorphonuclear leukocytes. In addition, deposition of immunoglobulins and activated complement is seen in a perivascular rosette pattern, corresponding to the astrocytic glia limitans and the distal astrocyte end feet (C9neo IHC; red chromogen).

outside their typical location in the spinal cord and optic nerve, the condition is called neuromyelitis optica spectrum disorder (NMOSD). Microscopic examination shows dense infiltrates of T cells, less often B cells, and macrophages, but in contrast to MS lesions, polymorphonuclear leukocytes are abundant in active lesions. At sites of active tissue injury, massive deposition of immunoglobulins and activated complement are seen on astrocytes and their processes in a rosette-like staining pattern that mainly targets the perivascular and subpial astrocyte foot processes. Astrocytes are in part destroyed through complement-mediated cellular injury mechanisms; they may survive in the periphery of the lesions but are devoid of aquaporin 4 expression. Demyelination and axonal loss, which is prominent in chronic, established NMO lesions, follow the destruction of astrocytes. Overall, NMO lesions are much more destructive than classical MS lesions, frequently resulting in cystic damage of the spinal cord tissue, as well as brain tissue, when affected. In chronic spinal cord lesions, remyelination by Schwann cells can occur.

7.6. MYELIN OLIGODENDROCYTE GLYCOPROTEIN AUTOANTIBODY-ASSOCIATED INFLAMMATORY DEMYELINATING DISEASE

Autoantibodies against MOG have long been thought to play a role in the pathogenesis of demyelination in a subset of patients with MS. However, when reliable immunological tests for such autoantibodies were developed, it turned out that they are seen mainly in children with monophasic or relapsing ADEM and in adults with a clinical presentation of ADEM, NMO, severe brainstem encephalitis, or very large, sometimes diffuse, sometimes multifocal, brain white matter lesions, but they were not seen in patients with classical MS. These data indicate that such anti-MOG antibodies may define a subset of patients with a disease distinct from MS. The pathology reflects an MS-like inflammatory demyelinating disease with T-cell–dominated inflammation; confluent, plaque-like primary demyelination; axonal preservation; and reactive gliosis. Inflammation is dominated by major histocompatibility complex class II restricted $CD4^{+}$ T cells, whereas $CD8^{+}$ T cells, B cells, and plasma cells are rare. The variable but low abundance of plasma cells corresponds with the absence of intrathecal immunoglobulins synthesis in the majority of cases. In accordance with an antibody-mediated process, active demyelination is associated with deposition of immunoglobulin and complement on myelin, but complement activation is less obvious in MOG autoantibody-associated inflammatory demyelinating disease (MOGAD) than in NMOSD. Demyelination starts around small veins and venules, and larger lesions are formed by confluence rather than by radial expansion. Chronic active and slowly expanding lesions are rare or absent, which mirrors the absence of clinically silent or overt disease progression in MOGAD.

7.7. DIAGNOSIS OF INFLAMMATORY DEMYELINATING DISEASES IN BRAIN BIOPSIES

Neuropathologists are sometimes called on to examine biopsy specimens containing lesions compatible with an inflammatory demyelinating disease. Patients who come to biopsy under these circumstances are individuals with single tumor-like mass lesions in the brain or spinal cord in whom a potential neoplasm is within the differential diagnosis. In addition to inflammatory demyelinating diseases and neoplasms, the differential includes virus-induced lesions of the white matter and a variety of vascular and metabolic diseases. Because it is difficult or sometimes impossible in atypical cases and small-needle biopsies to distinguish MS from ADEM, NMO, or MOGAD, analysis of the serum antibody status in the patient's serum is recommended. Intraoperative evaluation is often further complicated by the presence of marked atypia and/or Creutzfeldt–Peters cells mimicking malignancy.

As a first step, the cellular composition and any inflammation has to be assessed with H&E. The nature of the inflammatory infiltrate (perivenous, rich in lymphocytes and macrophages), with no sign of arterial wall involvement, supports the diagnosis of demyelinating disease. Demyelination has to be assessed with Luxol fast blue for myelin and with silver impregnation or IHC for axons. Double immunostaining against myelin and axons can also be used. The presence of naked axons and macrophage overload of myelin debris is decisive in determining demyelination. Then, the extent of demyelination (perivenous vs. confluent) can be studied. Vasculitic changes, B cell neoplasms, viral inclusions in astrocytes, and oligodendrocytes have to be excluded and intracellular accumulation of proteins or lipids, suggesting metabolic (storage) diseases, assessed. Only when all these conditions have been excluded can the diagnosis of an MS-like inflammatory demyelinating disease be considered. Dissociation between Glial Fibrillary Acidic Protein (GFAP) and AQP4 staining may provide arguments for NMO, but it will generally be difficult to differentiate between different types of demyelinating disease within the limits of a biopsy.

7.8. PATHOLOGICAL SUBSTRATE OF MAGNETIC RESONANCE IMAGING

During the past decade, MRI has become the most important paraclinical tool for diagnosis, monitoring the disease course, and assessing therapeutic effects in MS patients. In addition, the planning of a brain biopsy largely depends on lesion characterization by MRI. Multiple different imaging modalities and sequences have been developed with the aim of following the dynamics of inflammation, demyelination, neurodegeneration, and repair in the living patients. Pathological validation of the different MRI signal abnormalities is essential for their interpretation because most MRI sequences in essence detect water shifts in the tissue and their specificity for pathologically defined lesion types is poor.

White matter lesions can be easily detected in T2-weighted scans. However, they do not differentiate between active, inactive, or remyelinated lesions. In addition, approximately 30% of all focal T2 abnormalities in the white matter of MS patients do not have a clear pathological substrate but may reflect areas of edema, microglia activation, or secondary tissue degeneration. Active lesions are commonly detected through contrast enhancement, depicting blood–brain barrier leakage in fresh lesions. However, contrast enhancement is not specific for active inflammation but, rather, also seen in other conditions of blood–brain barrier disruption. Importantly, inflammation that is trapped in the brain or spinal cord behind a closed (or repaired) blood–brain barrier is not visualized by contrast enhancement. Thus, the equation of contrast enhancement and inflammation in MS is misleading. A feature that supports the diagnosis of MS is the presence of the so-called central vein sign, seen in iron-sensitive MRI sequences (Fig. 7.9). This reflects the development of lesions in MS around large veins, in contrast to the initiation of inflammation around small venules in the majority of other inflammatory diseases of the CNS.

The extent of tissue injury and loss is seen in T1-weighted scans. T1 hypo-intensity reflects the expanded extracellular space due to demyelination and axonal loss. Changes in myelin can be seen in short T2 sequences, which specifically measure the intra-myelinic water content. Remyelination is also in part reflected in the restoration of magnetization transfer ratio signals or in positron emission tomography using myelin markers.

More recently, research interest has focused on how to determine progressive tissue injury. One possibility is to quantitatively assess the voxel-based increase of the T1 signal, indicating progressive accumulation of neurodegeneration in established white matter lesions. Another possibility is to analyze the dynamic change of iron rings around slowly expanding lesions. The iron ring reflects iron-containing microglia at the edge of active lesions and offers a direct measurement of the lesion size (Fig. 7.9). To date, detection of cortical lesions is very incomplete. Cortical and subcortical lesions can in part be detected by double inversion recovery sequences, and their number provides an estimate of the global cortical lesion load in a given patient. However, despite the recent progress in pathological/MRI correlations, the gaps of knowledge are still significant and there is an urgent need for additional research in this field.

8

Pathology of Degenerative Diseases of the Nervous System

YUICHI RIKU, SUSANA BOLUDA, MEL FEANY, AND TOSHIKI UCHIHARA

8.1. INTRODUCTION

The concept of *neurodegeneration* can be defined as a disease process affecting neuronal groups (functionally related or anatomically connected) with diverse macroscopically and microscopically identifiable abnormalities and each correlated with variably definable neurological symptoms and signs. Although neurodegenerative diseases were once enigmatic conditions, their classification and evolving understanding have been aided by the identification of disease-related proteins and genetic abnormalities.

The neuropathologic findings of neurodegeneration include the following:

- Macroscopic findings: Neurodegenerative disorders affect specific neuronal groups, often spatially separated but functionally linked, and result in disease-specific regional atrophies and related neurological deficits.
- Microscopic findings: Histopathologic changes include neuronal loss in the affected regions, with variable astrocytic and microglial changes. Neurons are thought to die often through apoptotic processes.
- Molecular findings: Specific proteins accumulate in affected nervous tissues, including neurons, glia, and neuropil. Some disorders are associated with specific DNA abnormalities, including mutations or expansion of trinucleotide repeats.

Neurodegenerative diseases, such as Alzheimer disease (AD) or Parkinson disease (PD), may be sporadic or familial. The proportion of genetic-determined degenerative diseases in comparison to those that are apparently sporadic varies greatly in each category (e.g., Huntington disease [HD], generally hereditary; multiple system atrophy [MSA], generally sporadic).

Box 8.1 Classification of Neurodegenerative Diseases

Cortical Degenerations
Alzheimer disease
Frontotemporal lobar degeneration
Dementia with Lewy bodies

Movement Disorders

Akinetic/rigid syndromes
Parkinson disease
Progressive supranuclear palsy
Corticobasal degeneration
Multiple system atrophy (striatonigral degeneration)

Hyperkinetic syndromes
Huntington disease
Chorea-acanthocytosis

Cerebellar Ataxias
Hereditary
Sporadic

Diseases of Motor Systems
Motor neuron diseases
Hereditary spastic paraparesis

Autonomic Disorders
Parkinson disease
Multiple system atrophy (Shy–Drager syndrome)

8.2. CLASSIFICATION

8.2.1. Syndromic classification

There are several approaches to syndromic classification, each of which has its own advantages. The one adopted here is to classify disorders into five broad categories according to the dominant pattern of initial clinical manifestations: (1) dementias affecting the cerebral cortex, (2) movement disorders affecting the basal ganglia, (3) ataxia affecting the cerebellum, (4) motor neuron diseases, and (5) conditions associated with autonomic failure (Box 8.1). This arbitrary classification provides a pragmatic frame to bridge clinical and pathological domains. It is also noteworthy that there are often overlaps in the above categories, and distinctions may be blurred over the course of the disease. For example, a patient with PD, primarily a movement disorder, may develop dementia in the setting of a protracted clinical course (termed Parkinson disease with dementia). This clinical evolution may be related to extension of lesions from the extrapyramidal motor systems to the limbic and cortical areas.

8.2.2. Molecular classification

Identification of disease-associated protein deposits has made it possible to classify neurodegeneration based on the aggregated proteins or genetic abnormalities. In particular, identification of aggregated proteins as constituents of disease-specific lesions expanded our understanding, assigning them the designation of "proteinopathies." Although the exact pathogenetic roles of these intrinsic proteins and the mechanism of injury related to the aggregates remain to be clarified, they are sensitive and specific markers to classify the neuropathologic diagnostic categories:

- **Tauopathy**: This group is characterized by cytoplasmic, neuronal, or glial accumulation of tau protein, which is encoded by the *microtubule-associated protein tau* (*MAPT*) gene. Alternative splicing of *MAPT* yields six tau isoforms, which are classified into two groups based on the number of microtubule-binding domains, called "repeats." All six isoforms have either three repeats (3R) or four repeats (4R), and the isoforms of aggregated tau differ among the sporadic tauopathies: 3R tau inclusions in Pick disease; 4R tau inclusions in progressive supranuclear palsy (PSP), corticobasal degeneration (CBD), and argyrophilic grain disease (AGD); and both 3R and 4R tau in AD in combination with deposits of Aβ amyloid. In addition, mutations of *MAPT* are associated with familial tauopathies, which comprise various forms of frontotemporal lobar degeneration (FTLD) showing inclusions of 3R or 4R or both. Isoforms of aggregated tau can be identified using western blots or immunohistochemistry (IHC) with isoform-specific primary antibodies.
- **Aβ peptide**: The Aβ peptide is a fragment of 40–42 amino acids from a normal neuronal protein termed amyloid precursor protein (APP). The peptide is generated by sequential cleavage of APP in the extracellular domain (by a protease known as β-secretase or β-site amyloid precursor protein cleaving enzyme), followed by intramembranous cleavage (by an enzymatic complex known as γ-secretase, which includes presenilin). Aβ deposits in the neuropil and in senile plaques are a critical part of AD pathology.

Aβ also accumulates in the vessel walls, termed amyloid angiopathy. This condition can occur in isolation or in association with AD.

- **α-Synucleinopathy**: α-Synuclein is physiologically a membrane-associated, presynaptic protein. This group of diseases is characterized by aggregation of α-synuclein in the cytoplasm of neurons or glia. Aggregates may be visible on routine sections; many more are revealed by IHC. This group includes PD, other Lewy body diseases, and MSA.
- **TDP-43 proteinopathy**: Transactive response DNA-binding protein 43 kDa (TDP-43) is an RNA/DNA-binding protein implicated in alternative splicing, transcriptional regulation, messenger RNA (mRNA) stabilization, and microRNA processing. The full-length protein is normally present in the nucleus. In pathological conditions, the protein is fragmented, phosphorylated, and ubiquitinated; it accumulates in the cytoplasm of the cell body, not only principally of neurons but also of glia. It has also been found in neurites. Such accumulations define a subset of FTLDs and amyotrophic lateral sclerosis (ALS), referred to as FTLD-TDP and ALS-TDP, respectively.
- **Polyglutamine diseases**: Almost uniquely among the degenerative diseases, the polyglutamine disorders are invariably genetically determined. This group includes HD, spinal and bulbar muscular atrophy, and some of the dominantly inherited spinocerebellar ataxias (SCAs). Various cellular proteins contain a polyglutamine tract encoded by repeats of the trinucleotide, CAG, in the coding region of the corresponding gene. When one of these repeats expands, the protein contains an expanded polyglutamine tract. Typically, a longer repeat expansion in successive generations is associated with onset of clinical manifestation at a younger age and with increased severity (known as "anticipation"). The repeats or part of the repeats accumulate as neuronal intranuclear inclusions (NIIs). The mutated proteins are not structurally or functionally related to one another, apart from the presence of the polyglutamine tract.

It is important to note that the degree of the accumulation of tau, Aβ, α-synuclein, or TDP-43 is related to the clinical severity of the disease. In fact, accumulation of these proteins can also be observed in normal elderly individuals without neurological deficits. However, CAG (or any other) repeat expansions are not found in brains without the mutations, so the presence of repeat inclusions is a marker of disease.

8.3. PATHOLOGY OF DEGENERATIVE DISEASES OF THE CEREBRAL CORTEX AND DEMENTIAS

In dementing diseases, the clinical diagnosis is based on the decline in cognitive function across multiple modalities. In degenerative disease, cognitive decline is associated with processes affecting primarily the cerebral cortex. It can be complicated, particularly among the elderly, by concomitant cerebrovascular disease that may also involve the white matter. The main causes of dementia and an indication of their frequency are presented in Table 8.1.

8.3.1. Alzheimer disease

Alzheimer disease is the most common of the degenerative diseases. Its incidence increases with age (2.8/1,000 person-years in the 65- to 69-year-old age group to 56.1/1,000 person-years in the

Table 8.1 Main Causes of Dementia and Their Frequency

DISORDER	FREQUENCY
Alzheimer disease	
Sporadic	Very common
Familial	Uncommon
Vascular and mixed dementia	Very common
Dementia with Lewy bodies	
Pure without AD changes	Rare
Concomitant with AD changes	Common
Frontotemporal lobar degeneration	
Pick body disease	Uncommon
FTLD with *MAPT* mutations	Uncommon
FTLD-TDP	Not rare
FTLD with motor neuron disease	Not rare
FTLD-FUS	Uncommon
Argyrophilic grain disease	Common lesion
Uncommonly diagnosed clinically	

AD, Alzheimer disease; FTLD, frontotemporal lobar degeneration; FUS, fused-in-sarcoma; TDP, transactive response DNA binding protein.

older than 90 years age group). The prevalence of AD also depends on age: 5% in a population aged 70 years but over 20% after 80 years of age. The initial manifestation of the disease in most patients is memory failure, often with deficits in other cognitive modalities, including apraxia, aphasia, and agnosia.

8.3.1.1. MACROSCOPIC FINDINGS

Atrophy of cortical gyri and widening of sulci can be a striking finding. Atrophy involves predominantly the hippocampus (Fig. 8.1), the parahippocampal gyrus, and the amygdala, with parietal and frontal lobes being next most severely affected. The occipital lobe is generally spared. In some forms, especially late-onset types, the cerebral atrophy is inconstant and may be mild, marked by a symmetrical slight reduction in the volume of the temporal gyri. On cut surface, the ventricular dilation, generally of moderate degree, parallels the severity of the cortical atrophy. Depigmentation of the locus coeruleus in the face of relative preservation of the substantia nigra is also commonly observed.

8.3.1.2. MICROSCOPIC FINDINGS

The combination of (1) Aβ deposits in the neuropil, (2) neuritic plaques composed of a core of extracellular Aβ and of a crown of tau-positive neurites, and (3) neurofibrillary tangles containing 3R and 4R tau, with appropriate density and distribution, is required to make a neuropathological diagnosis of AD (see discussion in Section 8.3.1.3). IHC for Aβ and tau is a reliable method for making a diagnosis. Senile plaques and neurofibrillary tangles can also be identified with hematoxylin and eosin (H&E) staining or silver impregnation methods. Synaptic loss is early and constant, and it can be evidenced by a loss of synaptophysin immunoreactivity. By contrast, neuronal loss and gliosis in the hippocampus and cerebral cortex are often subtle during early phases of the disease.

Throughout the years, the clinical diagnostic criteria for the diagnosis of AD have evolved and do not necessarily rely on the demonstration of severe dementia. The diagnosis is now considered at earlier stages of the illness, with the onset of mild cognitive impairment; correspondingly, AD neuropathologic criteria now identify burden and distribution of lesions that are associated with the underlying disease process but are not typically associated with end-stage neurologic impairment.

8.3.1.2.1. Diffuse Aβ deposits. Aβ is highly prone to aggregate; small aggregates (termed *oligomers*) are the currently suspected critical mediator for eliciting cellular and synaptic dysfunction. Within the brain parenchyma, aggregates of Aβ appear in two forms: senile plaques and diffuse deposits. Senile plaques are composed of core and corona structures, showing argyrophilic and amyloid properties. By contrast, diffuse Aβ deposits are wispy, larger but less dense than plaques, and with convoluted shapes; they are not seen on H&E or Congo red stains but are immunolabeled by Aβ antibodies. The progression of Aβ deposits within the brain (termed *Thal phases*) typically follows a predictable sequence as follows: isocortex, hippocampus, basal ganglia, mesencephalon, and pons and cerebellum. Generation of Aβ from APP is considered critical for the initiation of AD pathogenesis because mutations in the APP gene, which accelerate generation of Aβ, cause familial forms of AD, as do mutations in presenilin, which increase the rate of generation of Aβ or shift its production

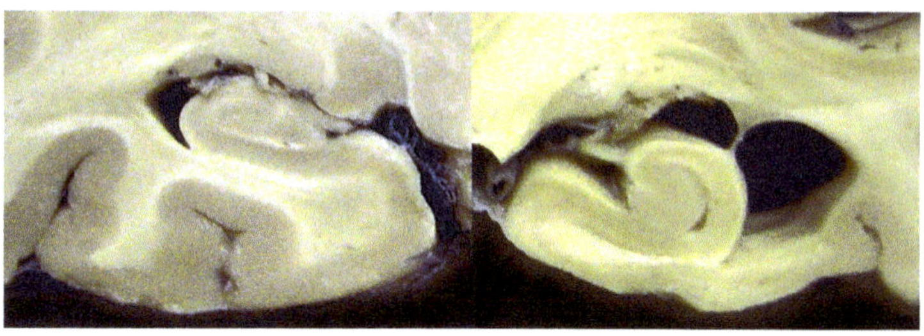

FIGURE 8.1 Alzheimer disease: On the right is the medial temporal lobe from a patient with AD; compare it to that on the left, which is from an age-matched patient with no cognitive abnormality. Note atrophy of parahippocampal cortex, shrinkage of white matter, and widening of the temporal horn of the left ventricle in the right image.

toward longer forms of Aβ (with 42 amino acids). The discovery that an APP mutation that hinders the generation of Aβ is protective against AD has further strengthened this argument.

8.3.1.2.2. Plaques. Senile (or neuritic) plaques (Fig. 8.2) consist of a core and a corona. The core is an extracellular deposit of Aβ, whereas the corona is made of enlarged degenerating neurites, mainly axons, immunoreactive for tau protein and ubiquitin (Fig. 8.2C) and highlighted on silver impregnation including Bielschowsky or Gallyas methods.

The Aβ peptide in the core of the senile plaque is misfolded, enriched in β-pleated sheets, and has all the features of amyloid (Fig. 8.2B); for example, it shows an apple-green birefringence under polarized light with Congo red stain, is fluorescent after thioflavin S staining, and appears fibrillar at electron microscopy examination. The neuritic plaque also elicits an astrocytic and microglial reaction. Neuritic plaques and diffuse deposits are typically found in neocortex, entorhinal cortex, and hippocampus, whereas the striatum and cerebellum show only diffuse deposits. Neuritic plaque burden in neocortical areas is typically reported in a semiquantitative method, separated into sparse, moderate, and abundant (Consortium to Establish a Registry for Alzheimer's Disease [CERAD] criteria).

8.3.1.2.3. Neurofibrillary tangles, neuronal and synaptic loss. Neurofibrillary tangles are intracellular inclusion bodies, primarily containing tau as well as other proteins (Fig. 8.3). Tau is a microtubule-binding protein, but in tangles it has separated from the microtubules and is hyperphosphorylated at a variety of serine and threonine residues. Tangles may be detected by immunostaining for tau protein, as well as silver impregnation techniques including Bielschowsky or Gallyas–Braak methods (Fig. 1.10). When nerve cells die, tangles may be left behind in the neuropil as so-called ghost tangles. Nerve cell processes (mainly dendrites) in the cortical neuropil may accumulate tau protein and are called *neuropil threads*. The corona of the senile plaque is made of tau-positive neurites, mainly axons, that are termed *degenerating neurites*. Both tangles and degenerating neurites contain a mixture of 3R and 4R forms of tau.

A scheme known as Braak and Braak staging is used to characterize the distribution of neurofibrillary pathology with good correlation to clinical status. Tangles and neuropil threads first occur in the transentorhinal (Stage I) and entorhinal (Stage II) cortices; the first sector of the hippocampus (CA1) is then affected as well as the occipitotemporal gyrus (Stage III). At Stage IV, the middle temporal gyrus is involved; at Stage V, the peristriate is involved; and at Stage VI, the striate cortex is involved. In addition, neurofibrillary changes are found in some other brain regions, including the amygdala, limbic nuclei of the thalamus (anterior complex, laterodorsal nucleus, and some intralaminar nuclei), nucleus basalis of Meynert, reticular formation of the mesencephalon, locus coeruleus, raphe nucleus, and selected subnuclei of the substantia nigra.

8.3.1.2.4. Amyloid angiopathy. Accumulation of Aβ peptide within the vessel walls causes amyloid angiopathy (Fig. 8.4). It is especially seen in the vessels of the neocortex (occipital, temporal, parietal, and frontal in decreasing frequency) and later in Ammon's horn and cerebellum. The amyloid accumulation results in irregular thickening of the terminal vascular bed. Two forms of amyloid angiopathy are defined by the presence or absence of Aβ accumulation in capillaries. In the Thal type 1 angiopathy (dyshoric type), the accumulation affects capillary walls and then extends into the adjacent parenchyma. The Thal type 2 angiopathy (macroangiopathy) does not affect the capillaries. Thal type 1 is less frequently seen and more strongly associated with the apolipoprotein E (apoE) ε4 genotype than Thal type 2. Aβ accumulation may also affect small arteries and veins in the meninges and superficial layers of the cortex. Cerebral amyloid angiopathy is frequent in patients with AD, although the vessel damage is seldom associated with hemorrhage or infarcts in this setting. Cerebral amyloid angiopathy is also found in nondemented, aged individuals; cerebral hemorrhages or microscopic infarcts often occur in cerebral amyloid angiopathy without AD (see Chapter 4).

8.3.1.3. DIAGNOSTIC CRITERIA AND STAGING OF ALZHEIMER DISEASE

The pathologic process of AD begins in the brain many years before the emergence of dementia. Hence, it is not surprising that AD-related changes (diffuse Aβ deposits, neuritic plaques, or neurofibrillary tangles) are seen in subjects without subjective or objective evidence of cognitive decline, although such cases typically show a low

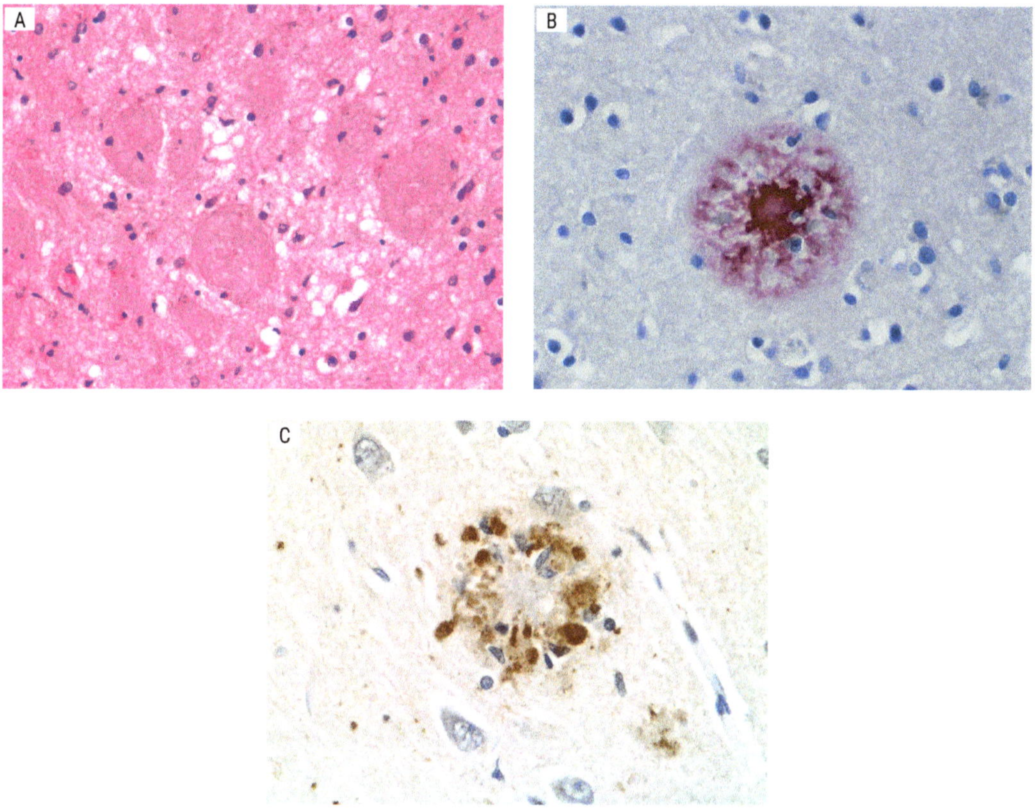

FIGURE 8.2 Alzheimer disease plaques. (**A**) Focal plaques can sometimes be seen as compact, rounded alterations in the texture of the neuropil (H&E). (**B**) Aβ peptide in the core of the plaque (Aβ IHC). (**C**) Neurites containing tau protein surround the central amyloid core material (tau IHC).

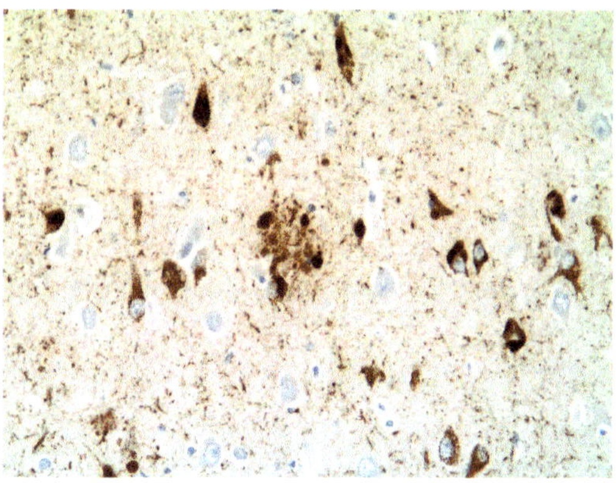

FIGURE 8.3 Alzheimer disease tangles. Tau immunostaining shows neurofibrillary tangles within neuronal cell bodies. In addition, dilated, so-called degenerating, neurites are seen around plaques. The immunolabeling also shows fine neurites, the neuropil threads, dispersed between neuronal cell bodies (tau IHC).

burden of lesions with a restricted distribution. This fact requires scoring of AD-related changes, with appropriate cutoff values, to conclude that the changes in an individual case are responsible for clinical manifestations of dementia. As indicated, there are three scales by which the lesions of AD are assessed: tangles and neuropil threads characterized by the Braak and Braak staging, diffuse Aβ deposits by the Thal phases, and neuritic plaques quantified by the CERAD system. With the most recent consensus proposal, by definition, Alzheimer disease neuropathologic changes (ADNCs) necessarily include Aβ aggregates with any combination of neuritic plaques and tangles. Progression and increasing burden along these histologic scoring scales are associated with greater probability of cognitive impairment in affected individuals. At one extreme are subjects with Thal Phase 1 Aβ deposits, with low Braak stages and sparse neuritic plaques (CERAD) that are most

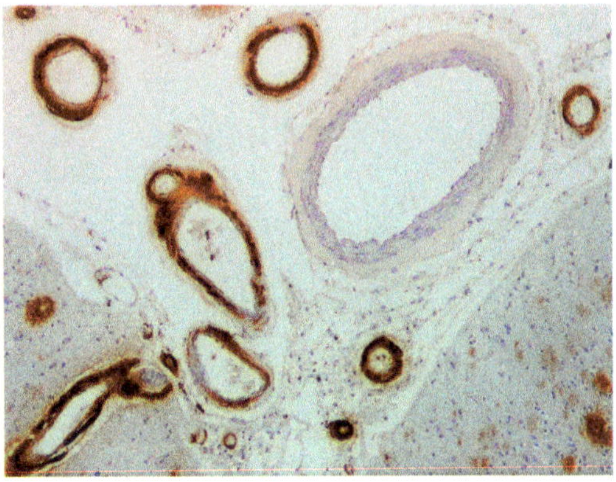

FIGURE 8.4 Alzheimer disease amyloid angiopathy: Aβ peptide deposits in vessel walls (Aβ IHC).

often cognitively intact. At the other extreme, cases with widespread Aβ deposits (Thal Phase 5), abundant neuritic plaques, and tangles throughout the neocortex and mesial temporal lobe (Braak V or VI) are associated with a high probability of cognitive impairment.

8.3.1.4. GENETIC RISKS

Recognition of the central pathogenetic role of Aβ in AD has been driven by observations from genetics. Several factors are recognized to promote or cause amyloid deposition. Rare early onset familial cases of AD are caused by mutations in—or duplication of—the APP gene on chromosome 21. It is believed that the association between Down syndrome and AD relates to the presence of three copies of the APP gene due to the trisomy 21. Mutations in genes coding for the presenilins (PS1, PS2), which are components of γ-secretase, are also recognized to cause early onset familial AD. These proteins are involved in the pathways of cleavage of APP with mutations giving rise to excess production of Aβ peptide. ApoE genotype influences the risk of AD: Individuals with one copy of the apoE4 allele have a 4- to 5-fold increased risk of developing AD, and those with two copies have a 10-fold increased risk, compared to those carrying apoE2 or apoE3 alleles. Genetic studies continue to identify other potential contributing risk factor alleles, although each of these makes only a small contribution to the risk of developing AD. Although neurofibrillary tangles (tau accumulation) form another essential part of the histologic lesions of AD, mutations in the *MAPT* gene do not result in AD.

8.3.2. Frontotemporal lobar degenerations

Several diseases are characterized by neurodegeneration distributed in the frontal and temporal lobes, with relative sparing of the parietal and occipital lobes. The clinical features relate to behavioral disturbances or language deficits, whereas memory dysfunction occurs only later in the course of the disease. This distinctive pattern of progression of clinical symptoms helps distinguish FTLD patients from those with AD. The clinical condition is typically referred to as frontotemporal dementia (FTD); pathologic substrate is termed FTLD. Among clinical phenotypes of FTD, the three best characterized are the behavioral variant FTD (bvFTD), primary progressive aphasia (PPA), and semantic dementia. However, correlations between clinical presentation and pathologic findings are not completely congruous; for instance, the cause of PPA is FTLD in approximately half the cases and AD in the other half.

Histologic and genetic findings have refined the classification of FTLDs. The classification of these diseases is now based on the type of protein inclusions observed in neurons and glia as well as mutational status, when known. The inclusions contain predominantly or exclusively one of three markers, shown by IHC: tau, in various combinations of 3R and 4R tau (FTLD-tau); TDP-43 (FLTD-TDP); and fused-in-sarcoma (FUS; FTLD-FUS). Within each entity of these groups, genetic markers and the distribution patterns of inclusions are heterogeneous. Clinical phenotypes of FTD may correspond to distribution of regional atrophy or neuronal loss rather than to the types of inclusions. A close relationship between FTLD (linked with TDP-43 or FUS) and ALS has been reported based of histologic findings, genetic causes, and clinical presentation.

8.3.2.1. FTLD-TAU

The FTLD-tau diseases are defined by the combination of lobar degeneration and inclusions containing 3R tau, 4R tau, or both forms. This group includes Pick body disease, tauopathies with mutation of the tau gene (*MAPT*), and other tauopathies without *MAPT* mutation. In addition, two disorders that are primarily classified as movement disorders (PSP and CBD) may also present with cognitive changes with lobar atrophy and tau-containing inclusions.

These are discussed with the movement disorders (see Sections 8.4.1.2 and 8.4.1.3).

8.3.2.1.1. FTLD-tau; Pick body disease. Pick body disease is a sporadic FTLD-tau dementia, characteristically beginning in the fifth and sixth decades of life. The behavioral changes are severe. This clinical pattern of symptoms corresponds to the distribution of lesions involving predominantly the frontal lobes early in the course of the disease. The term "Pick disease" as used in the literature has been applied to a broad spectrum of FTD even in the absence of postmortem observations or of Pick bodies. Hence, "Pick body disease" refers to a pathological phenotype with well-defined presence of Pick bodies.

8.3.2.1.1.1. Macroscopic findings. The circumscribed cortical atrophy, which is often so severe as to be described as "knife-edge" atrophy, is evident in the frontal lobes; when it involves the temporal lobe, it typically spares the posterior third of the superior temporal gyrus (Fig. 8.5). Memory disturbance is not the initial manifestation but can arise when involvement of the hippocampus becomes severe. The parietal cortex is seldom involved, and the occipital cortex is spared. In keeping with this pattern of lobar involvement, there is greater dilation of the anterior portion of the frontal and temporal horns of the lateral ventricles. This may be accentuated by concomitant involvement of the white matter and of striatal atrophy in some cases.

8.3.2.1.1.2. Microscopic lesions. Involved regions of cerebral cortex show extensive neuronal loss associated with dense astrocytic gliosis, usually accompanied by cortical microvacuolation. White matter in the involved gyri shows secondary attenuation. Pick disease is characterized by the presence of rounded, homogeneous neuronal cytoplasmic inclusions (NCIs), faintly visible on H&E staining (Fig. 8.6A). Pick bodies are strongly argyrophilic when using Bielschowsky and Bodian methods, but they are not demonstrable with the Gallyas method (Fig. 8.6B; see also Fig. 1.12). Immunohistochemical staining shows that these inclusions contain 3R tau (Fig. 8.7).

When deep gray matter structures are involved, there is comparable neuronal loss and gliosis without accumulation of Pick bodies. Such changes are most common in the head of the caudate nucleus, although they may also be found in the putamen, pallidum, and portions of the thalamus. Ballooned neurons (sometimes referred to as *Pick cells*) are also frequent (Fig. 8.8).

8.3.2.1.2. FTLD-tau with *MAPT* mutations. Mutations in the *MAPT* gene that encodes tau are found in some familial forms of FTLD-tau. These mutations can be grouped into those that alter the splicing of tau mRNA and those that are point mutations changing the amino acid sequence of the protein. The altered splicing results in a shift of the balance between 3R and 4R tau, and this disequilibrium is believed to contribute to the initiation of the cellular dysfunction. The underlying mechanisms relating point mutations to the disease are less clear but are thought to be related to altered microtubule binding, increased aggregation, or both.

The disease is characterized by diffuse atrophy of the frontal and temporal lobes, with corresponding

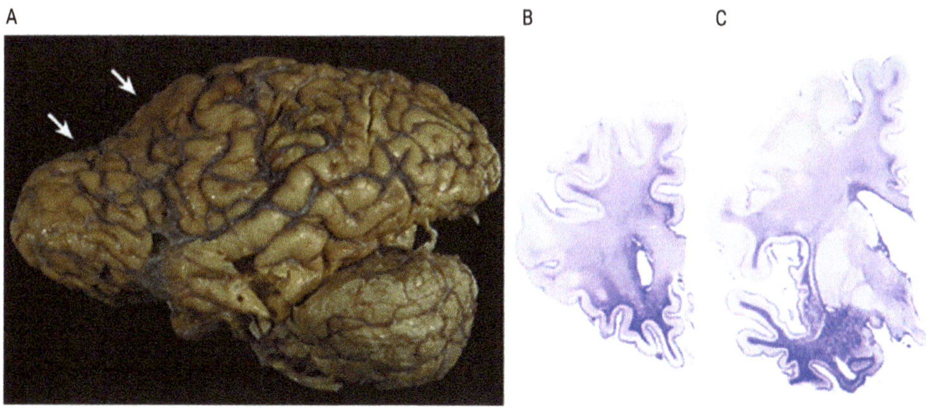

FIGURE 8.5 Macroscopic findings of Pick body disease. (**A**) The prefrontal area shows "knife-edge" atrophy (*arrows*). Holzer staining reveals atrophy and astrocytic gliosis prominently in the supraorbital prefrontal area (**B** middle panel) and the temporal lobe (**C** right panel).

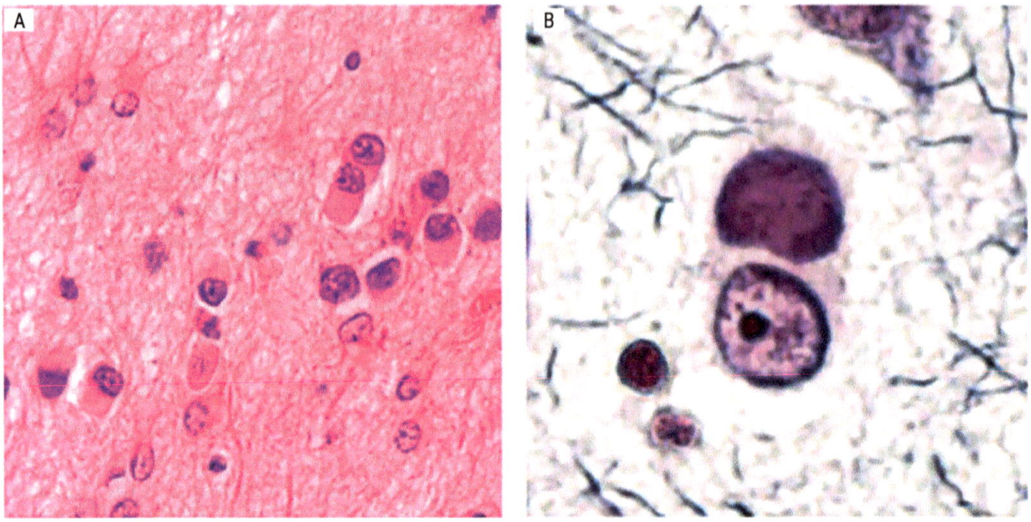

FIGURE 8.6 Pick body disease. (**A**) The hippocampal dentate gyrus shows severe neuronal loss with astrocytic gliosis, and cytoplasm of remaining neurons containing Pick bodies, which are subtle on routine stains (left panel, H&E). (**B**) Pick bodies are strongly labeled with silver impregnation, including Bodian staining (right panel, Bodian).

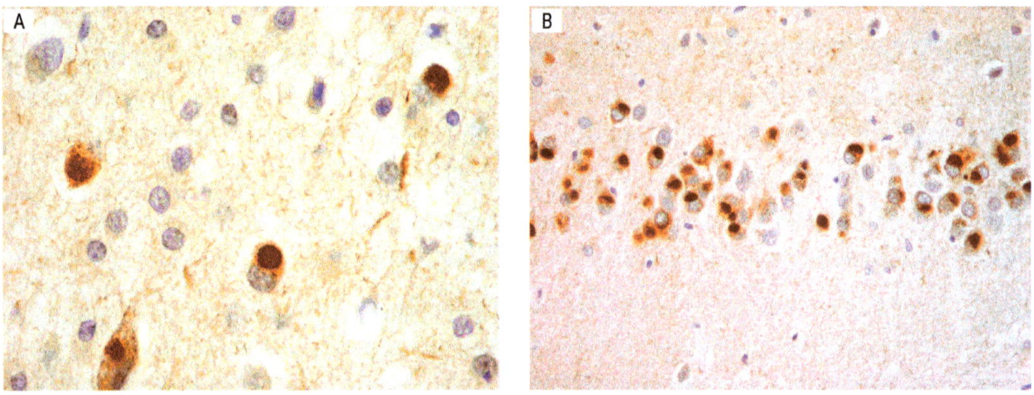

FIGURE 8.7 Pick bodies are spherical, tau-positive inclusions (**A**) in the neocortex (tau IHC) and (**B**) in the dentate gyrus of the hippocampus (tau IHC).

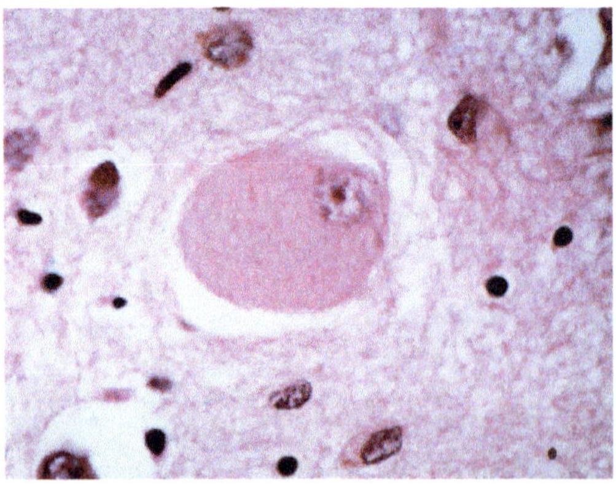

FIGURE 8.8 Ballooned neuron. Swollen cortical neurons are a characteristic feature of Pick disease, but they may be seen in other conditions (H&E).

cognitive changes. Parkinsonism may accompany the dementia (hence the older term *frontotemporal dementia with parkinsonism linked to chromosome 17* [FTDP-17], with *MAPT* being localized on chromosome 17).

8.3.2.1.2.1. Gross appearance. The frontotemporal atrophy and the ventricular dilation are of variable severity. The caudate nucleus may be atrophic. The substantia nigra is sometimes pale.

8.3.2.1.2.2. Microscopic lesions. The upper layers of cerebral cortex often show vacuolation, and extensive neuronal loss with reactive gliosis is observed. Remaining neurons contain tau aggregates appearing as tangles or "pretangles" that are a

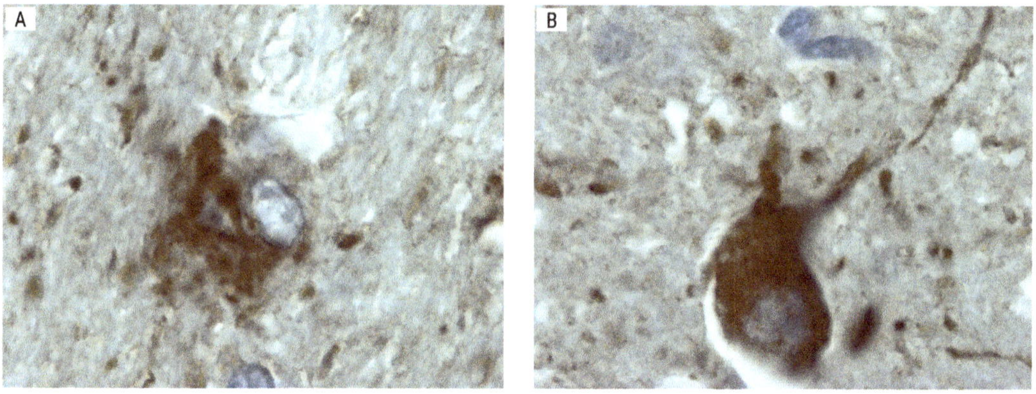

FIGURE 8.9 Tauopathy in a case with mutation of *MAPT*: P301L MAPT mutation, polyclonal anti-tau antibody. (**A**) Tau accumulation in an astrocyte (tau IHC); (**B**) Pretangle in the cerebral cortex (tau IHC).

diffuse cytoplasmic accumulation of tau in abnormal conformations (Fig. 8.9). Glial tau inclusions are quite common. These can occur diffusely, not only in white matter but also in astrocytes within gray matter. Neuropathologic findings may be quite heterogeneous, not well predicted by mutated sites in *MAPT*, and often cannot be classified into any single pathological entity seen in sporadic tauopathies.

8.3.2.1.3. FTLD-tau without tau mutation. Some cases of FTLD-tau are associated with neither *MAPT* mutations nor Pick pathology, although neither the gross nor the H&E microscopic appearance can differentiate them from cases with *MAPT* mutations.

8.3.2.2. FTLD ASSOCIATED WITH TDP-43-POSITIVE LESIONS

Frontotemporal lobar degeneration with tau-negative group was initially labeled as FTLD without distinctive pathology. Within this group, ubiquitin-positive inclusions in cortex or hippocampal dentate gyrus were identified (FTLD-U), and frequent association with ALS was described for FTLD-U. Although the component of ubiquitinated protein was not known initially, TDP-43 was identified as a pathological protein of both FTLD-U and ALS in 2006, and a close relationship between these two diseases was established. Currently, FTLD cases with TDP-43-positive inclusions are designated FTLD-TDP, and they may account for half the autopsy-confirmed FTLD cases. Several genetic loci harbor causative mutations for familial FTLD-TDP, which include *TDP-43*, *progranulin*, *valosin-containing protein* (*VCP*), and *C9orf72*. Sporadic forms of this disease also occur with comparable clinical features. As discussed above, FTLD-TDP is often associated with ALS. This is particularly true for those cases associated with mutations in *TDP-43* and the more frequent cases linked to expansion of the hexanucleotide (GGGGCC) repeat in *C9orf72*. In contrast, *progranulin*-linked FTLD-TDP is not associated with ALS. A genetic locus, *VCP*, has also been identified in the setting of familial FTLD (typically not linked to ALS), characterized by the combination of clinical syndromes comprising inclusion body myositis, Paget disease of the bone, and FTD.

8.3.2.2.1. Macroscopic findings. As with other forms of FTLD, the frontotemporal atrophy is frequently circumscribed in FTLD-TDP, as in Pick disease, and accounts for the clinically observed focal deficits. There is commonly ventricular dilation, and the caudate nucleus may be atrophic (Fig. 8.10). A subset of patients also show atrophy of subiculum in the anterior portion of hippocampus.

8.3.2.2.2. Microscopic findings. Superficial cortical vacuolation is commonly observed, particularly in layer II of the frontal cortex (Fig. 8.11). In some cases, the neuronal loss is severe, involving all the cortical layers with microvacuolation and astrocytic gliosis. TDP-43 is normally a nuclear protein. However, in these disorders, TDP-43 is phosphorylated and mislocalized. IHC shows ubiquitin- and TDP-43-immunopositive intraneuronal inclusions of various types and with variable distribution (Figs. 8.12–8.14). TDP-43-positive neuronal inclusions are located in the cell body (so-called NCIs) (Figs. 8.128.14), in the nucleus (NIIs) (Fig. 8.14), or in the neurites (Figs. 8.12 and

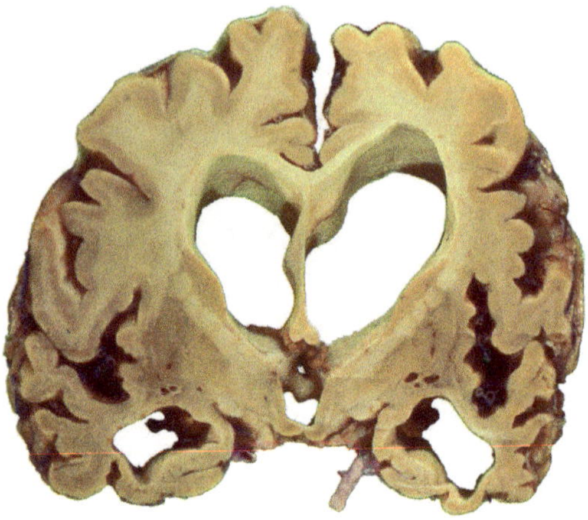

FIGURE 8.10 Frontotemporal lobar degeneration. There is severe cerebral atrophy with marked temporal lobe involvement, especially marked in its medial aspect (including hippocampus). Note enlargement of the lateral ventricles.

8.14); glial inclusions are also observed in affected regions. The inclusions are most abundant in the frontal and temporal cortices, in the striatum, and in the dentate gyrus of the hippocampus. In addition, *C9orf72*-linked FTLD-TDP and ALS-TDP show dipeptide repeat (DPR) inclusions derived by repeat-associated non-ATG (RAN) translation, which are ubiquitinated but negative for TDP-43 (Fig. 8.15). The DPR inclusions are typically abundant in the hippocampal dentate gyrus and cerebellar granule cell layer but sparse in motor neurons.

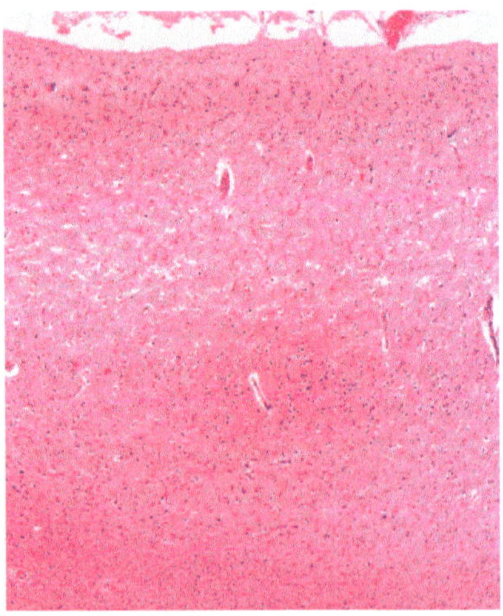

FIGURE 8.11 Frontotemporal lobar degeneration. Neuronal loss and microvacuolation predominate in the superficial layers of the neocortex. In more advanced cases (as here), the neuronal loss may be severe (H&E).

Different classification schemes have been proposed for FTLD-TDP, taking into account the appearance, abundance, and distribution of inclusions and correlating these with the underlying genetic alterations, but less so with the clinical phenotype:

- Type A shows the presence of many TDP-43-positive NCIs and short neurites, both mostly in upper cortical layers. These are accompanied by needle-like, or cat's eye–shaped, NIIs. This pattern is associated with sporadic cases or mutation in the *progranulin* gene.
- Type B shows predominantly NCI (not limited to upper cortical layers) with some neurites, but lacking NII. This pattern is commonly associated with bvFTD, with ALS, and with expansion of the hexanucleotide repeat in *C9orf72*.
- Type C shows many long dystrophic neurites, less abundant NCIs, and very few NIIs. This type is often associated with semantic dementia and rare among familial FTLD-TDP.
- Type D shows predominantly the lentiform NIIs, with abundant short neurites but scant NCIs. This pattern is associated with the rare mutations in *VCP*.

8.3.2.3. FTLD-FUS

In rare cases, the neuronal inclusions are negative for both tau and TDP-43 but are labeled by FUS IHC. This observation grew out of the demonstration that *FUS* mutations are associated with some familial forms of ALS (fALS). Some cases of FLTD-FUS were initially described as atypical FTLD-U (aFTLD-U) before the identification of FUS. Two other sporadic disorders are included in the category of FTLD-FUS: neuronal intermediate filament inclusion disease (NIFID) and basophilic inclusion body disease (BIBD). NIFID is characterized by Pick body–like spherical NCIs, approximately the size of the nucleus, in the cerebral cortex, basal nuclei, and brainstem; as the name implies, the inclusions contain neurofilament proteins as well as FUS. BIBD has a heterogeneous clinical phenotype that can include bvFTD, lower motor neuron (LMN) disease, and extrapyramidal signs. In NIFID and BIBD, NCIs are inconstantly ubiquitin immunopositive but intensely FUS positive (Fig. 8.16).

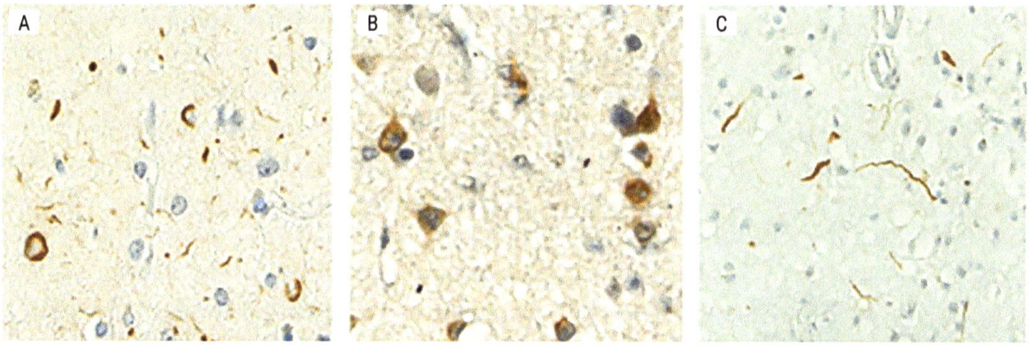

FIGURE 8.12 Sporadic FTLD-TDP. Phosphorylated TDP-43 is located within neuronal or neuritic inclusions. Sporadic cases can show any of three types of cortical TDP-43 pathology: (**A**) type A, with short neuritic aggregates and round or ring-shaped neuronal inclusions); (**B**) type B, with diffuse cytoplasmic inclusions and sparse neuritic aggregates; or (**C**) type C, with long and thick neuritic aggregates and sparse cytoplasmic inclusions (TDP IHC).

8.3.2.4. FTLD-UPS

In a few families with FTLD, the inclusions are detectable only by IHC directed against proteins belonging to the ubiquitin–proteasomal degradation system. The inclusions in these brains are characterized by the presence of ubiquitin and p62 (a protein that binds to polyubiquitinated proteins and assists in transporting them toward the proteasome and for autophagy). FTLD-UPS is associated with mutations in *CHMP2B* (charged multivesicular body protein 2B).

8.3.2.5. DEMENTIA LACKING INCLUSIONS

In a few cases of FTD, there is no cytoplasmic or nuclear inclusion detected. These cases were once classified as dementia without distinctive pathology and are now classified as FTLD-ni (for no inclusion).

8.3.3. Dementia with Lewy bodies

Dementia commonly occurs as an additional clinical manifestation in patients with PD (see Section 8.4.1.1). There is a somewhat arbitrary separation between dementia with Lewy bodies (DLB; formerly "diffuse Lewy body disease"), in which dementia develops within 1 year of the onset of parkinsonism (or in advance of it), and PD with dementia (PD dementia), in which the dementia develops after the PD diagnosis more than 1 year later. In either setting, the dementia is a progressive disorder with early hallucinations and prominent fluctuations in cognition. Neuropathological changes include the

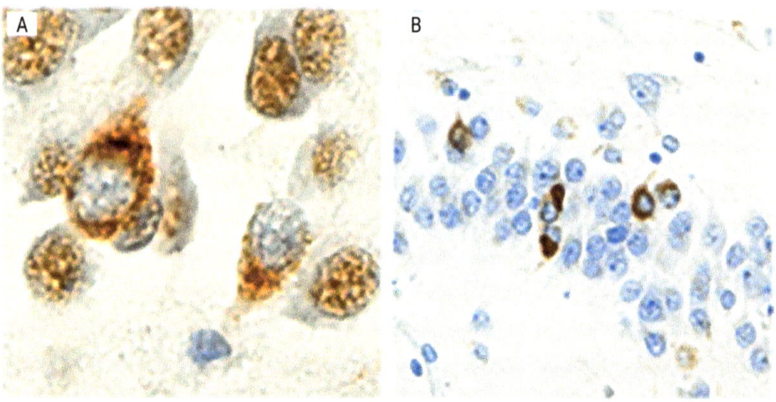

FIGURE 8.13 TDP-43 inclusions in hippocampal dentate gyrus of sporadic FTLD-TDP. (**A**) Full-length non-phosphorylated TDP-43 exhibits cytoplasmic inclusions and reduced immunostaining within the nuclei of affected neurons. (**B**) Anti-phosphorylated TDP-43 IHC visualizes aggregated TDP-43 cytoplasmic inclusions but not physiological intranuclear TDP-43(TDP IHC).

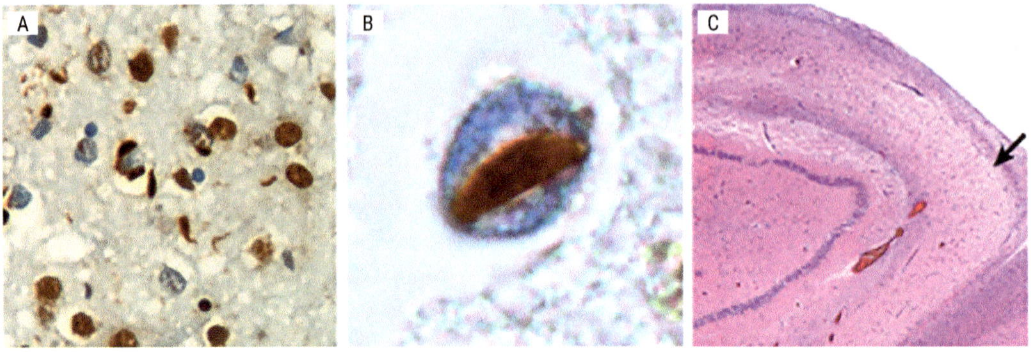

FIGURE 8.14 FTLD-TDP with mutation of the *progranulin* gene (*PGRN*). (**A**) Anti-TDP-43 IHC displays neuronal cytoplasmic and neuritic inclusions, showing type A pathology, in association with reduced intranuclear immunostaining. (**B**) TDP-43-immunopositive intranuclear inclusion with cat's eye appearance. (**C**) Neuronal loss in the hippocampus is often prominent in the CA1 (*arrow*) and subiculum, showing a pattern of hippocampal sclerosis.

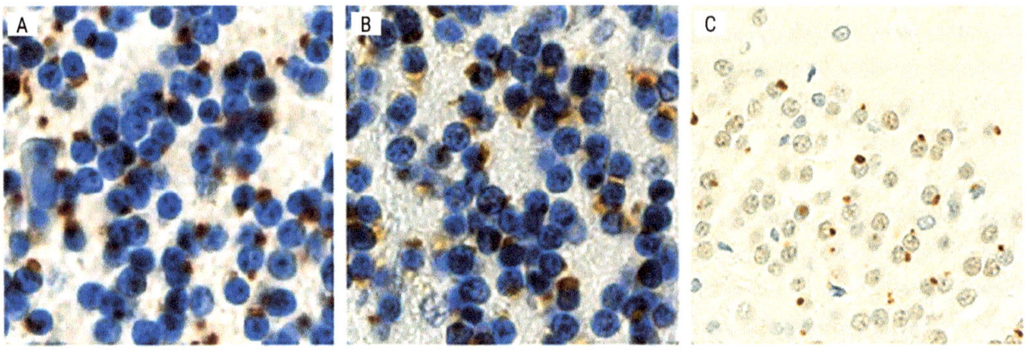

FIGURE 8.15 FTLD-TDP with hexanucleotide expansion of the *C9ORF72* gene. (**A**) The cerebellar granule cell layer shows numerous P62-immunopositive inclusions. (**B**) These inclusions are immunopositive for DPR (poly GA) but not for TDP-43. (**C**) DPR inclusions are also abundant in the hippocampal dentate gyrus.

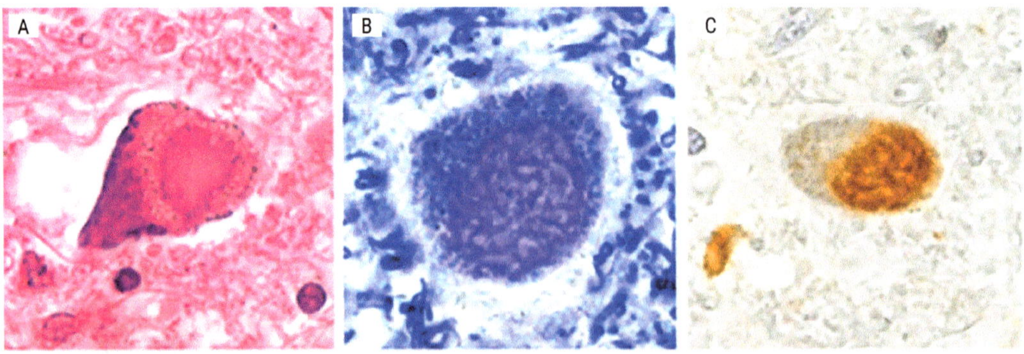

FIGURE 8.16 BIBD. (**A**) The lower motor neuron shows a well-circumscribed, basophilic inclusion in the cell body (H&E); the outline of the inclusion is emphasized by cresyl violet staining (**B**) and intensely immunopositive for FUS (**C**) (FUS IHC).

presence of Lewy bodies and Lewy neurites in the cerebral cortex as well as in the brainstem. These are often accompanied by some degree of ADNCs, often with a moderate plaque burden but relatively lower tangle burden. Although the etiologic relationship between the processes remains unclear, it is likely that each can contribute to cognitive impairment.

8.3.3.1. MACROSCOPIC FINDINGS

Cerebral atrophy is generally not as severe as that seen in AD of equivalent cognitive impairment, with brain weight often in the normal range. There is usually pallor of the substantia nigra and of the locus coeruleus, as would be seen in typical PD. Atrophy of the limbic system may be prominent.

8.3.3.2. MICROSCOPIC FINDINGS

Neuronal loss and gliosis are usually restricted to brainstem regions, particularly the substantia nigra and locus coeruleus. The severity of injury is typically comparable to that observed in PD, along with Lewy bodies: eosinophilic, laminated cytoplasmic neuronal inclusions surrounded by a clear halo. In contrast to these changes, the cerebral neocortex, hippocampus, and amygdala are usually unremarkable with routine H&E staining. With IHC directed against α-synuclein, another picture emerges. The brainstem Lewy bodies are highlighted, and their wider distribution in the reticular formation becomes evident, along with the presence of immunoreactive dystrophic neurites (Lewy neurites). In the deeper layers of the cerebral cortex (particularly temporal, insular, and cingulate cortices), there are ill-defined cytoplasmic inclusions that lack a clear halo (as surrounds the eosinophilic core in the brainstem-type Lewy body) but are immunostained comparably by α-synuclein antibodies (Fig. 8.17A, B). These are also accompanied by Lewy neurites in the cortical neuropil, and a superficial spongiosis involving the superficial cortical layers. In the amygdala, Lewy bodies are detected in neurons, whereas in the hippocampus Lewy neurites in CA2–3 can be the only finding (Fig. 8.18). As mentioned previously, most brains with DLB also show some plaques and tangles, although in most instances the lesions are not as severe as in AD.

8.3.3.3. DIAGNOSTIC CLASSIFICATION

Lewy body diseases (DLB and PD) are α-synucleinopathies and can be stratified into three groups: brainstem type, when Lewy bodies are restricted to brainstem structures; transitional, when there is involvement of limbic structures; and neocortical, when there is additional involvement of the neocortex. In the current diagnostic criteria, it is recommended to systematically assess Alzheimer pathology in order to evaluate the probability (high, intermediate, or low) that Lewy pathology is responsible for the cognitive deficit.

8.3.4. Argyrophilic grain disease

Lacking a distinctive clinical picture that reliably allows for its premortem diagnosis, AGD is largely defined on neuropathologic grounds. Argyrophilic grains are small, Gallyas-positive inclusions

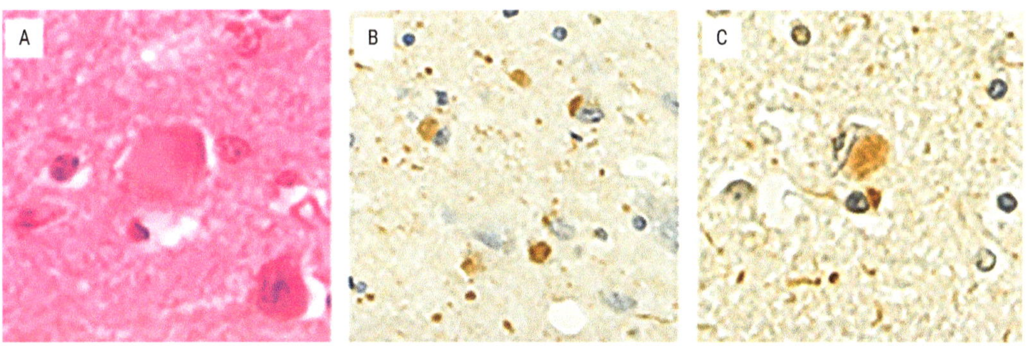

FIGURE 8.17 Dementia with Lewy bodies. (**A**) Cortical Lewy bodies are round-shaped cytoplasmic inclusions lacking clear halo and core structures and difficult to see on routine stains (H&E). (**B**) α-Synuclein immunohistochemistry labels many cortical Lewy bodies (α-synuclein IHC). (**C**) Cortical Lewy bodies also contain ubiquitin (ubiquitin IHC).

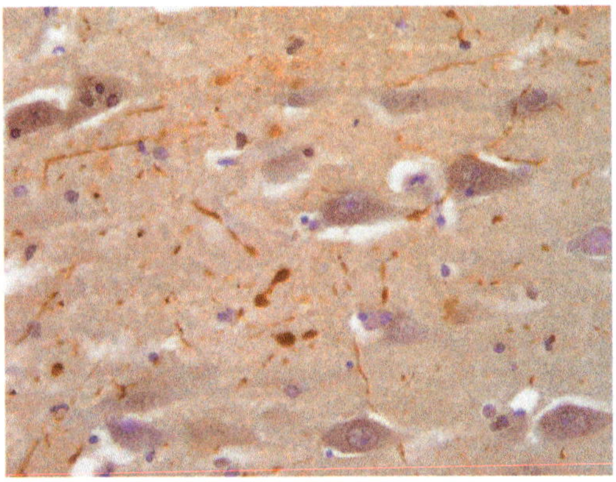

FIGURE 8.18 Dementia with Lewy bodies. Lewy neurites may be detected by ubiquitin immunostaining in both demented and nondemented patients with Lewy body diseases (ubiquitin IHC).

containing 4R tau in neurites. Argyrophilic, 4R tau inclusions are also frequent in oligodendrocyte perikaryon ("coiled bodies"). These pathologic findings in AGD are not consistently associated with clinical evidence of cognitive impairment. Recent studies have suggested that there can be localized atrophy of the ambient gyrus, and the accumulation of grains appears to begin there, with progressive involvement through medial temporal lobe structures and thence to other limbic regions, such as the cingulate and insular cortices (Fig. 8.19).

8.3.5. Hippocampal sclerosis

Hippocampal sclerosis (HS) has been largely described in patients with epileptic seizures, where it was first reported. However, in elderly patients, HS is associated with memory loss and dementia in the absence of seizures. HS is highly prevalent, particularly in the "oldest old" (>95 years). Clinically, the cognitive decline in HS may be indistinguishable from that in AD. HS is frequently associated with other neurodegenerative or vascular diseases, but it can be found in isolation. Macroscopic examination reveals a severe hippocampal atrophy. There is severe neuron loss and astrocytic gliosis limited to the CA1 sector and subiculum of the hippocampus, which explain the memory deficit. There is sparing of the CA4 sector and absence of dispersion of the dentate granule cell layer, in contrast to what is observed in younger patients with HS associated with epileptic seizures. In elderly subjects with dementia, HS can be seen unilateral, in one of the two hippocampi, or bilateral. Although the mechanisms of disease are largely unknown, there is a high prevalence of HS cases with TDP-43 inclusions in the granule cells of the dentate gyrus, suggesting a role of this protein in its pathogenesis.

8.3.6. Primary age-related tauopathy

Primary age-related tauopathy (PART) is a pathologically defined condition, characterized by the presence of neurofibrillary tangles with no or sparse Aβ deposits or senile plaques ("tangle-only pathology"). Spatial distribution and immunohistochemical properties of the neurofibrillary tangles are similar to those in AD. It is commonly observed in individuals with and without cognitive

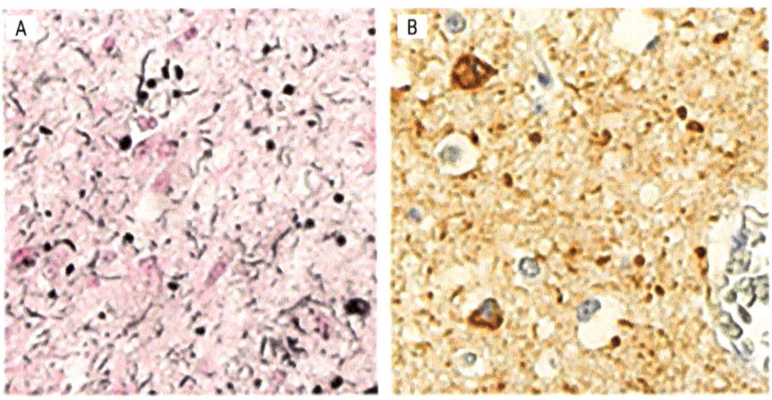

FIGURE 8.19 Argyrophilic grain disease. (**A**) Gallyas silver impregnation labels "grains" that are dot-shaped silver-positive granules spreading in the neuropil. (**B**) Grains are immunopositive for tau (tau IHC). It is sometimes difficult to distinguish argyrophilic grains from neuropil threads. Tau-immunopositive coiled bodies are also seen in the cytoplasm.

impairment; hence, the causation of cognitive changes due to PART is unclear. There are two interpretations for the neuropathologic finding of PART. One is that PART is a component of AD pathology, possibly reflecting an early pathological process. Another notion is that PART is a distinctive 3R and 4R tauopathy, which may lead to cognitive impairment in the absence of Aβ pathology, so-called tangle-only dementia.

8.3.7. Vascular dementia/vascular cognitive impairment

Injury to the brain parenchyma associated with vascular lesions may be a substrate for cognitive impairment and even dementia. The types of vascular lesions that can contribute to loss of normal cognition include infarcts involving multiple small or large territories with tissue destruction (multi-infarct dementia); small infarct(s) localized in strategic areas (e.g., thalamus); and diffuse white matter injury, as can be seen in the setting of poorly managed hypertension (a pattern sometimes referred to as Binswanger leukoencephalopathy), of amyloid angiopathy, or of diffuse small vessel diseases such as CADASIL (cerebral autosomal dominant arteriopathy with subcortical infarcts and leukoencephalopathy). Although pure vascular-based cognitive impairment is relatively infrequent, vascular comorbidity commonly contributes to dementia in individuals who also have neurodegenerative diseases, particularly AD.

8.3.8. Other causes of dementia

Dementia can be a component of neurodegenerative diseases, which are discussed elsewhere in this chapter because the primary burden of the disease process is borne by other functional systems. Examples encountered in subsequent sections include some of the movement disorders, such as the trinucleotide-repeat disorder HD as well as the tauopathies PSP and CBD. Dementia is also a prominent component of prion diseases (see Chapter 6); bacterial infections, including syphilis and Whipple disease (see Chapter 5); and viral diseases, such as the HIV-associated neurocognitive disorder (see Chapter 5). Various storage disorders can include cognitive impairment leading to dementia, such as Kufs disease and adult-onset Tay–Sachs disease (see Chapter 10).

8.4. MOVEMENT DISORDERS

Although numerous brain regions contribute to planning and execution of motor output, the term *movement disorders* is commonly reserved for diseases in which dysfunction of the basal ganglia circuitry results in either decreased or increased motor output. The functional organization of the basal ganglia (commonly defined to include the striatum, the globus pallidus, the subthalamic nucleus, the substantia nigra, and the white matter tracts that connect these structures) serves to modulate the planning and execution of movement through a pair of competing pathways. Because of this dynamic balance, loss of neurons that shifts the balance can allow the residual circuitry to either decrease motor capacity (akinetic movement disorders) or increase it (hyperkinetic movement disorders).

8.4.1. Akinetic rigid syndromes

Akinetic rigid syndromes are characterized by rigidity, bradykinesia, and tremor—a clinical triad known as *parkinsonism*—although not all affected individuals will manifest all features. The most common disorder underlying parkinsonism is PD. Other diseases may not only manifest a similar clinical picture but also show additional features; these are designated as "Parkinson plus" syndromes or atypical parkinsonism, for example. A critical component of these movement disorders is related to loss of striatal dopamine and associated abnormalities of the nigrostriatal system (Fig. 8.20).

8.4.1.1. PARKINSON DISEASE

The most common of the akinetic movement disorders, PD, is a degenerative disease mainly seen in older adults. The core of the clinical diagnosis is the presence of the parkinsonian triad (resting tremor, rigidity, and bradykinesia), progression, and symptomatic response to treatment with agents that increase striatal dopamine. In addition to the movement disorder, other common components of the illness include autonomic dysfunction, depression or behavioral changes, and sleep disturbances. Rapid eye movement sleep behavioral disorder is a relatively frequent antecedent to parkinsonism.

The annual incidence of PD ranges from approximately 7.0 to 19 per 100,000 and the prevalence from approximately 30 to 190 per 100,000; the majority of cases are sporadic, although there are rare

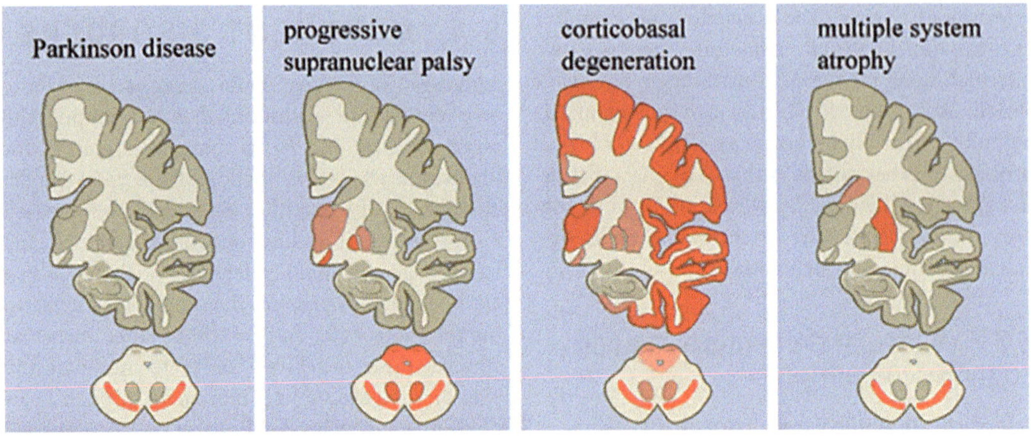

FIGURE 8.20 Typical distribution of regional atrophy in the basal ganglia of akinetic rigid disorders. Regions noted with dark red are more frequently involved than those colored with light red. Microscopic changes, including neuron loss and inclusion bodies, may extend more broadly than atrophic lesions.

familial forms. Patients with familial forms may have dominant or recessive inheritance patterns. From the study of these familial forms has come important insights into the pathways critical for development of PD and the nature of its diagnostic pathologic hallmark, the Lewy body (an intraneuronal cytoplasmic inclusion body containing α-synuclein already seen in DLB) (Fig. 1.13). With the recognition of α-synuclein as a marker of neuronal inclusions in PD, it has become clear that the disease involves much of the brainstem and can progress to involve cortical regions. This is based on the hypothesis that α-synuclein aggregations begin in the dorsal motor nucleus of the vagus nerve in the medulla, gradually progressing rostrally to the locus coeruleus of the pons and to the substantia nigra of the midbrain. Concomitant with the clinical onset of akinetic movement disorders, there is moderate involvement of the substantia nigra by neuronal loss and gliosis. A classification termed *Lewy body Braak stages (1–6)* has been introduced to describe the histopathologic progression of the severity of disease. The neuropathologic changes characteristic of the disease may extend to involve cortical regions, and the disease can be manifest clinically also as a dementia (PD dementia; the neuropathologic findings are the same as those for DLB; see Section 8.3.3), often with the characteristic fluctuations and visual hallucinations.

8.4.1.1.1. Macroscopic findings. The brain weight is ordinarily within normal limits for age in PD; the most striking findings are pallor of the substantia nigra (Fig. 8.21) and pallor of the locus coeruleus. Depigmentation is often more severe in the locus coeruleus than in the substantia nigra (Fig. 8.22).

8.4.1.1.2. Microscopic findings. Neuronal loss and astrocytic gliosis are seen in the pars compacta of the substantia nigra (Fig. 8.22), in the coeruleus–subcoeruleus area, and in the dorsal nucleus of vagus nerve. Neuromelanin pigment may be seen in

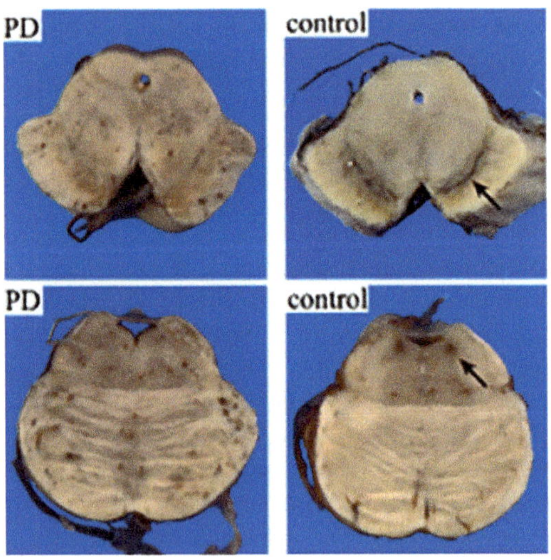

FIGURE 8.21 Parkinson disease. Macroscopic appearance: Midbrain (Top panel) shows pallor of the substantia nigra, compared with normal substantia nigra (*arrow*). Depigmentation is also observed in the locus coeruleus of the upper pons (Bottom panel) compared to control (*arrow*). These are the result of loss of neurons containing neuromelanin.

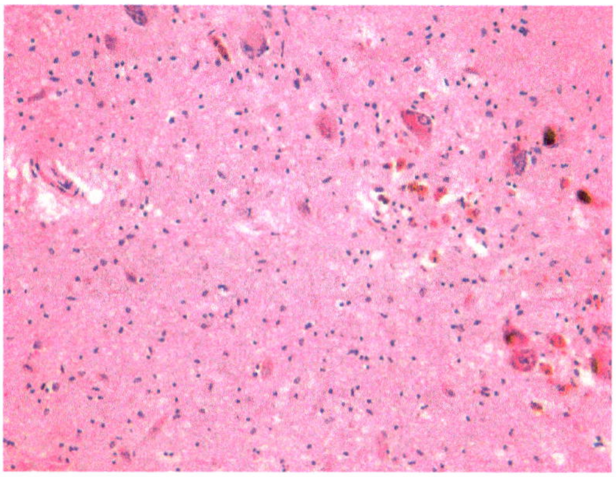

FIGURE 8.22 Histology of the substantia nigra showing loss of pigmented neurons and astrocytic gliosis. Pigment can be seen in macrophages (H&E).

macrophages or free in the neuropil. A few percent of the remaining neurons in these nuclei contain Lewy bodies.

Other regions may be affected by Lewy body pathology and may relate to other clinical features of disease. Changes in the dorsal motor nucleus of vagus nerve, commonly observed, may be associated with dysphagia. The nucleus basalis of Meynert and the amygdala are frequently affected. Lewy bodies may be seen in the cerebral cortex, and extensive pathology has been related to distinctive forms of dementia termed PD dementia and DLB, discussed above. Lewy bodies may also be encountered in the neurons of the intermediolateral cell columns of the spinal cord, sympathetic and parasympathetic ganglia, the enteric nervous system, the cardiac plexus, the pelvic plexus, skin, salivary glands, and the adrenal medulla; the involvement of these structures can be presumed to be the basis of the autonomic dysfunction (see Section 8.7).

In some affected brain regions, one may observe, in addition to the typical Lewy bodies situated in the neuronal perikarya, hyaline acidophilic inclusions, of which the outline and the halo may be less distinctly defined; these are elongated and are situated in cell processes (intraneuritic Lewy bodies or Lewy neurites) (Fig. 1.13C, D). Finally, the cortical (cerebral) Lewy bodies are situated in the perikaryon of cortical neurons, may not be spherical, and are less eosinophilic; they typically have neither central core nor peripheral halo (Fig. 1.13E, F). The presence of α-synuclein within these inclusions (Fig. 8.23) has led to the recommendation that IHC against this normal synaptic protein be used for the detection of Lewy bodies and Lewy neurites, which can otherwise be inconspicuous on routine stains.

8.4.1.1.3. Familial mutation-linked PD. Point mutations in α-synuclein (*SNCA*) or leucine-rich repeat kinase 2 (*LRRK2*) are well-known mutations linked to autosomal dominant familial forms of PD. There are also kindreds with PD caused by duplication or triplication of the *SNCA* locus. *SNCA* mutations are associated with Lewy body pathology, whereas a subset of *LRRK2* mutations lacks it. Mutations of the gene *PRKN*, encoding parkin (E3 ubiquitin ligase), and the gene *PINK1*, encoding a mitochondrial kinase, both encode proteins with a critical role in mitochondrial turnover. Mutations in DJ-1 (*PARK7*) and *ATP13A2* cause autosomal recessive parkinsonism, which usually presents before age 40 years and is sensitive to L-dopa therapy.

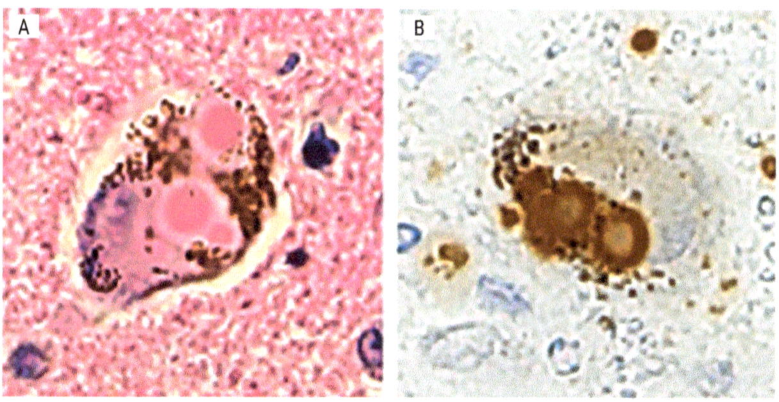

FIGURE 8.23 (**A**) The nigral neurons contain "brainstem-type" Lewy bodies with clear halo and core structures (H&E). (**B**) α-Synuclein immunostaining is prominent within the halo (α-synuclein IHC).

In these recessive forms, Lewy bodies are typically absent, although neuronal loss is severe in the substantia nigra.

The best characterized genetic risk factor for the development of PD is the presence of a mutated allele of the *GBA* gene, which encodes the enzyme β-glucocerebrosidase and is the recessive locus for Gaucher disease, a lysosomal storage disorder. Although the underlying mechanism of this relationship is not known, these mutations are found in 5–10% of cases of sporadic PD.

8.4.1.2. PROGRESSIVE SUPRANUCLEAR PALSY

Progressive supranuclear palsy, or Steele–Richardson–Olszewski disease, is clinically characterized by parkinsonism associated with supranuclear ophthalmoplegia. The parkinsonism is usually without tremor but with hypertonia, retrocollis (rather than flexion, as in PD), and axial rigidity (rather than greater involvement of the extremities, as in PD). Pseudobulbar palsy and cognitive abnormality leading to dementia are common. The average age of onset is approximately 64 years, with a prevalence of approximately 7 per 100,000. In general, these patients respond only with minimal symptomatic relief from therapeutic approaches to elevate striatal dopamine, in contrast to those with PD.

8.4.1.2.1. Macroscopic findings. The most striking abnormality is atrophy of the midbrain and pontine tegmentum. There is commonly pallor of the substantia nigra and locus coeruleus as in PD, but associated with atrophy of the globus pallidus and the subthalamic nucleus (Luys body) with variable severity (Fig. 8.24). The cerebral cortex is usually spared, although in cases with prominent cognitive impairment, there may also be frontotemporal atrophy.

8.4.1.2.2. Microscopic findings. The diagnostic features of PSP are the combination of regional neuronal loss and astrocytic gliosis, with neuronal and glial accumulation of tau protein (4R tau), as highlighted by IHC. The changes are prominent in basal ganglia (substantia nigra, the globus pallidus, and the subthalamic nucleus) as well as in the brainstem (superior colliculus, pretectal areas, periaqueductal gray matter, and the mesencephalic and pontine reticular formations). In addition, there may be moderate involvement of the cerebellar dentate nucleus, locus coeruleus, oculomotor nuclei, pontine nuclei, reticular formation in the medulla, inferior olivary complex, and thalamus.

In these affected regions, the neuronal loss and gliosis are accompanied by tau-containing inclusions in both neurons and glia. Within neurons, tau protein forms neurofibrillary tangles, which have a characteristic globose appearance (Fig. 8.25). Tufted astrocytes, highly characteristic of the disease, develop in affected areas, are usually abundant in the putamen, and are commonly found in the cerebral cortex, mostly motor and premotor areas of the frontal lobe (Fig. 8.26A). Aggregated tau accumulates in the proximal process of the tufted astrocyte. Thorn-shaped astrocytes (Fig. 8.26B) (see Chapter 1) may be seen but are not specific to PSP; rather, they are associated with increasing age and are features of aging-related tau astrogliopathy(ARTAG). Accumulation of tau protein in oligodendrocytes, known as a "coiled body," is also observed in PSP; it is less specific of PSP and may also be seen in other tauopathies.

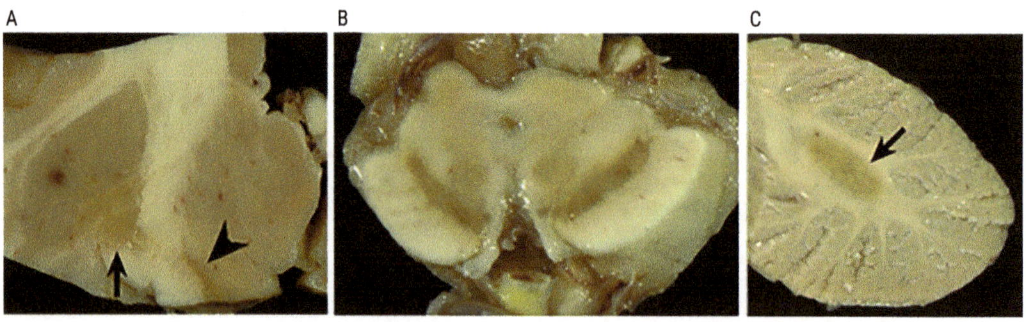

FIGURE 8.24 Macroscopic characteristics of progressive supranuclear palsy. Atrophy and brown discoloration are observed in the globus pallidus (**A**, *arrow*), subthalamic nucleus (**A**, *arrowhead*), substantia nigra and tegmentum of the midbrain (**B**), and cerebellar dentate nucleus (**C**, *arrow*).

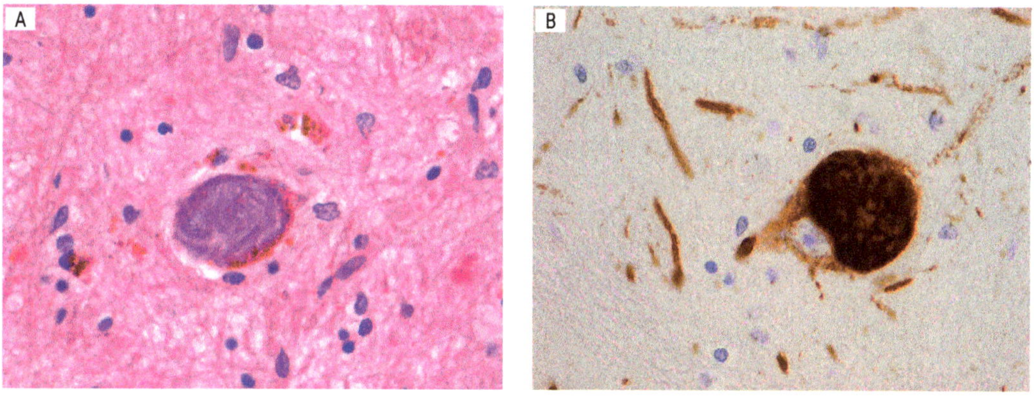

FIGURE 8.25 Progressive supranuclear palsy: (**A**) neuron containing a globose, slightly basophilic neurofibrillary tangle (H&E); (**B**) neuron containing a globose neurofibrillary tangle composed of tau protein (tau IHC).

8.4.1.2.3. Genetic risks. Nearly all cases of PSP are sporadic, although in rare cases *MAPT* mutations are present. There is also a strong risk association for the H1 haplotype of the *MAPT* locus. The H1 haplotype is defined by a series of genetic markers that are in strong linkage disequilibrium.

8.4.1.3. CORTICOBASAL DEGENERATION

Corticobasal degeneration is a clinicopathological entity characterized by degeneration of cortical areas and of the basal ganglia (including the substantia nigra). It is a rare 4R tauopathy and distinguished from PSP by neurological manifestations, distribution of regional atrophy, and histological findings. However, this distinction is not always clear premortem because of significant overlap in clinical features and inconsistent clinical–pathological correlations.

The disease is first clinically manifest with symptoms/signs of rigidity, clumsiness, stiffness, or jerking of arms or, less commonly, the legs. Early in the course of the illness, there is asymmetry of these movement abnormalities, and patients often develop progressive apraxia and the so-called alien limb phenomenon in which a limb moves without voluntary control and the patient has an associated illusion that the affected limb is not part of them. Walking difficulty develops due to apraxia of leg movement together with pyramidal deficits caused by upper motor neuron (UMN) involvement. Cognitive abnormalities occur in some patients with aphasia and dementia of frontotemporal type. In some patients, the cognitive abnormalities predominate over the movement disorder.

8.4.1.3.1. Macroscopic findings. Asymmetric atrophy of the hemisphere is the classical finding, most prominent around the Sylvian fissure or with

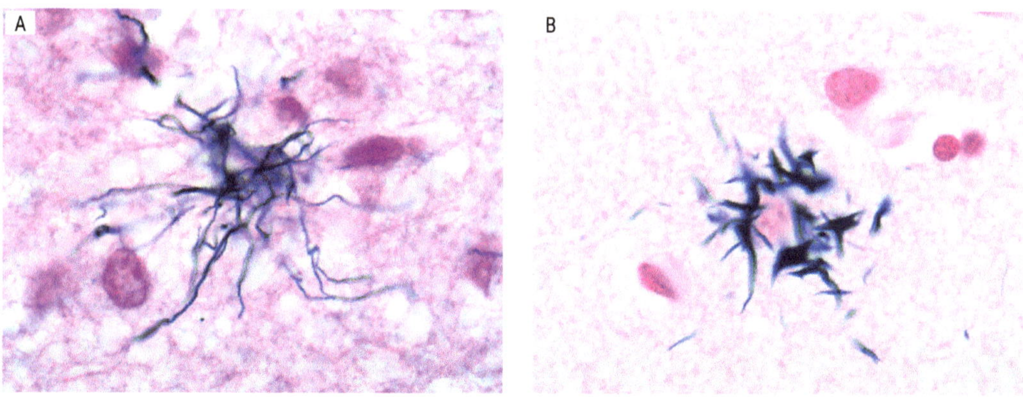

FIGURE 8.26 Glial pathology in progressive supranuclear palsy. (**A**) Tufted astrocytes in the gray matter are very suggestive of PSP (Gallyas silver impregnation). (**B**) Thorn-shaped astrocytes are commonly seen but are not specific and may be seen in other neurodegenerative conditions or in aging (Gallyas).

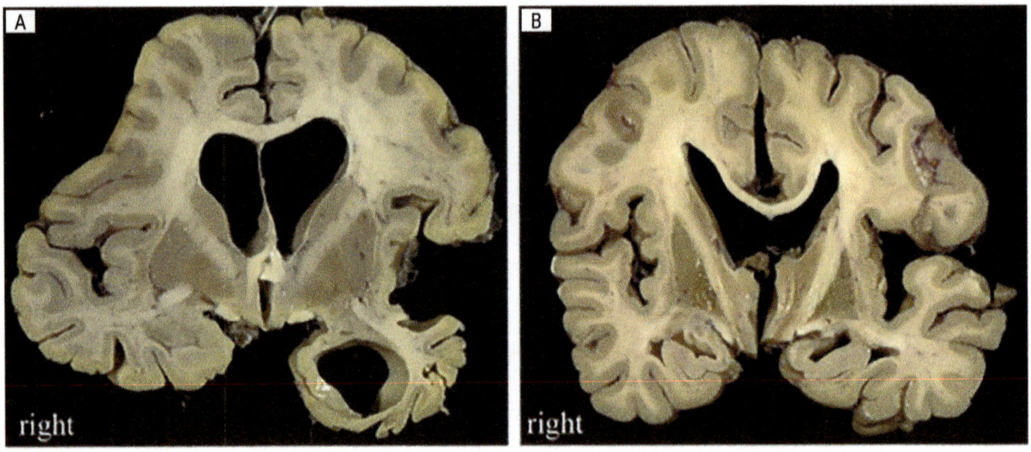

FIGURE 8.27 Gross appearance of corticobasal degeneration. Macroscopic findings may vary among cases. (**A**) One case shows asymmetric atrophy of the perisylvian and temporal cortices in the left hemisphere. (**B**) Another case shows bilateral atrophy of neostriatum, globus pallidus, thalamus, and corpus callosum.

a frontotemporal distribution. However, the asymmetry may not be clear in a subset of patients, and other diseases can be associated with the asymmetric atrophy (e.g., AD) (Fig. 8.27). The substantia nigra shows loss of pigment, and the basal ganglia are atrophic to variable degrees.

8.4.1.3.2. Microscopic findings. The characteristic features include the combination of neuronal loss, astrocytic gliosis, and 4R tau–containing inclusions in neurons and glia. In addition, there may be swollen neurons with effacement of the Nissl substance in the cortex, termed *achromatic* (Fig. 8.28). IHC for tau protein shows abundant pretangles that appear to be diffuse and fuzzy inclusions within the neuronal cytoplasm, lacking tangle structures visible on H&E staining. Globose neurofibrillary tangles are also found (Fig. 8.29). Accumulation of tau protein in astrocytes forms distinctive structures in gray matter areas termed *astrocytic plaques*. Astrocytic plaques are defined by tau accumulation in the distal portions of astrocytic processes, with the center of the plaque devoid of tau immunoreactivity (Fig 8.30); this makes a contrast with tufted astrocytes in PSP that demonstrates tau aggregation in the proximal portions of astrocytic processes. They are conspicuous in the cortex and in the putamen.

8.4.1.4. MULTIPLE SYSTEM ATROPHY

As the term *multiple* implies, MSA is a degenerative process that affects multiple functional systems and does not fit well into only one of the clinical

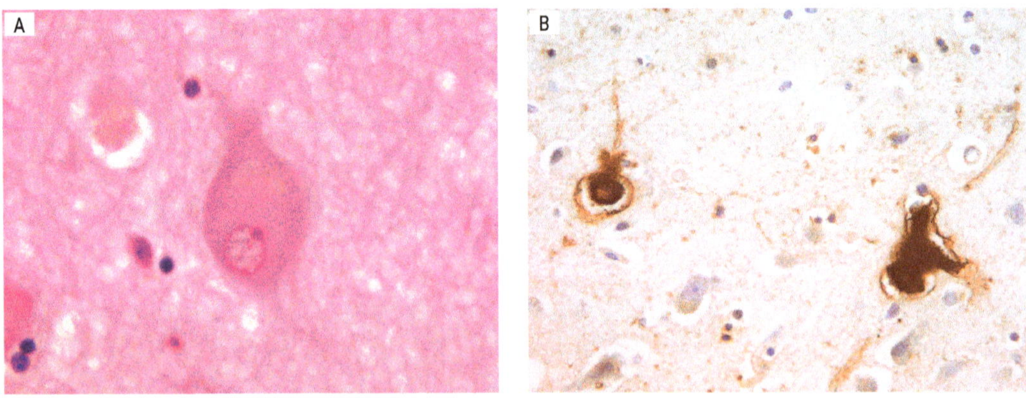

FIGURE 8.28 Corticobasal degeneration: (**A**) swollen achromatic neurons in the cerebral cortex (H&E); (**B**) swollen neurons contain αB crystallin, which is a useful method for detection (αB crystallin IHC).

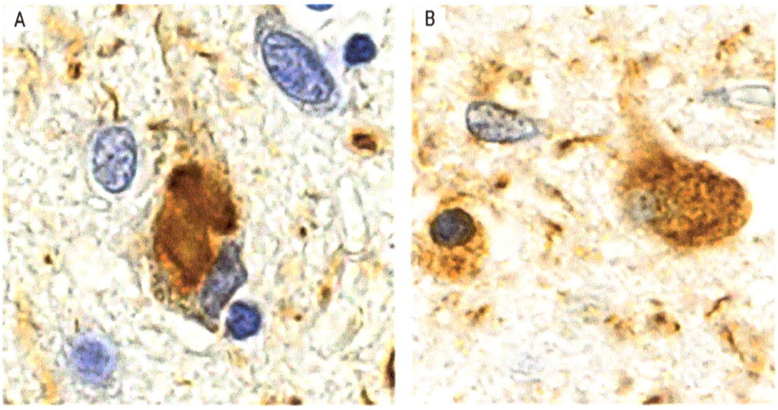

FIGURE 8.29 Corticobasal degeneration. Neuronal tau aggregations appear as globose neurofibrillary tangles (**A**) or pretangles that are diffuse and fuzzy within the cytoplasm or enhanced nearby the nucleus (**B**) (Tau IHC).

categories. Three disorders (striatonigral degeneration, responsible for a parkinsonism syndrome; olivopontocerebellar atrophy [OPCA], clinically associated with ataxia; and Shy–Drager syndrome, characterized by autonomic symptoms), which were originally thought to be distinct, were united after it was recognized that affected individuals often began with one symptom complex but gradually acquired the others. This clinicopathological association was further validated by the recognition that in these cases there was a common neuropathologic finding of distinctive inclusion bodies in glial cells. These inclusions were subsequently shown to contain α-synuclein, leading to the classification of MSA as an α-synucleinopathy, along with PD and DLB; no mutations in the gene for α-synuclein have been found in MSA.

The clinical features of MSA may show a predominance of the parkinsonism (MSA-P) or of the cerebellar ataxia (MSA-C); it is relatively rare to have the autonomic dysfunction as the sole manifestation of the illness, although some features of autonomic disturbances are seen in nearly all cases. In addition to the extrapyramidal motor symptoms, evidence of pyramidal involvement with hyperreflexia is commonly seen. The tempo of progression is not strikingly different across the patterns of presentation, with affected individuals typically dying within a decade of the onset of symptoms.

8.4.1.4.1. Macroscopic findings. As would be expected from the wide spectrum of clinical presentations, there can be a range of gross abnormalities observed in cases of MSA. The best correlate of MSA-P is the combination of pallor of the substantia nigra with atrophy of the putamen, often associated with a gray-green discoloration of the putamen (Fig. 8.31). When a prominent cerebellar

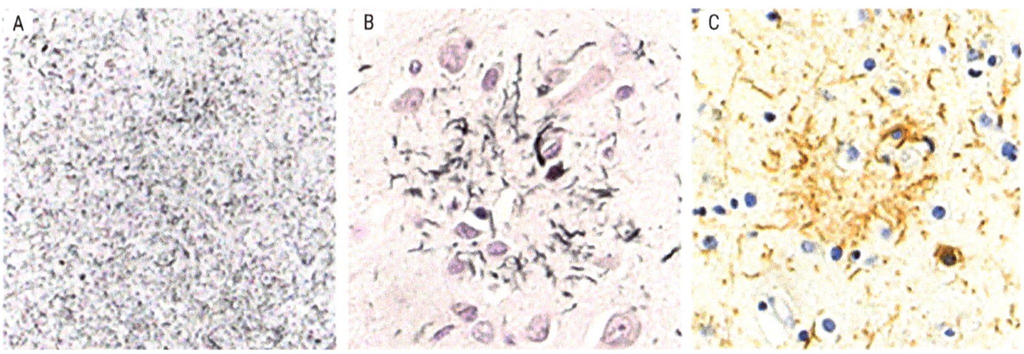

FIGURE 8.30 Corticobasal degeneration. (**A**) Silver impregnation exhibits dense neuropil threads across deep layers of cerebral cortex and white matter (Gallyas). Astrocytic plaques are labeled with silver stains (**B**, Gallyas) and anti-tau IHC (**C**).

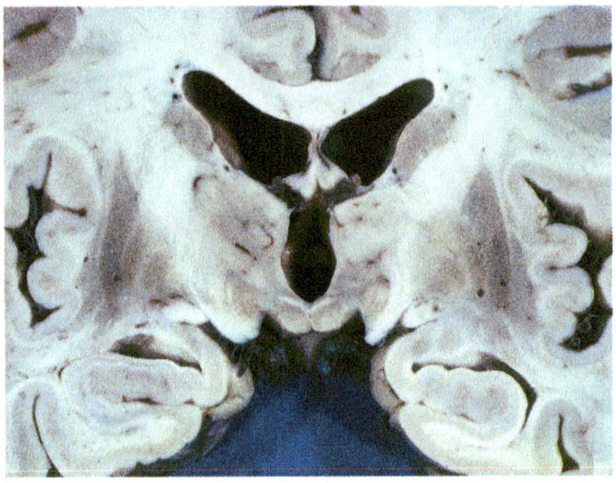

FIGURE 8.31 Multiple system atrophy. Macroscopic examination of the fixed brain shows shrinkage of basal ganglia and discoloration of the putamen, which adopts a gray-green color.

component has been present (MSA-C), the cerebellum, basis pontis, and inferior olivary complex are generally atrophied (see Section 8.5.1.2).

8.4.1.4.2. Microscopic findings. Involved brain regions show neuronal loss and astrocytic gliosis, and on routine stains (H&E, with or without Luxol fast blue), little else is evident. Use of silver impregnation, such as Gallyas or Bodian stains (Fig. 8.32), or IHC of α-synuclein or ubiquitin (Fig. 8.33) will show the characteristic glial cytoplasmic inclusions in oligodendroglia. They are widely distributed through the brain and appear as crescentic or sickle-shaped structures in glial cells, partially wrapping the nucleus and extending away from it. NCIs and neuronal nuclear inclusions are typically also present.

8.4.1.5. SECONDARY PARKINSONIAN SYNDROMES

Functional disruption of basal ganglia circuitry and, in particular, of nigrostriatal projections may result in the development of a parkinsonian syndrome. The diagnostic challenge is usually to separate these syndromes from the primary neurodegenerative diseases affecting the same brain regions.

8.4.1.5.1. Postencephalitic parkinsonism. Postencephalitic parkinsonism followed a pandemic of encephalitis lethargica (von Economo disease) between 1915 and 1927 (see Chapter 5). Half of the individuals who survived the acute encephalitic phase of the illness developed a parkinsonian syndrome after a latent period of approximately 9 years. Today, cases that fit this description are regarded as very rare. Macroscopic examination showed changes similar to those described in PSP. At microscopic examination, neurofibrillary tangles were found in widespread distribution, but particularly affecting the substantia nigra, the locus coeruleus, the nuclei of the reticular formation, the hypothalamus, and the nucleus basalis of Meynert. Affected regions showed cell loss with astrocytic gliosis.

8.4.1.5.2. Pharmacologic/toxic. Extrapyramidal disturbances are seen in the course of treatment with neuroleptics. The anatomic substrate is poorly defined. Toxic exposure to a by-product from illicit drug synthesis, 1-methyl-4-phenyl-1,2,3,6 tetrahydropyridine (MPTP), resulted in a parkinsonian syndrome with neuronal loss selectively involving the substantia nigra. Through this unfortunate rare episode, research efforts

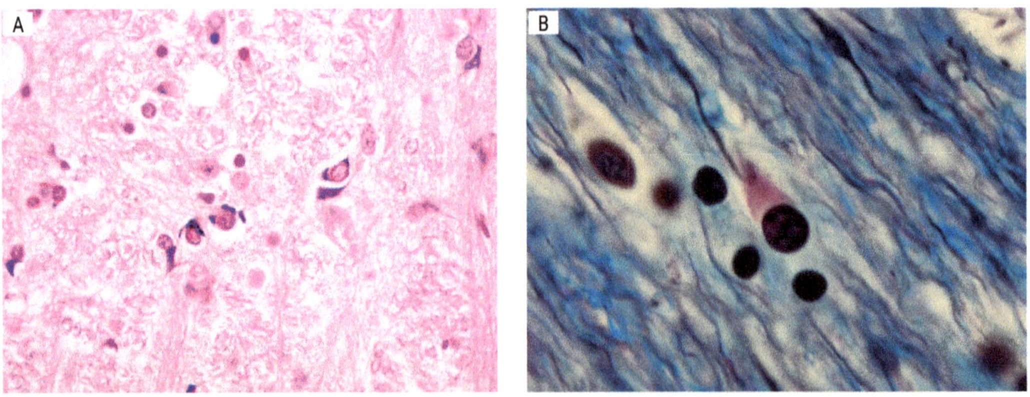

FIGURE 8.32 Multiple system atrophy. Glial cytoplasmic inclusions of multiple system atrophy, which have been termed Papp–Lantos inclusions, can be detected by silver staining, either Gallyas (**A**) or Bodian (**B**) silver impregnation.

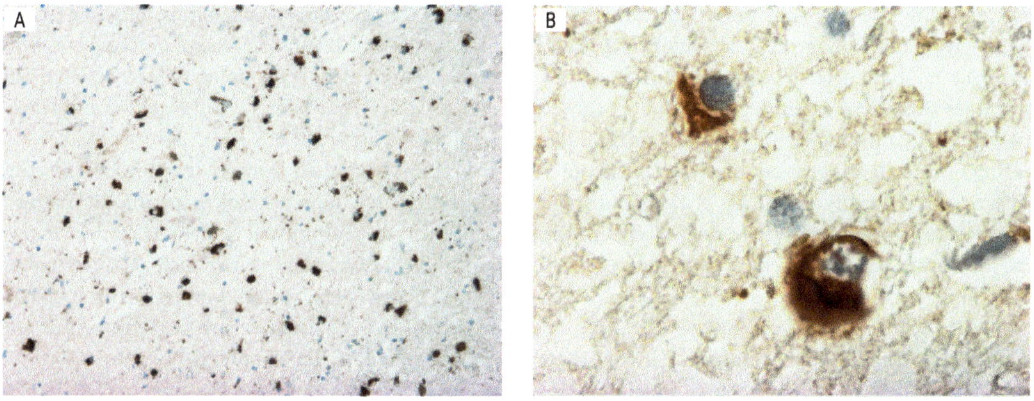

FIGURE 8.33 Multiple system atrophy. (**A**) α-Synuclein can be detected in a large number of glial cytoplasmic inclusions in the region of the substantia nigra (α-synuclein IHC). (**B**) Inclusions are seen in the cell body of an oligodendrocyte (upper left cell) and of an astrocyte (lower cell) (α-synuclein IHC).

led to the development of experimental animal models of PD using MPTP treatments.

8.4.1.5.3. Carbon monoxide poisoning. After sublethal exposure to carbon monoxide, there can be bilateral necrosis of the superomedial part of the pallidum (see Chapter 9). Lesions in the substantia nigra are inconstant and usually moderate and involve the pars reticulata of the nucleus rather than the dopaminergic pars compacta.

8.4.1.5.4. Vascular disease. The combination of hypertensive cerebrovascular disease involving the basal ganglia, with lacunae, and involvement of the brainstem and white matter projections essential for basal ganglia circuitry can result in parkinsonism. Marked clinical asymmetry is associated with the anatomic location of discrete lesions; a pseudobulbar palsy due to bilateral involvement of the pyramidal tract is frequent.

8.4.1.5.5. Trauma. As a delayed consequence of repeated traumatic injury (especially in boxers but also in other contact sports), a parkinsonism syndrome may develop; it may be a pure movement disorder or be associated with progressive dementia (dementia pugilistica) (see Chapter 3).

8.4.2. Hyperkinetic movement disorders

The clinical signs and symptoms of hyperkinetic movement disorders are chorea, ballism, myoclonus, dystonia, and tics. Chorea is characterized by "dance-like," non-rhythmic, rapid, involuntary movements. These disorders may be separated into two main groups, hereditary and sporadic, with a wide range of causes, the best studied being HD.

8.4.2.1. HUNTINGTON DISEASE

Huntington disease is an autosomal dominant disorder without a sporadic counterpart. The genetic basis of the disease is related to an expanded CAG repeat in the *HTT* gene, coding for the huntingtin protein, located on the distal portion of chromosome 4p. Its frequency varies in different populations, with levels of between 4 and 7 per 100,000. The disease usually becomes clinically manifest in middle or late life, but it may present earlier in life; patients with longer expansions of CAG repeat tend to develop symptoms at a younger age. HD is characterized clinically by chorea and mental deterioration leading to dementia. In some juvenile or early onset forms, hypertonia, rather than chorea, is the predominant symptom.

Huntingtin is widely expressed in a variety of tissues and contains a polyglutamine tract that normally varies in size from 9 to 35 copies of the amino acid, encoded by a trinucleotide (CAG) repeat in the gene. In patients with HD, the length of this repeat is expanded, with the average repeat length approximately 46 and a range of 36–86. There is a propensity for expansion of the CAG repeat during paternal transmission, such that this disease can occur at progressively younger ages in subsequent generations, a phenomenon referred to as *anticipation*. Unanswered questions remain in

HD, including the determination of anatomic specificity given that the protein is widely expressed throughout the nervous system as well as the processes that drive neurodegeneration. Proposed mechanisms contributing to pathology include loss of function of huntingtin because of the expanded repeat, gain of toxicity by mutant protein, transcriptional dysregulation caused by nuclear inclusions, excitotoxicity, oxidative stress, impaired proteolysis, and stimulated apoptosis.

8.4.2.1.1. Macroscopic findings. Grossly, there is mild to moderate cerebral atrophy. Sections reveal the main neuropathological abnormality of HD is atrophy of the caudate nucleus and putamen. Research studies have defined five grades of the disease: In some cases, the diagnosis is established genetically, in the absence of nonpathological abnormalities (Grade 0). In Grade 1, neuronal loss and astrocytosis are found microscopically, but the volume of the caudate nucleus remains normal. In Grade 2, the caudate nucleus is atrophic, but its ventricular border remains convex. In Grade 3, the medial outline of the caudate nucleus is flat and forms a nearly straight line. It is concave in Grade 4 (Fig. 8.34). Atrophy of the putamen follows the same overall gradient and time course, with changes seen in the globus pallidus during the later stages.

8.4.2.1.2. Microscopic findings. In the involved regions of the striatum, there is neuronal loss with astrocytic gliosis. The initial burden of degeneration is borne by the medium spiny neurons, although in late stages of the illness, most striatal neurons are lost. The cerebral cortex may show some degree of neuronal loss and gliosis, particularly in the setting of greater cognitive impairment.

Immunohistochemistry for huntingtin, for the expanded polyglutamine tract, or for ubiquitin shows accumulation of abnormal protein as nuclear inclusion bodies. Abnormal protein also accumulates in cortical neurites (Fig. 8.35). Intranuclear inclusions are relatively infrequent in striatal neurons but are more abundant in the cerebral cortex.

8.4.2.2. OTHER HYPERKINETIC DISORDERS

8.4.2.2.1. HD-like diseases. Individuals and families have been identified with clinical and neuropathologic features of HD but without expansion of the polyglutamine tract in the *HTT* gene for huntingtin. The best understood of these is known as HD-like 2 (HDL2), in which the genetic locus is an expansion of a CTG/CAG tract in the *JPH3* gene for junctophilin-3 (a protein involved in the complexes linking the plasma membrane with organelle membranes, particularly the endoplasmic reticulum).

8.4.2.2.2. Neurodegeneration with brain iron accumulation. The combination of behavioral changes with a progressive extrapyramidal syndrome typically combining rigidity with hyperkinesia, dystonia, and tremor is characteristic of the

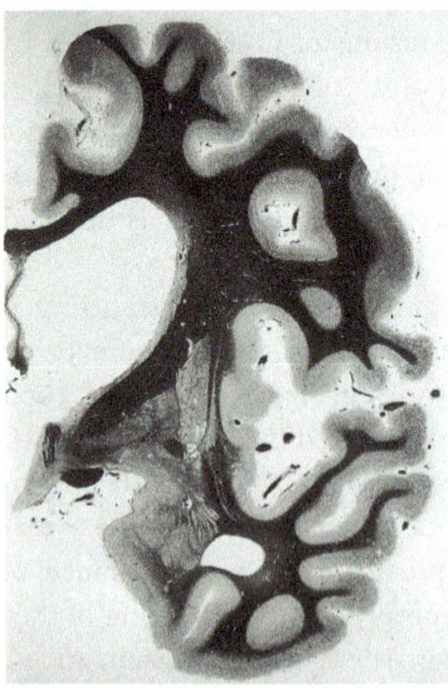

FIGURE 8.34 Huntington disease: Whole mount showing atrophy of the caudate nucleus and putamen with dilation of frontal horn and cortical atrophy (Loyez).

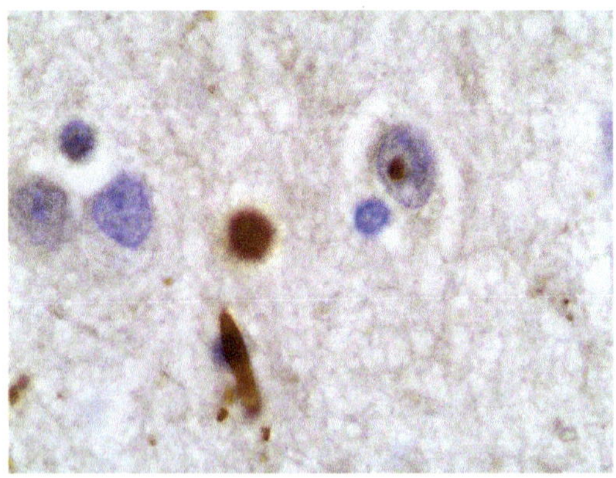

FIGURE 8.35 Huntington disease. Neurites can be detected in the cerebral cortex with immunostaining using anti-huntingtin or anti-ubiquitin antibodies. Neuronal nuclear inclusions are also identified by these immunostainings. A neuronal nuclear inclusion, approximately the size of a nucleolus, is seen in the neuron located in the upper right.

neurodegeneration with brain iron accumulation (NBIA) set of disorders, which can be caused by different mutations. There are common histologic features, including the presence of axonal spheroids predominantly in the internal globus pallidus and substantia nigra, as well as increased levels of brain iron, again primarily in these regions. Interestingly, coincident lesions such as Lewy bodies and tangles are often found in the basal ganglia. The ability to detect elevated iron levels through imaging methods has heightened the ability to suggest the diagnosis during clinical evaluation, based on the "eye-of-the-tiger" sign, a pattern resulting from iron deposition in the basal ganglia on T2-weighted imaging.

Mutations in the *PANK2* gene encoding an enzyme involved in the synthesis of coenzyme A (pantothenate kinase 2) are found in many of the cases of NBAI, particularly those with adult onset, now termed NBIA1. When the disease begins in early childhood, it is usually associated with more diffuse presence of axonal spheroids across the nervous system, hence the previous name of infantile neuroaxonal dystrophy. This form of the disease (NBIA2) is associated with regression of milestones, emergence of combinations of hypotonia and rigidity, as well as optic atrophy; a mutation of the gene *PLA2G6* (phospholipase A2 of the group 6) has been identified.

8.4.2.2.3. Chorea-acanthocytosis. The disorder of chorea-acanthocytosis is a clinical syndrome defined by the combination of chorea, dystonia, and tics with a hemolytic anemia, including the presence of acanthocytes ("thorny" red blood cells detectable on a blood smear) and a myopathy of variable severity. In these patients, acanthocytes may represent 5–30% of the red blood cell population, or the peripheral acanthocytosis may be lacking. Of recessive inheritance, the disease has been associated with mutations of the gene *VPS13A*, which encodes chorein. Acanthocytes may also be seen in association with movement abnormalities in McLeod syndrome, a disease due to mutations in the *XK* gene on the X chromosome; the encoded protein is required for generation of the Kell blood antigen.

8.5. CEREBELLAR DEGENERATIONS (ATAXIC DISORDERS)

The neurodegenerative diseases of the cerebellum can be classified either based on the pattern of inheritance and underlying genetic basis or according to the neuropathologic pattern of cellular degeneration (Boxes 8.2 and 8.3). Classification based on the topographic distribution of injury in now mostly of historical interest. The emergence of genetic information has allowed for more precise methods of classification (Box 8.3). Apart from neurodegeneration diseases, cerebellar degeneration may be seen in toxic, infectious, and metabolic disorders (Box 8.2). Knowledge of cerebellar circuitry continues to be useful for understanding the various patterns of cerebellar neurodegeneration; overlaps are frequent, and many of these disorders elude schematic descriptions.

Box 8.2 Classification of Ataxias

Primary Cerebellar and Spinocerebellar Degeneration
Inherited
Autosomal recessive
Autosomal dominant
Sex linked
Sporadic
Multiple system atrophy
Idiopathic cerebellar degeneration

Secondary Cerebellar and Spinocerebellar Degeneration
Neurometabolic
Prion disease
Toxic
Infectious
Vascular
Paraneoplastic cerebellar degeneration

Box 8.3 Classification of Some Inherited Spinocerebellar and Cerebellar Ataxias

Autosomal Recessive Cerebellar Ataxia
Friedreich ataxia
Ataxia with vitamin E deficiency
Ataxia–telangiectasia

Autosomal Dominant Cerebellar Ataxia
Spinocerebellar ataxias
Dentatorubral–pallidoluysian atrophy

X-Linked Cerebellar Ataxia
Fragile X tremor/ataxia syndrome

8.5.1. Types of cerebellar degeneration according to the topography of lesions

Based on the cerebellar circuitry, three main patterns of cerebellar degeneration are recognized:

- Cerebellar cortical atrophy
- OPCA
- Cerebellofugal atrophy

These are summarized in Figure 8.36. The classification is based on patterns of degeneration in the cerebellar cortex, cerebellopetal system (inferior olivary nucleus, pontine base, and inferior and middle cerebellar peduncle), or cerebellofugal system (dentate nucleus and superior cerebellar peduncle). Some cerebellar degenerations are accompanied by degeneration of the spinocerebellar tract in the spinal cord, forming a pathological phenotype of "spinocerebellar degeneration." The sensory tracts in the dorsal column or the corticospinal tract in anterolateral columns may be involved in some cerebellar degenerations, although these tracts do not have direct connections to the cerebellum.

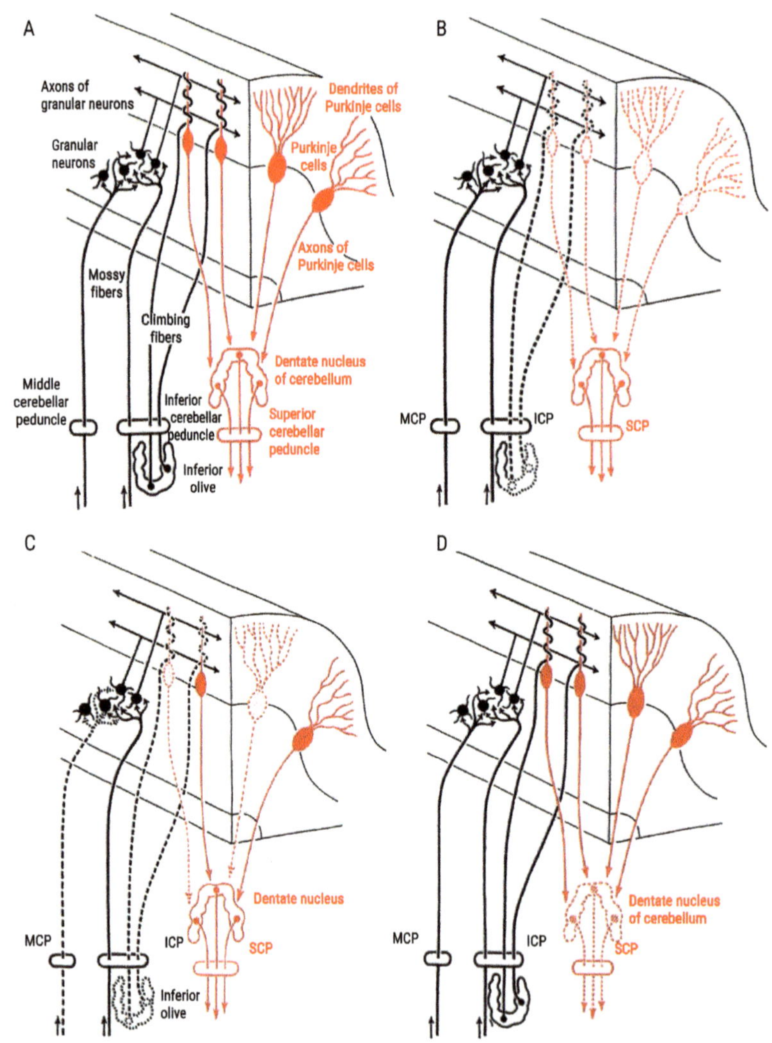

FIGURE 8.36 Prototypes of cerebellar atrophies: (**A**) normal cerebellum; (**B**) pure cortical atrophy, which may be accompanied by secondary degeneration of the inferior olivary nucleus after a protracted course; (**C**) olivopontocerebellar atrophy (cerebellopetal atrophy); (**D**) cerebellofugal atrophy. The main afferent pathways are in *black*; the main efferent pathways are in *red*; lost pathways are *stippled*. ICP, inferior cerebellar peduncle; MCP, middle cerebellar peduncle; SCP, superior cerebellar peduncle.

8.5.1.1. CEREBELLAR CORTICAL ATROPHIES

Within the group of cerebellar cortical atrophy disorders (Fig 8.37, left), some diseases manifest relatively consistent patterns of tissue injury, although some variability in the distribution and severity of the neuropathologic changes can be seen from case to case. The common denominator in all is degeneration of the cerebellar cortex with early, and eventually severe, loss of Purkinje cells. Loss of Purkinje cells is associated with Bergmann gliosis: reactive proliferation of astrocytes at the interface of the Purkinje cell layer and the molecular layer. Early and subtle evidence of Purkinje cell loss may be obtained with the use of silver impregnation to reveal the processes of basket cells, which normally wrap around the cell bodies of Purkinje cells; when Purkinje cells are lost, these processes remain as "empty baskets." As Purkinje cells die, their projections to the deep nuclei are lost, and this phenomenon is demonstrable as pallor in the fibers that wrap around the dentate nucleus (amiculum). Loss of Purkinje cells, after an extended period, is accompanied by loss of neurons in the inferior olivary nucleus.

8.5.1.2. OLIVOPONTOCEREBELLAR ATROPHIES

Olivopontocerebellar atrophy, classically regarded as the prototype of cerebellopetal atrophy, is characterized by the selective involvement of the afferent fibers of pontine and olivary origin (Figs. 8.36C and 8.37). The condition is characterized by pontine and cerebellar lesions, with variable degeneration of the inferior olivary nucleus.

- Atrophy of the basis pontis is evident on macroscopic examination. There is neuronal loss from the pontine nuclei and degeneration of the pontocerebellar fibers, which constitute the middle cerebellar peduncles. In myelin stains, there is pallor of the pontocerebellar fibers, which contrasts with preserved staining of the uninvolved superior cerebellar peduncles, tegmentum, and pyramidal tracts (Fig. 8.38).
- The cerebellar atrophy is characterized by severe degeneration of the cerebellar white matter with astrocytic gliosis (to a large extent due to loss of pontocerebellar fibers). The relative sparing of the amiculum of the dentate nucleus indicates the preservation of Purkinje cell axons.
- Inferior olivary involvement is characterized by neuronal cell loss and degeneration of the olivocerebellar fibers.

The neuropathological picture of OPCA is seen in MSA and several types of inherited spinocerebellar atrophy, such as SCA2 (Fig. 8.39; see Section 8.4.1.4).

8.5.1.3. CEREBELLOFUGAL ATROPHIES

Cerebellofugal atrophy is characterized by atrophy of the dentate nucleus and its efferent fibers in the superior cerebellar peduncles and of the red nucleus (Figs. 8.36D and 8.37). Spared Purkinje cell axons may form large growth cones in the dentate nucleus, visible on H&E stain and responsible for the aspect of "grumose degeneration." It may be observed in inherited conditions, including dentatorubral pallidoluysian atrophy (DRPLA), spinocerebellar

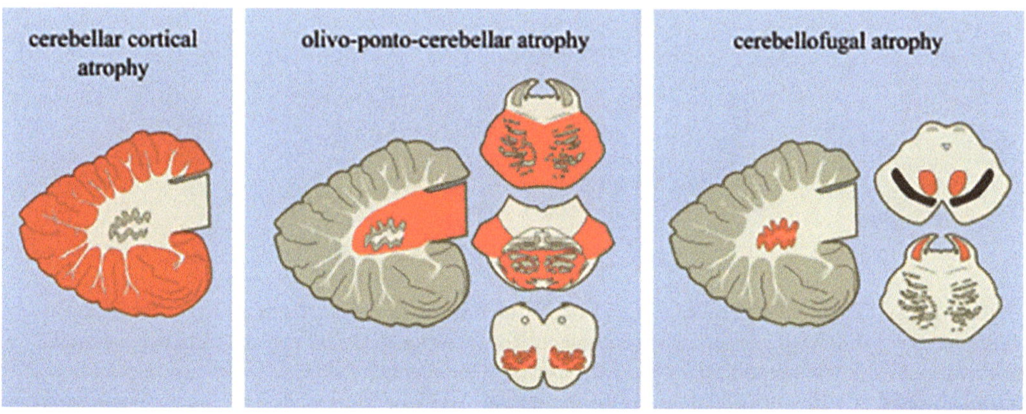

FIGURE 8.37 Distribution of lesions for patterns of cerebellar atrophies. Sections from the cerebellum, midbrain, upper and lower pons, and medulla oblongata are shown. Typical lesions are highlighted with red.

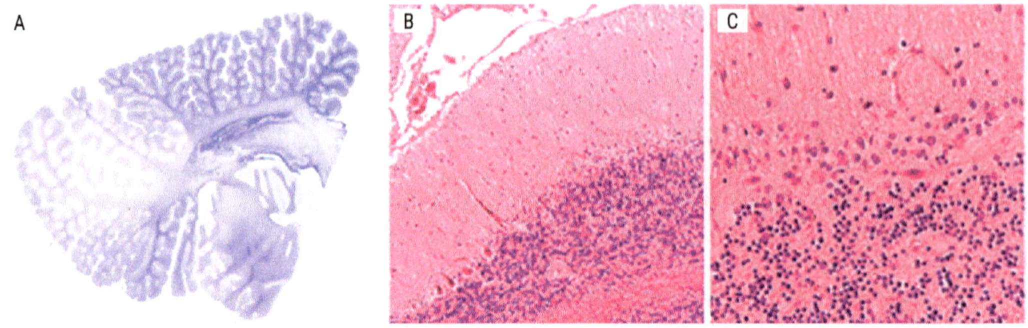

FIGURE 8.38 Cerebellar cortical atrophy. (**A**) Astrocytic gliosis with a range of severity among lobules (Holzer). (**B**) Loss of Purkinje cells is segmental (H&E). (**C**) In the portion showing Purkinje cell loss, proliferation of Bergmann glia is observed at the interface of the granule cell layer with the molecular layer.

atrophy type 3 (SCA3), and Friedreich ataxia (Figs. 8.40 and 8.41). Progressive supranuclear palsy, primarily a sporadic movement disorder, also shows cerebellofugal atrophy.

8.5.1.4. SECONDARY CEREBELLAR ATROPHIES

Although, strictly speaking, the patterns of pathology considered next are not degenerative disease, they are classically considered in this context.

8.5.1.4.1. Crossed cerebellar atrophy. Crossed cerebellar atrophy is unilateral general atrophy of all the neocerebellar structures; it is secondary to massive destruction of the efferent corticopontine pathways. It is a rare consequence of extensive contralateral cerebral hemispheric lesions and only seen when the survival after the initial lesions has been long. Crossed cerebellar atrophy, which has been occasionally described in adults, is particularly obvious when the responsible lesion has developed in utero or in the neonatal period.

8.5.1.4.2. Pseudohypertrophy of the inferior olive. Palatal myoclonus (rhythmical movements of the soft palate occurring 60–180 times a minute) is associated with pseudohypertrophy of the inferior olive, in which enlarged neurons may appear "fenestrated" (i.e., contain spaces in the perikaryon) after transsynaptic degeneration and the nucleus is gliotic. Inferior olivary hypertrophy is secondary to a long-standing, usually vascular, contralateral lesion involving the dentate nucleus or the superior cerebellar peduncle or to an ipsilateral lesion of the central tegmental tract.

8.5.2. Autosomal recessive cerebellar ataxias

Cerebellar ataxias with autosomal recessive inheritance are an important group of relatively rare

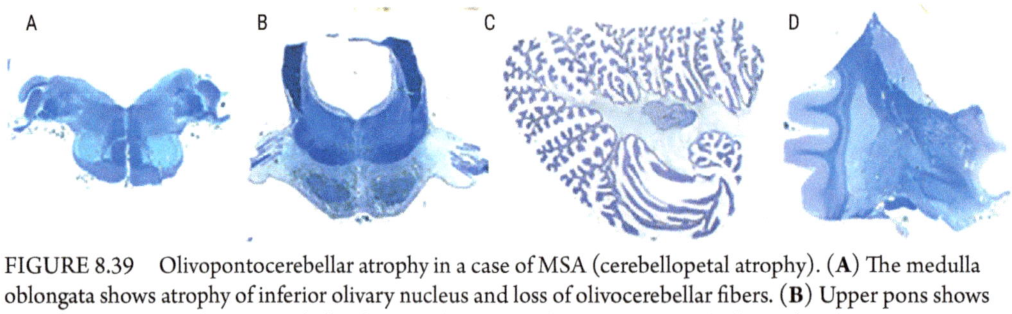

FIGURE 8.39 Olivopontocerebellar atrophy in a case of MSA (cerebellopetal atrophy). (**A**) The medulla oblongata shows atrophy of inferior olivary nucleus and loss of olivocerebellar fibers. (**B**) Upper pons shows massive myelin loss of pontocerebellar fibers with sparing of the superior cerebellar peduncles, tegmentum, and pyramidal tracts. (**C**) The cerebellum displays severe myelin loss of the white matter; myelin staining is barely retained in the fleece (amiculum) of the dentate nucleus. (**D**) The putamen is atrophic, which is a characteristic of MSA (whole mount, Klüver–Barrera stain).

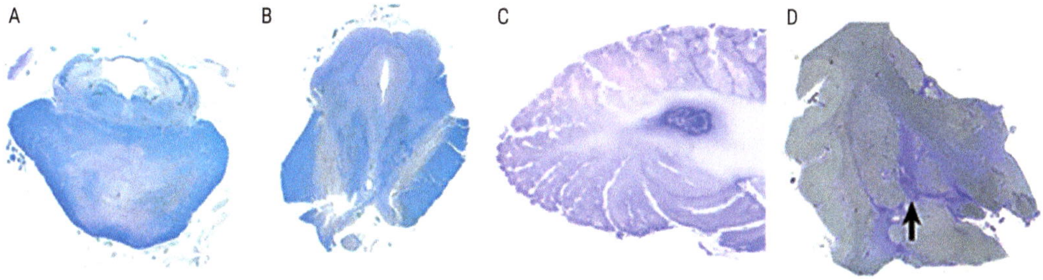

FIGURE 8.40 Dentatorubral pallidoluysian atrophy (cerebellofugal atrophy). (**A**) The superior cerebellar peduncle and (**B**) red nucleus are atrophic (whole mount, Klüver–Barrera stain). (**C**) Astrocytic gliosis is evident in the cerebellar dentate nucleus. (**D**) Astrocytic gliosis is also observed in the external segment of globus pallidus (GPe, *arrow*), which is a pathological characteristic of this disease (whole mount, Holzer).

disorders, with affected individuals commonly showing early age of onset and often with associated lesions outside the cerebellar system. The two most frequent diseases included (Friedreich ataxia [FA] and ataxia–telangiectasia [AT]) are considered here; a related rare disorder is caused by vitamin E deficiency.

8.5.2.1. FRIEDREICH ATAXIA

The disease typically begins in childhood with clinical manifestations that include clumsiness, gait ataxia, and signs of sensory peripheral neuropathy. Weakness and spasticity often emerge and can be a source of significant morbidity. Skeletal changes, including scoliosis and pes cavus (high instep) are common, as is hypertrophic cardiomyopathy (seen in up to 75% of cases) and diabetes (seen in one-third of cases).

FA is caused by mutations in the *FTX* gene on chromosome 9 coding for the protein frataxin. Normal frataxin is an 18-kDa mitochondrial protein with 210 amino acids involved in the regulation of iron homeostasis in mitochondria. The most common mutation is expansion of an intronic trinucleotide GAA repeat in the gene, which may reach 1,000 copies, with the normal length ranging from 6 to 34.

8.5.2.1.1. Macroscopic findings. The spinal cord and dorsal roots are consistently atrophic. The volume of the cerebellum is often unremarkable, but the degeneration of the dentate nucleus results in widening of the superior end of the fourth ventricle as the superior cerebellar peduncles atrophy. Outside the nervous system, there is often cardiomegaly and diffuse cardiac fibrosis, which is unlike the scarring seen after myocardial infarction.

8.5.2.1.2. Microscopic findings. Spinal cord sensory input is severely affected, with loss of dorsal root ganglion cells and degeneration of

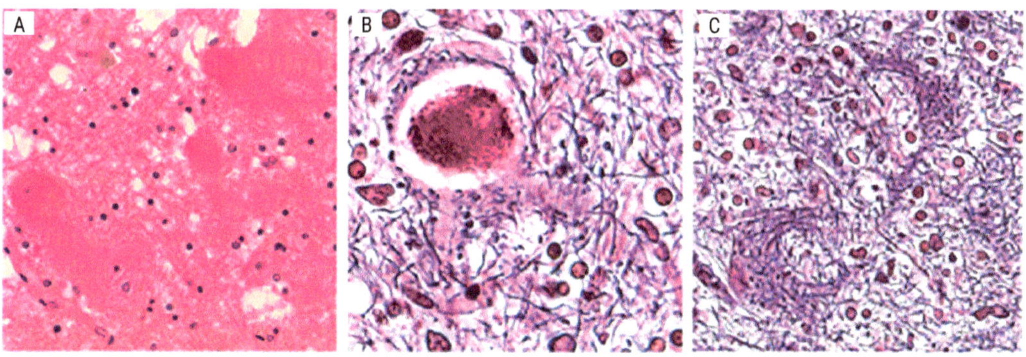

FIGURE 8.41 Grumose degeneration. (**A**) Cerebellar dentate nucleus of a DRPLA. Eosinophilic fuzzy changes cover the neuronal soma and neurites, reflecting hypertrophy of distal axons from Purkinje cells. (**B**) Bodian silver impregnation exhibits hypertrophic axons surrounding the neuron of dentate nucleus. (**C**) This hypertrophic change persists, even where the neurons have disappeared.

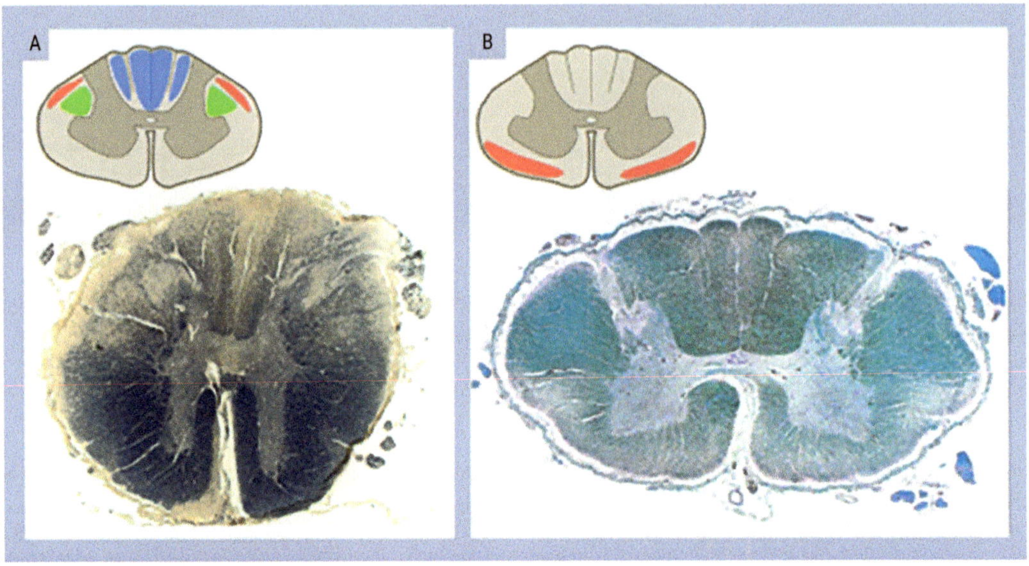

FIGURE 8.42 (**A**) Friedreich ataxia: Tract degeneration (color coded in diagram) is marked in the dorsal spinocerebellar tract (red) and dorsal column (blue), prominently in the gracile fasciculus. The pyramidal tract in the lateral column (green) is also involved (Loyez). (**B**) SCA3: Tract degeneration is prominent in the anterior spinocerebellar tract (red in diagram), whereas tracts in the posterior portion of the lateral funiculi are relatively spared (Klüver–Barrera stain).

the tract in the dorsal column. Involvement of the dorsal spinocerebellar tracts is also characteristic, although the ventral spinocerebellar tract is relatively spared (Fig. 8.42). Clarke's columns, from which the dorsal spinocerebellar tract arises, show neuronal loss. In the cerebellum, the dentate nuclei show severe neuronal loss and a grumose change, and the cerebellar white matter is generally gliotic. The cerebellar cortex and the inferior olivary nuclei are usually spared. The pyramidal tract often shows myelin pallor. Cardiomyopathy with fibrosis is frequently present and may lead to cardiac failure.

8.5.2.2. ATAXIA-TELANGIECTASIA

Ataxia–telangiectasia is the most common cause of progressive ataxia in infancy and is caused by mutations in a gene (ataxia–telangiectasia mutated or *ATM*) on chromosome 11q. The signs/symptoms that occur most often (in relative order of appearance) are the combination of oculomotor apraxia, cerebellar ataxia, and conjunctival telangiectasias. Systemic manifestations include increased sensitivity to injury from ionizing radiation, which can be attributed to the role of the ATM protein in the regulation of DNA repair mechanisms. This dysfunction is also associated with some degree of immunodeficiency as well as an increased risk of leukemia and lymphoma.

With progression of the disease, there is cerebellar degeneration typically involving the Purkinje cells as well as the dentate nucleus; dorsal column degeneration can be seen, as well as LMN degeneration. In addition, histological examination shows large, irregular, and hyperchromatic nuclei in various organs and also associated with vascular endothelial cells. This form of vascular abnormality appears to be independent of the telangiectasias that contribute to the name of the entity.

8.5.2.3. CEREBELLAR ATAXIA WITH ISOLATED VITAMIN E DEFICIENCY

Cerebellar ataxia with isolated vitamin E deficiency is a neurological condition that has been described in patients with mutations of the α-tocopherol transfer protein (*TTPA*) gene, leading to low availability of vitamin E. Symptoms are similar to those seen in FA. The disease has a relatively high prevalence in North Africa.

Neuropathological observations of the spinal cord show axonal spheroids and astrogliosis in the gracile and cuneate nuclei that are located at the rostral ends of the dorsal columns. Although neurons of dorsal root ganglia are almost spared in numbers, lipofuscin accumulation is marked in neurons. Purkinje cell loss and Bergmann gliosis are observed, but these may not be severe. Early treatment with vitamin E prevents the occurrence of lesions.

8.5.3. Autosomal dominant cerebellar ataxias

Approximately three dozen distinct forms of the complex set of autosomal dominant cerebellar ataxia diseases are now recognized; they are collectively termed *spinocerebellar ataxias*. Within this heterogeneous group of diseases, a set of disorders are polyglutamine (CAG trinucleotide repeat) diseases, similar to HD: SCA1, SCA2, SCA3, SCA6, SCA7, SCA17, and DRPLA. Among the other loci, a range of types of genetic mutation, including frameshift mutations, point mutations, deletions, expansion of noncoding repeats, and missense mutations, has been described; for some, a mapped locus but not an identified genetic alteration has been identified. A summary of the present classification of autosomal dominant cerebellar ataxias is presented in Table 8.2.

SCAs linked to expanded polyglutamine tracts show "anticipation" as HD, due to expansion of the repeat during genetic transmission (see Section 8.4.2.1). In addition, patients with SCA17 or DRPLA can also have a clinical presentation that mimics HD, such as choreoathetosis. A common histopathological finding among polyglutamine-linked SCAs is ubiquitinated intranuclear inclusions that contain an expanded polyglutamine portion of the mutated protein, which can be visualized using IHC directed against ubiquitin or CAG repeat. Table 8.3 summarizes patterns of lesion topography in CAG repeat-linked SCAs. Most SCAs, including polyglutamine-linked and other ones, have various lesions beyond the cerebellum, and lesion topography may be useful to predict SCA types in some cases, although genetic testing is required to confirm the diagnosis.

8.5.4. Fragile X tremor/ataxia syndrome

The fragile X syndrome is one of the causes of mental retardation caused by pathologic expansion of a noncoding trinucleotide repeat (CGG) in the fragile X mental retardation 1 (*FMR1*) gene. When the repeat length is in the "premutation" range (typically described as 55–200 copies), a cerebellar degenerative disease can emerge in males and, less frequently, in obligate carrier females. Characteristically, patients develop progressive ataxia with onset in adult life, often associated with tremor and parkinsonism. Sensory nerves are commonly involved as well. Although there may be gross atrophy of the cerebellum, microscopic findings include loss of Purkinje cells, widespread changes in white matter with volume loss and vacuolization, and the presence of ubiquitin-positive intranuclear inclusions in neurons and glia.

8.5.5. Sporadic degenerative ataxia

Cerebellar ataxia can arise as a neurological manifestation in sporadic neurodegenerative disorders. Some patients with MSA (see Section 8.4.1.4) show prominent cerebellar ataxia combined with parkinsonism or autonomic dysfunctions, which is termed MSA-C. Cerebellar degeneration in MSA-C corresponds to OPCA pattern. A subset of PSP patients also demonstrate cerebellar ataxia, which is associated with cerebellofugal degeneration. There remain other cases, typically with idiopathic late-onset cerebellar ataxia, that are associated with cerebellar cortical atrophy and some involvement of afferent and efferent paths and nuclei.

8.6. MOTOR NEURON DISEASES

Within the brain and spinal cord, sets of neurons are referred to as motor neurons: The LMNs are the cholinergic neurons in brainstem nuclei and the anterior horn of the spinal cord that project directly to muscle endplates. Conversely, the UMNs are the large glutamatergic pyramidal neurons of the precentral gyrus that descend from the cortex to innervate the LMNs. Although a range of other neurons contribute to motor output, involvement of UMNs or LMNs or both defines this category of illnesses, known as motor neuron diseases. In addition to neurodegenerative disorders, motor system degeneration may be seen in other conditions, including toxic, infectious, and metabolic disorders.

8.6.1. Amyotrophic lateral sclerosis

Amyotrophic lateral sclerosis is characterized by degeneration of both UMNs and LMNs. Although the relative extent and pace of involvement of these two

Table 8.2 Autosomal Dominant Cerebellar Atrophies

DISORDER	GENE	GENE PRODUCT	NO. OF CAG REPEATS IN DISEASE/MUTATION	TYPICAL NORMAL REPEATS	CLINICAL TYPE OF ADCA
SCA1	*ATXN1*	Ataxin 1	42–81 (CAG)	16–36	I (subclass 1)
SCA2	*ATXN2*	Ataxin 2	35–64 (CAG)	15–24	I (subclass 1)
SCA3/MJD	*ATXN3*	Ataxin 3	68–79 (CAG)	13–36	I (subclass 1)
SCA4	Unknown	Unknown	Unknown		I
SCA5	*SPTBN2*	Spectrin β, nonerythrocytic 2	In-frame deletion/missense		III
SCA6	*CACNA1A*	Voltage-gated calcium channel type p/q α 1 A subunit	20–33 (CAG)	4–18	III
SCA7	*ATXN7*	Ataxin 7	38–130 (CAG)	7–17	II
SCA8	*ATXN8OS*	Untranslated	16–37 (CTG)	107–127	I (subclass 2)
SCA10	*ATXN 10*	Untranslated	800–4,500 (ATTCT)	10–22	I (subclass 2)
SCA11	*TTBK2*	Tau tubulin kinase 2	Frameshifts		III
SCA12	*PPP2R2B*	Protein phosphatase 2 regulatory subunit B β	52–93	<32	I (subclass 2)
SCA13	*KCNC3*	Voltage-gated potassium channel, subfamily C, member 3	Missense		I (subclass 3)
SCA14	*PRKCG*	Protein kinase C γ	Missense		I (subclass 3)
SCA15/16	*ITPR1*	Inositol 1,4,5-triphosphate receptor 1	Exon deletions/missense		I (subclass 3)
SCA17	*TBP*	TATA box–binding protein	63 (CAG)	25–42	I (subclass 1)
SCA19/22	*KCND3*	Potassium voltage-gated channel, subfamily D, member 3	Missense		I (subclass 3)
SCA23	*PDYN*	Prodynorphin	Missense		I (subclass 3)
SCA26	*EEF2*	Eukaryotic translation elongation factor 2	Missense mutation		III
SCA27	*FGF14*	Fibroblast growth factor 14	Missense and frameshift mutation		I (subclass 3)
SCA28	*AFG3L2*	ATPase family gene 3-like 2	Missense mutation		I (subclass 3)
SCA31	*BEAN/TK2*	Untranslated	2.5- to 3.8-kb insertions containing (TGGAA), (TAAAA), (TAGAA), and (TAAAATAGAA)	1.5- to 2.0-kb insertions	III
SCA35	*TGM6*	Transglutaminase 6	Missense and in-frame mutation		I (subclass 3)
SCA38	*ELOVL5*	Elongation of very long-chain fatty acid like 5	Missense mutations		III
SCA42	*CACNA1G*	Calcium voltage-gated channel subunit α1 G	Missense mutation		I (subclass 3)
DRPLA	*ATN1*	Atrophin 1	48–93 (CAG)	7–35	I (subclass 1)

Disorder: ADCA, autosomal dominant cerebellar atrophy; DRPLA, dentatorubral–pallidoluysian atrophy; SCA, spinocerebellar ataxia.

Types of ADCA: In type I, the cerebellar atrophy is associated with other neurological signs and symptoms. Type II is characterized by pigmentary maculopathies and includes SCA7. Type III comprises pure cerebellar syndromes, although a subset of patients can present with mild non-cerebellar signs. ADCA type I is further subclassified into three groups based on genetical abnormalities. In subclass I, the CAG repeat expansion is located inside the protein-coding region and is responsible for an abnormally long polyglutamine tract in the expressed protein. In subclass II, trinucleotide repeat expansion is located outside the protein-coding region. Subclass III contains disorders caused by gene deletions, missense mutations, and nonsense mutations.

Table 8.3 Distribution of lesions in CAG repeat-linked SCAs

SCA TYPE	CLASSIFICATION OF CEREBELLAR DEGENERATION	DEGENERATION OF SPINAL CORD	DEGENERATION OF GLOBUS PALLIDUS	ADDITIONAL LESION
SCA1	Cerebellofugal atrophy	Spinocerebellar tract	External segment	Inferior olive Pontine base
SCA2	OPCA	Dorsal column	Mild	
SCA3	Cerebellofugal atrophy	Spinocerebellar tract	Internal segment	
SCA6	CCD	—	—	
SCA7	OPCA	—	Mild	Retina
DRPLA	Cerebellofugal atrophy	—	External segment	

CCD, cerebellar cortical degeneration; DRPLA, dentatorubral-pallidoluysian atrophy; OPCA, olivopontocerebellar atrophy; SCA, spinocerebellar ataxia.

sets of neurons vary from case to case, the combined damage to both systems is characteristic of ALS. In many cases, the disease begins with involvement of spinal cord LMNs, manifesting as weakness in the arms or legs. In others, ALS begins with bulbar symptoms, termed progressive bulbar palsy.

Reflecting the pathological characteristics, typical ALS patients show combined signs or symptoms indicating both UMN and LMN involvement. However, infrequent clinical variants are known to occur in ALS. The UMN signs or symptoms may be predominant in the absence of LMN impairment; this phenotype is referred to as primary lateral sclerosis, drawing its name from the changes in the descending corticospinal tracts of the lateral column of the spinal cord. In contrast, LMN signs or symptoms may arise exclusively, initially with preservation of UMNs, which is referred to as progressive muscular atrophy.

Although the disease is sporadic in most patients, familial forms account for approximately 5–10% of cases, with an ever-increasing spectrum of mutations and genetic loci being identified. Autosomal dominant inheritance is most common; autosomal recessive or X-linked patterns of inheritance may also occur. Mutations of superoxide dismutase 1 (SOD1) were the first recognized to cause fALS, with different point mutations associated with a range of disease spectrums, including both age of onset and rate of progression. Following the discovery of SOD1 mutations, various pathogenic mutations have been identified in ALS cases. Hexanucleotide expansion of *C9orf72* is the most common genetic cause of fALS. Mutations in the gene encoding TDP-43 (*TARDBP*) are less frequent but are notable given the presence of TDP-43-immunoreactive inclusions in most cases of ALS.

8.6.1.1. MACROSCOPIC FINDINGS

The brain appears macroscopically normal in most cases. Atrophy of the precentral gyrus can occur with long periods of survival, particularly in patients provided with nutritional and ventilator support. In patients who have developed clinical dementia, atrophy of frontal and temporal lobes may be present. Reflecting UMN involvement, degeneration of the descending corticospinal tracts is observed in the medullary pyramids or lateral column of the spinal cord; these regions show atrophy and discoloration on axial sections. The most striking finding on macroscopic observation is atrophy of nerve roots of the hypoglossal nerve or anterior roots of the spinal cord, which reflects LMN involvement (Fig. 8.43). By contrast, posterior roots of the spinal cord or cranial nerves associated with extraocular muscles (III, IV, and VI) are usually spared until very late in the course of the disease in some cases.

8.6.1.2. MICROSCOPIC FINDINGS

The most prominent finding is neuronal loss with associated astrogliosis and microgliosis in the anterior horn of spinal cord, some brainstem motor nuclei, and the motor cortex (Fig. 8.44). The injury is relatively restricted to motor neurons within these structures. Loss of LMNs is evident in the spinal cord anterior horn and the brainstem motor nuclei (hypoglossal nucleus, nucleus ambiguus, motor nucleus of trigeminal nerve, and facial nerve). The surviving neurons occasionally have eosinophilic inclusions in the cytoplasm, termed Bunina bodies. Conversely, loss of UMNs is observed in the primary motor cortex (precentral gyrus); the large

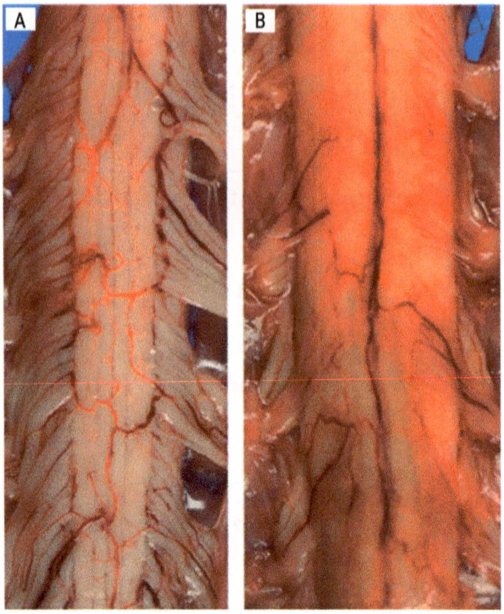

FIGURE 8.43 Macroscopic findings of the spinal cord in a case of ALS. (**A**) From the dorsal aspect of cord, the dorsal (sensory) roots appear normal. (**B**) In contrast, from the ventral aspect, there is marked atrophy of the anterior (motor) roots; the dorsal roots can be seen behind the atrophied anterior roots.

projecting pyramidal neurons of layer V (Betz cells) are involved. Although it is sometimes difficult to determine whether Betz cells are reduced, gliosis at the gray–white matter junction of the precentral gyrus is commonly observed.

Myelin staining of spinal cord white matter shows pallor in corticospinal tracts within the lateral and anterior columns, associated with the loss of UMNs. Similar changes can be observed in these tracts at more rostral levels, including the medullary pyramids (Fig. 8.45A), the basis pontis, and the cerebral peduncles. It is uncommon to be able to detect the loss of these descending fibers at higher levels than the upper brainstem, such as within the posterior limb of the internal capsule. Pallor of myelin staining may not be confined to the corticospinal tracts and may involve the anterior and lateral columns to a lesser extent (Fig. 8.45B).

Protein aggregates may be detected by IHC to aid in the pathological diagnosis of ALS. The aggregates are often ubiquitinated and can be recognized using anti-ubiquitin IHC in the cytoplasm of surviving motor neurons. In most cases of sporadic ALS, the ubiquitinated aggregates appear as collections of thread-like structures (or *skein-like inclusions*) or as round inclusions, and they are immunopositive for TDP-43 (Fig. 8.46). Although TDP-43 is normally a nuclear protein, the nuclear immunostaining is often reduced in the neurons having cytoplasmic inclusions, as shown in FTLD-TDP (see Section 8.3.2.2.2 and Fig. 8.13). TDP-43 aggregates are also found in fALS cases associated with *TDP-43* mutations, expansion of the hexanucleotide repeat in *C9orf72*, or some rare gene mutations. Although it is

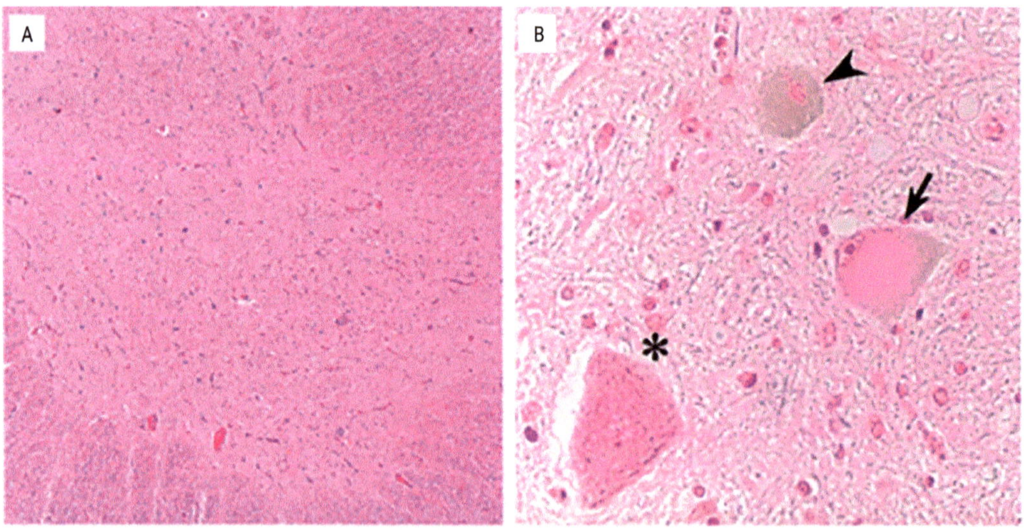

FIGURE 8.44 Lower motor neuron changes in ALS. (**A**) This low-magnification view shows severe loss of motor neurons from the anterior horn of the lumbar cord (H&E). (**B**) In the spinal cord anterior horn, surviving neurons show chromatolysis (*arrow*) and contain abundant lipofuscin. Some may have Bunina bodies (*arrowhead*). The neuron noted with an *asterisk* shows relatively normal appearance of lower motor neuron, showing a polygonal outline and dense Nissl bodies.

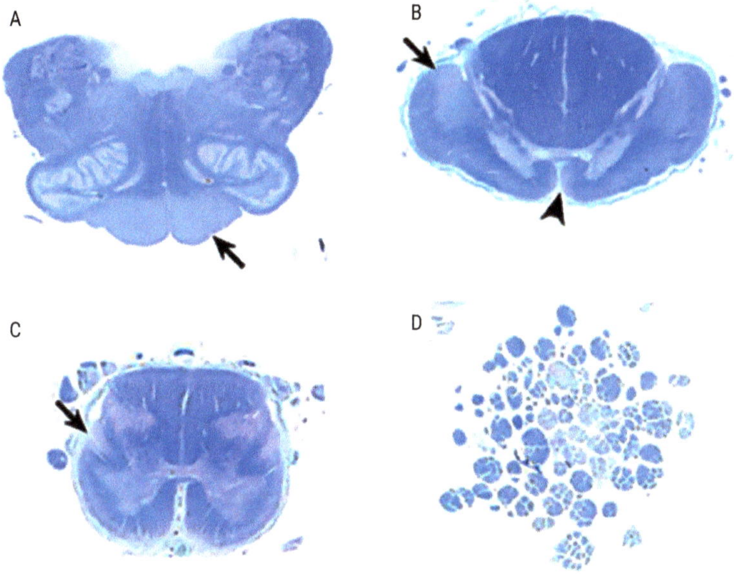

FIGURE 8.45 Tract degeneration in ALS. (**A**) The medullary pyramid (*arrow*), (**B**) the lateral column of the cervical cord (*arrow*), and (**C**) the lateral column of the lumbar spinal cord (*arrow*) show pallor of myelin staining secondary to degeneration of the corticospinal tract. (**B**) The uncrossed anterior corticospinal tract (*arrowhead*) is also involved. (**D**) In the cauda equina, fascicles of the anterior roots display less myelin staining than those of dorsal roots (Klüver–Barrera stain).

difficult to predict a mutation in each patient based on morphological characteristics of TDP-43 pathology, DPR inclusions of *C9orf72* can be detected using anti-ubiquitin or anti-DPR IHC (see Section 8.3.2.2.2). In contrast, TDP43-negative, FUS-immunopositive inclusions are observed in a minor subset of sporadic ALS and in fALS with FUS mutations. *SOD1*-linked fALS does not show TDP-43 aggregates but, rather, misfolded SOD1 aggregates prominently in LMNs. In some cases harboring *SOD1* mutations, surviving neurons have conglomerate inclusions composed of neurofilament within the cytoplasm.

8.6.2. Spinal muscular atrophy

In spinal muscular atrophy (SMA; types 1–4), spinal motor neurons progressively degenerate. with resulting severe weakness. The age of onset varies, with earliest onset in the most severe phenotypes. The two most well-recognized patterns are SMA 1 (Werdnig–Hoffmann disease), with onset during the first 6 months of life, often as a "floppy" baby, or as the failure to achieve the developmental milestone of sitting; and SMA 3 (Kugelberg–Welander disease), with onset around the second birthday, in which children walk before the onset of motor weakness. As would be expected, there is atrophy of skeletal muscles and of anterior nerve roots along with loss of motor neurons from the anterior horns of the spinal cord.

These different phenotypes of the disease are linked to mutations in the pair of survival motor neuron genes, *SMN1* and *SMN2*, which sit as an inverted repeat on the long arm of chromosome 5 (5q13). In addition to the few single amino acid differences between the protein products of the two genes, there is also a difference that decreases the efficiency of splicing into the mRNA of exon 7 from *SMN2*. As a result, the *SMN2* gene is far less efficient at generating functional SMN protein compared to the *SMN1* gene. The severity of the phenotype is associated with the number of copies of *SMN2* present in the setting of homozygous loss of *SMN1*. Currently, novel therapeutic approaches to this disorder are focused on alteration of the splicing of *SMN2* mRNA or mutagenic conversion of the *SMN2* gene into an *SMN1* gene.

8.6.3. X-linked spinal and bulbar muscular atrophy (Kennedy disease)

X-linked spinal and bulbar muscular atrophy (Kennedy disease) involves LMNs of the spinal cord and brainstem, with typical onset of symptoms in

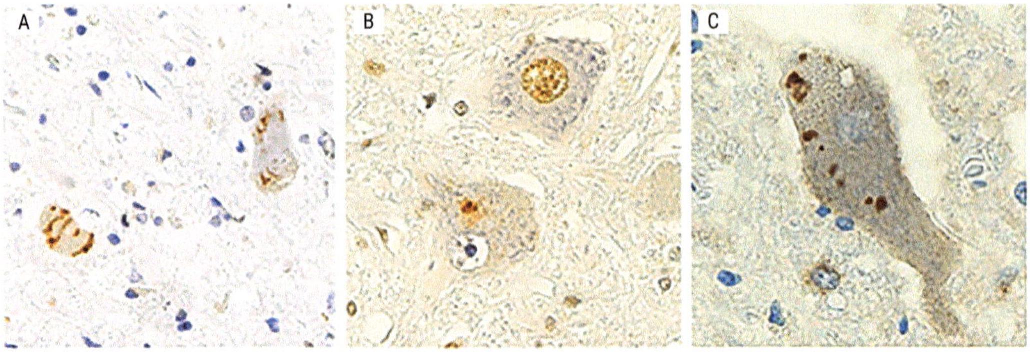

FIGURE 8.46 TDP-43–related ALS, anterior horn of spinal cord. (**A**) Cytoplasmic TDP-43 inclusion typically appears to be "skein-like" (anti-TDP-43 IHC). (**B**) Anti-full-length TDP-43 IHC reveals reduced nuclear immunoreactivity as well as cytoplasmic aggregation. (**C**) Bunina bodies are labeled with anti-cystatin-C IHC.

early to mid-adult life. Men are predominantly affected, as the causative mutation is an expansion of a polyglutamine tract (trinucleotide CAG repeat) in the androgen receptor, which is encoded by the *AR* gene on the X chromosome. Neurologic involvement typically includes weakness, muscle atrophy with fasciculations, and decreased tone without spasticity. Systemic findings such as gynecomastia and testicular atrophy may develop as well, as a consequence of relative androgen insensitivity. Grossly, there can be evidence of motor root atrophy in both the brainstem and the spinal cord. Microscopic examination reveals the corresponding loss of motor neurons from these motor nuclei, with the appearance of ubiquitinated polyglutamate-containing intranuclear inclusions in remaining neurons.

8.6.4. Hereditary spastic paraparesis

Hereditary spastic paraparesis is a genetically and clinically heterogeneous set of disorders in which patients develop slowly progressive paraparesis, beginning with the legs and having more spasticity than weakness. These symptoms reflect a length-dependent axonal injury process involving the descending corticospinal tracts. There is variability in age of onset (even within kindreds), variability in severity, and variability in associated symptoms (sensory changes, cerebellar ataxia, epilepsy, and intellectual deficit). Despite the heterogeneity, autosomal dominantly inherited forms predominate, with the most common, type 4 (SPG4), resulting from mutations in the gene encoding spastin (*SPAST*).

The disease results in the degeneration of corticospinal tracts, most marked in the lumbar and lower thoracic spinal cord, with preservation of anterior horn cells. In cases with clinical evidence of sensory changes, degeneration of dorsal columns may also be observed. In keeping with the length-dependent pattern of the disease, degeneration of the dorsal columns is most severe in the upper thoracic and cervical cord.

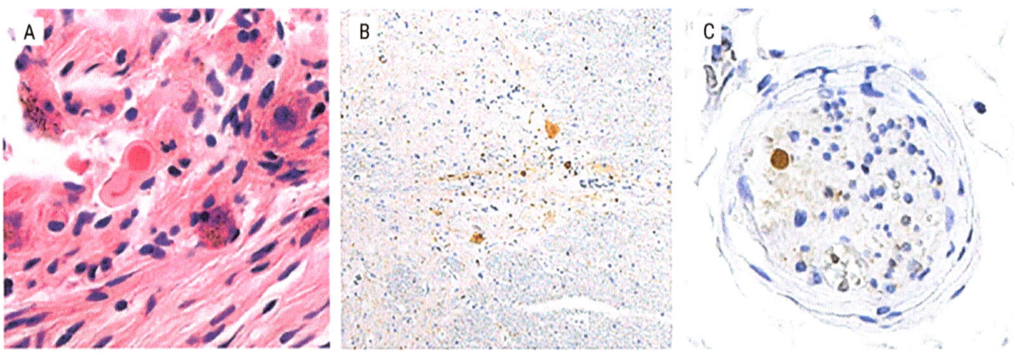

FIGURE 8.47 Lewy body pathology in the autonomic system in Parkinson disease: (**A**) Lewy bodies in the sympathetic ganglia (H&E); (**B**) in the spinal cord, accumulation of α-synuclein in the intermediolateral nucleus (α-synuclein IHC); (**C**) aggregates of α-synuclein in the axons of cardiac sympathetic nerves (α-synuclein IHC).

8.7. INVOLVEMENT OF THE CENTRAL AUTONOMIC SYSTEMS IN DEGENERATIVE DISORDERS

Neurodegenerative disorders can be associated with autonomic failure. Autonomic failure often arises together with other neurological symptoms, including parkinsonism or ataxia, but can appear in isolation. MSA with autonomic failure (formerly Shy–Drager syndrome) is the most common cause of this type of autonomic failure, but dysautonomia may also occur in some patients with Lewy body disorders. Loss of preganglionic, sympathetic neurons in the intermediolateral column of the spinal cord appears to be the cause of this type of autonomic failure. However, neurons in the sympathetic ganglion or postganglionic fiber are also involved, particularly in Lewy body diseases (Fig. 8.47).

9

Acquired Metabolic Diseases of the Nervous System

MICHAEL PUNSONI, LUCIANO NEDER, ISABELLE PLU, AND DOUGLAS C. ANTHONY

A WIDE range of acquired systemic conditions, including metabolic derangements such as hypoxia, hypoglycemia, disorders of serum electrolytes, vitamin deficiencies, and exogenous intoxications, cause neurologic symptoms and have neuropathologic manifestations. In this chapter, we address the neuropathology associated with these systemic disorders. Although the disorder is systemic in nature, the impact in the nervous system may show selective involvement of specific brain regions or subsets of cells, with complete preservation of others, a phenomenon referred to as *selective vulnerability*. The predisposition to injury for a particular anatomic region or specific set of cells depends on the type and duration of the insult. It varies considerably from one disease to another but is relatively consistent between individual patients. Differences in the vascular anatomy and blood flow regulation may explain the phenomenon of selective vulnerability in some disorders. On the other hand, neuronal necrosis may occur within subsets of neurons damaged due to a systemic injury, with relative sparing of other neurons and glia cells. Variations in the biochemical properties of neuronal populations, their specific metabolic processes, or the amount and distribution of receptors for various excitatory and inhibitory amino acids also play a role in some conditions.

9.1. CEREBRAL HYPOXIA AND ISCHEMIA

The brain normally receives approximately 15% of the cardiac output, consumes approximately 20% of the blood oxygen, and utilizes approximately 10–20% of the blood glucose, while comprising only approximately 2% of the body weight. Due to this high oxygen and energy utilization, the brain is particularly vulnerable to hypoxemia, ischemia, or hypoglycemia. Neurons are the most sensitive cells to deprivation of oxygen or blood flow, followed by glial cells (especially oligodendrocytes in infants) and endothelia. Glutamate (and other excitatory amino acids) may be released in the extracellular fluid of the brain due to neuronal injury or by reversal of astrocytic glutamate transporters in the setting of hypoxic–ischemic conditions. This release of excitatory neurotransmitters can amplify the magnitude of neuronal damage and death, a phenomenon termed *excitotoxicity*. Various states of deficient oxygen supply, blood flow, and deficient substrate may produce prominent cerebral pathologic changes, a category often referred to as hypoxic–ischemic encephalopathy, with subcategories:

- *Anoxic or hypoxic hypoxia* results from decreased access to oxygen. This may be due to insufficient oxygen in the inspired air, upper airway obstruction, drowning, or pulmonary disorders that impede the uptake of oxygen. In rare instances (i.e., hyperthermia and excessive effort), it may be due to increased metabolic demand.
- *Anemic hypoxia* results from decreased oxygen transport, either from reduced blood hemoglobin levels, such as in hemoglobinopathies, or from reduced capacity of the hemoglobin to transport oxygen, as occurs in carbon monoxide (CO) poisoning.
- *Stagnant hypoxia* results from global or focal reduction or cessation of blood flow. This can be the result of impaired cardiac output producing global ischemia or be localized, as is the case in brain infarcts. The cerebral lesions that result from stagnant hypoxia are due to a combination of an inadequate supply of oxygen and glucose, plus lactic acid accumulation. Differences in patterns of injury may be seen with reduction in flow, as in hypotensive episodes, and complete cessation of flow for an interval of time.
- *Histotoxic hypoxia* results from impaired tissue utilization of oxygen caused by exposure to intoxicants, such as cyanide, azide, or hydrogen sulfide, that render the neural parenchyma incapable of utilizing oxygen and substrates.
- *Severe hypoglycemia* may generate a form of hypoxia in which oxygen is not utilized because of severe metabolic substrate deficiency.

9.1.1. Basic cellular reactions to injury

The basic cellular reactions to injury seen in cerebral hypoxia involve neurons most severely (ischemic neuronal change, see Chapter 1). Glial cells may also be affected, with manifestations such as reactive gliosis or rod-shaped microglia. With complete tissue infarction, glial necrosis subsequently occurs.

9.1.2. Selective vulnerability

The cellular changes resulting from global hypoxia are maximal in certain areas of the brain that are regarded as susceptible to selective vulnerability. Which neuronal populations are most vulnerable is dependent on the type of injury.

In the *cerebral cortex*, the neuronal changes resulting from global hypoxic or ischemic injuries in adults are more pronounced in the third, fifth, and sixth layers of the neocortex. In addition, the changes are more severe in the depths of sulci than along the crests of the gyri. Widespread, severe destruction of the deeper layers of the cortex leads to *laminar* (or *pseudolaminar*) *necrosis* (Fig. 9.1). This descriptive term applies to a phenomenon whereby the distribution of the necrosis predominantly involves one or more layers of the midportion of the isocortex, especially affecting the cortical layer 3, whereas layers 2 and 4 are more resilient. It may be especially evident in the parietal and occipital lobes, where impaired perfusion of the posterior circulation may exacerbate the effects of hypoxia. In the most severe cases, the cortical necrosis is not selective and there is destruction of all cortical layers.

The hippocampus (*Ammon's horn*) often shows selective involvement by hypoxia. This is most evident in the CA1 sector (an area that corresponds to what is anatomically defined as Sommer's sector) (Fig. 9.2A, B). The CA3 area is often affected less severely, and the CA2 sector tends to be relatively resistant to hypoxic changes. The regional variation in the susceptibility of the pyramidal hippocampal

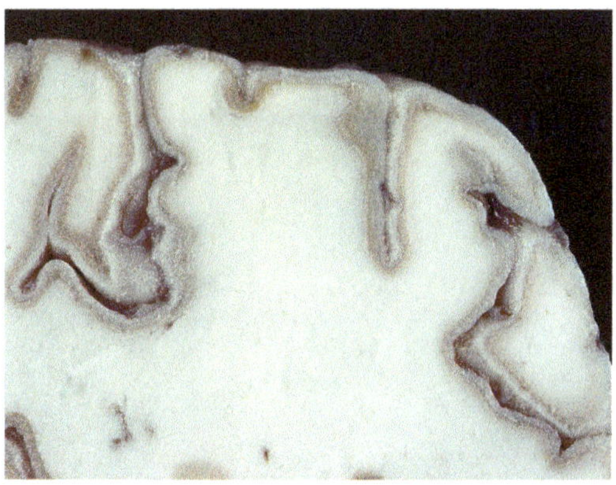

FIGURE 9.1 Laminar cortical necrosis. The necrotic layers are partially cystic and discolored brown; forming a band, they weave between neuronal layers 3 and 6, generally sparing the more superficial layers, which appear a paler shade of white.

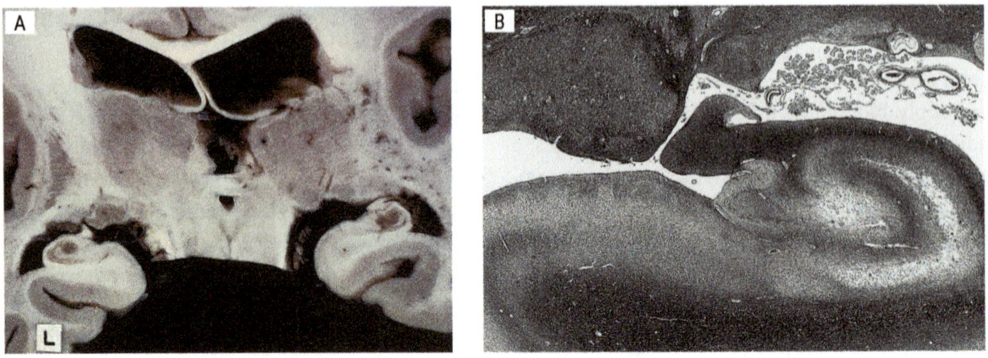

FIGURE 9.2 Involvement of the hippocampus following short-term global anoxia: (**A**) gross discoloration; (**B**) microscopic demonstration of cell loss from the CA1 sector and CA3 (Loyez stain for myelin).

neurons is now best explained by the distribution of excitatory receptors, with excitotoxicity being an important pathogenetic factor.

Neurons with High Susceptibility to Global Hypoxic–Ischemic Injury

Hippocampus, most severe in CA1 (Sommer sector), following global hypoxia; CA3 affected less severely

Neocortical layers 3, 5, and 6; injury may create pseudolaminar pattern of cortical necrosis

Cerebellar Purkinje cells: reactive proliferation of Bergmann glia and relative sparing of granule cells

Among the *basal ganglia*, the pallidum (especially the medial portion or globus pallidus internus [GPi]) (Fig. 9.3), the striatum (especially the lateral portion of the putamen), and the thalamus are vulnerable to hypoxia. The mammillary bodies may be especially vulnerable when hypoxia occurs in infancy.

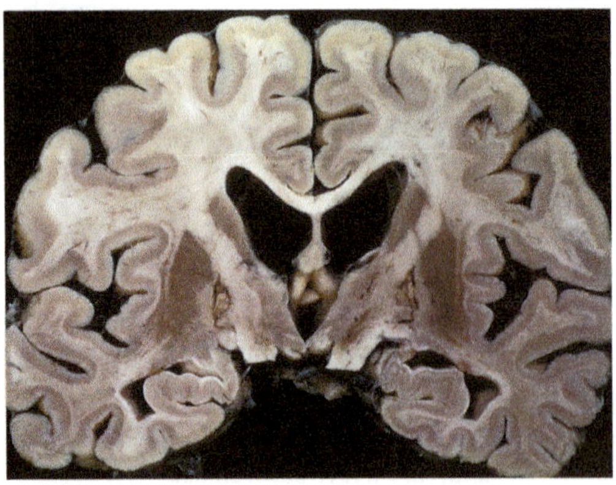

FIGURE 9.3 Bilateral necrosis of the pallidum (GPi), gross appearance.

In the *cerebellum*, cortical involvement is frequent and affects chiefly the Purkinje cells, with secondary proliferation of Bergmann glia. The dentate nucleus is also often involved.

In the *brainstem*, the medullary olives are vulnerable areas. In children, the brainstem is sometimes severely damaged, especially the medial and lateral reticular formations and the adjacent cranial nerve nuclei.

Various types of *white matter* lesions may be seen in isolation in response to anoxia or in association with gray matter damage. Some white matter lesions consist predominantly of extravasation of edema fluid due to physiologically increased vascular permeability but with preservation of the morphological integrity of the microcirculation. These lesions currently are designated as *reversible leukoencephalopathy* and may be seen in hypoxia and other acquired metabolic disturbances or intoxications. Other white matter lesions occur in *hypoxic–ischemic encephalopathy* that consist of varying proportions of loss of myelin and white matter necrosis. The severity of these lesions ranges from small, perivascular foci of demyelination to focal plaque-like areas of demyelination and necrosis and up to large confluent areas of demyelination and necrosis. The lesions tend to be most severe deep in the white matter and often show relative preservation of the subcortical U-fibers (Fig. 9.4).

The pattern of injury is different in the perinatal period than in adults. Hypoxic–ischemic injury in newborn infants leads to white matter injury (perinatal leukoencephalopathy), neuronal loss in the pontine nuclei and subiculum (pontosubicular necrosis), and selective granule cell loss in the cerebellum. Perinatal hypoxic–ischemic injury in premature and term infants is discussed in Chapter 11.

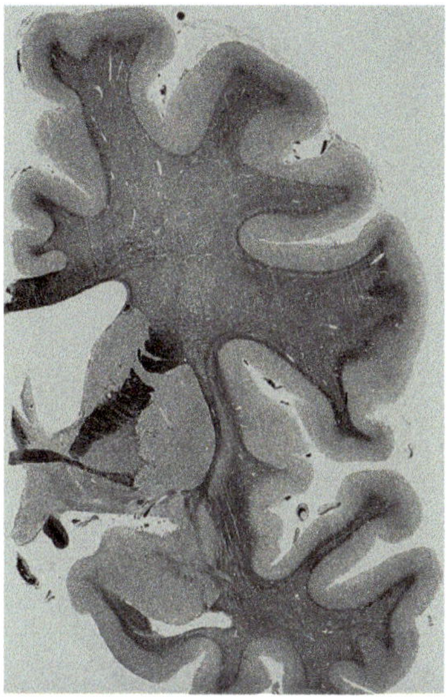

FIGURE 9.4 Whole-brain section showing extensive white matter injury with preservation of the U-fibers in hypoxic leukoencephalopathy (Loyez stain).

9.1.3. Variation of lesions according to etiology

A survival time of approximately 48 hours is necessary for macroscopically visible lesions of cerebral hypoxia to be apparent on gross examination. Before that interval, a variable degree of cerebral swelling may be observed. In cases of sudden death or where only moderate cerebral hypoxia has occurred, unquestionable signs of hypoxia may only be discerned on histological examination; these changes consist of ischemic neurons in the most vulnerable areas, where they are difficult to detect before 24 hours of survival after the onset. Depending on the mechanism of cerebral hypoxia/ischemia, separate and distinctive patterns of ischemic changes are recognized.

9.1.3.1. CEREBRAL INFARCTS

Cerebral infarcts are the result of localized ischemic hypoxia due to vascular occlusion (see Chapter 4). Infarcts or ischemic lesions in the boundary zone areas between major arterial territories, or "watershed" areas, are the result of global oligemic hypoxia, especially in the setting of low cerebral blood flow of sudden onset, even of short duration. These lesions are one of the possible adverse consequences of acute heart failure (cardiogenic shock), drug-induced hypotension, or general anesthesia. Boundary-zone infarcts are not typically seen in the setting of complete cardiac arrest.

9.1.3.2. CARDIOVASCULAR ARREST

Cardiovascular arrest exceeding 3 or 4 minutes at normal temperature ordinarily causes diffuse cortical lesions and hippocampal (Sommer sector) involvement; the distribution and extent of damage in the basal ganglia and in the brainstem are variable (Fig. 9.5).

Comparable lesions are caused by profound hypoglycemia (see Section 9.1.3.5) and status epilepticus under some circumstances.

9.1.3.3. CARBON MONOXIDE POISONING

Carbon monoxide is produced by incomplete combustion of carbon-containing substances. Humans are exposed to CO mainly through improperly ventilated stoves or heaters, automobile exhaust (accidental or with suicidal or homicidal intent), and tobacco smoke. The toxic effects of CO result primarily from the displacement of O_2 molecules from hemoglobin due to the high affinity of CO for hemoglobin, which decreases the capacity of blood to transport oxygen.

At autopsy of an individual who dies within a few hours of intoxication, the skin is often bright red, and the brain is diffusely swollen and congested. The blood within vessels has a characteristic cherry red color of carboxyhemoglobin, and as a result, that discoloration is also imparted to the external and cut

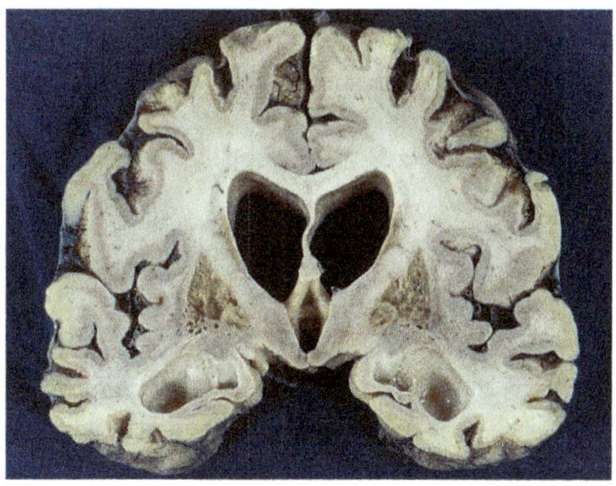

FIGURE 9.5 Diffuse cortical and basal ganglia lesions in a patient who was resuscitated after cardiovascular arrest and survived for an extended period after the episode.

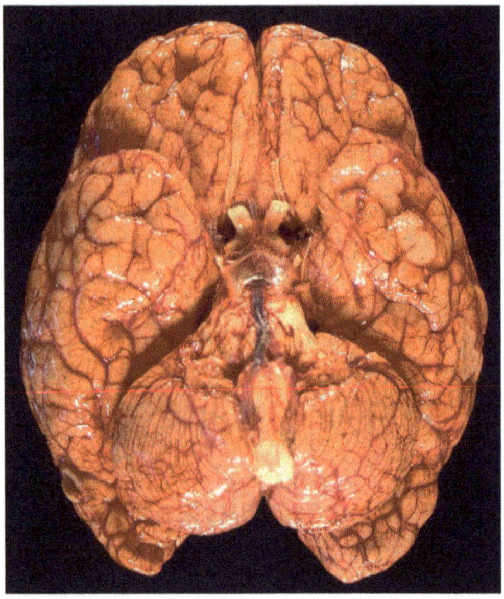

FIGURE 9.6 The brain from a patient with acute carbon monoxide poisoning. The postmortem blood carbon monoxide saturation was 60%. The cherry red color of the carboxyhemoglobin imparts a red hue to the entire brain.

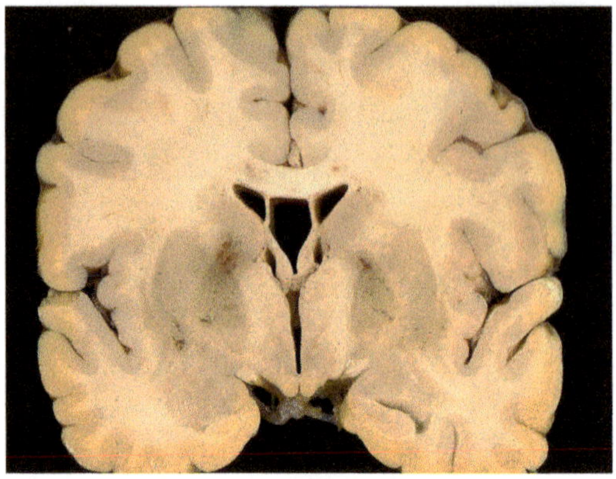

FIGURE 9.7 Coronal section showing bilateral pallidal necrosis, involving internal and external globus pallidus and extending into the internal capsule. This can be seen following a protracted period from the initial carbon monoxide or other hypoxic insult.

surface of the brain (Fig. 9.6). Scattered petechial hemorrhages also may be present. With formalin fixation, the red discoloration fades.

Some individuals who seem to recover clinically from acute toxic exposure to CO may develop a neurologic syndrome days to weeks later that includes neuropsychiatric manifestations, including personality changes, parkinsonism, dementia, incontinence, and frank psychosis. In these cases, different combinations of the neuropathological abnormalities described next may occur.

Pallidal necrosis is most often observed in fatal cases of CO intoxication, occurring 6 or more days after exposure. Microscopic foci of ischemic or hemorrhagic necrosis may develop even sooner. The pallidal lesions are usually bilateral but are often asymmetrical. The necrosis usually involves the anterior portion and inner segment of the pallidum but may extend into the outer segment or dorsally into the internal capsule. Although pallidal necrosis is characteristic of, and frequently seen in, delayed deaths from CO (Fig. 9.7), it may also be seen in other conditions associated with hypoxia or anoxia (Fig. 9.3). The selective involvement of the globus pallidus in CO poisoning has been attributed to selective vulnerability of pallidal neurons, the result of hypotension and impaired circulation through the pallidal branches of the anterior choroidal arteries, or to the relatively high iron content of this portion of the brain, which may render the structure especially susceptible.

Other gray matter regions that may be involved include the neocortical and hippocampal neurons and the cerebellar Purkinje cells and granule cells, where there may be focal neuronal loss.

Lesions of the white matter may also be encountered in individuals who die after CO poisoning. These lesions consist of varying degrees of demyelination and associated necrosis. There may be small perivascular foci found in the deep white matter, large confluent areas that extend from the frontal to occipital poles in the periventricular white matter, or sharply demarcated foci of demyelination with relative sparing of axons in the deep white matter ("Grinker myelinopathy") (Fig. 9.8). All these lesions tend to spare the subcortical U-fibers.

9.1.3.4. CYANIDES

Cyanides are histotoxic or cytotoxic agents, the toxicity of which is due to bonding between the cyanide ion and the ferric iron of intracellular cytochrome oxidase (complex IV of the respiratory electron chain). This reaction leads to cessation of cellular respiration (oxidative phosphorylation). Acute intoxication can result from either ingestion or inhalation of cyanides. Rarely, survivors of cyanide intoxication may develop parkinsonism or dystonia.

When death is acute in cyanide intoxication, the brain may be edematous, and in some cases focal subarachnoid hemorrhages develop. If death occurs

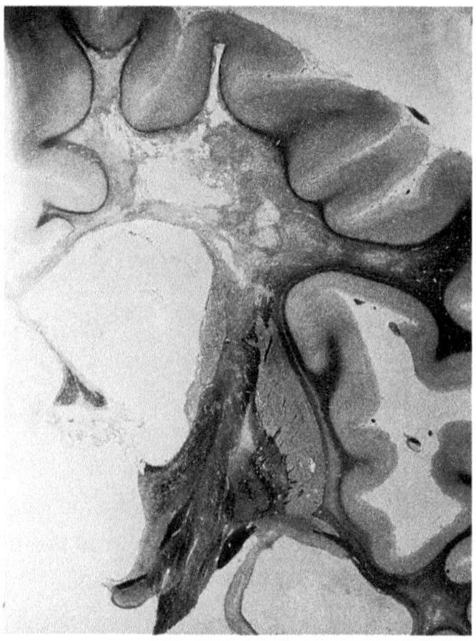

FIGURE 9.8 Carbon monoxide poisoning. Necrosis of the white matter with sparing of the subcortical U-fibers in a case of Grinker myelinopathy (Loyez stain).

following an extended period, the brain may show foci of necrosis in the basal ganglia and white matter and loss of Purkinje cells.

9.1.3.5. HYPOGLYCEMIA

Glucose is the principal source of energy in the central nervous system (CNS). Neuronal and astrocytic stores of glucose and glycogen are relatively small and need practically continuous replenishment. A decrease of glucose level under 1.5 mmol/L (25–30 mg/100 mL) leads to brain damage within 1 or 2 hours.

The most common cause of severe hypoglycemia is an excess of exogenous insulin. The effects of hypoglycemia are not due just to the energy deficits. Release of aspartate, and to a lesser extent glutamate, probably contributes to neuronal damage through excitotoxic mechanisms.

In acute hypoglycemia, the lesions are similar to those of acute hypoxia but not identical. In general, the pattern of injury is that of selective cell death of neurons rather than frank necrosis of all other cellular components. Affected neurons are shrunken with hypereosinophilic cytoplasm. Initially, the nucleus is pyknotic, as seen in anoxia, but later may become eosinophilic and appears to blend in with the cytoplasm (nuclear dropout). The topography of the lesions is roughly similar to that in hypoxia, but Purkinje cells may be relatively spared.

In long-term survivors of severe hypoglycemia who later come to postmortem examination, the cerebral cortex may appear thinner than normal and the hippocampi shrunken and discolored. The white matter is reduced in bulk, and the ventricles are dilated. There may be marked atrophy of the caudate nucleus and putamen. On microscopic study, the cerebral cortex shows laminar neuronal loss and gliosis associated with capillary proliferation. There is often dense subpial gliosis. The hippocampal pyramidal cell layer and subiculum are replaced by a loose meshwork of glial tissue. The white matter is usually rarefied and gliotic. The caudate nucleus and putamen are diffusely gliotic. The globus pallidus is relatively spared. Moderate neuronal loss and gliosis may be evident in the thalamus. As in acute hypoglycemia, the cerebellar cortex, including the Purkinje cells, is relatively spared.

9.1.3.6. HYPERTHERMIA

Acute hyperthermia or heat stroke is a thermal insult to the cerebral thermoregulatory system controlling heat production and heat dissipation. The thermal insult may be endogenous, as in "exertional heat stroke," or environmental, as in "classic heat stroke." It is also a feature of malignant hyperthermia, which occurs in patients with an autosomal dominant disorder of skeletal muscle characterized by a hypermetabolic response to commonly used inhalation anesthetics (halothane, isoflurane) and depolarizing muscle relaxants (succinylcholine). Clinically, *heat stroke* is defined as a syndrome characterized by nonfebrile elevated core body temperature over 40°C and accompanying neurologic dysfunction. Neuropathological studies are rare. Abnormalities similar to those of hypoxic–ischemic damage, probably resulting from a combination of cardiovascular collapse and an increased metabolic rate, have been described. Severe diffuse loss of Purkinje cells associated with expression of heat shock protein 70 by Bergmann glia, with consequent degeneration of the cerebellar efferent pathways, is known to occur, usually in the absence of injury to Ammon's horn and other areas susceptible to hypoxia.

9.2. ELECTROLYTE DISTURBANCES

9.2.1. Central pontine myelinolysis

Central pontine myelinolysis is a monophasic demyelinating disease that predominantly involves

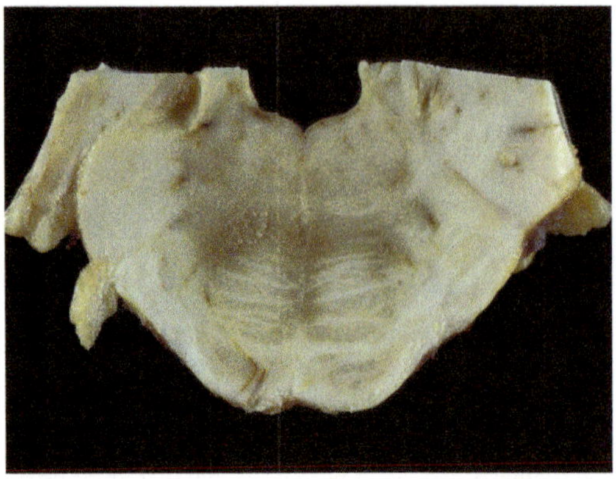

FIGURE 9.9 Transverse section of pons from patient with central pontine myelinolysis. Note the ill-defined brown discoloration of the demyelinated lesion.

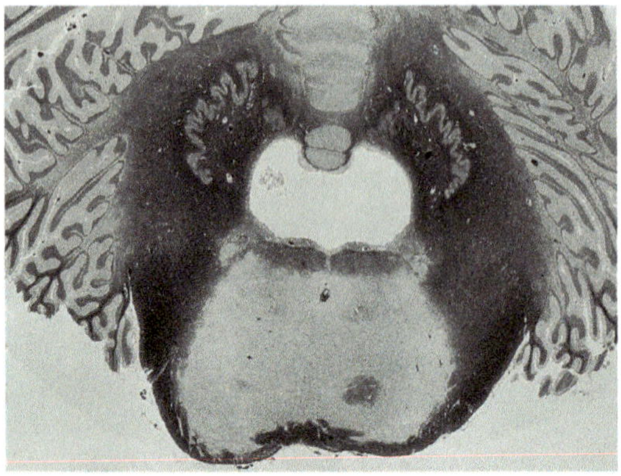

FIGURE 9.11 Large demyelinated lesion of pons from a patient with extensive central pontine myelinolysis (Luxol fast blue myelin stain).

the basis pontis. It usually occurs as a complication of rapid correction or overcorrection of chronic hyponatremia. The clinical manifestations of central pontine myelinolysis vary from asymptomatic to severe neurologic compromise, depending on the size and severity of the lesion. In life, the diagnosis can be made by magnetic resonance imaging (MRI).

At autopsy, the typical lesion of central pontine myelinolysis appears as a discolored, destructive area in the basis pontis that may be centrally cavitated (Fig. 9.9). The lesions are often triangular, T-shaped, or diamond-shaped, and vary from a few millimeters across (Fig. 9.10) to involving nearly the entire basis pontis. Even when the lesion is extensive, generally at least a thin rim of intact tissue with myelin preservation is present at the lateral and ventral margins of the basis pontis (Fig. 9.11). Demyelination is usually maximal in the middle and rostral portions of the pons. Lesions may extend to the middle cerebellar peduncles.

Histologically, the lesion of central pontine myelinolysis is characterized by demyelination with relative preservation of axons and neuronal perikarya (Fig. 9.12). Acute lesions contain numerous lipid-laden macrophages but few or no inflammatory cell infiltrates. Occasionally, foci of necrosis and cavitation are present in the center of the more severe lesions. Sometimes, especially in more severe cases, central pontine myelinolysis

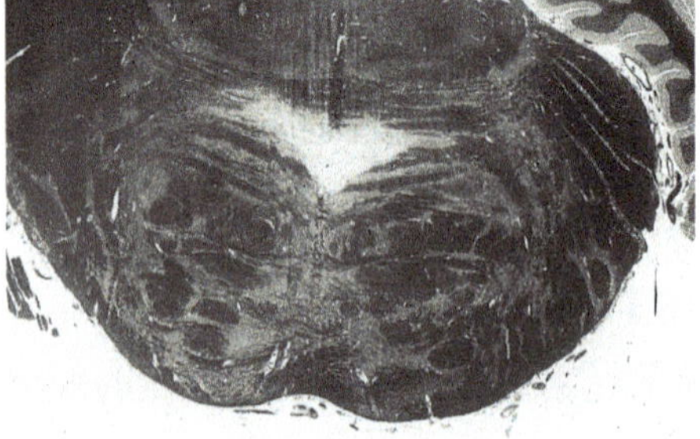

FIGURE 9.10 Limited triangular lesion of central pontine myelinolysis (Loyez stain).

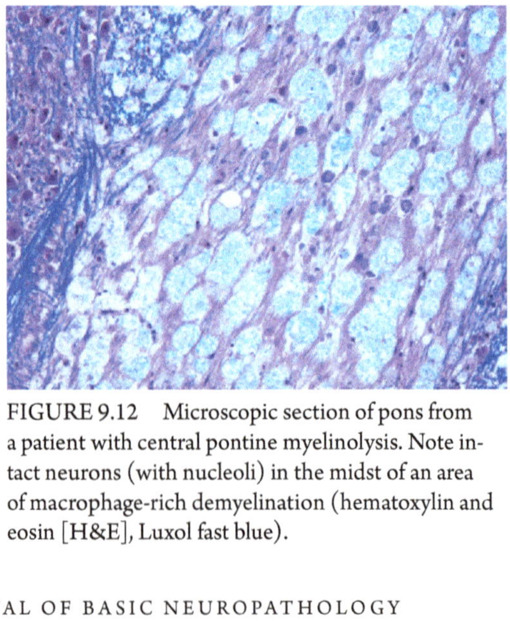

FIGURE 9.12 Microscopic section of pons from a patient with central pontine myelinolysis. Note intact neurons (with nucleoli) in the midst of an area of macrophage-rich demyelination (hematoxylin and eosin [H&E], Luxol fast blue).

is accompanied by extrapontine demyelinated lesions. These may involve the subcortical white matter, striatum, anterior commissure, internal and external capsules, lateral geniculate bodies, and cerebellar folia.

9.2.2. Disorders of iron metabolism

In primary or secondary *hemochromatosis,* the blood–brain barrier provides effective protection against the diffusion of protein-bound iron into the CNS. Therefore, hemosiderin iron deposits are limited to regions of the CNS devoid of the blood–brain barrier, including the choroid plexuses; area postrema; pineal gland; adenohypophysis; dorsal root ganglia; and vestigial remnants, such as the paraphysis and the subfornical organ. Macroscopically, these regions have a gross rusty appearance and show marked Prussian blue reaction with ferrocyanide on tissue sections.

9.2.3. Disorders of calcium metabolism

Massive perivascular deposits, including not only calcium (Fig. 9.13A) but also iron (Fig. 9.13B) and other minerals, may be observed in the basal ganglia and sometimes in the dentate nucleus, the white matter, and Ammon's horn. This type of mineralization may also be seen as a feature of hereditary neurodegeneration with brain iron accumulation (see Chapter 10) but may also be seen in several other acquired disorders, including hypoparathyroidism and conditions accompanied by hypercalcemia.

9.3. VITAMIN DEFICIENCY DISORDERS

9.3.1. Thiamine deficiency

The Wernicke–Korsakoff syndrome is caused by thiamine (vitamin B_1) deficiency from inadequate intake or nutritional deficit as in fasting or famine, or from a lack of gastric absorption as may occur in *hyperemesis gravidarum*, gastrointestinal neoplasms, and gastric plication for morbid obesity. Thiamine is a cofactor for key enzymes in the citric acid cycle, glycolysis, and pentose phosphate pathways that allow the production of ATP.

An acute psychotic encephalopathy, known as Wernicke encephalopathy, has characteristic periventricular lesions and accounts for symptoms that include disturbances of consciousness, ataxia, and ocular palsies. The lesions are found in the medial aspect of the thalamus, hypothalamus, and mammillary bodies and also in the periaqueductal region of the midbrain at the level of the oculomotor nuclei (Figs. 9.14 and 9.15). The reticular formation of the midbrain, the caudal portion of the corpora quadrigemina, and the floor of the fourth ventricle may also be involved. The mammillary bodies are the most frequently affected structures.

The morphologic changes vary with the stage and severity of the disease. On gross examination, following death in the acute stages of the disease, petechial hemorrhages involve predominantly the mammillary bodies (Fig. 9.16) and sometimes may extend to involve more extensive periventricular areas (Fig. 9.15). Patients with less severe, chronic, or previously treated disease may have mildly atrophic mammillary bodies that are gray to brown

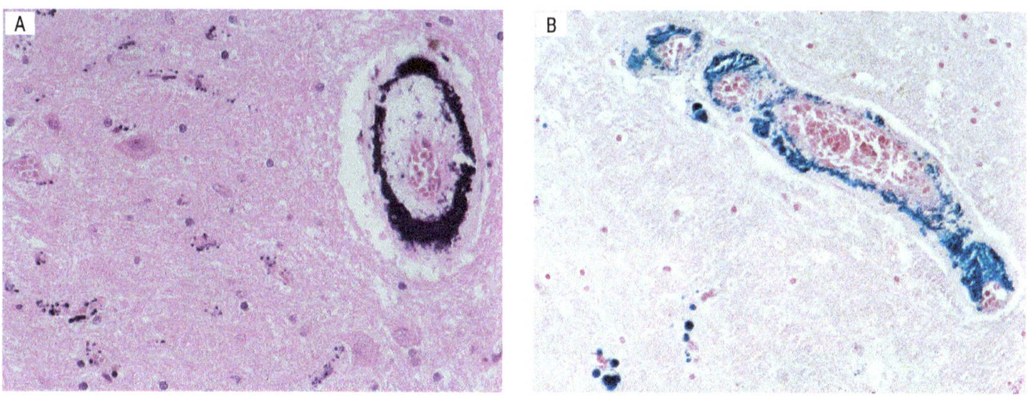

FIGURE 9.13 (**A**) Extensive perivascular mineral deposits in a case of idiopathic basal ganglia calcification (H&E). (**B**) Iron perivascular deposits in the same patient revealed by Perl's method for iron (Perl).

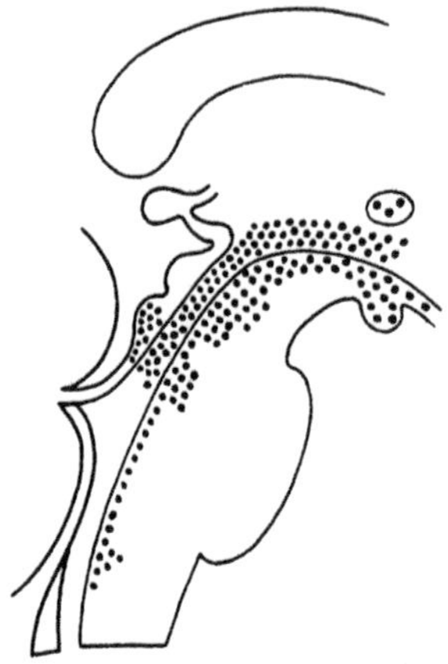

FIGURE 9.14 Diagram showing topographical distribution of the lesions in Wernicke encephalopathy.

in color as a result of hemosiderin deposition (Fig. 9.17). A narrow band of tissue immediately adjacent to the ventricular system and around the aqueduct usually remains unaffected.

On microscopy, the acute lesions display edema, petechial hemorrhages, myelin loss, and reactive astrocytosis. Neurons are generally preserved. Swelling and hyperplasia of endothelial cells make the capillary network abnormally prominent (Fig. 9.18). The perivascular spaces may contain lipid-laden macrophages. Extravasated erythrocytes and hemosiderin-laden macrophages are seen in cases with grossly discernible petechial hemorrhages. In the chronic stages of the disease and in treated patients, the affected regions may show little more than mild loss of neurons and gliosis.

Korsakoff psychosis is defined clinically as retrograde amnesia and an impaired ability to create new memories; it usually is encountered in alcoholic patients with chronic thiamine deficiency. The pathological basis of Korsakoff syndrome is debated. It does not seem to result from the lesions of the mammillary bodies only. According to some authors, involvement of the medial dorsal nuclei (Figs. 9.15A and 9.19) or

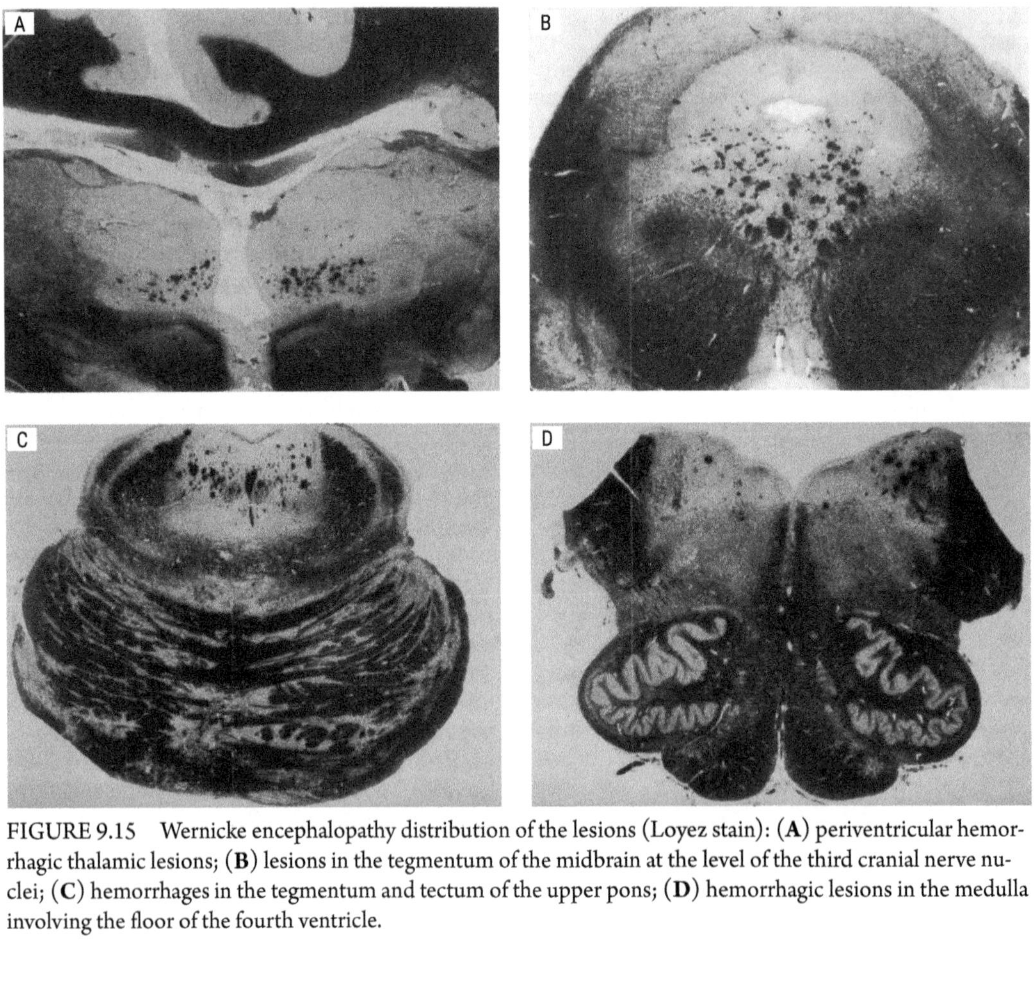

FIGURE 9.15 Wernicke encephalopathy distribution of the lesions (Loyez stain): (**A**) periventricular hemorrhagic thalamic lesions; (**B**) lesions in the tegmentum of the midbrain at the level of the third cranial nerve nuclei; (**C**) hemorrhages in the tegmentum and tectum of the upper pons; (**D**) hemorrhagic lesions in the medulla involving the floor of the fourth ventricle.

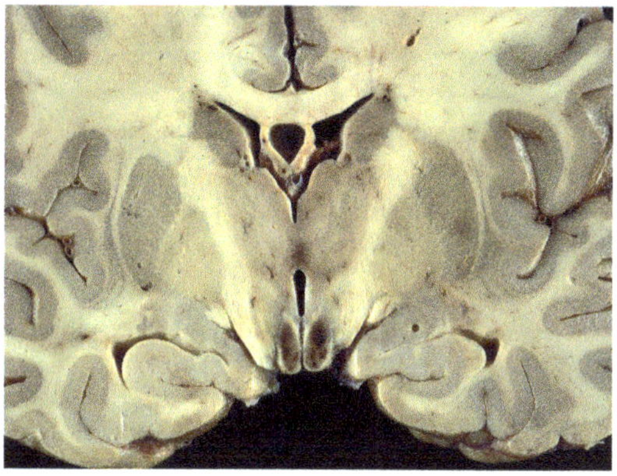

FIGURE 9.16 Acute Wernicke encephalopathy. Note the hemorrhages in the mammillary bodies and, to a lesser extent, the walls of the third ventricle.

midline region of the thalamus plays an important causative role.

Chronic thiamine deficiency also produces peripheral neuropathy, known as beriberi neuropathy, and may account for some cases of so-called alcoholic polyneuropathy ("dry beriberi"). When cardiac symptoms are prominent, there may be generalized edema, and the term "wet beriberi" is sometimes used. In the absence of cardiac failure, chronic thiamine deficiency may be described as dry beriberi.

Thiamine (Vitamin B_1) Deficiency

- Beriberi: cardiac involvement (sometimes with heart failure) and peripheral neuropathy
- Acute psychosis (Wernicke encephalopathy) with ophthalmoplegia, confusion, and ataxia
- Petechial hemorrhage most frequently involving the mammillary bodies
- Chronic encephalopathy (Korsakoff syndrome) with retrograde amnesia, impaired new memory formation, and confabulation

9.3.2. Pellagra

Typical clinical manifestations of pellagra are dermatitis, diarrhea, and dementia. The disease has long been recognized among malnourished individuals who depended on corn as a major part of their diet. It results from lack of nicotinic acid or niacin in the diet, causing vitamin B_3 deficiency. It is now known that deficiency of either niacin or tryptophan, an amino acid precursor of niacin that is deficient in corn, leads to pellagra. The disease has become very rare as the result of enriching common foods, such as bread, with niacin. This vitamin deficiency is now encountered most often in patients with chronic alcoholism. In these patients, the disease may be clinically atypical, lacking the characteristic skin lesions.

The neuropathologic changes resulting from niacin deficiency consist of neuronal changes of central chromatolysis type (Fig. 9.20) without associated glial or vascular alterations. They affect, in decreasing order of frequency, the Betz cells of the cerebral motor cortex, the pontine nuclei, the dorsal nucleus of the vagus, the gracile and cuneate nuclei, the nucleus ambiguus, the trigeminal nerve nuclei, the oculomotor nuclei, the reticular formations, and the anterior horn motor neurons of the spinal cord. In some cases of niacin deficiency, there may be degeneration of the posterior columns and corticospinal tracts.

9.3.3. Vitamin B_{12} deficiency

Vitamin B_{12} is obtained primarily from meat and dairy products. The vitamin must be bound to "intrinsic factor," a glycoprotein produced by the gastric parietal cells, prior to being absorbed in the ileum. Most cases of vitamin B_{12} deficiency result from inadequate production of intrinsic factor. In pernicious anemia, this is due to autoimmune atrophic gastritis and more rarely to gastric neoplasms or gastrectomy. Vitamin B_{12} deficiency also can result from impaired ileal absorption in individuals with malabsorption syndromes, intestinal tuberculosis, regional enteritis, or lymphomas. Rarely, the cause of the deficiency is the result of competitive utilization of the vitamin within the intestine by the fish tapeworm (*Diphyllobothrium latum*) or bacterial overgrowth in intestinal blind loops or diverticula. Very similar changes, "vacuolar myelopathy," have been observed in patients with AIDS, resulting from abnormalities of vitamin B_{12} metabolism.

Vitamin B_{12} deficiency affects the hematopoietic (megaloblastic anemia), gastrointestinal (glossitis, anorexia, diarrhea, and weight loss), and nervous systems. Neurological complications develop in 40% of untreated cases and can occur in the absence of hematologic abnormalities. The neuroanatomical/clinical syndrome of nervous system involvement has been termed *subacute combined degeneration of the spinal cord.*

The spinal cord from patients with long-standing severe vitamin B_{12} deficiency may be mildly shrunken with discolored posterior and lateral

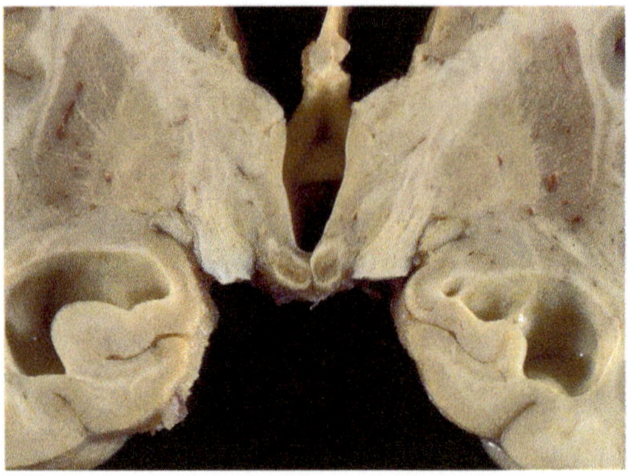

FIGURE 9.17 Shrunken, discolored mammillary bodies in a patient who had been treated for previous episodes of Wernicke encephalopathy.

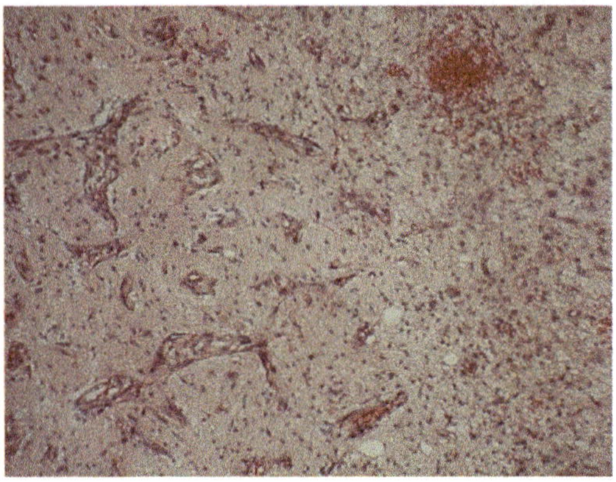

FIGURE 9.18 Microscopic appearance of the mammillary bodies from a patient with acute Wernicke encephalopathy. Note the petechial hemorrhages and the swelling of the endothelial cells (H&E).

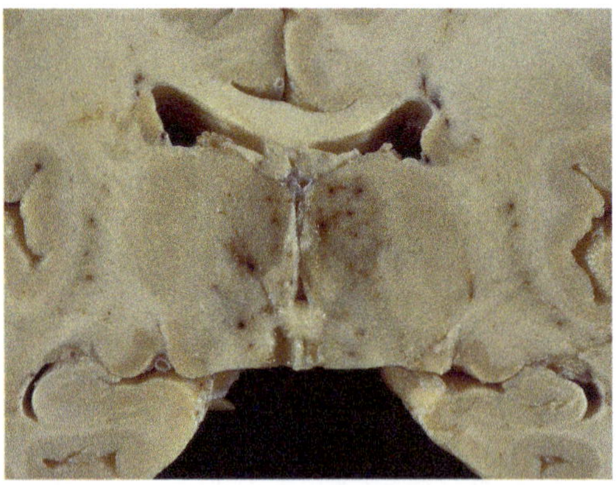

FIGURE 9.19 Petechiae and myelin loss in the medial thalamus from a patient with Korsakoff syndrome.

columns. Histologically, the earliest lesions consist of vacuolar distension of myelin sheaths, resulting in a characteristic spongy appearance of the affected white matter. With progression, lipid-laden macrophages become scattered throughout the lesions. Some of the axons traversing the lesions undergo Wallerian degeneration. Initially, astrocytic proliferation is not severe, but dense gliosis may be seen in patients who have had the disease for a protracted period of time. The distribution of the lesions is remarkably constant. They are bilateral and symmetrical and involve both the ascending and descending long tracts of the spinal cord ("combined" degeneration). Initial lesions are found in the central part of the posterior column of the thoracic cord from where they extend peripherally and affect the corticospinal and spinocerebellar tracts in the lateral columns. In severe cases, the lesions may involve virtually all the white matter, including the anterior columns, only sparing the fibers adjacent to the gray matter. The severity of the lesions usually decreases toward the cervical and lumbar levels, in which they are restricted to the dorsal and lateral columns, often sparing a small peripheral zone (Fig. 9.21). However, secondary changes of ascending and descending tract degeneration may be seen at those levels. Rarely, the lesions may extend rostrally into the medulla. Occasionally, similar mixed demyelinating and destructive lesions may be seen in the optic nerve and cerebral white matter.

9.4. TOXIC ENCEPHALOPATHIES

The nervous system is particularly susceptible to toxic compounds. There are several reasons for this. Neurons are highly vulnerable to energy deprivation; in addition, they are postmitotic cells and cannot regenerate as a response to toxic insults. It is also important to recognize that the susceptibility of neurons to toxic substances in different anatomic regions is quite variable. These differences are attributable in part to the selective blood–brain barrier susceptibility to some toxic substances. The type of exposure, dose, age, gender, and inherent genetic factors also determine the extent and severity of the toxic insult. Accordingly, the neuropathological picture is highly variable, reflecting the selective vulnerability of some brain structures and the diversity of the underlying mechanisms (e.g., energy deficiency,

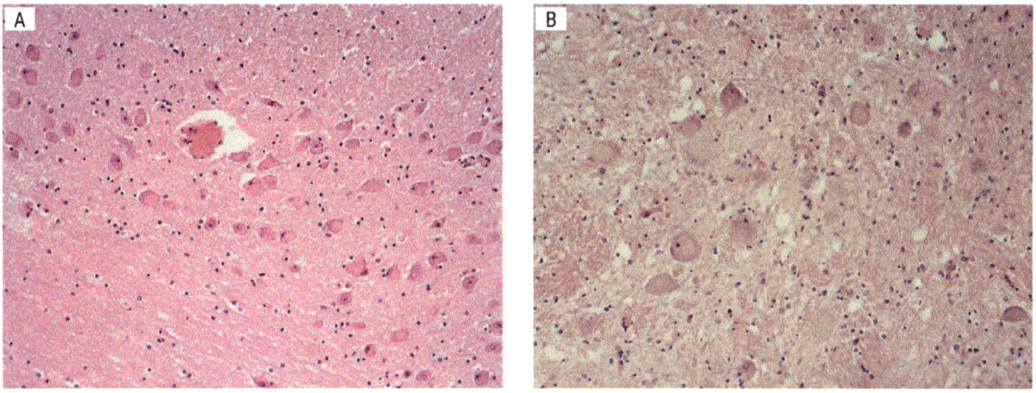

FIGURE 9.20 Pellagra encephalopathy. Microscopic picture of chromatolysis (H&E): (**A**) in pontine nuclei; (**B**) in the gracile nucleus.

excitotoxicity). Some lesions may also result from systemic toxicity. In some neurotoxic syndromes, the peripheral nervous system (PNS) may also be affected. The following sections describe the most widely recognized toxic substances known to produce lesions of the nervous system.

9.4.1. Ethanol

Ethanol has many effects on the CNS. It is well known that alcoholism potentiates infections; contributes to traumatic injuries; and may increase the risk of strokes, especially hemorrhagic stroke.

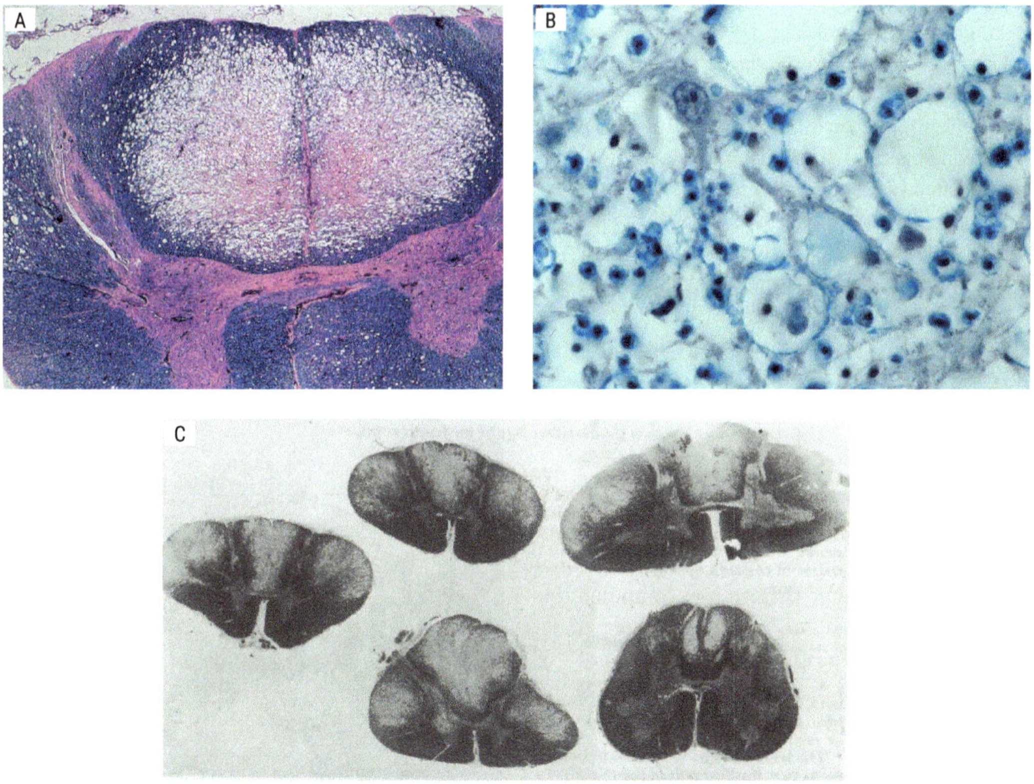

FIGURE 9.21 Subacute combined degeneration of the spinal cord: (**A**) Klüver–Barrera stain showing spongy appearance of the white matter in the central part of the posterior columns of the thoracic cord; (**B**) Bodian Luxol stain showing vacuolar distension of myelin sheaths surrounding the axon; (**C**) Loyez myelin stain showing pallor of the posterior and lateral columns of the spinal cord.

9.4.1.1. ACUTE ALCOHOL INTOXICATION

Ingestion of large quantities of alcohol can lead directly to death from cardiorespiratory arrest. Blood alcohol levels over 450–500 mg/dL are generally considered potentially lethal, although there is considerable individual variation. Autopsy examination of the brain in fatal cases of acute alcohol intoxication usually shows only cerebral edema.

9.4.1.2. CEREBRAL LESIONS IN CHRONIC ALCOHOLISM

Patients suffering from chronic alcoholism develop a wide range of lesions, with some remaining uncertainty about which lesions result from direct neurotoxicity of ethanol and which lesions arise indirectly from nutritional or other systemic effects of chronic alcoholism.

- *Hepatic encephalopathy* may result from decompensated cirrhosis, leading to hepatic coma or occurring in the setting of a portocaval shunt (see Section 9.5.2).
- *Cerebral lesions due to vitamin deficiency* include Wernicke–Korsakoff encephalopathy secondary to deficiency of vitamin B_1 and pseudopellagra encephalopathy, with which it is frequently associated (see Section 9.3.2).
- *Alcoholic cerebellar degeneration* may occur as an isolated lesion or in association with other alcohol-related lesions, such as Wernicke encephalopathy. Its pathogenesis is unclear. Morphologically similar but generally milder cerebellar vermal atrophy can also occur as an age-related phenomenon independent of alcoholism.

The clinical manifestations evolve slowly over months to years and include truncal instability, a wide-based stance, and an ataxic gait. The vermal atrophy can be demonstrated by computed tomography (CT) and MRI, but the degree of atrophy does not correlate well with the severity of the clinical manifestations. The lesions involve the rostral vermis (Fig. 9.22) and, to a lesser extent, the superior surface of the cerebellar hemispheres (Fig. 9.23). The folia are pale and sclerotic and separated by widened sulci. The atrophy affects the crests of the folia more severely than the depths of the interfolial sulci. Microscopically, the lesions

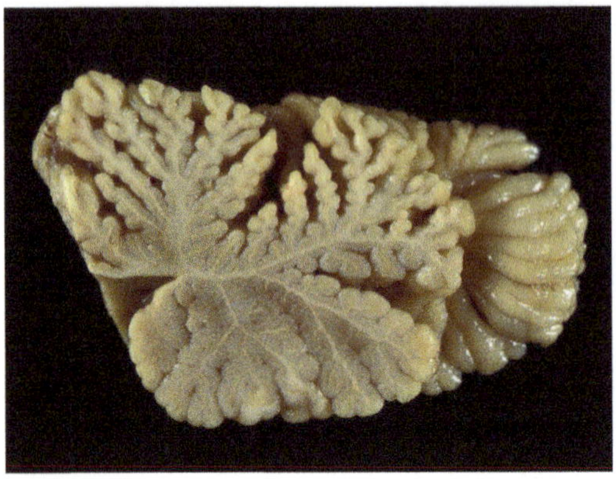

FIGURE 9.22 Superior vermal atrophy from a patient with chronic alcoholism.

consist of loss of Purkinje cells with proliferation of Bergmann glia and variable depopulation of the internal granular cells. They are associated with lesions of the dorsal laminae of the inferior olives. The cerebellar white matter remains relatively unaffected.

- *Central pontine myelinolysis* was first described in individuals with chronic alcoholism but may also be seen in other conditions in which severe electrolyte disturbances are present (see Section 9.2.1).
- *Marchiafava–Bignami disease* is a rare disorder, the pathophysiology of which is unknown. It is observed in the setting of chronic alcoholism of long duration and great severity. Rarely, Marchiafava–Bignami disease has been described in association with Wernicke encephalopathy or with central pontine myelinolysis. The diagnosis

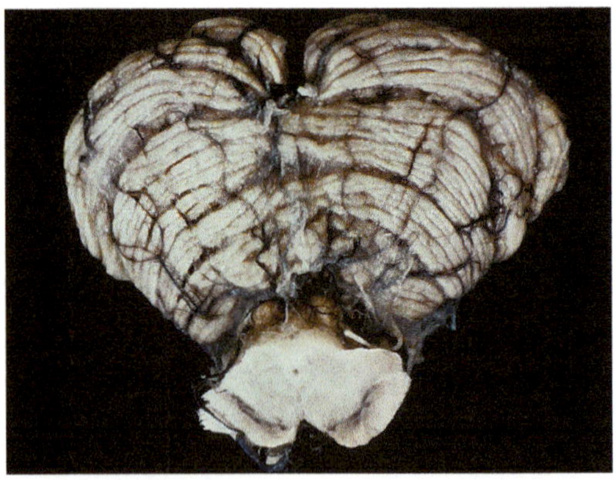

FIGURE 9.23 Atrophy of the rostral vermis and superior surface of the cerebellar hemispheres in a patient with chronic alcoholism.

is usually established at autopsy, but the lesions may be seen by CT and MRI.

The macroscopic appearance of the lesions is that of partially necrotic areas of damage in the central portions of the corpus callosum, with relative preservation of a thin strip of myelinated fibers on its dorsal and ventral surfaces. The involvement is maximal in the genu and body of the corpus callosum (Fig. 9.24) and may be accompanied by similar involvement of the optic chiasm, anterior commissure (Fig. 9.24B), centrum semiovale (Fig. 9.24A), and middle cerebellar peduncles. Histologically, the lesions show loss of myelin with abundant lipid-laden macrophages and relative sparing of axons.

- *Morel laminar sclerosis* is known to occur in chronic alcoholism. It is characterized by a glial astrocytic band-like proliferation localized to the third cortical layer, especially in the lateral frontal cortex. This disease is usually associated with, and probably secondary to, the callosal lesions of Marchiafava–Bignami disease.

9.4.2. Methanol

Methanol poisoning results most often from oral intake as a substitute for ethanol, and it may cause acute cerebral and ocular lesions. Methanol catabolites, especially formic acid, are thought to be the primary toxic agent. Formic acid and formates block cellular respiration and contribute to the metabolic acidosis and anion gap that are characteristic of this intoxication.

The ocular pathology of the blindness has been investigated extensively. The lesions include principally optic disc edema and optic nerve necrosis. Pathologic changes in the brain include cerebral edema, demyelination, and necrosis of the subcortical white matter, the lateral aspect of the putamen, and the claustrum (Fig. 9.25). The putaminal

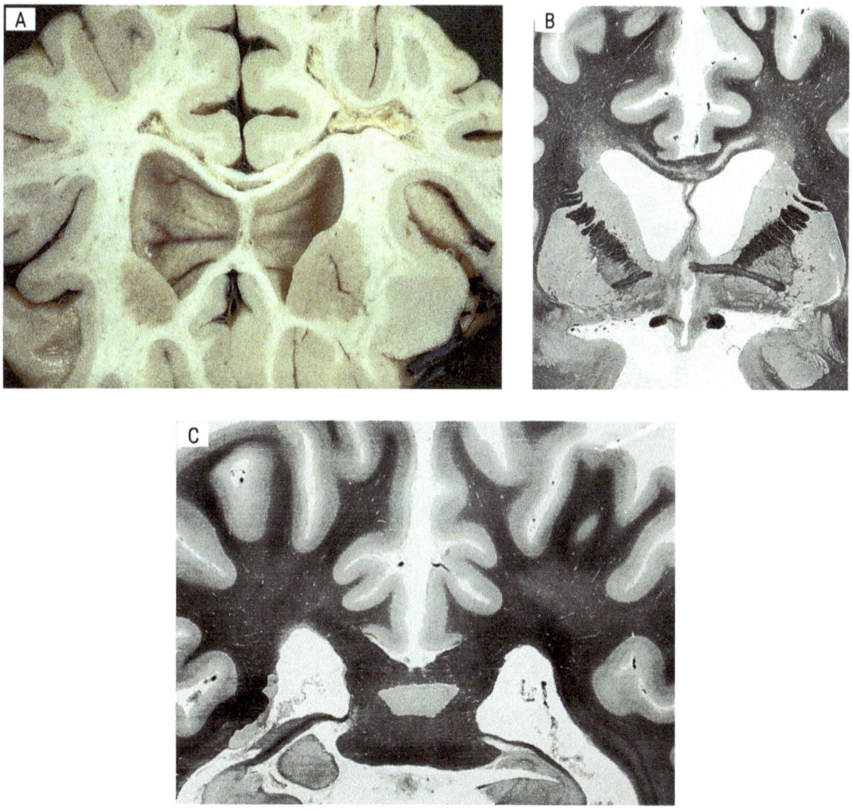

FIGURE 9.24 Marchiafava–Bignami disease. (**A**) Gross appearance showing necrosis of the central portion of the corpus callosum. Note involvement of the adjacent white matter. Whole-brain section showing necrosis and pallor of the corpus callosum and anterior commissure (**B**) and splenium of corpus callosum (**C**) (Loyez).

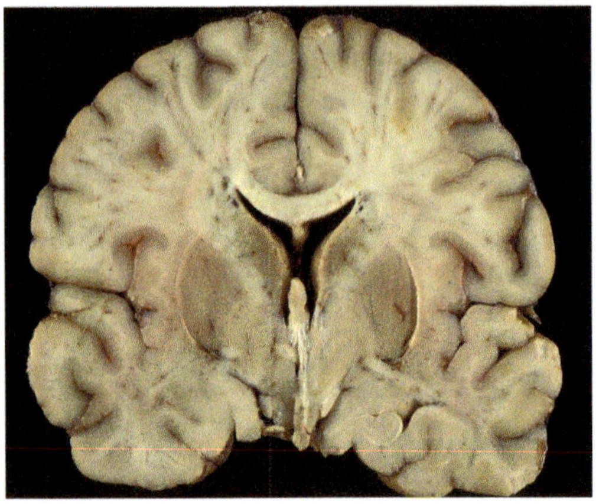

FIGURE 9.25 Methanol intoxication. Note the necrosis of the lateral putamen and claustrum present bilaterally.

necrosis is often hemorrhagic and may evolve into a massive hematoma, whereas the necrosis of the claustrum is generally nonhemorrhagic. The white matter lesions and the retrolaminar demyelination of the optic nerves are believed to be due to histotoxic myelinoclastic damage caused by formates. The pathogenesis of the putaminal lesions remains unclear.

9.4.3. Ethylene glycol

Ethylene glycol is a dihydroxy alcohol that is widely used as a solvent and component of certain antifreezes and coolants. Intoxication with this compound is encountered most often when it is consumed as a substitute for ethanol or with suicidal intent. Ethylene glycol is progressively oxidized to more toxic compounds, including glycoaldehyde, glycolic acid, and glyoxylic acid. A small proportion is also oxidized to oxalic acid. The clinical manifestations include encephalopathy, severe metabolic acidosis, cardiopulmonary failure, and acute renal failure.

Macroscopic examination of the brain in fatal cases shows edema, meningeal congestion, and, occasionally, petechial hemorrhages. Microscopically, acute inflammatory cells may be seen in the meninges and around intraparenchymal blood vessels. Deposits of calcium oxalate may be seen as refractile material in and around blood vessels in the meninges, brain parenchyma, and choroid plexus. These crystals are birefringent under polarized light (Fig. 9.26A, B).

9.4.4. Phenytoin

Patients with seizure disorders who have been treated with phenytoin for prolonged periods of time may develop cerebellar cortical atrophy, which can be documented by CT and MRI during life or at autopsy. Histopathological studies have shown folial atrophy, loss of Purkinje cells throughout the cerebellum, and mild loss of internal granular layer cells (Fig. 9.27). Whether the drug itself is the sole factor that causes toxic damage to Purkinje cells has been difficult to establish because loss of Purkinje cells may also be the result of hypoxia during seizures or from preexisting brain damage. Reports of patients with seizure control under long-term phenytoin

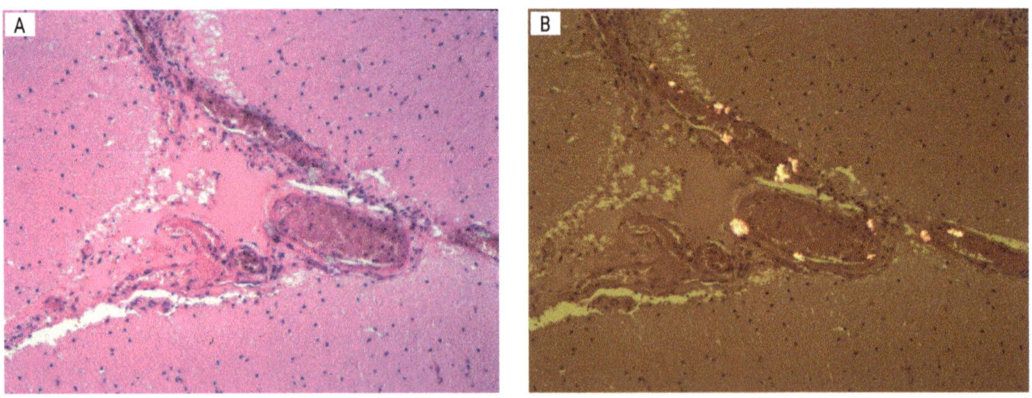

FIGURE 9.26 Microscopic sections showing cerebellar cortex and leptomeninges from a patient with ethylene glycol intoxication. (**A**) Note the refractile calcium oxalate crystals in the vessel walls (H&E). (**B**) Birefringence of the same crystals is evident when viewed with polarized light.

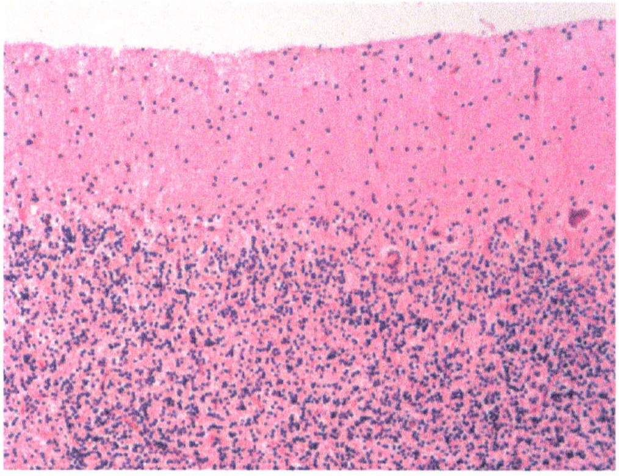

FIGURE 9.27 Microscopic section of cerebellar cortex from a patient who had been on long-term treatment with high-dose phenytoin. Note the loss of Purkinje cells with Bergmann gliosis, and the mild loss of internal granule cell layer neurons (H&E).

treatment who develop cerebellar atrophy support the view that phenytoin itself may be neurotoxic.

9.4.5. *N*-methyl-4-phenyl-1,2,3,6-tetrahydropyridine

Acute-onset L-dopa–responsive parkinsonism may be caused by exposure to pesticides, particularly 1-methyl-4-phenyl-1,2,3,6-tetrahydropyridine (MPTP), a contaminant in preparations of methyl-4-phenyl-4-propionoxypiperidine (desmethylprodine), which is a synthetic opioid used illegally. The pathological changes include nigral degeneration and Lewy bodies. MPTP acts by causing inhibition of complex I of the mitochondrial respiratory chain. Depletion of neurons in other brain areas is also present, with loss of dopaminergic neurons and accompanying gliosis in the hypothalamus and locus coeruleus.

9.4.6. 3-Nitropropionic acid

3-Nitropropionic acid, a fungal metabolite of the genus *Arthrinium*, is a structural analogue of succinic acid and irreversibly inhibits succinate dehydrogenase, complex II of the mitochondrial respiratory chain. It may cause poisoning through consumption of contaminated sugar cane. Affected patients develop convulsions, followed by coma and death, but those who recover show low-density lesions on CT scans, predominantly in the putamen. There is vascular breakdown, a decrease in endothelial cell cytoplasmic density, thrombin accumulation, aggregates of perivascular protein, and petechial hemorrhages, in addition to a selective loss of medium-size neurons in the putamen and occasionally in the globus pallidus and caudate. A more diffuse lesion may occur. Internal capsule axonal swelling and myelin splitting may occur, like that observed in hypoxic–ischemic damage.

9.4.7. Organophosphorus compounds

Insecticides belonging to the organophosphorus group are widely used not only in agriculture but also sometimes in the home and as agents of chemical warfare. Although acute neurotransmission effects due to inhibition of acetylcholinesterase are well recognized, most of the toxic symptoms are delayed after long-term low level exposures and result in distal polyneuropathy (see Chapter 13); neuropsychiatric symptoms may also occur.

9.4.8. Intoxication by heavy metals and certain metalloids

Many different metals and some metalloids, in sufficient concentration and specific chemical form, are toxic to humans. It is usually difficult to correlate a particular type of neuropathologic lesion with a specific etiologic agent. In some hyperacute fatal forms of intoxication, the clinical course may be so rapid that at the time of autopsy examination, histological changes have not yet become evident. Some of the morphologic changes that may be seen in such cases include edematous or hemorrhagic lesions. Furthermore, in most cases, brain lesions are secondary to a range of visceral disturbances caused by the intoxication.

9.4.8.1. ALUMINUM

Many instances of aluminum toxicity were described in patients undergoing chronic hemodialysis. This neurotoxicity was due to exposure to aluminum in the dialysate and the use of oral phosphate-binding compounds containing aluminum; these are no longer in use. The clinical syndrome of dialysis dementia includes dyspraxia, asterixis, myoclonus, and dementia. The neurotoxicity of environmental aluminum is not well-established. Various aluminum compounds applied directly onto or injected into the cerebral cortex of certain laboratory animals produce seizures and neurofibrillary tangles, but these are different from the Alzheimer neurofibrillary tangles seen in humans. Epidemiological studies have not found a clear association between aluminum exposure and neuropathologic changes of Alzheimer disease.

9.4.8.2. ARSENIC

Arsenic intoxication is encountered most often as the result of occupational exposure or after ingestion with homicidal or suicidal intent. Individuals suffering from acute trivalent arsenic poisoning develop clinical manifestations that include abdominal pain, nausea, vomiting, and diarrhea, followed by renal failure. Death may occur in severe cases. Chronic arsenic intoxication is manifest by gastrointestinal and dermatological symptoms. Mixed sensory and motor neuropathy is a well-known and often disabling consequence of both acute and chronic arsenic intoxication. Encephalopathy also has been reported with acute and chronic arsenic intoxication. Acute hemorrhagic leukoencephalopathy has been reported in patients treated with organic pentavalent arsenicals. This manifestation of the intoxication may have been the result of a hypersensitivity reaction to the drug.

9.4.8.3. LEAD

The heavy metal lead can enter the body through the gastrointestinal and respiratory tracts and, when in organic compounds, through the skin. Lead encephalopathy is now encountered predominantly in young children who chew on items coated with lead paint. Acute encephalopathy produces irritability, seizures, altered consciousness, and evidence of increased intracranial pressure. The intoxication usually responds to sedation and chelation therapy but can lead to permanent damage. Many authors have attributed the encephalopathy to vascular injury, which seems to be more severe in the immature nervous system.

At autopsy examination of affected individuals, the brain is diffusely swollen. The histological changes include congestion, petechial hemorrhages, and foci of necrosis. Intraparenchymal capillaries may show necrosis, thrombosis, and swelling of endothelial cells. There is a proteinaceous exudate in the perivascular space extending into the adjacent brain tissue. Periodic acid–Schiff–positive globules may be seen within the exudates and within astrocytes. Diffuse astrocytosis has been reported even in the absence of capillary changes.

9.4.8.4. MANGANESE

Manganese exposure may result from inhaling dust in manganese mines or vapor released during ferromanganese smelting. The clinical manifestations include headaches, transient psychiatric disturbances, and a hypokinetic extrapyramidal dysfunction resembling Parkinson disease but nonresponsive to L-dopa.

Pathologic studies in humans are limited, but they document degenerative lesions in the pallidum and subthalamic nucleus and, to a lesser extent, the striatum. The substantia nigra is involved in some cases.

9.4.8.5. MERCURY

Acute poisoning from inorganic mercury compounds is manifest clinically predominantly by gastrointestinal tract and renal tubular injury. Pulmonary injury is caused by inhalation of metallic mercury vapors. Neurotoxicity is also a prominent manifestation of chronic inorganic mercury poisoning. Patients manifest behavioral changes, intention tremor, and movement disorders; peripheral neuropathy may also develop.

Organic mercury intoxication is usually caused by ingestion of contaminated food. Some years ago, reports from Japan described a large number of cases that developed chronic organic mercury intoxication by eating fish contaminated by methyl mercury in the ocean near Minamata (Minamata disease). Other large outbreaks have resulted from the consumption of grain treated with an organic mercury fungicide. The clinical manifestations in these cases included cortical blindness, impaired proprioception, movement disorders, mental retardation, and quadriparesis.

The neuropathology of organic and inorganic mercury poisoning is essentially indistinguishable. The slight differences between cases may reflect variations in the rate of entry of mercury into the nervous system. The lesions observed involve neurons predominantly. There is cerebral atrophy involving mainly the anterior portions of the calcarine fissures with loss of neurons, especially the outer cortical layers, and gliosis. Cerebellar atrophy is also frequent, notably with loss of granule cell neurons, loss of Purkinje cells, and proliferation of Bergmann glia (Fig. 9.28).

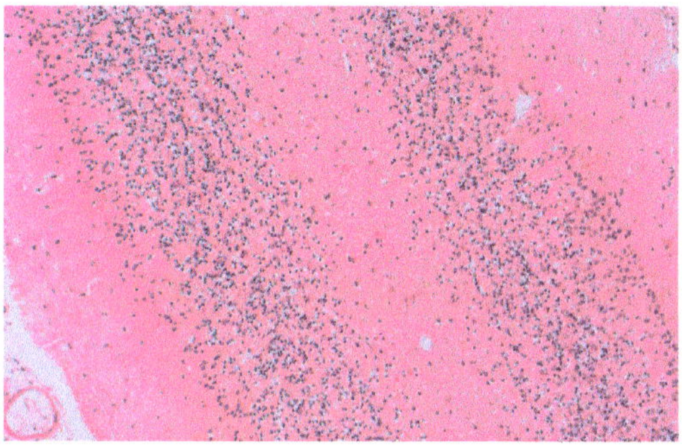

FIGURE 9.28 Massive loss of Purkinje cells, Bergmann gliosis, and granule cell loss in the cerebellum in cerebellar injury due to mercury (H&E).

9.4.8.6. THALLIUM

Most cases of thallium intoxication result from accidental or deliberate ingestion of thallium pesticides used for insect and rodent control. The clinical picture resembles that of trivalent arsenic poisoning. The only consistent abnormalities in the CNS are chromatolysis of spinal motor neurons and degeneration of the posterior columns related to the sensorimotor distal axonopathy.

9.4.8.7. TIN

Inorganic tin is not neurotoxic, but two organic tin compounds, triethyl-tin and trimethyl-tin, are neurotoxic. Triethyl-tin causes striking white matter edema due to accumulation of fluid in vacuoles within the myelin sheaths, which are separated along the intraperiod lines (see Chapter 1 and Fig. 1.26C). Trimethyl-tin does not cause intramyelinic edema but is toxic to neurons in the hippocampus, the entorhinal cortex, and the amygdala.

9.5. CENTRAL NERVOUS SYSTEM CHANGES SECONDARY TO SYSTEMIC DISEASES

9.5.1. Respiratory encephalopathies

The neuropathology of respiratory encephalopathy is characterized by diffuse vasodilation, microscopic perivascular hemorrhages, and anoxic neuronal changes of variable intensity, most often secondary to chronic bronchopulmonary disease and its related hypoxia and hypercapnia.

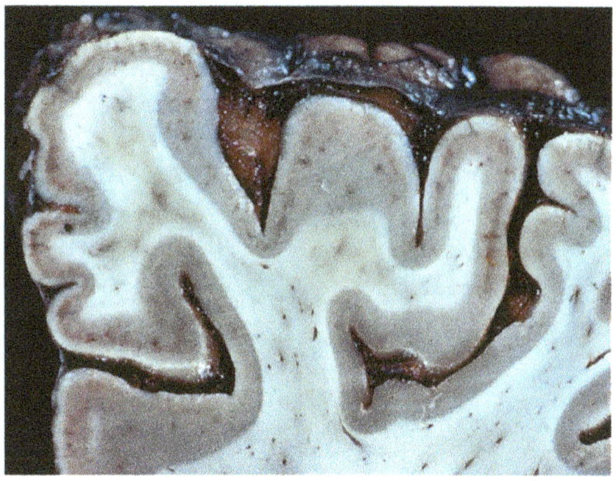

FIGURE 9.29 Petechial hemorrhages and laminar necrosis, sparing the most superficial layers, in the brain of a patient who died from asphyxia.

At postmortem examination, the brains of patients who die soon after acute asphyxia show congestion of the meninges and cortex due to venous and capillary dilation (Fig. 9.29). Perivascular hemorrhages predominating in the white matter may be seen. Later effects of hypoxia were summarized previously (see Section 9.1).

9.5.2. Hepatic encephalopathy

Hepatic encephalopathy occurs in the course of severe hepatic insufficiency in cases of hepatic cirrhosis or hepatitis, in association with portocaval anastomosis and in individuals with Wilson hepatolenticular degeneration. It is characterized by the presence of Alzheimer type II glia (see Chapter 1 and Fig. 1.21). The lesions predominate in the pallidum but may also involve the cerebral cortex and the cerebellar dentate nuclei.

9.5.3. Kernicterus

Kernicterus or nuclear jaundice is a condition in which unconjugated bilirubin penetrates the blood–brain barrier in the perinatal period and causes toxic damage to neurons and other cells in the hippocampus, globus pallidus, and subthalamic nucleus and also in other nuclear groups in the diencephalon, brainstem, and cerebellum. Macroscopically, these areas are abnormally tinged with a yellowish-orange hue (Fig. 9.30), and microscopically there is evidence of neuronal injury, vascular proliferation, and gliosis. The disease is currently rare but may still occur throughout the world as a result of inadequate perinatal care. The

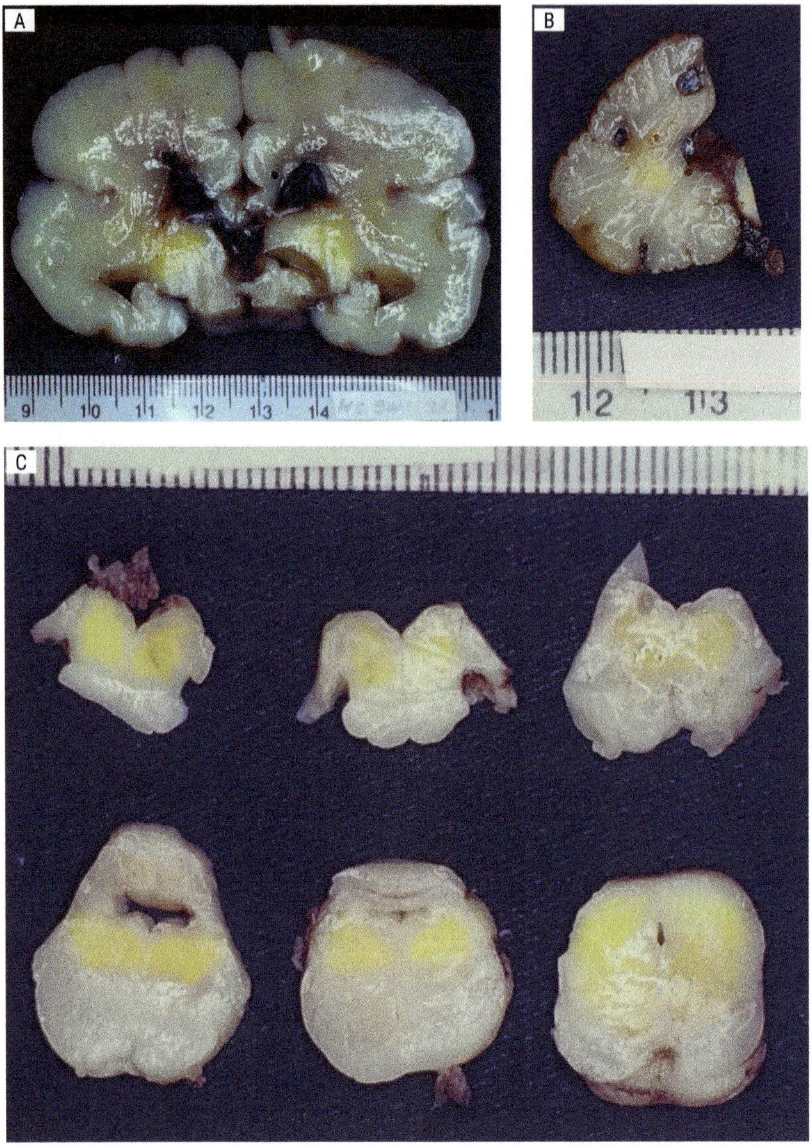

FIGURE 9.30 Kernicterus: Yellow discoloration in the CNS of a premature baby, including the (**A**) globus pallidus and hemispheric white matter; (**B**) dentate nucleus of the cerebellar hemisphere; and (**C**) brainstem nuclei, including cranial nerve nuclei. Intraventricular (**A**, **B**) and parenchymal (**B**) hemorrhages are also common in premature infants.

primary risk factor is hyperbilirubinemia during the neonatal period. There are a number of predisposing conditions, including extreme prematurity, hemolytic diseases, hereditary diseases such as glucose-6-phosphate-dehydrogenase deficiency, breastfeeding, sepsis, intestinal disorders, and hypothyroidism. Also, at risk are the infants of diabetic mothers, individuals of East Asian or Mediterranean descent, or babies born in a setting of excessive maternal bleeding in the newborn period.

9.5.4. Multifocal necrotizing leukoencephalopathy

Multifocal necrotizing leukoencephalopathy is characterized by the development of multiple, usually microscopic, foci of necrosis in the white matter. It often affects the basis pontis (focal pontine leukoencephalopathy). The pathogenesis is unclear. Affected individuals are predominantly those who are found to have increased levels of circulating pro-inflammatory cytokines (e.g., patients with AIDS, neoplasms treated with radio- and chemotherapy, or sepsis). In most cases, it is discovered at autopsy.

In general, the lesions are only visible on microscopic examination and consist of well-demarcated areas of necrosis disseminated in the white matter but particularly involving the transverse pontine fibers (Fig. 9.31A). There is loss of myelin staining, proliferation of macrophages, and lesions of axons, which appear swollen and fragmented and tend to calcify (Fig. 9.31B).

9.5.5. Paraneoplastic encephalomyelopathies

Paraneoplastic CNS syndromes are neurologic disorders associated with systemic malignancies and are unlikely to be the direct result of involvement by the neoplasm, such as by compression, invasion, or metastasis. Excluded, by definition, are iatrogenic complications of radiotherapy or chemotherapy and also opportunistic infections related to immunosuppression or secondary to the neoplastic process itself. Also set apart are the metabolic or deficiency disorders and vascular disorders associated with the development of malignant disease.

Paraneoplastic syndromes can affect the central, peripheral, or autonomic nervous systems. The neurological symptoms of the paraneoplastic syndrome may be the initial manifestation of the neoplastic process. Comparable idiopathic autoimmune disorders of the CNS in which no systemic cancer is found have also been described.

Many paraneoplastic syndromes have been shown to develop from autoimmune mechanisms, with antibodies directed against an oncoantigen expressed by the tumor that mimics antigens normally present in the nervous system.

In recent decades, specific autoantibodies (immunoglobulin [Ig] Gs) and their antigens have been identified. They are often, but not exclusively, associated with specific neoplasms and specific neurological syndromes (Tables 9.1 and 9.2).

In some of these syndromes, the patient develops antibodies against neuronal cell surface receptors or channels. The antibodies have a pathogenic role, and there can be clinical improvement after early immunotherapy. In this group (Table 9.1), many patients may have a neurological syndrome and autoantibodies without cancer.

In other conditions, the antigens are not superficial but intracellular, and the immune reaction is cellular through major histocompatibility complex class 1 molecules and cytotoxic T-cell mechanisms. Neuronal degeneration is then mediated by cytotoxic T cells. In this group, cancer is almost always present. These disorders (Table 9.2) are accompanied by autoantibody markers of neuronal peptide-specific cytotoxic effector T cells, and they are generally poorly responsive to immunotherapy.

The main neuropathological entities encountered in CNS paraneoplastic syndromes are paraneoplastic cerebellar degeneration, paraneoplastic encephalomyelitis, and opsoclonus–myoclonus syndrome. A novel tauopathy associated with antibodies against the neuronal adhesion protein IgLON5 has been recently described in a few patients in the absence of cancer.

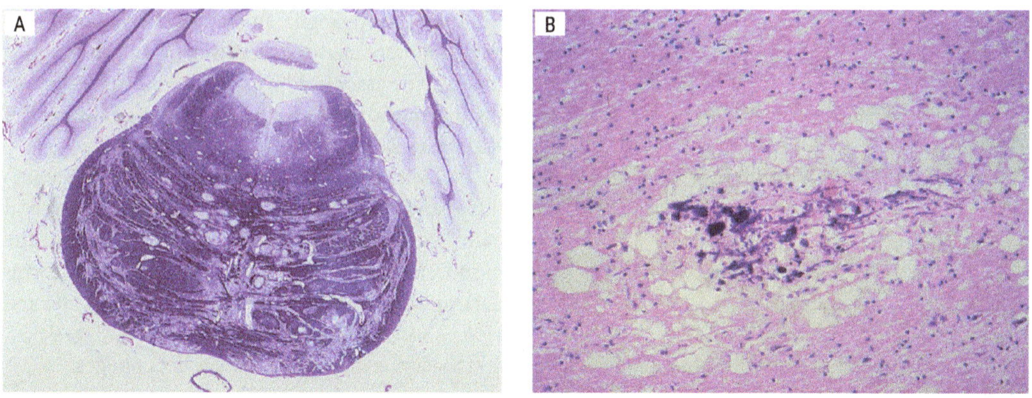

FIGURE 9.31 Multifocal necrotizing leukoencephalopathy: (**A**) whole-mount section of the pons showing disseminated necrotic foci in the transverse pontine fibers (Klüver–Barrera); (**B**) microscopic section showing a necrotic lesion with vacuolation and central calcification (H&E).

Table 9.1 Antibodies Recognizing Superficial Neuronal Antigens: Antigen, Associated Neoplasm, and Neurologic/Neuropathologic Aspects

ANTIGEN	TUMOR	NEUROPATHOLOGY
NMDAR	Ovarian teratoma Small cell lung cancer Testicular teratoma	Encephalitis
AMPA R	Thymic tumors Carcinoma of breast, lung	Limbic encephalitis
$GABA_BR$	Small cell lung carcinoma Other neuroendocrine tumors	Limbic encephalitis
LGI1	Small cell lung carcinoma	Limbic encephalitis
CASPR2	Thymoma	Morvan syndrome
GlycineR	No tumor association	Progressive encephalitis with rigidity and myoclonus
mGluR5	Hodgkin lymphoma	Limbic encephalitis
IgLON5	No tumor association	Sleep disorders, bulbar involvement Brainstem tauopathy
mGluR1	Hodgkin lymphoma Prostate adenocarcinoma	Cerebellar ataxia
VGCC	Small cell carcinoma	Lambert–Eaton syndrome Paraneoplastic cerebellar degeneration

AMPAR, α-amino-3-hydroxy-5-methyl-4-isoxazolepropionic acid receptor; CASPR2, contactin-associated protein-like 2; $GABA_BR$, γ-aminobutyric acid–B receptor; GlycineR, glycine receptor; Ig, immunoglobin; LGI1, leucine-rich glioma inactivated 1; mGluR, metabotropic glutamate receptor; NMDAR, N-methyl-D-aspartate receptor; VGCC, voltage-gated calcium channel.

9.5.5.1. PARANEOPLASTIC CEREBELLAR DEGENERATION

The clinical course of paraneoplastic cerebellar degeneration is generally subacute and manifests as gait ataxia, incoordination, dysarthria, and often nystagmus. The cerebellum may be atrophic but is usually macroscopically normal. Histologically, there is massive, diffuse loss of the Purkinje cells, with proliferation of the Bergmann glia (Fig. 9.32A, B) and sparing of the basket fibers and, to a lesser extent, the granular layer neurons (Fig. 9.32C). The degeneration of Purkinje cell axons often produces myelin pallor surrounding the dentate nucleus (Fig. 9.33). Microglial nodules and perivascular mononuclear cuffs in the leptomeninges and parenchyma are frequent, but inflammation may be sparse or absent.

9.5.5.2. PARANEOPLASTIC ENCEPHALOMYELITIS

Subacute polioencephalomyelitis lesions involve predominantly the gray matter and include, in variable proportions, neuronal loss, nodules of neuronophagia, proliferation of rod-shaped microglia, astrocytic gliosis, and infiltration by B and T lymphocytes. The latter are mainly of the CD4 helper type in the perivascular cuffs and of the CD8 cytotoxic type in the parenchymal infiltration. B cells may predominate in disorders accompanied by neuronal plasma membrane–reactive autoantibodies. The lesions have a characteristic distribution and show a predilection for the medial temporal cortex (limbic encephalitis), the rhombencephalon (medullary pontine encephalitis), the cerebellum, the gray matter of the spinal cord (poliomyelitis), and the spinal root ganglia. In some patients, lesions in these different anatomic locations may coexist; they may also be associated with inflammatory lesions in the myenteric plexuses, the peripheral nerves, or the skeletal musculature.

Patients with paraneoplastic limbic encephalitis display behavioral changes, memory loss, and hallucinations. Limbic structures, including the hippocampi, cingulate gyri, insular cortex, amygdala, and parts of the temporal lobe, may be affected (Fig. 9.34A, B). The midbrain, medulla (Fig. 9.35), and thalamus may also show similar changes.

Sensory neuropathy is a frequent component of an encephalomyeloneuropathy. Clinically, it is manifest by numbness, paresthesias, dysesthesias, and reduced or absent reflexes. The peripheral nerves

Table 9.2 Antibodies Recognizing Intraneuronal Antigens: Antigens, Associated Neoplasm, and Clinical/Neuropathological Aspects

ANTIGEN	TUMOR	NEUROPATHOLOGY
Hu (ANNA-1)	Small cell lung carcinoma	Peripheral and autonomic neuropathy Paraneoplastic encephalomyelopathy
Ri (ANNA-2)	Small cell lung carcinoma Breast carcinoma	Brainstem encephalitis Opsoclonus–myoclonus
SOX-1 (AGNA)	Small cell carcinoma	Encephalomyelitis Cerebellar degeneration
Ma	Testicular tumors Small cell carcinoma	Cerebellar degeneration Brainstem encephalitis
Yo (PCA-1)	Müllerian adenocarcinoma Breast carcinoma	Cerebellar degeneration Paraneoplastic encephalomyelopathy Peripheral neuropathy
Tr (DNER)	Hodgkin lymphoma	Cerebellar degeneration
CV2 (CRMP5)	Small cell carcinoma Thymoma	Cerebellar degeneration Paraneoplastic encephalomyelopathy Peripheral and autonomic neuropathy
Amphiphysin	Small cell carcinoma Breast adenocarcinoma	Stiffness Paraneoplastic encephalomyelopathy Peripheral neuropathy
GAD65	Thymoma, renal, breast, or colon adenocarcinoma	Stiffness Paraneoplastic myelopathy

AGNA, anti-glial nuclear antibody; ANNA, anti-neuronal nuclear antibody; CRMP5, collapsin response mediator protein; DNER, delta/notch-like epidermal growth factor–related receptor; GAD65, glutamic acid decarboxylase 65; PCA, Purkinje cell autoantibody.

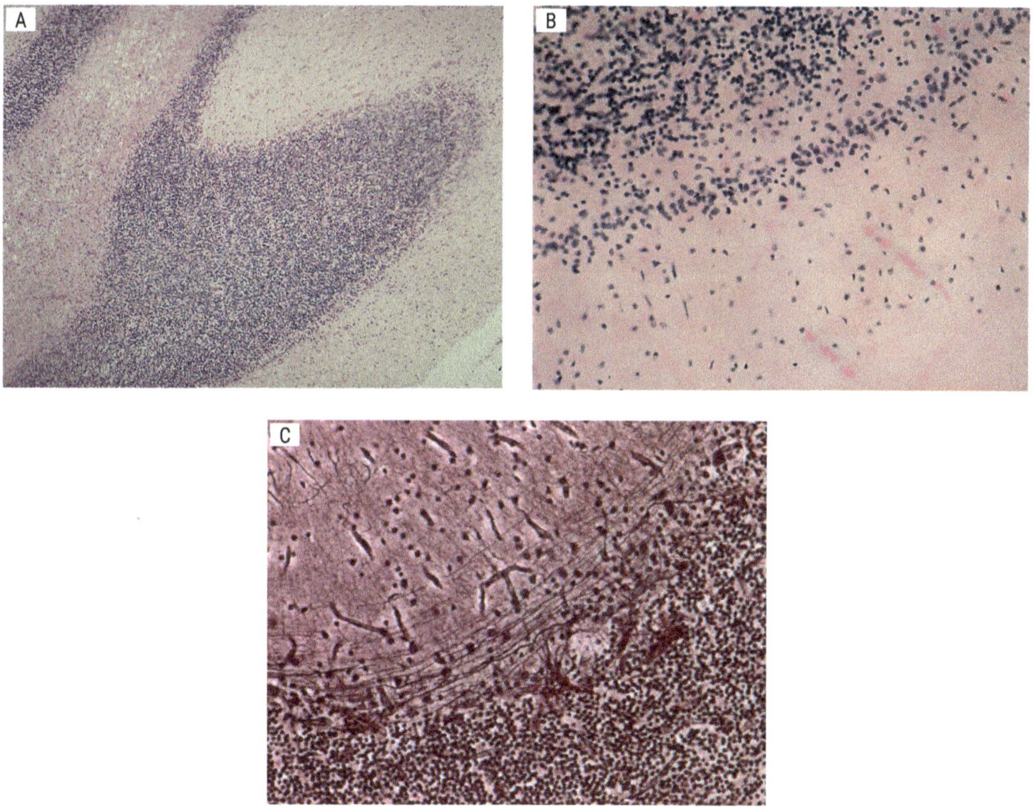

FIGURE 9.32 Paraneoplastic cerebellar degeneration: (**A, B**) massive loss of Purkinje cells and proliferation of Bergmann glia (H&E); (**C**) loss of Purkinje cells and preservation of superficial basket cell neurons (Bielschowsky).

show axonal degeneration with varying degrees of secondary segmental demyelination. Additional pathological changes include degeneration of posterior roots, degeneration and pallor of the posterior columns of the spinal cord (Fig. 9.36A), and degeneration of dorsal root ganglia. Mild perivascular and intraparenchymal infiltrates of mononuclear inflammatory cells are often present. In the sensory ganglia, inflammatory cell infiltrates may be especially prominent. The number of ganglion cells is reduced, and nodules of Nageotte are found where the ganglion cells have been lost (Fig. 9.36B). Autonomic ganglia may be involved as well as dorsal root ganglia, but show less severe changes.

9.5.5.3. PARANEOPLASTIC OPSOCLONUS–MYOCLONUS SYNDROME

The opsoclonus–myoclonus syndrome is rare but is best known in association with neuroblastomas in children. Even more rarely, the syndrome occurs in adults in association with small cell carcinoma of the lung, breast carcinoma, or Hodgkin disease. Autopsy

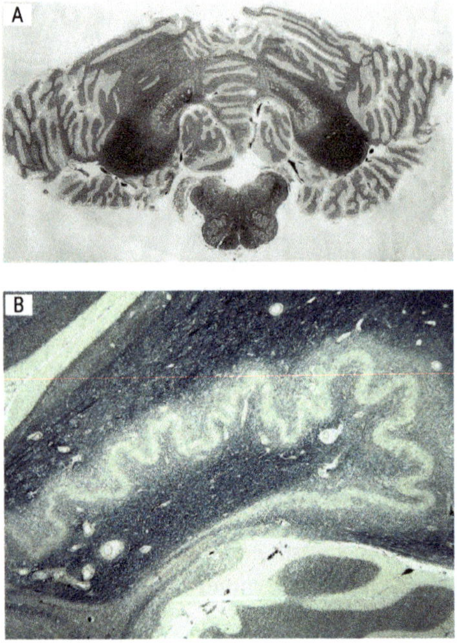

FIGURE 9.33 Paraneoplastic cerebellar degeneration: there is myelin pallor surrounding the dentate nucleus (A, B), which is the site of convergence of Purkinje cell axons (Loyez).

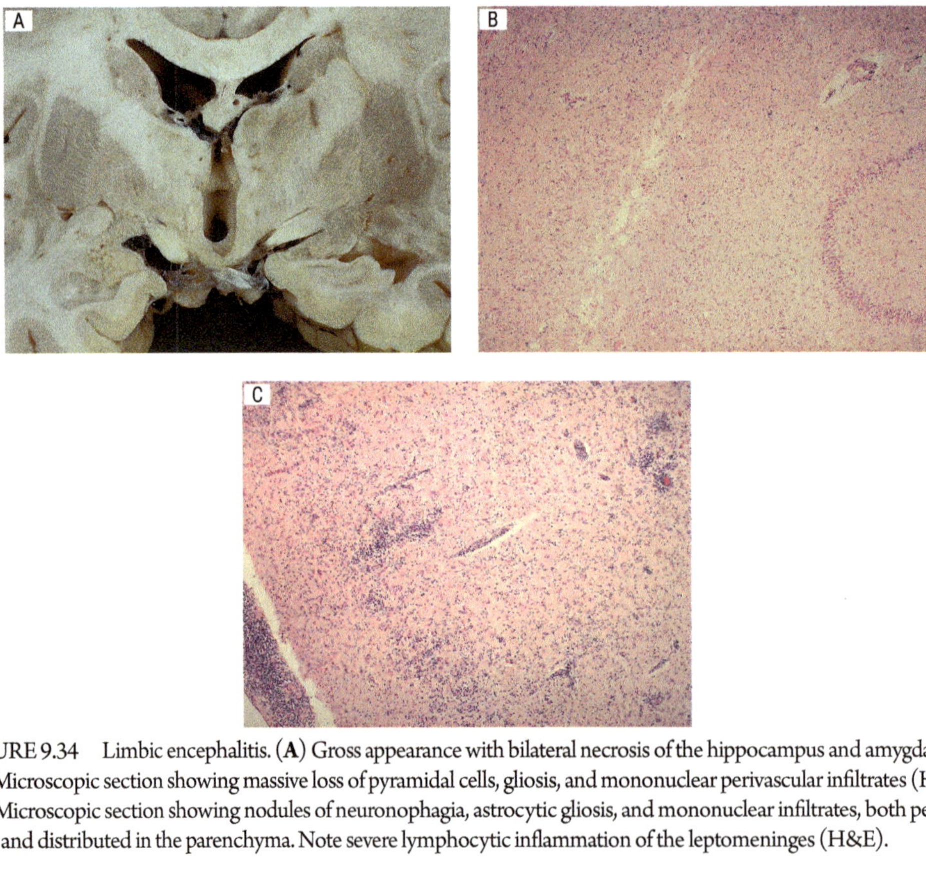

FIGURE 9.34 Limbic encephalitis. (**A**) Gross appearance with bilateral necrosis of the hippocampus and amygdala. (**B**) Microscopic section showing massive loss of pyramidal cells, gliosis, and mononuclear perivascular infiltrates (H&E). (**C**) Microscopic section showing nodules of neuronophagia, astrocytic gliosis, and mononuclear infiltrates, both perivascular and distributed in the parenchyma. Note severe lymphocytic inflammation of the leptomeninges (H&E).

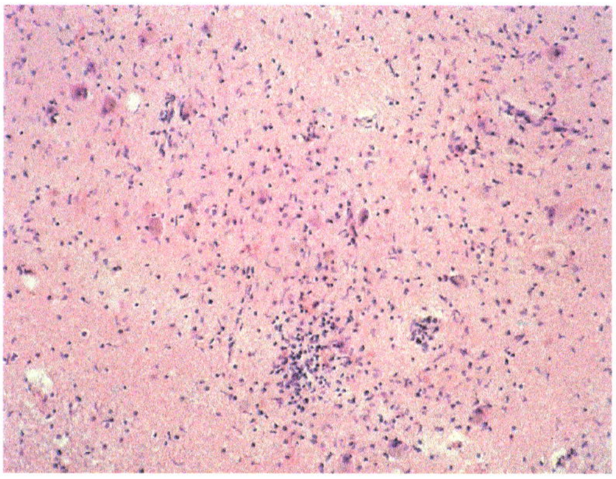

FIGURE 9.35 Medullary pontine paraneoplastic encephalitis. Microscopic section showing nodules of neuronophagia, proliferation of microglia, astrocytic gliosis, and mononuclear infiltration in the medullary inferior olive.

examination of the brain of affected individuals may show no histopathologic abnormalities or may have Purkinje cell loss or mild periaqueductal infiltrates of inflammatory cells.

9.5.5.4. ANTI-IGLON5–RELATED TAUOPATHY

Anti-IgLON5–related tauopathy is characterized by a unique non–rapid eye movement (NREM) and REM parasomnia with sleep apnea and stridor, accompanied by bulbar dysfunction and specific association with antibodies against the neuronal cell adhesion protein IgLON5. Neuropathological examination shows degenerative changes, including neuronal loss and gliosis in the absence of inflammation, with remarkable neuronal accumulation of hyperphosphorylated tau composed of both three-repeat (3R) and four-repeat (4R) isoforms. These changes involve preferentially the hypothalamus and more severely the tegmental nuclei of the brainstem, with a craniocaudal gradient of severity to the level of the upper cervical cord.

9.5.6. Neurological complications in stem cell transplantation recipients

Central nervous system complications occur commonly in the course of the first year post-hematopoietic stem cell transplantation (HCST), resulting in increased morbidity. Opportunistic infections (see Chapter 5) are frequent in patients receiving multiple immunosuppressive agents to control chronic graft-versus-host disease (GvHD); nocardiosis, aspergillosis, toxoplasmosis, and viral infections are the more frequent offending agents. Drug-related toxicity arising from conditioning regimens and GvHD prophylaxis also occur. Intracranial hemorrhage is a life-threatening complication after allogeneic HSCT. Some years into the clinical course, patients may also develop primary CNS lymphoma, particularly liver and heart recipients, or a post-transplant lymphoproliferative disorder involving the brain in liver allograft, heart, and heart–lung recipients.

Graft-versus-host disease is a common and difficult-to-manage complication of allogeneic bone marrow transplantation or HCST. Neurological complications are part of the spectrum of the disease and result from involvement of the CNS, PNS, as well as the muscle, although strict documentation in a number of reported cases is lacking.

Immune-mediated demyelinating disease after allogeneic HSCT is rare, and the pathogenesis of the

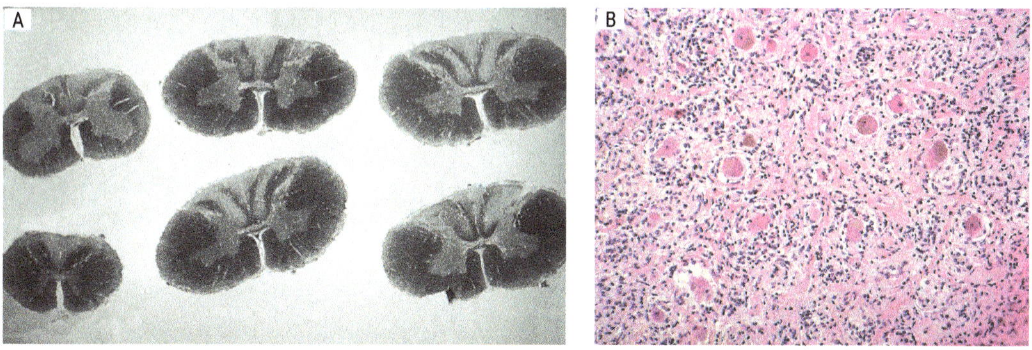

FIGURE 9.36 Paraneoplastic sensory neuropathy: (**A**) note degeneration in the posterior columns, resulting from degeneration of the centrally directed axon of the dorsal root ganglion cell (Loyez); (**B**) spinal ganglion with loss of ganglion cells, proliferation of satellite cells, and interstitial lymphocytic infiltration (H&E).

disorder is unclear. Instances of acute demyelination, encephalomyelitis, and tumefactive multiple sclerosis have been reported in patients who had chronic GvHD after allogeneic HSCT. In these patients, the clinical course most often includes alterations of consciousness and seizures. The precise underlying basis of the disorder is often unknown because biopsies of the involved tissues are difficult to obtain safely. The clinical differential diagnosis is broad and includes infection, drug toxicities (see Section 9.4), metabolic encephalopathy, and disease relapse.

Acute, subacute, or chronic sensorimotor polyneuropathy, sometimes with autonomic nerve involvement, may occur in association with chronic GvHD in patients with a long-standing disease course. Biopsy specimens from skin and skeletal muscle in reported cases have shown perivascular lymphocytic infiltrates expressing T-cell markers. Examination of sural nerves has shown a loss of myelinated nerve fibers with epineurial fibrosis and rare T cells, but without vasculitis. Inflammatory muscular disease and disorders of neuromuscular transmission are also reported complications of HSCT.

9.5.7. Posterior reversible encephalopathy syndrome

Posterior reversible encephalopathy syndrome (PRES) is a clinical syndrome characterized by symptoms that can include seizures, headache, altered mental status, focal neurological signs, impaired vision, and hypertension. Neuroimaging reveals foci of vasogenic edema, particularly in the posterior occipital lobes, which is often reversible.

Posterior Reversible Encephalopathy Syndrome

Characterized by seizures, headache, altered mental status, focal neurological signs, impaired vision, and hypertension

Vasogenic edema in the posterior occipital lobes on MRI, often reversible

Triggers: hypertension, cancer, chemotherapy, preeclampsia, autoimmune disorders

The risk factors for PRES include hypertension, sepsis, organ or stem cell transplantation, preeclampsia, malignancy, autoimmune disorders, and certain medications. Medications linked to PRES include both traditional antineoplastic and immunosuppressive drugs and newer biologic agents. Among the small-molecule drugs, cisplatin, cyclophosphamide, vinblastine, doxorubicin, daunorubicin, methotrexate, and corticosteroids have been described. Biologic agents associated with PRES include those that target the vascular endothelial growth factor pathway (bevacizumab, sunitinib, and pazopanib), androgen receptor antagonist (enzalutamide), and supportive care medications (granulocyte colony-stimulating factors, erythropoietin, tacrolimus, sirolimus, and azathioprine). The underlying mechanism is thought to be failed cerebral autoregulation within the posterior circulation. Neuropathological descriptions are rare. Vasogenic edema without vascular damage or infarct has been reported in a biopsy, and dilated perivascular spaces with proteinaceous exudates, macrophages, fibrinoid necrosis, and acute hemorrhage reminiscent of acute hypertensive encephalopathy were described in a fatal case.

10

Hereditary Metabolic Diseases

DOUGLAS C. ANTHONY, YANN NADJAR, AND HANS H. GOEBEL

10.1. INTRODUCTION

Hereditary metabolic diseases were first identified utilizing biochemical methods to demonstrate accumulation or deficiency of one or more metabolites, often related to the decrease of specific enzyme activities in specific metabolic pathways. Decreased enzyme activity may be due to different mechanisms, bringing some complexity to the identification of the underlying gene defect. The enzyme itself may be altered with a mutation in the gene encoding that enzyme. Alternatively, there may be an abnormality of the metabolism of a cofactor required by the enzyme, with the result being a similar enzyme activity but with a different gene involved (examples include a defect of vitamin absorption and transport or a defect of synthesis of a cofactor from the vitamin). Another mechanism involves intracellular transport defects when the enzyme, substrate, or a cofactor needs to be transported to a given intracellular compartment for the biochemical reaction to occur. Biochemical studies and classification of enzymes or other factors involved in metabolic pathways have led to the identification of many of the genes involved in metabolic pathways. In addition to identification of impaired metabolic pathways, more recently, some disease-associated phenotypes have been linked to specific genetic loci, and by identifying the involved genes, the DNA and protein sequences have been identified and putative protein functions have been predicted. This genetic diagnostic approach, now widely accessible due to the recent development of methods such as whole-exome or whole-genome sequencing, has increased the speed of discovery of the genetic basis of inherited diseases considerably and has also increased the number of the categories of disease.

Currently, there is some uncertainty about the relationships between a specific gene sequence variant and the disease phenotype. Designations have been developed that specify the level of certainty that individual variants are associated with the disease phenotype. To assess the level of uncertainty, several features are considered, including similar variant findings in patients with a similar phenotype, in silico prediction of the impact of the variant on protein function, frequency of the variant among large genome databases (e.g., gnomAD), conservation among species, and in vitro or in vivo studies of the function of the involved gene. For this last point, when the gene involved participates in a metabolic function, some biochemical investigations (metabolite dosages, enzymatic study) in patient samples (blood, urine, and cerebrospinal fluid [CSF]) or in vitro (usually cultured fibroblasts derived from skin biopsy of the patients) may help clarify whether a specific gene sequence variant is pathogenic or not. According to a combination of these variant features, the variant can be categorized as *pathogenic, likely pathogenic, likely benign*, or *benign*. When the relationship is unclear or the evidence is conflicting, the sequence variants may be designated as *variants of uncertain significance (VUS)*.

In this chapter, we present two classification systems to organize the neuropathology of genetic diseases. We first separate groups of disorders linked to abnormalities of the function of cellular organelles. These disorders may have increased intracellular levels of intermediate metabolites and may have a structural abnormality of the organelle, including abnormalities of lysosomes, peroxisomes, and mitochondria. The metabolic disorders may involve a specific catabolic pathway and result in the accumulation of metabolites whose catabolic pathways are impaired. These diseases have traditionally been designated "storage diseases" and are particularly characteristic of lysosomal disorders. Second, we discuss separately the hereditary metabolic disorders from the perspective of analyzing the metabolic pathway affected, because this is a better way to categorize disorders that are associated with altered serum levels, rather than intracellular accumulation of metabolic products. These disorders may be viewed as systemic biochemical disorders in which biochemical abnormalities are most evident in the blood or urine (e.g., abnormalities in the metabolism of amino acids, metals, or organic acidurias). These disorders are classified by the biochemical pathways involved and are characterized by identification of circulating small molecules or by genetic testing. Furthermore, some disorders under discussion are not associated with either a known metabolic pathway or metabolite or with altered serum levels but, rather, result in accumulation of complex lipids within the brain or from altered cellular structural proteins. The disorders of structural proteins are covered in the last section of this chapter.

10.1.1. Biochemical abnormalities in metabolic pathways

Depending on the metabolic pathway involved, inherited metabolic diseases can be divided into several categories of biochemical abnormality, many being manifest by similarities in clinical presentation, diagnostic methods, and treatment strategies. These disorders include abnormalities in energy metabolism, impaired lipid synthesis or catabolism, syndromes characterized by the effects of abnormally elevated metabolic intermediaries (the inherited "intoxication" syndromes), abnormalities of neurotransmitter function, abnormalities of metal metabolism, and abnormalities of small molecule metabolism such as those of amino acids and organic acids. In this last category, the substrate may accumulate and cause a subacute syndrome often with encephalopathy, referred to as intoxication syndrome, as seen sometimes in porphyrias. Some diseases related to vitamin metabolism may involve several metabolic pathways due to pleiotropic vitamin functions (e.g., biotinidase deficiency).

10.1.1.1. ABNORMALITIES IN ENERGY METABOLISM

Energy metabolism disorders include those that directly affect the respiratory chain and others that involve metabolic pathways required for energy production. Included are defects in the respiratory chain (including coenzyme Q synthesis defects); pyruvate dehydrogenase deficiency and related disorders involving thiamine (e.g., thiamine and biotin-responsive basal ganglia disease); deficiencies of enzymes in the Krebs cycle; glucose transport (*GLUT1*) deficiency; and β-oxidation defects, including disorders involving cofactors such as electron transfer flavoprotein deficiency, glycogenosis, and creatine deficiency syndromes. Mitochondrial respiratory chain defects, also called mitochondrial cytopathies, are also classified as an organelle defect (see below). Acute manifestations of impaired energy metabolism may be triggered by infections and include Leigh syndrome, acute optic neuropathy, acute cerebellar ataxia, rhabdomyolysis, and hypoglycemia. The clinical evolution of the disease may have a protracted course, with muscle weakness, cerebellar or basal ganglia (parkinsonism) dysfunction, symptoms indicating involvement of the cerebral cortex (epilepsy, myoclonus) or the peripheral nervous system (PNS; axonal polyneuropathy), neurosensorial disorders, and diabetes mellitus. In adults, these diseases rarely involve the brain white matter, and spastic paraparesis is very uncommon.

10.1.1.2. DISORDERS OF LIPID METABOLISM

Lipid metabolism disorders include some lysosomal diseases and peroxisomal diseases also classified as organelle dysfunction. Lysosomal diseases mainly include the sphingolipidoses (Krabbe disease, metachromatic leukodystrophies, Niemann–Pick A–C, Fabry disease, and Gaucher disease). Peroxisomal disorders include X-linked adrenoleukodystrophy/adrenomyeloneuropathy (X-ALD), Refsum disease and disorders of phytanic and pristanic acid metabolism, and peroxisome biogenesis disorders. Tangier disease and cerebrotendinous xanthomatosis (CTX) are also lipid metabolism disorders.

Given the high content of lipids in the nervous system, these diseases often have severe neurologic symptoms. Leukodystrophies and demyelinating polyneuropathies are characteristic of disorders interfering with myelin formation or maintenance. A patient history of prolonged neonatal jaundice may indicate disorders of cholesterol and bile acid metabolism. Splenomegaly is highly suggestive of some lipid storage diseases, such as Gaucher disease, Tangier disease, and Niemann–Pick disease types A–C. Other clinical manifestations are less specific for lipid metabolism disorders: cerebellar ataxias, dementia, psychiatric disorders, epilepsy, and spastic paraparesis. A slow progression of symptoms, which corresponds to progressive lipid storage, is highly suggestive of these disorders.

10.1.1.3. METABOLIC INTOXICATION SYNDROMES

Some metabolic disorders are associated with variable clinical symptoms that correlate with the serum levels of a small molecule or metabolite. These include porphyrias, urea cycle defects, organic acidurias, and amino acidopathies. Onset of acute symptoms that accompany the metabolic crisis is characteristic of these disorders and has led to their designation as intoxication syndromes. However, in mild adult forms, symptoms can be progressive, giving rise to white matter syndromes, epilepsy, psychiatric disorders, or spastic paraparesis.

10.1.1.4. DISORDERS OF NEUROTRANSMITTER METABOLISM

The best-described disorders of neurotransmitter metabolism are those caused by defects in the synthesis of serotonin and dopamine. Clinical signs are related to dopamine deficiency (dystonia, parkinsonism, and oculogyric crisis), noradrenergic deficiency (ptosis, myosis, and hypotension), or serotonin deficiency (sleep disturbance, dysthermia, and behavioral disturbance). Dopa-responsive dystonia or parkinsonism (Segawa syndrome) is highly suggestive of the disorder. Diurnal fluctuations of symptoms are also characteristic, with improvement in the morning and worsening during the day. Diagnosis of these disorders relies on analysis of neurotransmitter metabolism in the CSF and/or molecular genetic testing of relevant genes such as GTP cyclohydrolase 1, tyrosine hydroxylase, and others. Cerebral folate deficiency is included in this group because it shares several clinical features, although the clinical manifestations of the syndrome are heterogeneous.

10.1.1.5. DISORDERS OF METAL METABOLISM

Metal storage disorders include Wilson disease, aceruloplasminemia, a recently identified disorder of manganese metabolism, and neurodegeneration with brain iron accumulation (NBIA) disorders (neuroferritinopathy/*FTL* associated, *PANK2*-associated neurodegeneration, and PLA2G6-associated neurodegeneration). The hallmark of these diseases is an abnormality in metal metabolism that may result in metal deposits, often in the basal ganglia, sometimes visible on brain magnetic resonance imaging (MRI). The most commonly observed clinical manifestations are movement disorders due to involvement of the basal ganglia. The available treatment modalities are mainly based on metal chelators.

10.1.2. Subcellular classification

Many of the biochemical pathways involved in inherited metabolic diseases are associated with a specific cellular organelle, either totally or partially, as a metabolic pathway may only have a few biochemical steps in one or more organelles. There are three organelles commonly associated with the metabolic disorders: lysosomes, peroxisomes, and mitochondria. As a general rule, *disorders involving lysosomal proteins* tend to involve catabolic pathways, and the lack of a lysosomal enzymatic function is often associated with accumulation of a metabolite for which the catabolic pathway is defective. The disorder resulting in the accumulation of the nondegraded metabolite in lysosomes is often referred to as a "storage disease"; the accumulation may lead to distention of nerve cell bodies and their processes, glia, blood vessel walls, or cells outside the nervous system. When that occurs in the liver and spleen, for example, it leads to hepatosplenomegaly.

Other disorders involve a different cellular organelle, the *peroxisome*. Like the lysosome, the peroxisome is involved in specific catabolic pathways; serum levels of metabolites associated with disorders of these pathways can be elevated in peroxisomal disorders. However, in contrast to lysosomal disorders, intracellular storage of the metabolite is not usually present. Anabolic pathways also take place in the peroxisomes, and their impairment may result in deficiency of metabolites.

Mitochondria are the third organelle associated with specific metabolic disorders. In these disorders, serum levels of intermediary metabolites are often normal, although impairment of oxidative phosphorylation may lead to elevation of lactic acid. The mode of inheritance has a Mendelian pattern for the mitochondrial proteins encoded in nuclear DNA, but a maternal pattern of inheritance for genes encoded in mitochondrial DNA (mtDNA).

10.1.3. Clinical findings

In hereditary metabolic disorders, the clinical symptoms and physical findings of affected patients often correlate with the anatomic site of involvement. Some disorders tend to affect neurons and may do so within certain regions or nuclei. Disorders that involve gray matter, or neurons, have been termed *poliodystrophies*, whereas those involving white matter are called *leukodystrophies*. The latter disorders are characterized by loss of myelin (demyelination) or diminished myelin formation (hypomyelination), which is often evident on MRI of the brain. Hereditary leukodystrophies, in which the production of myelin may be impaired due to abnormalities in the synthesis of myelin, are often considered "dysmyelinating" disorders rather than "demyelinating" diseases. The dysmyelinating diseases, similar to demyelinating disorders, are characterized pathologically by the absence of myelin with relative preservation of axons, but they differ in that myelin is not formed normally, whereas demyelinating diseases represent the loss of myelin formed normally and later damaged due to a pathologic process.

As a consequence of the many metabolic pathways involved and different structures and regions affected, the clinical presentation of hereditary metabolic disease is highly variable. Patients can come to medical attention with complex neurological syndromes involving multiple areas of the nervous system (simultaneously or sequentially in the course of the disease). However, some typical patterns of involvement can elicit the initial diagnostic considerations:

1. Involvement of white matter in metabolic leukodystrophies may concern lysosomal diseases (Krabbe disease and metachromatic leukodystrophy), peroxisomal diseases (X-ALD, Zellweger spectrum disorders), polyglucosan body disease (the adult form of type 4 glycogenosis), CTX, Canavan disease, and phenylketonuria.
2. Progressive involvement of the basal ganglia, especially when mineral deposits and/or necrosis are detected by MRI, is common in disorders of metal metabolism such as Wilson disease, NBIA1, *PANK2*-associated neurodegeneration, aceruloplasminemia, phospholipase A2 group VI (*PLA2G6*) mutation, and neuroferritinopathy (*FTL* associated), in addition to energy defects (e.g., mitochondrial disease and pyruvate dehydrogenase deficiency, often in a context of Leigh syndrome). Disorders of dopamine synthesis also lead to clinical manifestations such as parkinsonism and dystonia but with no basal ganglia lesion.
3. Degeneration of the cerebellar or hemispheric cortex implies a neuronal storage disease or neuronal metabolic disorder; differential diagnostic considerations include gangliosidoses, neuronopathic Gaucher disease, Niemann–Pick disease, neuronal ceroid lipofuscinoses, or mucopolysaccharidoses.
4. Predominant involvement of the PNS is common in a subset of disorders, including Tangier disease, Refsum disease, the porphyrias, certain lysosomal diseases, and mitochondrial diseases.

5. Predominant involvement of the vascular system may be seen in Fabry disease and homocystinuria.
6. Weakness and muscle atrophy are common in metabolic myopathies and may be seen in glycogenoses and mitochondrial myopathies.
7. Acute encephalopathy is an uncommon presentation in hereditary metabolic diseases but may occur in MELAS (mitochondrial encephalopathy, lactic acidosis, and stroke-like episodes), Leigh syndrome, urea cycle disorders, or nonketotic hyperglycinemia.

10.2. LYSOSOMAL DISORDERS (LYSOSOMAL STORAGE DISEASES)

The lysosomal disorders are mainly due to a deficiency of a specific lysosomal enzyme required for the lysosomal catabolism of a particular substrate, usually a complex lipid or sphingolipid, and are often accompanied by the accumulation of the lipid ("storage disease"). Current classifications most often refer to the lipid involved or to the enzyme deficiency responsible for their accumulation, rather than to clinical features. However, distinct clinical syndromes are recognized and often carry the eponyms of the author of the early clinical description.

The abnormalities commonly affect both the cerebrum and the cerebellum; they often consist of neuronal storage, with enlargement of the neuronal cell body initially, but ultimately neuronal loss and gliosis. When involvement of white matter is the predominant abnormality, the disorder may be referred to as a leukodystrophy. In some lipid disorders, especially those involving myelin lipids, the brain lesions are accompanied by peripheral nerve disease due to involvement of Schwann cells and peripheral myelin sheaths. Accumulation of the substrate in lysosomal storage diseases also often occurs in the heart, liver, kidney, spleen, or eye. Ocular storage may be seen on ophthalmic examination as a "cherry red" spot, resulting from discoloration due to storage within retinal ganglion cells with sparing of the macula; involvement of viscera may be detected as hepatosplenomegaly or cardiomyopathy.

Deficiencies in specific lysosomal proteins cause the accumulation of sphingolipids (gangliosides, cerebrosides, and sulfatides), mucopolysaccharides, and complex neutral lipids.

10.2.1. Sphingolipidoses

Sphingolipidoses are the most common neuronal lysosomal storage diseases. The catabolic enzyme defect impairs the lysosomal catabolism of the sphingolipid, and accumulation of the sphingolipid is the most common result. Sphingolipids are defined by the presence of a ceramide (*N*-acylsphingosine) and either a sugar or a phosphocholine moiety. When a sugar moiety is present (galactose or glucose), the metabolites are cerebrosides; when a phosphocholine is present, the metabolite is sphingomyelin; when a sulfated sugar is present, the metabolite is a sulfatide; and when multiple sugar moieties are present, including sialic acid (*N*-acetylneuraminic acid [NANA]), the metabolites are gangliosides.

10.2.1.1. GAUCHER DISEASE (GLUCOCEREBROSIDASE DEFICIENCY)

Gaucher disease (or glucocerebrosidase deficiency) is an autosomal recessive disease due to a deficiency of acid β-glucosidase (glucocerebrosidase), which catabolizes glucosylceramide into ceramide and glucose. The disease is characterized by the accumulation of glucosylcerebroside within lysosomes and involves the bone marrow, liver, and spleen. The most common form (type 1) is also known as nonneuronopathic Gaucher disease because there is no involvement of the nervous system; it often presents in adults. The rarer neuronopathic form (type 2) often begins in infancy and is associated with early death. An intermediate form (type 3) often presents in children or young adults. The gene (*GBA*; glucosidase, beta, acid) is located on chromosome 1q22, and mutations in this gene are responsible for all clinical forms of the disease. Although specific mutations are associated with specific clinical phenotypes, there is no correlation with enzyme activity measured in vitro.

In the typical form (type 1 Gaucher disease), hepatosplenomegaly is common, and pancytopenia results from replacement of the marrow with storage cells. The storage cells are predominantly macrophages and are known as Gaucher cells. They are found in large numbers outside the nervous system, sometimes appearing to have almost replaced the normal parenchyma of the liver, lymph nodes, marrow, and spleen. These large (30- to 40-μm) Gaucher cells are distended with cerebrosides, and the parallel clefted vacuoles give the cells a distinct appearance that has been described as resembling "crumpled tissue paper." By electron microscopy, the cells contain tubular, sickle-shaped profiles measuring 12–30 nm.

The infantile-onset neuronopathic form (type 2 Gaucher disease) presents with a rapidly progressive clinical course and prominent neurologic symptoms, whereas the neuronopathic form with a later onset (type 3 Gaucher disease) has a more prolonged course and is characterized by motor, cognitive, and epileptic manifestations. In both type 2 and type 3 forms, Gaucher cells are present in the brain, where they are distributed chiefly around blood vessels. Accumulation of glucocerebroside within the neurons is variable.

Survival in type 1 Gaucher disease has dramatically improved due to utilization of enzyme replacement therapy; however, enzyme therapy is not effective in neuronopathic Gaucher. Type 2 neuronopathic Gaucher disease has a severe and rapidly progressive course, with death usually occurring before age 2 years, whereas survival may be much longer in type 3 neuronopathic Gaucher disease.

10.2.1.2. KRABBE DISEASE (GALACTOCEREBROSIDASE DEFICIENCY)

Krabbe disease (globoid cell leukodystrophy, galactosylceramide β-galactosidase deficiency) is an autosomal recessive leukodystrophy due to a deficiency of the enzyme galactosylceramidase (*GALC*), which is necessary for the catabolism of galactosylceramide (galactocerebroside), an integral component of myelin. The gene, *GALC*, is located on chromosome 14q31.3 and encodes the enzyme. It is a rare condition and is the only sphingolipidosis in which accumulation of the metabolite (galactocerebroside) does not occur. Rather, the block in catabolism of galactocerebroside leads to shunting of galactocerebroside to psychosine (galactosylsphingosine), with elevated levels of psychosine. The elevated levels of psychosine have a toxic effect on oligodendrocytes in tissue culture experiments, and it has been postulated that psychosine impairs the maintenance of myelin. Instead of neuronal storage, there is destruction of white matter, resulting in a leukodystrophy. The onset is usually before age 6 months, and the clinical course is usually rapidly progressive, with death usually occurring before age 2 years, but later onset forms exist (even adult onset).

Demyelination is widespread, resulting in atrophy of the white matter of the cerebrum and cerebellum and marked fibrillary gliosis. A common feature of the disease is the presence of rounded macrophages with a large amount of cytoplasm, known as "globoid" cells. They may measure up to 40 μm, with more irregular outlines and are often multinucleated. Globoid cells occur throughout the white matter of the CNS (but are not present in the PNS) and may be found singly, but are more often grouped to form perivascular collections (Fig. 10.1A, B). By electron microscopy, globoid cells contain intracytoplasmic inclusions, which appear as elongated cleft-like empty spaces, sometimes bordered by an osmiophilic limiting membrane; they are variably needle- or splinter-shaped or gently curved (10–100 nm wide) and of indeterminate length.

Involvement of the PNS may also occur. The clinical manifestation referable to the PNS is hyporeflexia, particularly in the childhood variants of the disease. Loss of myelinated fibers and relative preservation of unmyelinated axons are the principal findings, although segmental demyelination and remyelination also occur. By electron microscopy, inclusions similar to those seen in globoid cells may be seen in histiocytes and Schwann cells (Fig. 10.1C). There is no storage of galactocerebroside in the liver or spleen and no visceral enlargement or dysfunction.

10.2.1.3. NIEMANN-PICK DISEASE (SPHINGOMYELIN LIPIDOSIS)

Niemann–Pick disease is an autosomal recessive, multiorgan storage disease with several forms, each form sharing the defining feature of accumulation of sphingomyelin (sphingomyelin lipidosis). Sphingomyelinase is the enzyme that catalyzes the breakdown of sphingomyelin to phosphocholine and ceramide. There are at least three distinct genetic loci and multiple distinct clinical forms of the disease at the different loci. Clinical forms A and B are caused by mutations in the gene for acid sphingomyelinase (*SMPD1*, chromosome 11p15.4) and are the forms of "classic" Niemann–Pick disease with sphingomyelinase deficiency. Type C is caused by mutations in *NPC1* (chromosome 18q11.2) or *NPC2* (chromosome 14q24.3) genes, both of which are involved in lipid catabolism, but without complete biochemical characterization. In both of these forms (C1 and C2), there

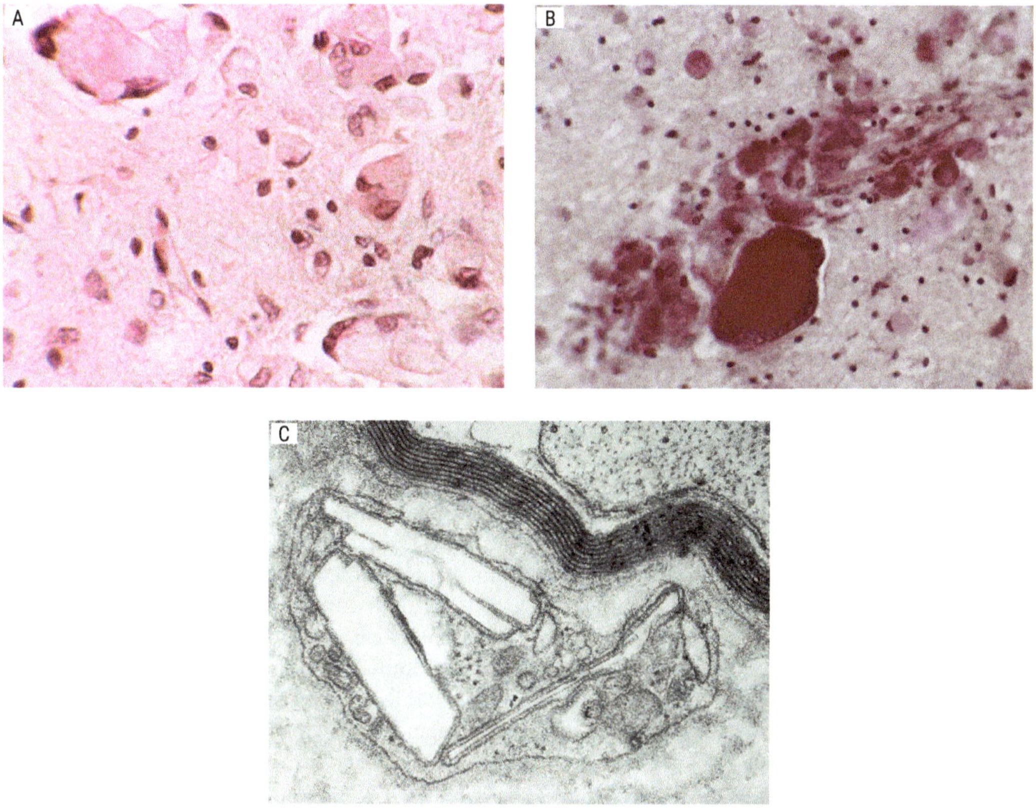

FIGURE 10.1 Krabbe disease: (**A**) globoid cells (H&E); (**B**) globoid cells with a perivascular distribution (PAS); (**C**) electron microscopy (EM) of peripheral nerve showing characteristic electron-lucent inclusions in a Schwann cell.

is sphingomyelin storage (sphingomyelin lipidosis), but sphingomyelinase enzyme activity is normal. Historically, a type D was described in a Nova Scotia genetic isolate and recognized as caused by the *NPC1* gene.

The nervous system is prominently involved in the acute infantile form (type A), which is most common in families of Ashkenazi Jewish heritage. Patients manifest severe hepatosplenomegaly, a retinal cherry red spot, diffuse reticular infiltration of the lungs, and rapidly progressive encephalopathy. Hypotonia may be present in the early course, but there is gradual loss of motor function and intellectual deterioration. Death usually occurs by age 3 years.

Type B is variable in presentation and progression but much less severe than type A. Patients do not have neurologic involvement (nonneuronopathic form) but develop massive hepatosplenomegaly, detected on routine physical exam. Survival into adulthood is common.

Type C1, including former type D described in families from Nova Scotia, has a slower clinical course; it may also involve the nervous system. However, the neurological manifestations appear later in the course of the disease. Type C2 is a rare infantile form of Niemann–Pick type C and, like type C1, has similar abnormalities of cholesterol homeostasis, sphingomyelin accumulation, and normal sphingomyelinase activity.

Histopathologically, all forms of Niemann–Pick disease, regardless of the gene involved, are characterized by the presence of large macrophages with distended cytoplasm. These large cells have round, clear vacuoles by light microscopy and electron microscopy and have been called "foam cells" (Fig. 10.2), regardless of location. They are often detected on bone marrow biopsy, but they also occur in the liver, spleen, and lymph nodes. Involvement of the nervous system occurs in the neuronopathic forms—types A, C1/D, and C2. Types A and C2 show marked atrophy of the brain, with severe

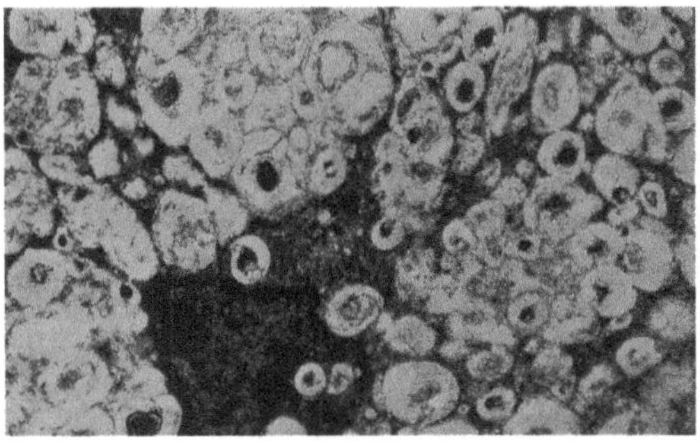

FIGURE 10.2 Niemann–Pick disease: EM of a foam cell.

gliosis. Type C1/D may show atrophy, but the finding is more variable. In all three neuronopathic forms (types A, C2, and C1/D), there are abundant large neurons with distended cytoplasm and many small, round, clear vacuoles. Histochemical studies performed on frozen sections may demonstrate the presence of neutral lipids. Patients with onset of the disease in infancy, who have severe involvement of the CNS, sometimes show evidence of PNS involvement. When PNS involvement is present, it is characterized morphologically by the presence of lamellated inclusions and empty vacuoles in the cytoplasm of Schwann cells and in endoneurial and perineurial fibroblasts.

10.2.1.4. FARBER LIPOGRANULOMATOSIS (CERAMIDASE DEFICIENCY)

Farber lipogranulomatosis (ceramidase deficiency, Farber disease) is an autosomal recessive disorder resulting from deficiency of acid ceramidase, a lysosomal enzyme required for the catabolism of ceramide into sphingosine and fatty acids. Ceramide accumulates in various tissues, including the CNS and PNS. The *ASAH1* gene (*N*-acylsphingosine amidohydrolase 1), located on chromosome 8p22, encodes the acid ceramidase protein.

The characteristic feature of the disease is the development of periarticular and perivascular nodules that are composed of lipid-filled macrophages, typically accompanied by a granulomatous inflammatory reaction. The nodules are often first detected within the skin, where they form readily visible subcutaneous nodules. Similar lipogranulomas may also involve the joints, bones, and kidneys. In the CNS, the large neurons of the anterior horns of the spinal cord and their homologues in the brainstem are the main structures affected, which appear distended with lipid inclusions. Peripheral (sensory and autonomic) ganglion cells are also affected. Characteristic inclusions (curvilinear tubular structures) are also seen in capillary endothelial cells in the CNS.

10.2.1.5. FABRY DISEASE (A-GALACTOSIDASE A DEFICIENCY, ANGIOKERATOMA CORPORIS DIFFUSUM)

Fabry disease (α-galactosidase A deficiency, angiokeratoma corporis diffusum) is a rare X-linked disorder due to a deficiency of the hydrolase enzyme α-galactosidase. This enzyme is encoded by the *GLA* gene on the long arm of the X chromosome (Xq22.1). α-Galactosidase A deficiency results in the accumulation of glycosphingolipids, particularly globotriaosylceramide, forming abnormal intracellular lipid inclusions (foam cells), especially in vascular endothelial and smooth muscle cells.

Clinically, Fabry disease is characterized by the development of angiokeratomas of the skin and mucous membranes and by corneal changes (cornea verticillata). The disease commonly results in life-threatening pathologic changes in the kidneys, heart, and cerebral blood vessels, leading to renal or cardiac failure or multiple strokes. Gastrointestinal dysfunction is likewise frequent; this has been attributed to lipid inclusions in the myenteric plexus. Common symptoms suggesting involvement of the PNS are recurrent attacks of severe pain in the hands or feet (especially in the presence of heat) and the absence of sweating.

Foam cells are found in the liver, spleen, and lymph nodes as well as in renal and cutaneous tissues. The storage material is sudanophilic, periodic acid–Schiff (PAS) positive, and birefringent with a Maltese cross shape under polarized light. By electron microscopy, the inclusions often have a myelin-like lamellated structure, sometimes in parallel arrays, sometimes in concentric layers, with a periodicity of 5 nm. Some of them are membrane bound, others not. Some, instead of being lamellated, are in the form of dense osmiophilic aggregates.

CNS involvement is limited to the amygdala, hypothalamus, hippocampus, entorhinal cortex, and brainstem nuclei. Neurons in these areas have reticular foamy cytoplasm with abundant storage material. Storage is also seen in astrocytes, endothelial cells, and smooth muscle cells in blood vessel walls. In peripheral nerves, inclusions may be found in the cytoplasm of perineurial cells, vascular endothelial cells, and smooth muscle cells in the tunica media of arteries.

10.2.1.6. GANGLIOSIDOSES

The gangliosidoses are disorders characterized by the accumulation of gangliosides, which are composed of ceramide linked to an oligosaccharide (up to four hexose saccharides, either galactose or glucose) and one or more sialic acids (NANA). Gangliosides stain intensely with myelin stains in histologic sections (e.g., Luxol fast blue stain [LFB]) but do not stain appreciably with routine hematoxylin and eosin (H&E), so swollen neurons usually appear to have clear vacuoles on H&E-stained sections (Fig. 10.3A). By electron microscopy, the perikaryon of neurons contain storage inclusions which may have two appearances: circular concentric profiles formed by alternating concentric electron-lucent and electron-dense bands 5 or 6 nm wide, known as membranous cytoplasmic bodies (MCBs), or oblong profiles with alternating linear electron-lucent and electron-dense bands, known as zebra bodies (Fig. 10.3B, C).

10.2.1.6.1. Tay–Sachs disease (hexosaminidase A deficiency, GM2-gangliosidosis B variant). Tay–Sachs disease is an autosomal recessive disease, formerly known as amaurotic idiocy (to emphasize the blindness and intellectual deterioration). It is caused by mutations in the α-subunit gene of hexosaminidase A (*HEXA*, chromosome 15q23), with deficiencies in hexosaminidase A and S activities. Hexosaminidase A is composed of α and β subunits (encoded by the *HEXA* and *HEXB* genes, respectively). Hexosaminidase B is composed of two β subunits (*HEXB* gene), and hexosaminidase S is composed of two α subunits (*HEXA* gene). Mutations of the α gene, therefore, lead to deficiencies of both hexosaminidase A and S activities.

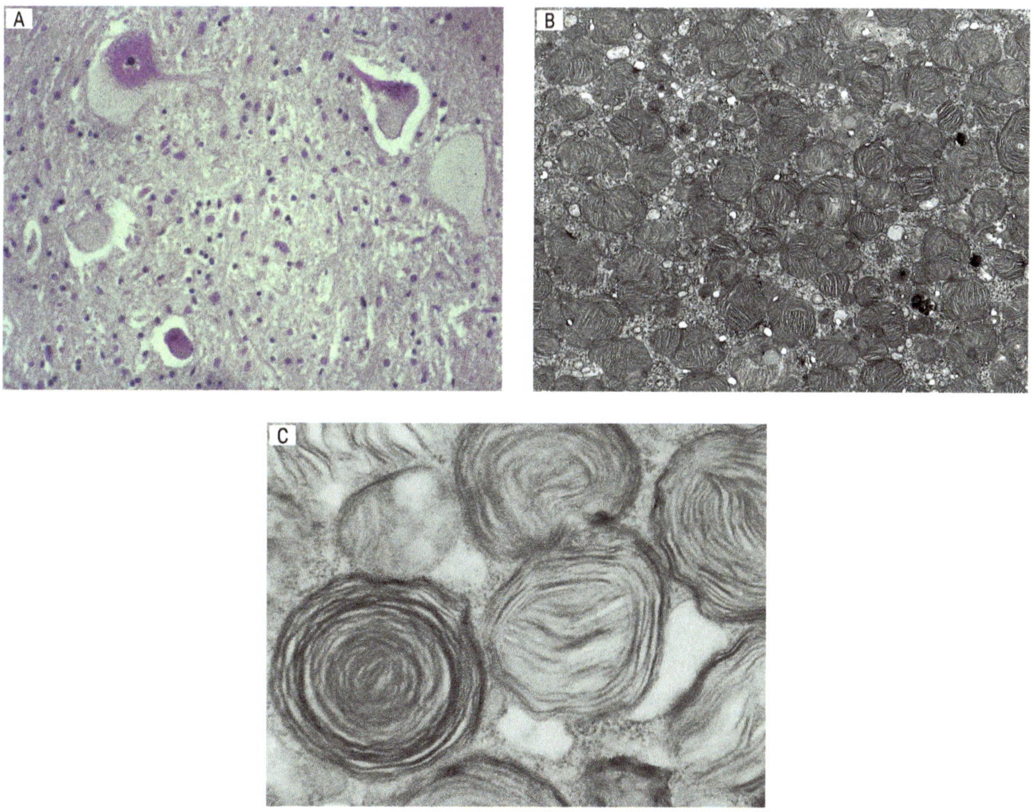

FIGURE 10.3 Tay–Sachs disease: (**A**) swollen neurons with clear peripheral vacuolization (H&E); (**B**, **C**) membranous cytoplasmic bodies (EM).

Tay–Sachs disease occurs predominantly in families of Ashkenazi Jewish heritage, with a high mutation frequency in that population. The onset is most often in infancy, usually within the first few months of life, but later-onset forms exist, even of adult onset. Affected children present with poor head control and other symptoms of psychomotor decline. In the early stages, the head and brain are enlarged, but there is no hepatosplenomegaly. Gradual decline occurs, and death usually occurs within 2 years. The neuropathology is that of a neuronal storage disease, with greatly enlarged neurons with distended cytoplasm and large, clear vacuoles on H&E. The microscopic features are the same as in other gangliosidoses (PAS positive on frozen sections, PAS negative on routine sections, and strongly LFB positive and membranous cytoplasmic bodies on electron microscopy).

10.2.1.6.2. GM2-gangliosidosis type II (Sandhoff disease) and GM2-gangliosidosis AB variant. Sandhoff disease (GM2 gangliosidosis type II) results from mutations involving the *HEXB* gene (chromosome 5q13.3), causing deficiency of hexosaminidase A and B activities; hexosaminidase S activity is preserved. Sandhoff disease does not show any particular ethnic predominance and is clinically indistinguishable from Tay–Sachs disease.

The GM2-gangliosidosis AB variant, which is rare, is clinically and histologically identical with Tay–Sachs disease; however, there is normal hexosaminidase A and B activity. The disease is caused by mutations in the GM2 activator protein (*GM2A*, chromosome 5q33.1).

10.2.1.6.3. GM1 gangliosidosis type I (β-galactosidase 1 deficiency). GM1 gangliosidosis type I is an autosomal recessive neuronal storage disease caused by a deficiency of β-galactosidase (*GLB1*, chromosome 3p22.3). Similar to Tay–Sachs disease, the onset of the disease is most often seen in infancy, where affected individuals show early onset of hypotonia and cherry red spots. However, there are also signs of systemic involvement, including corneal opacities, depression of the nasal bridge, and hepatomegaly—features that are similar to Hurler disease, a mucopolysaccharide storage disorder. The disorder is therefore sometimes known as pseudo-Hurler disease. The staining properties of the gangliosides are similar to those in Tay–Sachs disease; however, storage material may also be found in the liver, spleen, kidney, and bone marrow, where it may appear vacuolar.

10.2.1.7. METACHROMATIC LEUKODYSTROPHY (ARYLSULFATASE A DEFICIENCY) AND RELATED DISORDERS

Metachromatic leukodystrophy (MLD) is an autosomal recessive disorder resulting from a deficiency of lysosomal arylsulfatase A activity, which catalyzes the catabolism of the sphingolipid galactocerebroside sulfate (sulfatide) to the corresponding nonsulfated sphingolipid. These lipids are integral components of myelin sheaths in both the CNS and PNS; deficiency of the enzyme activity creates an excessive accumulation of sulfatides, which in turn results in breakdown of myelin and phagocytosis of its disintegration products.

These sulfatides have an unusual staining property known as *metachromasia*. When certain dyes bind to sulfatides, the absorption spectrum of the dye shifts to a different color. This chemical property led to the distinction between MLD and the majority of leukodystrophies, in which, on the contrary, the color is the same as the original dye, and therefore they are called "orthochromatic" leukodystrophies. These have also been referred to as "sudanophilic" leukodystrophies because of the staining of the lipid products with Sudan stains.

MLD most often occurs due to mutations in the arylsulfatase gene (*ARSA*), located on chromosome 22q13.33. Differences in severity and age of onset are thought to be related to residual enzyme activity associated with the two mutations affecting each allele, with the least enzyme activity associated with the late infantile form of the disease. The onset of symptoms in the disease may be during the infantile or juvenile periods or in adulthood. In the late infantile form, clumsiness and spasticity are often early findings, with onset between ages 2 and 3 years. Progression is relentless, and death usually occurs in early childhood.

On macroscopic examination, the brain may be atrophic, especially in long-standing cases. Microscopically, the entire white matter shows loss of myelin, with sparing of the subcortical fibers (Fig. 10.4A). Myelin is largely absent throughout the entire centrum semiovale, and gliosis is severe, with scattered macrophages. In the PNS, there is demyelination, and there may be some onion bulb formation. Schwann cells, macrophages, and

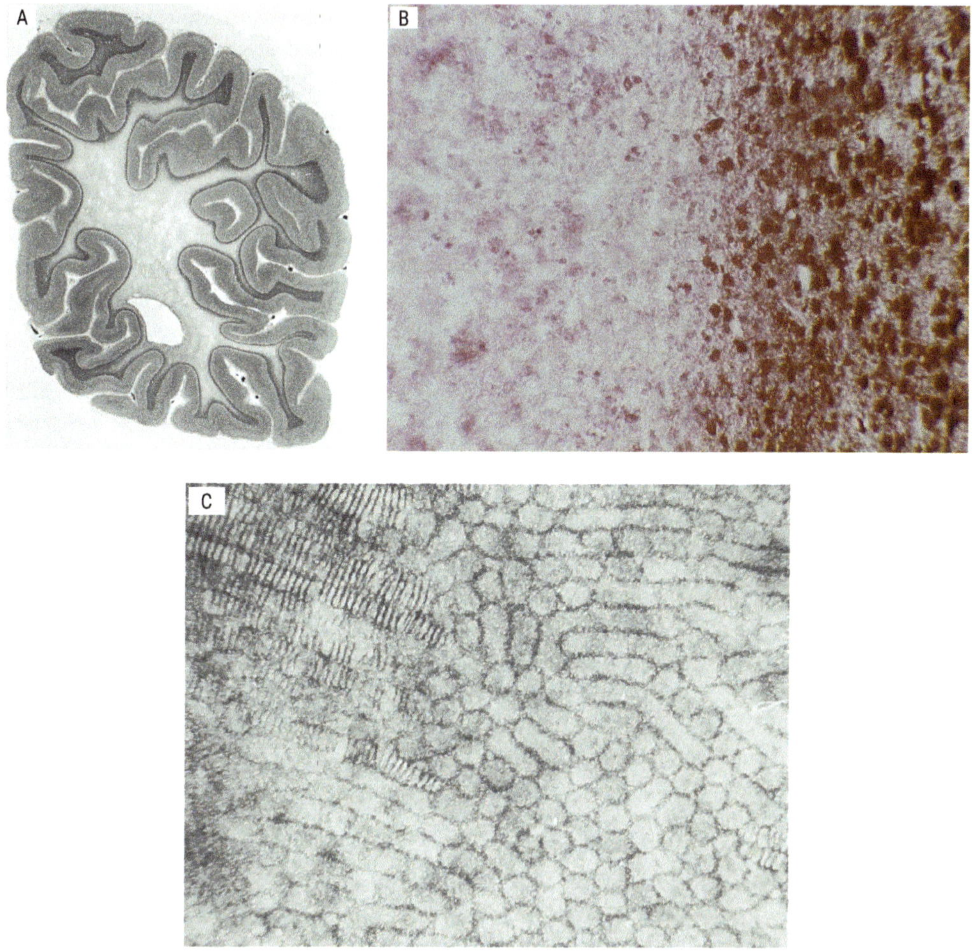

FIGURE 10.4 Metachromatic leukodystrophy: (**A**) whole mount section with extensive demyelination of the white matter and sparing the U-fibers in the right parieto-occipital region (Loyez); (**B**) metachromasia within white matter, which stains brown with acidic cresyl violet stain; (**C**) sulfatide herringbone inclusion (EM).

occasionally axons may contain metachromatic material. Electron microscopy in peripheral nerves shows characteristic inclusions.

Sulfatides accumulate in many tissues, and the deposits may be up to 20–30 μm in diameter. They are PAS positive and metachromatic (stain brown with acidic cresyl violet [Fig. 10.4B] and pink with toluidine blue). Metachromasia is identified principally in macrophages, which tend to have a perivascular location. By electron microscopy, these lysosomal inclusions have a lamellar structure with a periodicity of 5.8 nm. They may be arranged concentrically, but parallel prismatic bodies, or rectilinear "tuffstone" bodies (Fig. 10.4C), are characteristic.

Two important variants are known that involve separate genetic loci: activator protein saposin B and sulfatase-modifying factor 1. Mutations involving the activator protein saposin B (prosaposin gene, *PSAP* gene located on chromosome 10q22.1) lead to a clinical appearance that is indistinguishable from arylsulfatase A deficiency but in which arylsulfatase activity is normal (MLD due to saposin B deficiency). Multiple sulfatase deficiency (sulfatidosis, juvenile Austin type) is caused by mutations in the sulfatase-modifying factor 1 gene (*SUMF1*) and leads to an absence of arylsulfatase A, B, and C activity. The sulfatide accumulation is accompanied by an accumulation of mucopolysaccharides, and patients have some facial and bony features that resemble those of Hurler disease. There are also benign mutations in the arylsulfatase A gene, which lead to pseudodeficiency of arylsulfatase A activity. These mutations, although characterized biochemically by greatly reduced in vitro enzyme activity, are not associated with neurologic disease, and pseudodeficiency of arylsulfatase activity may be present in up to 2% of some populations.

10.2.2. Mucopolysaccharidoses

The nervous system and especially neurons are involved only in certain forms of mucopolysaccharidosis. In such cases, a systemic disturbance of acid mucopolysaccharides, or glycosaminoglycans (which are excreted in the urine), is accompanied by a neuronal lipid storage disorder that closely resembles the gangliosidoses. Because of the secondary nature of the gangliosidoses, this group of diseases is not a form of neurolipidosis, but it should be stressed that in some forms the neuronal changes dominate the pathological findings.

The histopathological findings consist of an association of nervous system changes with alterations in the blood vessel walls. In the cerebral cortex and cerebellum, the appearance of the swollen neurons is comparable to that seen in gangliosidoses, with the presence of zebra bodies (Fig. 10.5A) and other structures that are intermediary to the membranous cytoplasmic bodies of Tay–Sachs disease. Capillary pericytes may show marked vacuolation (Fig. 10.5B), which corresponds to the excessive accumulation of glycosaminoglycans. Vacuolization is found in the CNS, in various visceral organs (including the liver, myocardium, and bone marrow), and in lymphocytes. The vacuoles appear to be of lysosomal origin, as suggested by the demonstration of acid phosphatase.

The following mucopolysaccharidoses involve the CNS to the greatest extent:

- Hurler syndrome (type IH mucopolysaccharidosis; α-L-iduronidase deficiency; dermatan sulfate and heparan sulfate storage; *IDUA* gene locus 4p16.3) with facial and skeletal deformities (gargoylism), corneal opacities, and nervous system lesions
- Hunter syndrome (type II mucopolysaccharidosis; iduronate-2-sulfatase deficiency; dermatan sulfate and heparan sulfate storage; *IDS* gene locus Xq28), similar to Hurler disease, with similar deposition of glycosaminoglycans, but with X-linked inheritance and absence of corneal opacities
- Type III A mucopolysaccharidosis (Sanfilippo disease; heparan sulfate storage; heparan sulfate *N*-sulfoglucosamine sulfohydrolase deficiency; gene locus 17q25.3), which is histologically similar to types I and II, but in which only heparan sulfate accumulates in excessive amounts, whereas dermatan sulfate does not.

10.2.3. Enzymes involved in metabolism of cholesterol, other lipids, and lipoproteins

10.2.3.1. WOLMAN DISEASE (LYSOSOMAL ACID LIPASE DEFICIENCY)

Wolman disease (lysosomal acid lipase deficiency) is an autosomal recessive infantile disease with hepatosplenomegaly, gastrointestinal signs, and progressive neurologic deterioration caused by mutations of the lysosomal acid lipase gene (*LIPA*, chromosome 10q23.31) and accumulation of cholesterol and triglycerides. Calcification of the adrenals is accompanied by lesions in the intestinal mucosa and by the presence of foam cells in the liver,

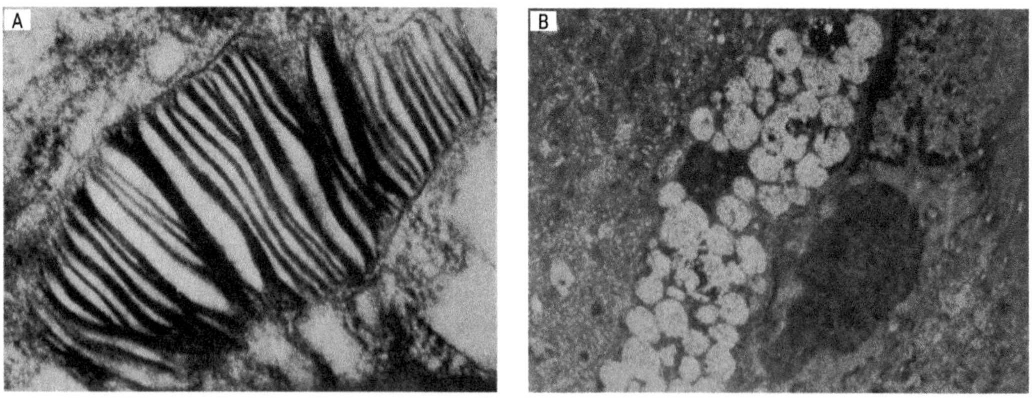

FIGURE 10.5 Mucopolysaccharidosis: (**A**) zebra body in Hurler disease (EM); (**B**) vacuoles in a pericyte (EM).

spleen, and lymph nodes. The foam cells are derived from macrophages and have large, clear vacuoles. In the CNS, choroid plexus, leptomeninges, and Purkinje cells are often affected. Death usually occurs before age 1 year.

10.2.3.2. TANGIER DISEASE

Tangier disease (high-density lipoprotein deficiency type I, analphalipoproteinemia) is an autosomal recessive multiorgan disease affecting cells of the lymphoreticular type, cornea, and PNS due to mutations in the adenosine triphosphate (ATP)–binding cassette 1 (*ABCA1*) gene. The gene is located on chromosome 9q31.1 and encodes an ATP-binding cassette transporter, an important protein involved in regulating the intracellular transport of cholesterol.

The disease is characterized by near or total absence of circulating α lipoproteins. Histiocytes, which may be encountered in lymphoid tissues and bone marrow, transform to foam cells due to cholesterol ester accumulation. Tonsil hypertrophy, hepatomegaly, and splenomegaly are common, and nearly all patients have some degree of neuromuscular dysfunction during the course of the illness. Approximately one-third of patients come to medical attention because of peripheral neuropathy.

Neuropathologic features vary with each of three fairly distinct clinical syndromes. Sural nerve biopsies from patients with peripheral neuropathy, characterized by remittent and relapsing asymmetric polyneuropathy, have shown striking evidence of segmental demyelination and remyelination and very little overall fiber loss. Patients with a distal symmetric polyneuropathy have loss of large myelinated fibers and a relative increase in very small fibers, with evidence of remyelination and fiber regeneration (sprouting). In patients with a syringomyelia-like syndrome, mostly middle-aged adults, there has been severe loss of small myelinated and unmyelinated fibers, with a tendency for the large myelinated fibers to be relatively spared. Accumulation of lipid droplets in Schwann cells is a constant feature.

10.2.3.3. ABETALIPOPROTEINEMIA (BASSEN–KORNZWEIG DISEASE)

The rare autosomal recessive syndrome abetalipoproteinemia (Bassen–Kornzweig disease) is characterized by a combination of malabsorption of lipids, chronic progressive peripheral neuropathy, pigmentary degeneration of the retina, and acanthocytosis (burr cells) affecting red blood cells. Signs of cerebellar dysfunction (intention tremor, nystagmus) are frequently seen in association with peripheral neuropathy characterized by prominent sensory impairment, muscular weakness, and atrophy (leading to kyphoscoliosis and pes cavus in some cases).

The disease results from mutations of a gene on chromosome 4q23 that encodes the microsomal triglyceride transfer protein (*MTTP*). This protein catalyzes transport of lipids between membrane surfaces and is required for assembly of very low-density lipoprotein particles in the liver, and in the absence of functional MTTP, the apolipoprotein is never assembled and released from the liver.

The peripheral neuropathy is characterized by marked loss of myelinated axons, especially large ones, and involvement of the posterior horns of the spinal cord. Retinal pathology entails loss of photoreceptors and pigmentary retinopathy with mobilization of retinal pigment epithelial cells, which enter the sensory retina to produce brownish pigmentation. The formation of finely granular lipopigments in peripheral nerve and skeletal muscle fibers resembles that seen in vitamin E or α-tocopherol deficiencies, and tocopherol therapy has been found beneficial for patients with Bassen–Kornzweig disease.

10.2.3.4. CEREBROTENDINOUS XANTHOMATOSIS

Cerebrotendinous xanthomatosis is an autosomal recessive disorder of sterol metabolism that results in extensive lipid deposition, mainly in large tendons (Achilles tendons and elbow regions) and in the CNS, where it is associated with ataxia, spasticity, accelerated atherosclerosis, and impaired intellect. The disease generally becomes manifest in young adult life and progresses slowly. The disease is caused by mutations of the *CYP27A1* gene or chromosome 2q35, which encodes polypeptide 1 of the cytochrome P450, subfamily XXVIIA, required for sterol 27-hydroxylase activity. This enzyme activity is required for hydroxylation of a variety of sterols at the 27 position. In a few cases of CTX, there has been evidence of a peripheral neuropathy clinically and pathologically on nerve biopsy. The changes in the nerves have been those of relative loss of large myelinated fibers and segmental demyelination and remyelination with some onion bulb formation.

10.2.3.5. NEURONAL CEROID LIPOFUSCINOSIS (BATTEN DISEASE, KUFS DISEASE)

The ceroid lipofuscinoses, neuronal (CLNs), are the most frequent type of neurodegenerative disease in children and are marked by neuronal loss and ubiquitous accumulation of intracellular lipopigments. Juvenile and late infantile forms of the disease are the most common, but there are also rare adult forms (including Kufs disease, characterized by the absence of visual defect). The frequency is 0.1–7/100,000 live births. They are mainly autosomal recessive progressive disorders of uniformly fatal outcome and are characterized by lysosomal accumulation of lipopigments that are positive for acid phosphatase and autofluorescent by light microscopy.

Infantile, late infantile, juvenile, and adult forms are defined based on the age of onset of clinical symptoms. Whereas the juvenile form is the most frequent one in northern Europe and North America, the late infantile form is the most frequent one in southern Europe and South America. The infantile form predominates in Finland as one of the hereditary diseases of Finnish heritage and, though more rarely, may be encountered worldwide. The former classification of CLNs, according to clinical subtypes, has been replaced by one based on genetic defects, now numbering CLN1 to CLN14 loci (Table 10.1). With progress in genotyping, it is now clear that the mutations of the same gene may lead to different clinical subtypes. For example, mutations in CLN1 may lead to infantile, late infantile, juvenile, or adult-onset phenotypes. In the four infantile/early childhood forms (CLN1, CLN2, CLN10, and CLN14), three different proteases (palmitoyl protein thioesterase 1 [PPT1], tripeptidyl peptidase 1 [TPP1], and cathepsins D) are the deficient gene products. Four other genetically identified forms (CLN3, CLN5, CLN6, and CLN8) are marked by deficiencies of structural transmembrane proteins, perhaps of lysosomal location; the CLN3 protein has been named *battenin*. For in vivo and prenatal diagnoses, biochemical activities of PPT1, TPP1, and cathepsins D and F may be measured and are severely reduced or absent in CLN1, CLN2, CLN10, and CLN13, respectively. Putative CLN9 is a juvenile form, without a disease-specific gene or protein. Several adult CLN patients have been found to have autosomal recessive mutations in genes associated with childhood onset (CLN1, CLN5, and CLN6). Recently, mutations in a new gene, *DNAJC5*, have been identified in a few families with adult autosomal dominant CLN, also named Parry disease, now assigned to CLN4. CLN11 and CLN13 are adult autosomal recessive forms, whereas CLN12 is a juvenile variant with parkinsonism, and CLN14 is an infantile form (Table 10.1).

The CLNs are uniformly fatal disorders, with the late infantile form resulting in death during the second decade of life. Patients with juvenile forms may survive to the third or even fourth decade of life. Patients who have adult forms usually succumb within less than 10 years after onset. In affected children, the clinical tetrad of visual disturbance (ending in blindness due to retinal degeneration), ataxia, seizures, and dementia may be encountered in each form, although with a different onset of first symptoms and sequence of subsequent clinical findings. The ocular fundi show thinning of the degenerating retina and brownish pigmentation. However, visual disturbances or blindness are not a clinical component of the adult form, and the electroretinogram is largely normal.

Lesions in CLN involve predominantly the cortex (cerebral and cerebellar), resulting in almost complete depletion of nerve cells in the infantile form at autopsy, less depletion in the late infantile form, and some neuronal depletion in the juvenile form, whereas there is relatively little neuronal loss in the adult form. Macroscopically, there is variable brain atrophy, which correlates with onset and duration of the disease. It is particularly severe in the infantile and late infantile forms (Fig. 10.6A), whereas the juvenile CLN cortex may display a brownish hue. Secondary loss of axons and myelin, shrinkage of the white matter, and dilation of the ventricles and the subarachnoid space are also common.

Two microscopic features define CLN: (1) loss of nerve cells followed by cellular and fibrillar astrocytosis and proliferation of macrophages; and (2) the intracellular, especially intraneuronal, accumulation of lipopigments. This may lead to enlargement of nerve cell perikarya (Fig. 10.6C, D) and proximal axonal segments, albeit usually not to the degree as seen in the gangliosidoses. The lipopigments are autofluorescent (Fig. 10.6B) and rich in acid phosphatase. They are PAS positive and are stained by LFB (Fig. 10.6C). Varying in degree, the lipopigments may also contain the subunit C of mitochondrial ATP synthase and sphingolipid activator proteins that are demonstrable by immunohistochemistry. Immunohistochemical

Table 10.1 Current Classification of the Ceroid Lipofuscinoses, Neuronal (CLNs)

GENE	CLINICAL FORM/*EPONYM*	CHROMOSOME	GENE PRODUCT	ULTRASTRUCTURE OF LIPOPIGMENTS	PROTEINS ACCRUED
CLN1/PPT1	Infantile CLN (ICLN)/*Santavuori–Haltia* (autosomal-recessive)	1p34.2	Lysosomal palmitoyl-protein thioesterase 1 (PPT1)	GROD	SAPs
CLN14/KCTD7		7q11.21	Potassium channel tetramerization domain-containing protein 7	RP, FP	SCMAS
CLN2/TPP1	Late infantile CLN (LICLN)/*Jansky-Bielschowsky* (autosomal recessive)	11p15.4	Lysosomal tripeptidyl peptidase 1 (TPP1)	CP, FP	SCMAS
CLN1/PPT1		1p34.2		GROD	SAPs
CLN10/CTSD		11p15.5	Cathepsin D	GROD	SAPs
CLN3	Juvenile CLN (JCLN)/*Spielmeyer–Sjögren–Vogt* (autosomal-recessive)	16p12.1	Transmembranous CLN3 protein (battenin) in lysosomes	RP, CP, FP	SCMAS
CLN1/PPT1	*Kufor–Rakeb, juvenile parkinsonism*	1p34.2	PPT1	GROD	SAPs
(CLN9)		Unknown	Unknown	CL, FP	SCMAS
CLN10/CTSD		11p15.5	Cathepsin D	GROD	SAPs
CLN12/ATP13A2		1p36.13	P-type ATPase	GROD, lamellar	Unknown
CLN1/PPT1	Adult CLN (ACLN)	1p34.2		GROD	SAPS
CLN6	*Kufs* (autosomal recessive)	15q23		CP, FP	SCMAS
CLN11/GRN	*Parry* (autosomal dominant)	17q21.31	Progranulin	FP	Unknown
CLN13/CTSF		11q13.2	Cathepsin F	GROD	Unknown
CLN4/DNAJC5		20q13.33	Cysteine-string protein, alpha	GROD, FP	SAPs
CLN5	Finnish variant CLN (vLICLN) (autosomal recessive)	13q22.3	Soluble . . . . protein in lysosomes	RP, CP, FP	SCMAS
CLN6	Early juvenile Indian/Czech Roma variant CLN (eJCLN/vLICLN)/*Lake–Cavanagh* (autosomal recessive)	15q23	Transmembranous CLN6 protein in ER	RP, CP, FP	SCMAS
CLN7/MFSD8	Late infantile Turkish variant CLN (vLICLN) (autosomal recessive)	4q28.2	Transmembranous CLN7 protein in lysosomes	RP, CP, FP	SCMAS
CLN8	"Northern epilepsy" (autosomal recessive)	8p23.3	Transmembranous CLN8 protein of ER and ER–Golgi complex	GROD, CP, FP	SCMAS
CLN9	Juvenile CLN (JCLN)	Unknown	Unknown	CP, FP	SCMAS
CLN10/CTSD	Congenital + juvenile CLN (CCLN) (autosomal recessive)	11p15.5	Cathepsin D in lysosomes	GROD	SAPs

CP, curvilinear profiles; ER, endoplasmic reticulum; FP, fingerprint profiles; GROD, granulo-osmiophilic deposits; RP, rectilinear profiles; SAPs, sphingolipid activator proteins; SCMAS, subunit C of mitochondrial ATP synthase.

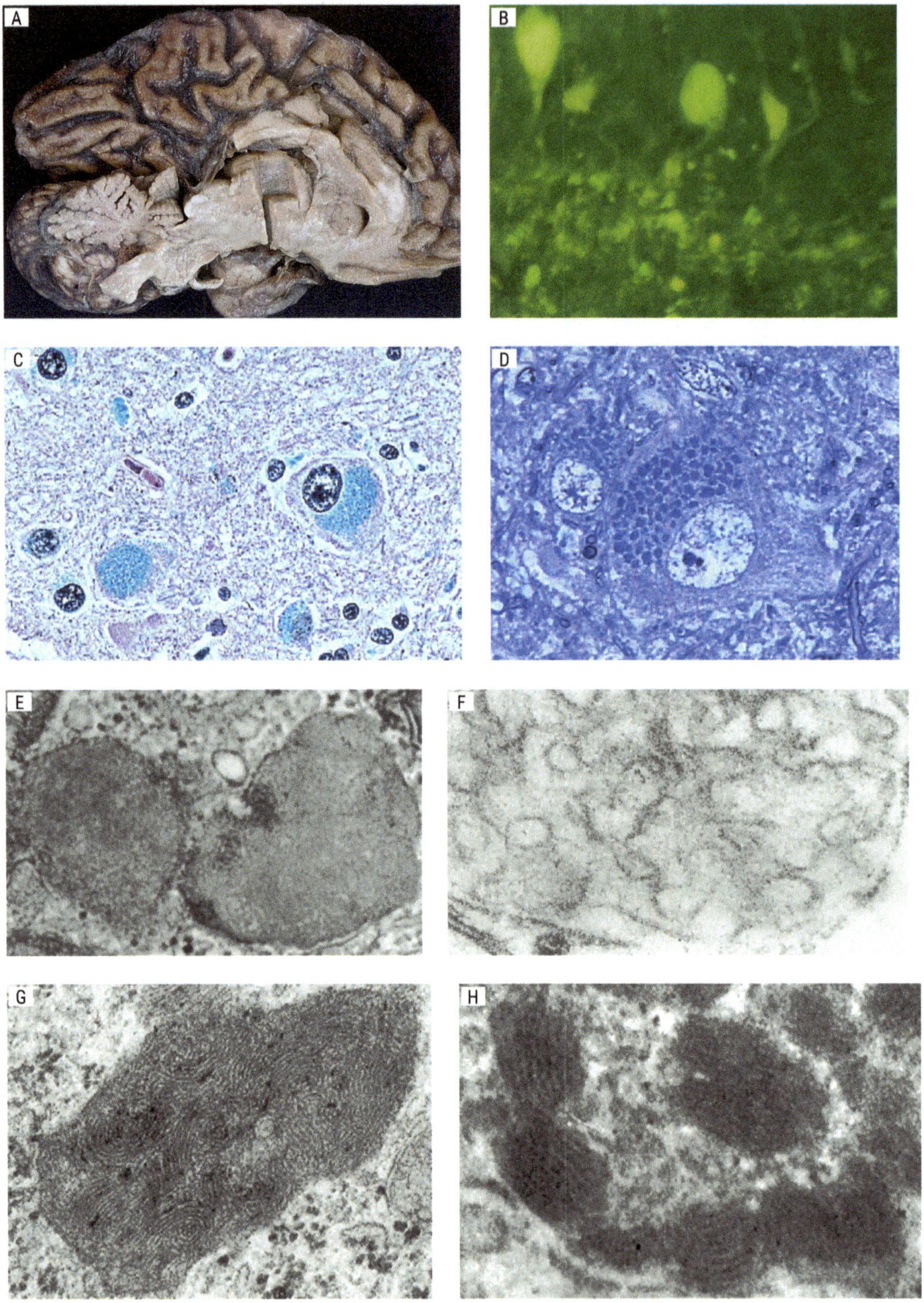

FIGURE 10.6 Neuronal ceroid lipofuscinosis: (**A**) gross appearance with severe atrophy of the cerebral and cerebellar cortices; (**B**) cerebellar cortex with autofluorescent pigment in the Purkinje cells (H&E by fluorescence microscopy); (**C**) intraneuronal accumulation of pigment positive on Luxol fast blue stain (LFB H&E); (**D**) semithin section showing intraneuronal accumulation of ceroid lipofuscin (toluidine blue); (**E–H**) ultrastructural appearance of the ceroid lipofuscin pigment: (**E**) granular osmiophilic deposits in infantile CLN; (**F**) curvilinear profiles in late infantile CLN; (**G**) fingerprint profiles in juvenile CLN; and (**H**) fingerprint profiles in granular matrix in adult CLN.

absence of the genetically deficient *TPP1* enzyme protein in late infantile CLN2 has been documented.

Because the lipopigments in CLNs show different ultrastructural patterns, conventional diagnosis of individual CLN forms may be achieved by electron microscopic examination of blood lymphocytes in which, in addition to numerous other cell types (skin, appendix, and skeletal muscle), lipopigments accrue. A granular pattern may be seen in infantile CLN (Fig. 10.6E); curvilinear bodies are a hallmark of late infantile CLN (Fig. 10.6F); fingerprint profiles within membrane-bound lysosomal vacuoles are indicative of juvenile CLN (Fig. 10.6G); and genetic late infantile variants show a granular matrix and fingerprint profiles within the blood lymphocytes. In adult CLN, lymphocytes have not been found to be affected by lipopigment formation. Apart from granular material, fingerprint profiles have been identified in neuronal lipopigments (Fig. 10.6H) and curvilinear/rectilinear lipopigment profiles within skeletal muscle fibers in Kufs disease. Prenatal electron microscopy may reveal granular lipopigments in the infantile type and lamellar inclusions in juvenile CLN within mural cells of chorionic vessels, whereas late infantile CLN is prenatally marked by curvilinear bodies within amniotic fluid cells.

The nosographic spectrum of the NCL has recently been expanded in that mutated forms have been described without the characteristic ubiquitous deposition of NCL-specific lipopigments—for example, pure retinopathy with *CLN3* mutations, spinocerebellar ataxia 7 with *CLN2/TPP1* mutations, and mutations in the *KCTD7* gene (CLN14).

10.3. PEROXISOMAL DISORDERS

Peroxisomes are intracellular organelles with a single membrane and a granular matrix by electron microscopy. Initially identified as "microbodies" by electron microscopy, peroxisomes contain catalase, and their ability to cleave hydrogen peroxide via the enzymatic activity of catalase allowed their initial localization and is the basis for their name. They are involved in a number of metabolic pathways, including the initial pathway for breakdown of very long-chain fatty acids (VLCFAs), and the catabolism of several organic acids (phytanic acid, glutaric acid, and pipecolic acid). Defects in the assembly of the organelle may lead to more or less complete deficiency of the global peroxisomal enzymatic function, with the clinical correlate named Zellweger spectrum disorder (ZSD), encompassing previously described Zellweger syndrome, neonatal Refsum disease, and neonatal adrenoleukodystrophy. The other genetic defects leading to a more restrictive peroxisomal function—for example, single enzymatic function defect or transport defect of a substrate catabolized in the peroxisome—are responsible for other peroxisome syndromes than ZSD.

10.3.1. Zellweger syndrome (peroxisomal biogenesis disorder)

Zellweger syndrome is a peroxisomal biogenesis disorder (PBD); it is an autosomal recessive systemic syndrome caused by mutations in any of 13 genes involved in the biogenesis of the peroxisome. They are noted as PBDs, with specific disorders sublabeled with numbers and letters, such as PBD1A or PBD9B. The genes identified so far in PBD have all been named "peroxins," or peroxisome biogenesis factors, and mutations in each (*PEX1*—*PEX26*) have been identified in PBD. In the most severe phenotype, often referred to as Zellweger syndrome (PBD1A), patients are symptomatic at birth, with dysmorphic features, severe hypotonia ("floppy baby"), and often have cataracts, retinitis pigmentosa, deafness, hepatomegaly, small renal cysts, pulmonary hypoplasia, and cerebral malformations. Death usually occurs before age 6 months.

Electron microscopy of cells from patients with Zellweger syndrome has demonstrated an absence of peroxisomes, usually identified by special techniques that localize catalase in the peroxisome of control patients. Absence of peroxisomal function is identified by elevated serum levels of VLCFA, pipecolic acid, and phytanic acid.

The neuropathologic findings in patients with Zellweger syndrome are principally those of a neuronal migration disorder. The cortex may show polymicrogyria, pachygyria, or subcortical neuronal heterotopias, all findings that are associated with abnormalities of neuronal migration. Closely related to Zellweger PBD1A, but less severe, is the clinical phenotype of neonatal adrenoleukodystrophy (NALD) and infantile Refsum disease (IRD), due to mutations in several *PEX* genes and also known as PBD1B. These disorders share the early onset and cerebral malformation findings of Zellweger disease but are less severe phenotypes with longer survival. NALD also has the inflammatory demyelination of

ALD, and IRD shares the high phytanic acid levels with Refsum disease.

10.3.2. Adrenoleukodystrophy and Adrenomyeloneuropathy

Adrenoleukodystrophy encompasses three different clinical forms that may be found isolated or overlapping in the same individual and that may coexist within the same family: X-linked adrenoleukodystrophy (X-ALD), adrenomyeloneuropathy, and isolated adrenal insufficiency. Only the adrenomyeloneuropathy form has a full penetrance at age 50 years for men; the two other forms may not occur in patients with the X-ALD genotype (either hemizygous males or heterozygous females). X-ALD is an X-linked recessive disease with a defect in the peroxisomal catabolism of VLCFAs. The affected gene (*ABCD1*), located on chromosome Xq28, encodes a member of the ATP-binding cassette, subfamily D, member 1, which is located in the peroxisome and is involved in transporting VLCFAs into the peroxisome for catabolism. In the absence of functional *ABCD1*, VLCFAs accumulate in the blood and brain. Accumulation is also evident in the adrenal glands and may lead to functional hypoadrenalism.

In the classic juvenile leukodystrophy form, young males often present with behavioral problems associated or not with adrenal insufficiency (Addison disease). The adrenal insufficiency often includes hyperpigmentation of the skin. The disorder is rapidly progressive; initial demyelination is detected in the occipital lobes (Fig. 10.7B), but it progresses to eventually involve the entire cerebral hemispheres (Fig. 10.7A). Demyelination in the CNS is the predominant neuropathologic finding and is extensive and symmetrical. Midline structures (corpus callosum, fornix) and the optic nerves and tracts are severely affected (Fig. 10.7A), and at late stages, the demyelination may be accompanied by axonal loss and cavitary leukomalacia with secondary degeneration of the descending pathways. Myelin stains show the complete absence of myelin in the areas of chronic involvement, and the older central portion of the demyelinated lesion shows severe fibrillary gliosis. Scattered macrophages contain myelin degradation material, which stains with neutral lipid stains and is PAS positive. In chronic lesions, macrophage infiltration is intense and is accompanied by a marked inflammatory infiltrate (Fig. 10.7C).

Adrenomyeloneuropathy affects only adults. These patients present with slowly progressive spastic paraplegia and proprioceptive ataxia, which result from involvement of the long tracts of the spinal cord and peripheral nerve. The disease may occur in either hemizygous males or heterozygous females in families with *ABCD1* gene mutations. Adrenal insufficiency is also common. The pathology in peripheral nerves is predominantly demyelinating neuropathy, with thin myelin sheaths and segmental demyelination on teased fibers. By electron microscopy, membrane-bound, cleft-like intracytoplasmic inclusions are seen, usually in cells of the adrenal cortex, interstitial cells of the testis, and Schwann cells. By electron microscopy, storage material forms cleft-like inclusions composed of two lamellae that measure 2.5–3.5 nm in thickness and are separated by a clear space measuring from 4 to 10 nm (Fig. 10.7D). These inclusions are sometimes associated with lipid droplets. They are most readily identified in cells of the adrenal cortex but may also be found in macrophages in the CNS, in Schwann cells in peripheral nerves, and in interstitial cells of the testis.

10.3.3. Refsum disease (phytanic acid oxidase deficiency)

Refsum disease is an autosomal recessive disease caused by mutations in the *PHYH* gene (chromosome 10p13) encoding the peroxisomal enzyme phytanoyl–coenzyme A (CoA) hydroxylase (phytanic acid oxidase). The disease is characterized by progressive distal motor and sensory impairment, ataxia of trunk and limb movements, blindness (from pigmentary degeneration of the retina), and deafness of the sensorineural type. Additional clinical manifestations of varying degree include anosmia; pupillary abnormalities; nystagmus; ichthyosis; skeletal deformities; and a cardiomyopathy that can lead to arrhythmias, cardiac failure, and early death. The disease begins in late childhood, adolescence, or early adult life and, untreated, progresses gradually, although with occasional remissions.

The biochemical abnormality is a marked increase in the serum levels of phytanic acid, a branched 20-carbon fatty acid. Accumulation of phytanic acid is due to the deficiency of phytanoyl–CoA hydroxylase, the enzyme responsible for the first step in the catabolism of phytanic acid via α-oxidation within the peroxisome.

The PNS shows severe demyelinating neuropathy. The nerves (including the spinal nerve roots) are considerably larger than normal. Microscopically, there are prominent concentrically arranged Schwann cells interspersed with collagen fibers, creating a striking onion bulb pattern. There is also an increase of

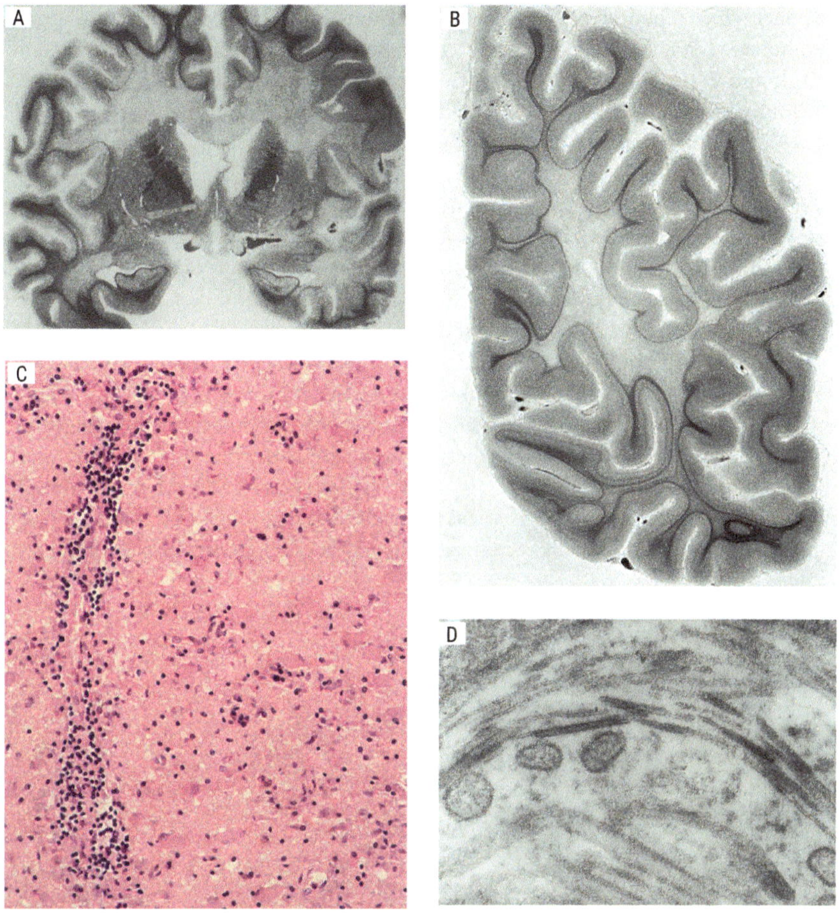

FIGURE 10.7 Adrenoleukodystrophy: (**A**) whole mount coronal section of the cerebral hemispheres showing symmetrical severe demyelination (Loyez); (**B**) extensive demyelination partly sparing the U-fibers in the right occipital lobe (Loyez); (**C**) white matter with severe myelin loss, macrophages, reactive astrocytosis, and perivascular inflammatory infiltrate (H&E); (**D**) EM showing characteristic membrane-bound cleft-like inclusions in a macrophage of the CNS.

endoneurial and epineurial connective tissue. Axons, myelinated and unmyelinated, are decreased in numbers. In the CNS, cerebellar system degeneration is often present, with neuronal loss in the inferior olivary nucleus and dentate nucleus and loss of fibers in the cerebellar peduncles. Posterior column degeneration and loss of neurons in the gracile and cuneate nuclei also have been observed.

10.4. MITOCHONDRIAL DISEASES (MITOCHONDRIAL ENCEPHALOMYELOMYOPATHIES)

The mitochondrial encephalomyelomyopathies (MEs) are a group of clinically heterogeneous disorders with multiorgan involvement caused by dysfunction of the mitochondrial respiratory chain. Most cases involve muscle, for which the morphological and biochemical analyses often allow the diagnosis (see Chapter 12). But abnormalities are not always present in skeletal muscle, especially when the CNS is predominantly involved. Some mitochondrial syndromes have a strong phenotype–genotype correlation (MELAS), and others have very heterogeneous genetic defects (Leigh). However, many patients within this group do not have a clear syndrome but, rather, a complex syndrome with some manifestations suggestive of a mitochondrial disease (e.g., chronic external ophthalmoplegia, ptosis, sensory neuronopathy, and associated diabetes mellitus).

Mitochondria contain their own DNA, mtDNA, containing 37 genes and encoding 13 polypeptides, including subunits of the respiratory chain (complexes I, III, IV, and V), 22 transfer RNAs (tRNAs), and 2 ribosomal RNAs. The remainder of the mitochondrial proteins are encoded by nuclear genes. Mitochondrial disorders may thus be caused by mutations in either the mitochondrial or the nuclear genome; defects of intergenomic signaling have also been identified and are classified as mitochondrial disorders. There are two main types of mtDNA mutations: those that affect mitochondrial protein synthesis in toto and those that affect protein-coding genes. Disorders related to mtDNA mutations are sporadic or due to maternal transmission. Mendelian transmission characterizes nuclear DNA mutations and defects of intergenomic signaling.

The abnormalities of the brain in patients with most forms of the MEs are characterized histologically by sponginess affecting gray and white matter, capillary proliferation, and some degree of neuronal loss and gliosis.

10.4.1. Leigh disease (subacute necrotizing encephalopathy)

Leigh disease (subacute necrotizing encephalopathy) is seen most often in early childhood, but variants with late onset have been described. The condition is characterized by the presence of symmetrical spongy necrotizing lesions that affect both the gray and the white matter; the lesions are predominantly located near midline structures. The striatolenticular nuclei (especially the putamen), thalamus (Fig. 10.8A), substantia nigra, subthalamic nucleus, tegmentum of the midbrain (Fig. 10.8B), inferior olives, and posterior columns of the spinal cord

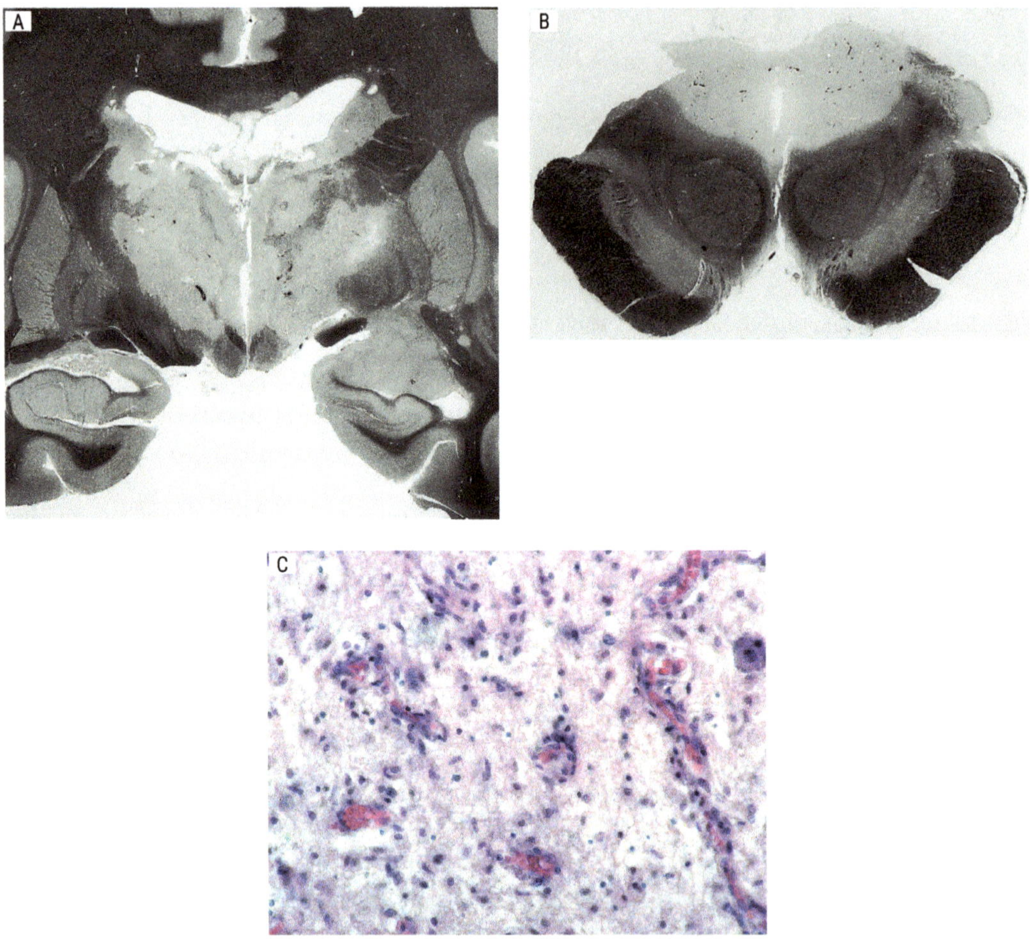

FIGURE 10.8 Leigh disease: (**A**) necrosis of the walls of the third ventricle and of the basal ganglia; note sparing of the mammillary bodies (Loyez); (**B**) periaqueductal necrosis within the midbrain tectum (Loyez); (**C**) microscopic appearance of necrosis, macrophage reaction, capillary proliferation, and relative neuronal sparing (H&E).

may be involved. The relative sparing of the neurons, the presence of gliosis, and especially the capillary proliferation (Fig. 10.8C) closely resemble the lesions of Wernicke encephalopathy (see Chapter 9). Sponginess and myelin loss are subsequently replaced by cystic cavitation, necrosis, and cortical pseudolaminar destruction. Sensory neuropathy occurs in rare instances. Ultrastructural studies show alterations of mitochondria in a few cases, but most cases have no mitochondrial structural abnormalities in brain, peripheral nerve, or skeletal muscle.

Recent data have demonstrated extensive genetic heterogeneity of the disease that may be related to mutations of mitochondrial genes, nuclear autosomal genes, or an X-linked gene (pyruvate dehydrogenase complex, subunit E1α, deficiency). Among the nuclear autosomal genes, there are abnormalities of the nuclear genes of complex I, II, and IV (mutations of assembly genes of cytochrome C oxidase, such as *SURF1*). Among the mitochondrial-encoded genes are genes coding for adenosine triphosphatase (ATPase) 6 and tRNA (Lys). Enzyme defects have been demonstrated in muscle biopsy material in a low percentage of cases and fewer in the brain. Congenital lactic acidosis may likewise cause necrotizing lesions in the hemispheric white matter.

10.4.2. Mitochondrial encephalopathy with lactic acidosis and stroke

The definition of MELAS results from the association of mitochondrial encephalomyopathy, lactic acidosis, and stroke-like episodes. Other CNS signs include dementia, seizures, and deafness. Pathologically, infarcts are present in the cerebral cortex and subcortical white matter, often located in the parieto-occipital lobes, the cerebellum, and rarely the brainstem. The spinal cord may be involved. Calcifications of basal ganglia are common. Enlarged mitochondria, present in pericytes, smooth muscle cells, and endothelial cells of the terminal arterioles, have been considered responsible for the recurrence of transient cerebral ischemia. Ragged red fibers (RRFs) are usually abundant in muscle, and structural abnormalities of mitochondria may be seen by electron microscopy (Fig. 10.9). MELAS was first associated with a point mutation in the tRNA Leu$^{(UUR)}$ (3243 A-G), *MT-TL1* gene, but it has also been described with mutations in mitochondrial genes encoding complexes I and IV. It is transmitted maternally in most cases.

10.4.3. Myoclonic epilepsy with ragged red fibers

Myoclonic epilepsy with ragged red fibers (MERRF; Fukuhara disease) is defined by the association of myoclonic epilepsy with RRFs. Other signs include dementia, cerebellar ataxia, and deafness. Pathologically, the CNS, PNS, and skeletal muscle are involved. The topographical distribution of lesions is reminiscent of neuronal system degeneration: degeneration of the dentatorubral and pallidoluysian system; spinal cord lesions resembling Friedreich ataxia; and degeneration of the substantia nigra, cerebellar cortex, inferior olivary nucleus, locus coeruleus, gracile and cuneate nuclei, and pontine tegmentum. Many RRFs are found in muscle. MERRF was first associated with point mutations in the tRNA *Lys* gene (8344 A-G; 8356 T-C); deficiencies in complexes I, III, and IV

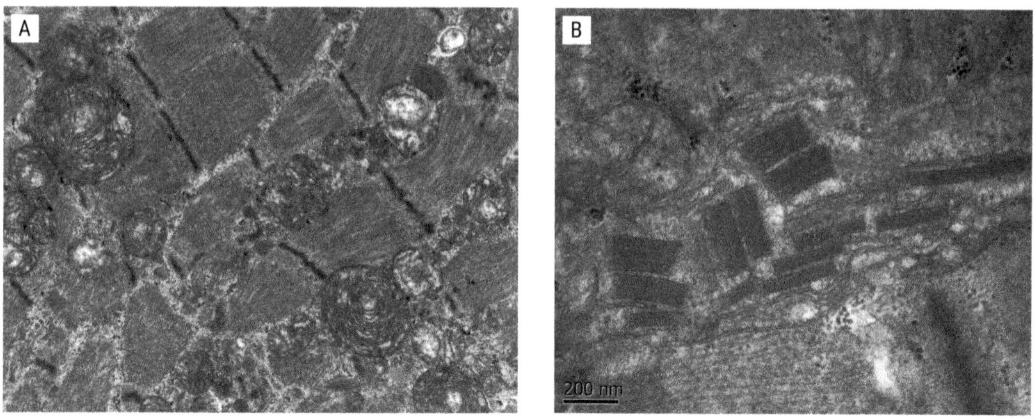

FIGURE 10.9 Mitochondrial encephalopathy, lactic acidosis, and stroke-like episodes (MELAS): (**A**) mitochondria with concentric cristae (EM); (**B**) paracrystalline mitochondrial inclusions (EM).

(Cox II) have been reported subsequently. Most often it is transmitted maternally.

10.4.4. Kearns–Sayre syndrome

Kearns–Sayre syndrome (KSS) is defined as progressive external ophthalmoplegia and pigmentary retinopathy with onset before age 20 years. Cardiac conduction block is important for prognosis. The disease progresses slowly and often develops more severe multisystem involvement. In the CNS, its pathological hallmarks are spongy or vacuolar myelinopathy of the brainstem and cerebellum with neuronal loss. The lesions may extend to the cerebral white matter with mineralization of basal ganglia and thalamus. Skeletal muscle nearly always displays RRFs (see Chapter 12). Large-scale deletions of mtDNA are present in some patients with KSS ("common deletion of 4977 bp"). Most cases are sporadic.

10.4.5. Alpers syndrome (mitochondrial DNA depletion syndrome 4A)

Alpers syndrome (mitochondrial DNA depletion syndrome 4A) is an autosomal recessive disorder characterized by progressive neurologic deterioration, seizures, cortical blindness, and liver failure (progressive neuronal degeneration of childhood with liver disease). The disease is caused by mutations in the gene encoding mtDNA polymerase gamma (*POLG*), a nuclear gene located on chromosome 15q.26.1. Survival is not usually beyond age 3 years. The hepatic involvement is initially fatty change and midzonal necrosis, but it often progresses rapidly to nodular cirrhosis. The neuropathology shows spongy changes in less affected areas of the brain, but in severely affected areas, there is widespread neuronal loss and extensive gliosis. Although the changes are diffusely distributed, they tend to be the most severe in the occipital visual cortex.

10.5. DISORDERS OF THE METABOLISM OF GLYCOGEN AND OTHER CARBOHYDRATES

10.5.1. Glycogenoses

The glycogenoses are glycogen storage diseases (GSDs) that result in the intracellular accumulation of glycogen. Some, such as McArdle disease and Forbes disease, involve chiefly the skeletal musculature (see Chapter 12); the CNS is affected only exceptionally. Pompe disease (or GSD II), which is caused by acid maltase deficiency (acid α-1,4-glucosidase deficiency), however, may involve the CNS. The neurons of the anterior horns, of some brainstem nuclei, of the cerebellum, and, to a lesser extent, of the cortex may be vacuolated and swollen and may show excessive lysosomal storage of glycogen when examined by electron microscopy or stained with PAS. Glia may also have excess glycogen content. A unique feature of acid maltase deficiency among the GSDs is the lysosomal localization of the enzyme, related to its role in lysosomal degradation of glycogen; its deficiency results in the intralysosomal storage of glycogen. The glycogen is surrounded by a lysosomal membrane on electron microscopy (Fig. 12.25C) and is associated with histochemical acid phosphatase activity in light microscopic sections. The disease often presents as a "floppy" infant and is rapidly progressive, with death by age 1 year. Enzyme replacement therapy has allowed improved survival.

10.5.2. Lafora disease and adult polyglucosan body disease

Lafora disease (myoclonic epilepsy of Lafora) is an autosomal recessive disorder characterized by progressive myoclonic seizures. It is caused either by mutations of the laforin gene (*EPM2A*, chromosome 6q24.3) or by mutations of the malin gene (*NHLRC1*, chromosome 6p22.3). The laforin gene encodes a protein phosphatase that hydrolyzes phosphorylated tyrosine, serine, or threonine residues; laforin also plays a role in glycogen metabolism. The malin gene encodes a single subunit E3 ubiquitin ligase. Both genetic defects result in an abnormality of carbohydrate metabolism that causes an accumulation of polyglucosan bodies, the Lafora bodies (Fig. 1.18), in a number of cell types. The onset of the disease is usually during childhood, and there is progressive degeneration of the nervous system, along with progressive myoclonic epilepsy.

In adults, storage of glucose polymer inclusions (polyglucosan bodies) has been described in the axons of the CNS and PNS, in astrocytic processes, and in some of the viscera, associated with progressive involvement of central and peripheral motor neurons, sensory disturbances, sphincter disturbances, and dementia. This form of "adult polyglucosan body disease" (APBD) can be distinguished from the nonspecific presence of corpora amylacea—which may be numerous in the elderly—by the distribution of the inclusions in the cortex (Fig. 10.10B) and in the axons in peripheral nerves (Fig. 10.10D, E) and by the presence of a diffuse or focal myelin pallor in the cerebral white matter, with accumulation of polyglucosan bodies especially in the perivascular regions (Fig. 10.10A, C). Reduced glycogen-branching enzyme (GBE) activity has been found in APBD, and mutations in the *GBE1* gene have been identified. As a result, the disease may be considered a form of glycogen storage disorder, GSD IV (amylopectinosis or Andersen disease). Most patients, however, have no family history.

10.6. ENZYME DEFICIENCIES WITHOUT INTRACELLULAR STORAGE

In addition to enzyme deficiencies that lead to intracellular accumulation of a metabolic product ("storage diseases"), some metabolic disorders are due to a deficiency of the activity of a cytoplasmic enzyme without storage or elevation of intracellular metabolites. This section includes neuroaxonal dystrophies, the disorders of DNA repair, and defects in heme biosynthesis (porphyrias).

10.6.1. Neuroaxonal dystrophies

10.6.1.1. INFANTILE NEUROAXONAL DYSTROPHY (SEITELBERGER DISEASE AND SCHINDLER DISEASE)

Infantile neuroaxonal dystrophy (INAD; Seitelberger disease and Schindler disease) is a recessive autosomal disorder of infancy characterized by axonal enlargement with a dystrophic appearance (axonal dystrophy). The disease affects only the nervous system and has a wide distribution of spheroid bodies throughout the nervous system, which correspond to the axonal dilations. The classic form of the disease, Seitelberger disease, INAD type 1 (INAD1), known as neurodegeneration with brain iron accumulation (NBIA type 2A), is characterized by intellectual disability, paralysis, and epilepsy; it is caused by mutations in the *PLA2G6* gene (located on chromosome 22q13.1), a phospholipase (type A2, group 6). A similar form of INAD, Schindler disease (types I and III), results from a deficiency of *N*-acetyl-α-D-galactosaminidase (NAGA, chromosome 22q13.2). NAGA is a lysosomal enzyme that cleaves acetylgalactosaminyl moieties from complex carbohydrates. But there is still an unclarified discrepancy between the morphology in Schindler disease, the abundance of central and peripheral intra-axonal spheroids, and the biochemical and molecular data which may be associated with vacuolar lysosomal storage that has not been morphologically identified. Also, separate additional mutations in INAD-associated genes are not known in Schindler disease. The pure NAGA deficiency, also called Kanzaki disease, shows vacuolar lysosomal pathology only, no spheroids.

On macroscopic examination in INAD, the globus pallidus may be orange-yellow, and the white matter has a chalky appearance (Fig. 10.11A). The ventricles may be dilated, and there is frequently cerebellar atrophy. Microscopic studies have shown the presence of dystrophic axons, which have given the disease its name and which consist of rounded structures, measuring 10–20 μm. These axonal "spheroids" are argentophilic and weakly eosinophilic, and they stain strongly with PAS stain. They are especially numerous in the gray matter of the spinal cord and the medulla, and fewer are present in the cerebellum, the pontine nuclei, the white matter of the spinal cord, the medulla, and the pons; they are rare in the cerebral hemispheres. Severe and diffuse cerebellar atrophy is common and includes almost total loss of Purkinje cells and granule cells, as well as glial proliferation.

Axonal swellings are also seen in the peripheral nerves and in the nerve fascicles of the dental pulp, the skin, the conjunctiva, and the perirectal plexuses, thus permitting the diagnosis to be made with biopsies. By electron microscopy, the axonal swellings are composed of tubulomembranous material, in contrast to other axonal swellings (Fig. 10.11B).

10.6.1.2. NEUROAXONAL DYSTROPHY WITH IRON ACCUMULATION TYPE 1

Pantothenate kinase–associated neurodegeneration (PKAN), or NBIA1, is an autosomal recessive disorder that results from a mutation in the pantothenate kinase gene, *PANK2*, located on chromosome 20p13. PKAN is the most frequent genetic cause of NBIA. Onset is in the first or second decade with a typical survival of 15–20 years, although

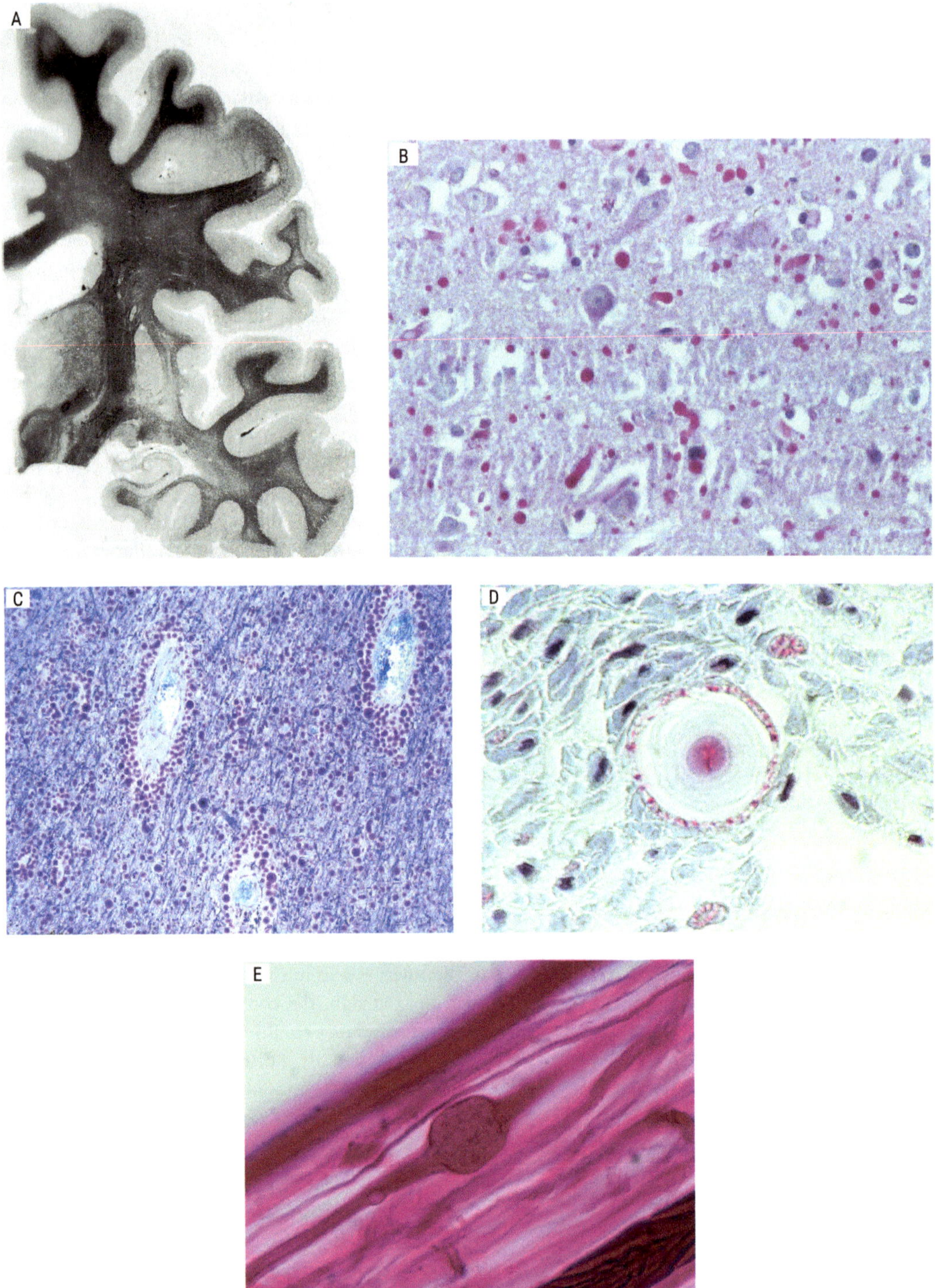

FIGURE 10.10 Adult polyglucosan body disease: (**A**) presence of multiple foci of myelin pallor in the cerebral white matter (Loyez); (**B**) cerebral cortex with numerous polyglucosan bodies present in the neuropil (PAS); (**C**) hemispheric white matter with accumulation of polyglucosan bodies especially in the perivascular regions (cresyl violet–Luxol fast blue); (**D**, **E**) peripheral nerve with intra-axonal inclusions stained with trichrome (**D**) and with PAS after teasing (**E**).

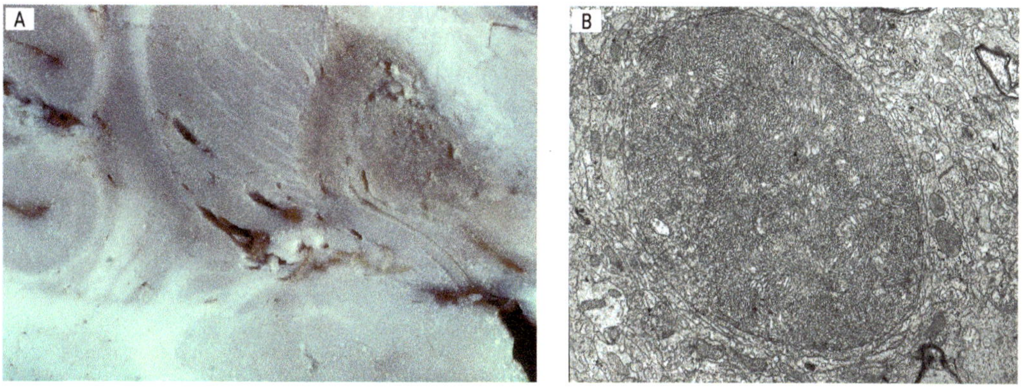

FIGURE 10.11 Neuroaxonal dystrophy: (**A**) orange-yellow discoloration of the globus pallidus seen grossly; (**B**) EM of a swollen axon containing tubulomembranous material.

adult cases have been reported. Progressive rigidity is accompanied by involuntary movements involving limbs, face, and tongue; mental deterioration and pigmentary retinitis occurs later. MRI enables antemortem diagnosis of the disease, showing iron deposition in the globus pallidus and pars reticulata of substantia nigra. Gross examination of the brain shows orange-yellow discoloration of the globus pallidus and substantia nigra and iron deposition in the basal ganglia, which results from intracytoplasmic accumulation of iron pigment in neurons, astrocytes, and macrophages or free in the parenchyma, surrounding the blood vessels. Neuronal loss and gliosis are marked in the globus pallidus and inconstant in the cerebral cortex. The red nucleus and the subthalamus may also be involved. Axonal spheroids are abundant in the globus pallidus and substantia nigra. Ultrastructurally, the spheroids consist of packed membranes, dense bodies, tubules, and mitochondria. There are other rare forms of NBIA, with at least 15 genes involved altogether.

10.6.2. Disorders associated with defective DNA repair

10.6.2.1. XERODERMA PIGMENTOSUM

Xeroderma pigmentosum (XP) is a genetically heterogeneous autosomal recessive disorder that is characterized by exaggerated sensitivity of the skin and eyes to ultraviolet (UV) radiation and a greatly increased susceptibility to sun-induced malignant epithelial neoplasms. Neurologic abnormalities occur in 18% of patients; among these, the most frequent abnormality (in 80%) is intellectual impairment, which is often progressive. In a smaller proportion of patients, there is evidence of involvement of peripheral neuropathy: absence of stretch reflexes, ataxia, muscular wasting, and distal sensory impairment. Examination of peripheral nerves shows both demyelination and axonal degeneration with endoneurial and perineurial fibrosis. The molecular basis for the disease is a lack of normal mechanisms to protect or repair UV-induced damage to DNA. The disease may be caused by mutations in any of several genes involved in the nucleotide excision repair mechanism. Group A patients have mutations in the *XPA* gene (located on chromosome 9q22.33); group B patients have mutations in the *ERCC3* gene (located on chromosome 2q14.3); and group C patients, the most common form, have mutations in the *XPC* gene, which encodes a protein involved in the detection of DNA damage, a first step in nucleotide excision and repair. Additional groups of patients (D–G) have recognized mutations; all affect genes involved in DNA nucleotide excision and repair.

10.6.2.2. COCKAYNE SYNDROME

Cockayne syndrome is a very rare autosomal recessive disorder with intellectual disability and photosensitivity. There are multiple genes that can give rise to the Cockayne syndrome. *ERCC8* and *ERCC6* are the genes affected in Cockayne syndrome, types A and B, respectively. Overlap syndromes between mild forms of XP and Cockayne syndrome have been recognized; XP group B (with mutations in *ERCC3*) and group G (with mutations in *ERCC5*) include some families initially described as Cockayne syndrome. Similar to XP, the genes involved in Cockayne syndrome are involved in the repair of DNA following UV radiation, but there is no association with increased incidence of malignancies.

Classic Cockayne syndrome, with a gene locus on chromosome 5q12.1 (*ERCC8*), is associated with dwarfism, microcephaly, retinitis pigmentosa, deafness, and peripheral nerve involvement. The brain is atrophic, especially the cerebellum and brainstem. The demyelination, which is often subcortical, is a "tigroid" demyelination. Calcifications are present in the basal ganglia and the dentate nuclei. A demyelinating peripheral neuropathy can be demonstrated electrophysiologically and pathologically.

10.6.2.3. ATAXIA-TELANGIECTASIA

Ataxia–telangiectasia (AT; Louis–Bar disease) is a rare autosomal recessive disorder that combines progressive neurologic symptoms, including cerebellar ataxia, and extrapyramidal and oculomotor disturbances with telangiectatic vascular proliferation in the skin and conjunctiva and defects in the immune system (involving both B-cell and T-cell function). Patients with AT are prone to neoplastic diseases, particularly non-Hodgkin lymphomas and carcinoma of the stomach. It is caused by a defect in DNA repair, and AT cells are abnormally sensitive to ionizing radiation.

The gene, *ATM*, is located on chromosome 11q22.3 and encodes a phosphatidylinositol-3 kinase protein, a member of the group of proteins that respond to DNA damage by phosphorylating the substrates involved in DNA repair.

Neuropathological examination shows constant and usually diffuse atrophy of the cerebellar cortex. The atrophy involves predominantly the Purkinje cells and the granule cells and may be accompanied by neuronal cell loss in the dentate nuclei and the inferior olives. Nerve cell loss in the anterior horns and degeneration of the posterior columns are common, especially in long-standing cases. In the spinal root ganglia, neurons are small, the number of satellite cells is reduced, and the residual satellite cells may show marked nuclear abnormalities, as do the nuclei of Schwann cells in peripheral nerves.

10.6.3. Porphyrias

Porphyrias are a group of disorders of heme biosynthesis. Acute intermittent porphyria is a neurologic disorder characterized by acute psychotic episodes and acute-onset peripheral neuropathy. The disorder is due to a deficiency of porphobilinogen deaminase (hydroxymethylbilane synthase; *HMBS* gene), and onset of symptoms is abrupt, typically with gastrointestinal symptoms and neuropathy. Patients are healthy between episodes. In the PNS, there is an axonopathy; in the CNS, neuronal chromatolysis in the anterior horn cells and in the motor nucleus of the vagus may be associated with cerebellar lesions.

10.7. DISORDERS OF COPPER METABOLISM

10.7.1. Wilson disease

Wilson disease (hepatolenticular degeneration) is an autosomal recessive disorder of copper metabolism with accumulation of copper in the liver and brain and prominent hepatic and neurologic symptoms. It is due to mutations of the Wilson gene (*ATP7B* gene, chromosome 13q14.3). The protein product of *ATP7B* is a plasma membrane cation-transporting, P-type ATPase with six copper-binding domains. Characteristic brain lesions are found in the basal ganglia. These culminate, in advanced stages, in necrosis of the putamen with cavitation (Fig. 10.12A), whereas the globus pallidus, the thalamus, and the cerebral cortex are involved to a lesser extent. Less severe lesions consist of a spongy state, with glial changes that involve the astrocytic nuclei. These nuclei are large, pale, and multilobulated and present the picture of Alzheimer type II glia. Large cells of macrophage/microglial origin with eccentric nuclei, Opalski cells, are also found scattered in the basal ganglia (Fig. 10.12B–D). Microscopic copper deposits are found at the periphery of astrocytes but are difficult to visualize. The disorder is also accompanied by cirrhosis of the liver with elevated copper levels and Kayser–Fleischer rings (copper-colored rings at the periphery of the cornea). Mitochondrial dysfunction has been demonstrated in the liver but not in the brain.

Low serum levels of ceruloplasmin are a diagnostic feature of Wilson disease but are secondary to the decreased fixation of copper on apoceruloplasmin. The ceruloplasmin gene, *CP*, located on chromosome 3, is not affected in Wilson disease. In contrast, in cases of hereditary ceruloplasmin deficiency linked to a mutation of the ceruloplasmin gene, the major morphological

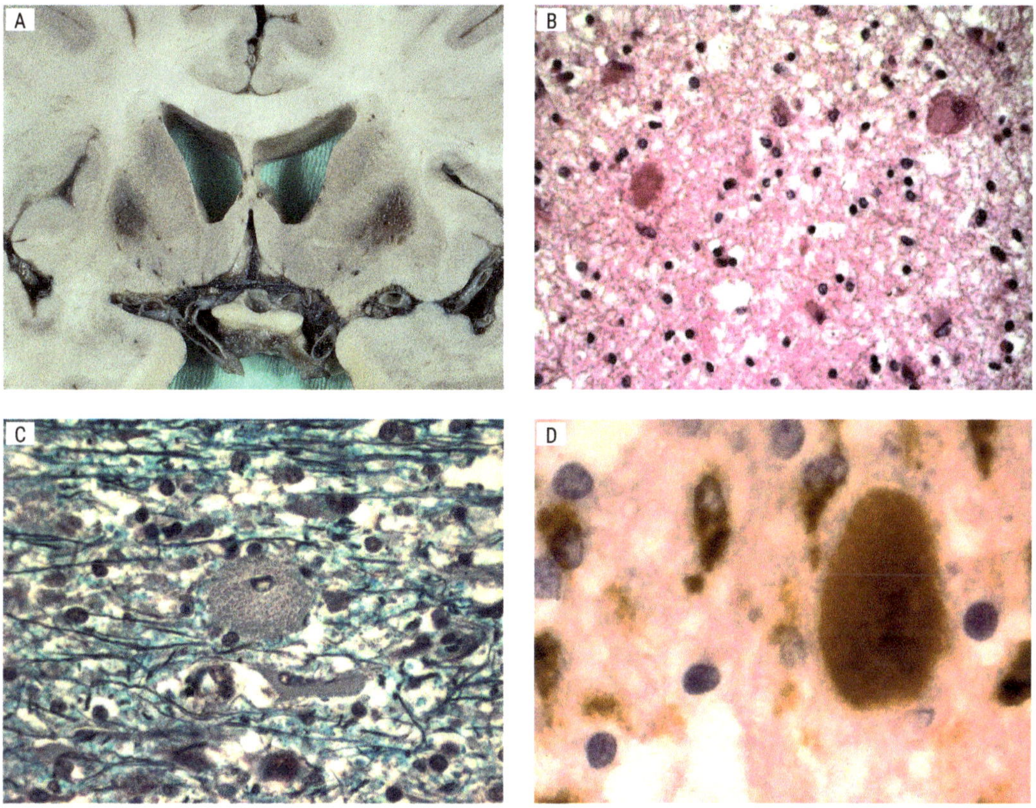

FIGURE 10.12 Wilson disease: (**A**) bilateral necrosis of the putamen; (**B–D**) Opalski cells with eccentric nucleus and granular cytoplasm (**B**, H&E; **C**, Bodian–Luxol stain; **D**, immunolabeling with CD68 macrophage marker).

feature is the deposition of iron in the basal ganglia, particularly the putamen, thalamus, and dentate nuclei.

10.7.2. Menkes disease (kinky/steely hair disease)

Menkes disease (trichopoliodystrophy) is an X-linked disorder of copper metabolism. The disease is due to mutations of the gene *ATP7A* on chromosome Xq21.1, which encodes the copper-transporting ATPase, α polypeptide. There are low levels of copper and ceruloplasmin in the blood. The disease causes abnormalities in the hair (kinky/steely hair disease) and neuropsychiatric manifestations. Pathologically, there are changes in the hemispheric myelin (temporal lobes) and lesions in the cerebellar cortex (granule and Purkinje cells) and blood vessel walls (thickening and splitting of elastic fibers).

10.8. DISORDERS OF AMINO ACID AND UREA METABOLISM

The disorders of amino acid and urea metabolism are the cause of many syndromes of intellectual disability in childhood and may be associated with a number of neurological manifestations. Most of the disorders of amino acid metabolism are autosomal recessive disorders and are characterized pathologically by a prominent spongiosis or cavitation of the white matter with accompanying gliosis. Different mechanisms are involved in the pathogenesis of the neurologic disorders, as amino acids have a role in neurotransmission, protein synthesis, lipid metabolism, and mitochondrial function. A direct toxic effect may be induced by abnormal accumulation of by-products. The diagnosis is usually made by identification of elevated amino acids or their by-products in serum or urine.

10.8.1. Canavan disease (spongy leukodystrophy, van Bogaert–Bertrand disease)

Canavan disease is an autosomal recessive leukodystrophy caused by mutations of the gene encoding the enzyme aspartoacylase (*ASPA*; gene locus 17 p13.2). Aspartoacylase is the enzyme that cleaves *N*-acetylaspartate into aspartate and acetate, and its absence leads to elevated levels of *N*-acetylaspartate. Missense point mutations involving the *ASPA* gene are the most common, but deletions have also been detected.

The symptoms include mental deterioration and megalencephaly. The onset is usually in the first 6 months of life, with death occurring by age 18 months. The abnormality is exclusively in the CNS and consists of spongy degeneration creating an increased volume of the brain with a soft, gelatinous consistency. The spongiosis often involves the subcortical white matter of the cerebral hemispheres and cerebellum (Fig. 10.13A) with intramyelinic edema (Fig. 10.13B). Proliferation of Alzheimer type II astrocytes is common, and the severity of demyelination usually parallels that of the spongiosis. Macrophages are infrequent.

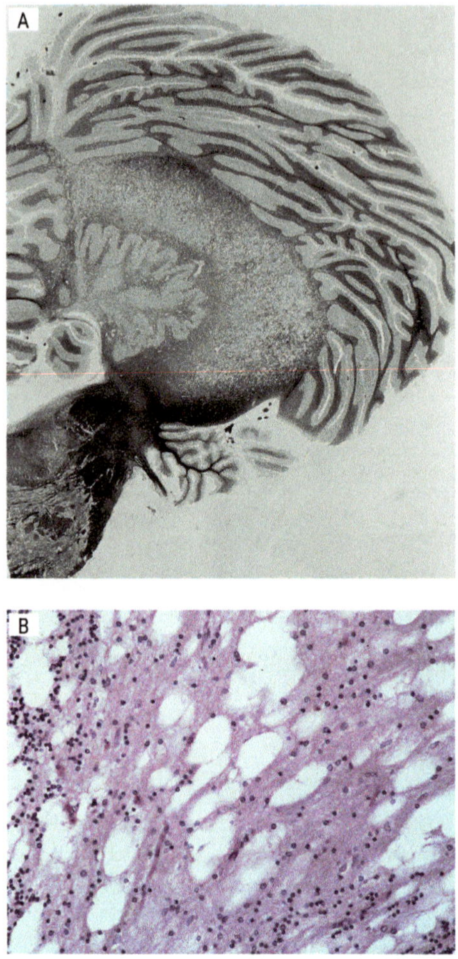

FIGURE 10.13 Spongy degeneration of the CNS (Canavan disease): (**A**) spongiosis of the cerebellar white matter (Loyez); (**B**) microscopic appearance of intramyelinic edema (H&E).

10.8.2. Phenylketonuria

Phenylketonuria, the most common amino aciduria, is due to the absence of phenylalanine hydroxylase, encoded by the *PAH* gene on chromosome 12q23.2, which hydroxylates phenylalanine to tyrosine. Elevated levels of phenylalanine result in abnormalities in neural development with subsequent intellectual disability if not treated (low protein regimen), and there is a relative deficiency of tyrosine, which becomes a dietary essential amino acid. The neuropathological findings are variable but include microcephaly; spongiosis of the white matter; atrophic neurons with poorly developed dendritic trees; and pallor of the myelin of hemispheric and cerebellar white matter, optic tracts, and fornices, resembling a leukodystrophy.

10.8.3. Maple syrup urine disease (branched-chain ketoaciduria)

Maple syrup urine disease (branched-chain ketoaciduria) is a neonatal disorder caused by mutations of genes (*BCKDHA, BCKDHB, DLD,* and *DBT*) encoding enzymes involved in the catabolism of the branched-chain amino acids leucine, isoleucine, and valine. These amino acids are catabolized by an α-keto acid dehydrogenase specific for branched-chain amino acids, and mutations in the individual subunits of the complex cause the disorder. The disease may be identified by the presence of sotolone in the urine, which has a characteristic odor that has been likened to maple syrup. Plasma concentrations of branched-chain amino acids are increased, with a particularly elevated level of leucine. The disorder is characterized by spongy lesions in the white matter resembling those of Canavan disease without evidence of myelin breakdown.

10.8.4. Homocystinuria

Homocystinuria is an autosomal recessive disorder characterized by ocular abnormalities (lentis ectopia and myopia), intellectual disability, and a propensity for thromboembolic events. The disorder is due to mutations of the cystathionine β-synthase gene (*CBS* gene located on chromosome 21q22.3); the gene product is the enzyme of the same name that normally couples homocysteine to serine to form cystathionine. The disease may cause alterations in blood vessel walls, with fibrosis of the intima, degeneration of the elastic fibers, and thromboses. Foci of cerebral necrosis of vascular origin are often found, and although the onset is typically in the first or second decade of life, it may also present in young adulthood.

10.8.5. Hartnup disease

Hartnup disease is due to an abnormality in tryptophan metabolism and produces a picture that resembles pellagra, with clinical features of skin lesions, dementia, and diarrhea. The neuropathologic features include cortical atrophy and neuronal loss, especially in the occipital cortex and cerebellum. The gene (*SLC6A19*) is located on chromosome 5p15.33 and encodes the amino acid transporter protein that transports neutral amino acids across the apical membrane in the kidney and gastrointestinal tract.

10.8.6. Hyperglycinemia

Hyperglycinemia arises in two forms. In the ketotic form of hyperglycinemia (also known as propionic acidemia), the disease is caused by a defect in the catabolism of propionic acid. The deficiency of propionyl–CoA carboxylase results in elevation of glycine and propionic acid, with episodes of lethargy, vomiting, and leukopenia and progressive developmental intellectual disability. The nonketotic form of hyperglycinemia (hyperglycinemia, transient neonatal) is due to a defect of the mitochondrial glycine cleavage enzyme system and leads to encephalopathy in the newborn characterized by hypotonia, lethargy, and seizures. Agenesis of corpus callosum and gyral malformations are associated with vacuolation of the white matter and loss of myelin.

10.8.7. Urea cycle disorders

Urea cycle disorders are genetic disorders in the conversion of ammonia to urea; a block in this detoxification pathway is associated with hyperammonemia and its complications. The most common deficiency is that of ornithine carbamoyltransferase, which is an X-linked disorder. Other forms include arginase deficiency, arginosuccinic aciduria, citrullinemia, and carbamoyl phosphate synthetase deficiency. Alzheimer type II astrocytes, related to hyperammonemia, are frequent; in severe cases, the cerebral cortex and the deep gray matter may be involved.

10.9. ORTHOCHROMATIC LEUKODYSTROPHIES

The orthochromatic leukodystrophies are a heterogeneous group of rare disorders characterized by abnormalities largely limited to the white matter of the brain. Some of the disorders are infantile, with presentation before age 5 years, often with a rapidly progressive course. Other disorders present in adults and have a slower evolution. They represent the most frequent leukodystrophies in adults. The lesions involve the CNS only. Demyelination is diffuse, ill-defined, and often irregular (Fig. 10.14); it tends to predominate in the frontal lobes, which accounts for the frequency of neurobehavioral symptoms. Axonal involvement is frequent. Macrophage reaction is discrete, and there is no inflammation.

In a subset of young patients, an autosomal recessive orthochromatic leukodystrophy is known as leukoencephalopathy with vanishing white matter (or childhood ataxia with central hypomyelination). It is characterized by cavitary orthochromatic leukoencephalopathy with increased oligodendrocyte density. It is caused by mutations in any of the five genes encoding the subunits of the translation initiation factor EIF2B: *EIF2B1, E1F2B2, E1F2B3, E1F2B4,* or *E1F2B5* (with chromosomal loci of 12q24.31, 14q24.3, 1p34.1, 2p23.3, and 3q27.1, respectively).

In a few adult cases of orthochromatic leukodystrophy, sporadic or familial, the macrophages and glial cells contain a brown, autofluorescent, and PAS-positive pigment (pigmentary orthochromatic leukodystrophy [POLD] of van Bogaert and Nyssen). A similar, apparently allelic form is HDLS, autosomal-dominant hereditary diffuse leukoencephalopathy with spheroids, sharing

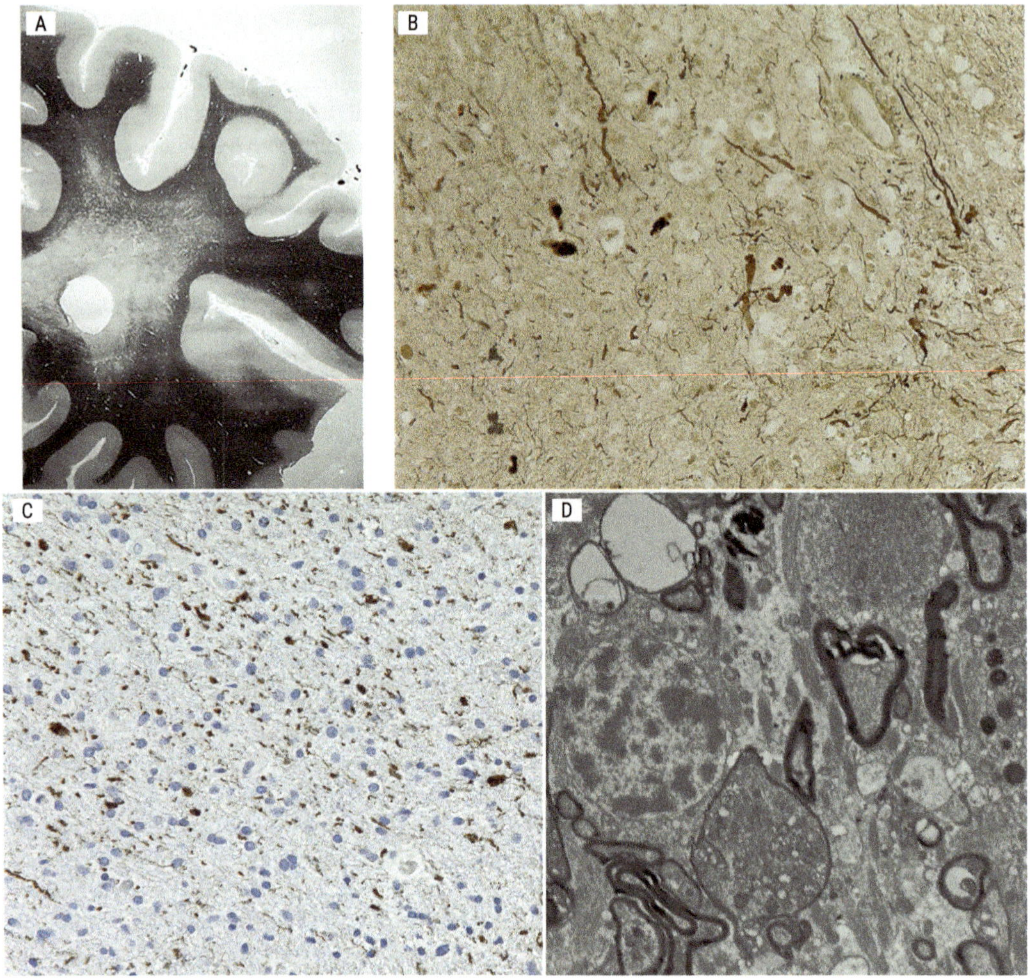

FIGURE 10.14 Orthochromatic leukodystrophy: (**A**) whole mount of brain with ill-defined area of demyelination (Loyez); (**B–D**) hereditary diffuse leukoencephalopathy with axonal spheroids (HDLS1) with familial heterozygous c2330G>A, p.R777Q mutation in the *CSF1R* gene: (**B**) enlarged neuronal processes (Bielschowsky stain); (**C**) swollen axons (neurofilament IHC); and (**D**) EM of an enlarged axon with attenuated myelin sheath.

POLD mutations in the *CSF1R* gene (Fig. 10.14B–D). Spheroids may also be present in dermal axons. Cavitary forms presenting as highly destructive white matter lesions (Fig. 10.15) with increased density and "clustering" of oligodendrocytes have been described in children and adults. Overlapping disorders between cavitary and pigmentary forms have been observed occasionally.

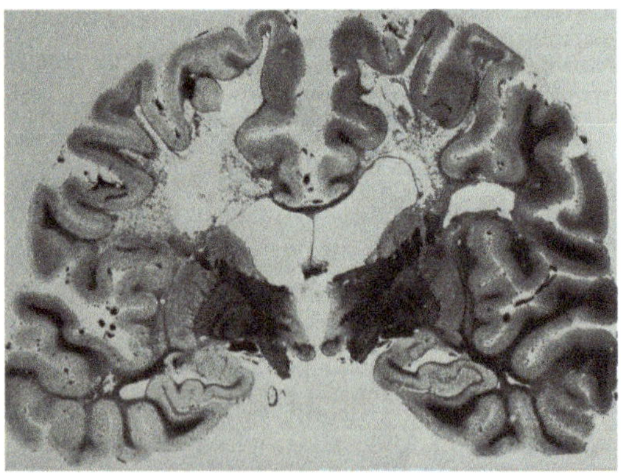

FIGURE 10.15 Cavitating sudanophilic leukodystrophy on whole mount section (Loyez).

10.10. DISORDERS OF STRUCTURAL PROTEINS

Unlike the hereditary metabolic disorders described thus far, some inherited diseases are caused by genetic mutations of genes encoding structural proteins. Because they have no known role in cellular metabolism, their classification as "metabolic" diseases could be questioned. However, they share the genetic inheritance and clinical progression of other metabolic diseases and were classified with the other inherited metabolic diseases prior to the identification of the genes involved.

10.10.1. Alexander disease

Alexander disease is an autosomal dominant megalencephalic leukodystrophy caused by mutations of the *GFAP* (glial fibrillary acidic protein) gene. GFAP is the intermediate filament protein of astrocytes, with individual subunits assembled into 10-nm intermediate filaments. Point mutations are typically found and may be inherited or occur as de novo mutations.

In the typical clinical form, the onset of symptoms is usually with seizures and megalencephaly in the early infantile period. Death usually occurs within 10 years of the age of onset. On gross examination, the white matter is softened and friable, and the abnormality is especially prominent in the frontal lobes. There is massive demyelination involving the cerebral hemispheres (Fig. 10.16A), cerebellum, and, to a lesser degree, the brainstem and spinal cord. A unique histologic feature that sets Alexander disease apart from other leukodystrophies is a prominent accumulation of Rosenthal fibers. Rosenthal fibers are densely eosinophilic astrocytic processes, which by electron microscopy are filled with glial intermediate filaments and electron-dense structures composed of αB-crystallin (Fig. 10.16C). In Alexander disease, Rosenthal fibers are particularly numerous around blood vessels (Fig. 10.16B), adjacent to the ventricular walls, and in the subpial zone where

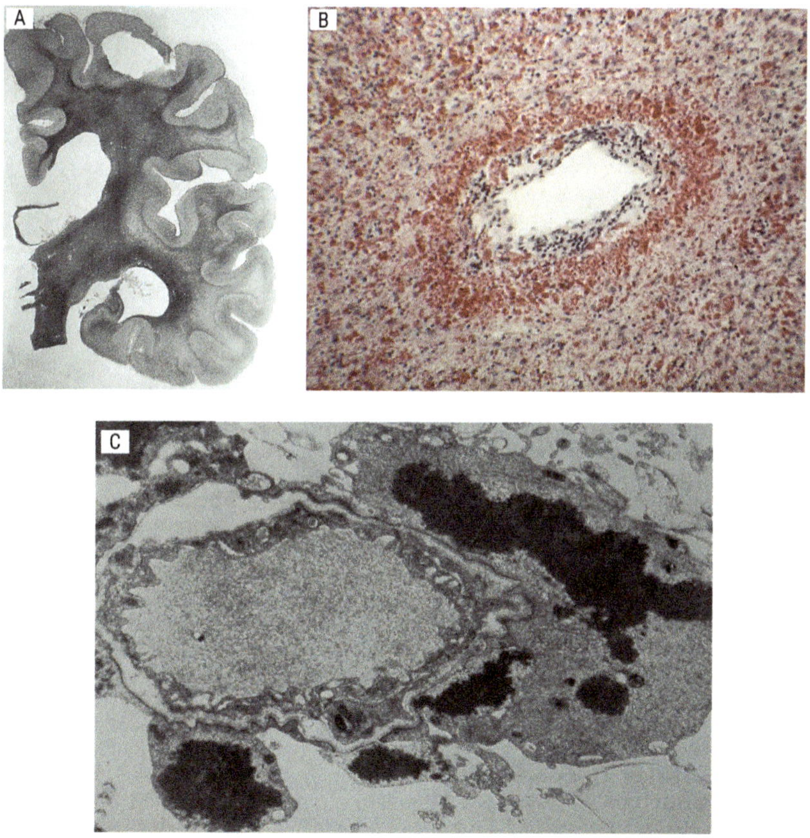

FIGURE 10.16 Alexander disease: (**A**) the massive demyelination of the cerebral hemispheres is less obvious as the numerous Rosenthal fibers are stained by the Loyez method; (**B**) hemispheric white matter with numerous Rosenthal fibers especially dense around a blood vessel (H&E); (**C**) EM of Rosenthal fibers, which appear as electron-dense masses in pericapillary astrocytic processes.

astrocytic foot processes are located. A very similar pattern of abundant Rosenthal fibers is present in the brain of patients with autosomal recessive giant axonal neuropathy, but this condition also shows spheroids and profound involvement of peripheral nerves with giant axons due to mutations in the gigaxonin-encoding *GAN* gene.

10.10.2. Pelizaeus–Merzbacher disease

Pelizaeus–Merzbacher disease is an X-linked recessive leukodystrophy caused by mutations in the proteolipid protein 1 gene (*PLP1*) located on chromosome Xq22.2. Proteolipid protein 1 is a structural protein of CNS myelin, and point mutations, deletions, and gene duplications in *PLP1* have all been described in Pelizaeus–Merzbacher disease. In the classic infantile form, infants have rotary movements of the head and eyes and develop spasticity of the limbs, cerebellar ataxia, and parkinsonian symptoms during childhood. Death usually occurs in late adolescence. As in other leukodystrophies, the disease is characterized by the loss of myelin in the white matter. Due to the sparing of a few small islands of normal myelin, often in perivascular distribution, the "striped" appearance of perivascular myelin sparing has been known as a "tigroid leukodystrophy" (Fig. 10.17A, C, D). The cerebral and cerebellar white matter appears atrophic. Axons are relatively preserved, and there is severe gliosis. The abnormalities of myelin are limited to the CNS; the PNS is usually spared, and visceral involvement is absent.

Whereas the usual form of the disease presents in the first 3 months of life, a connatal form (congenital form of Seitelberger) is characterized by a nearly complete absence of CNS myelin (Fig. 10.17B) and

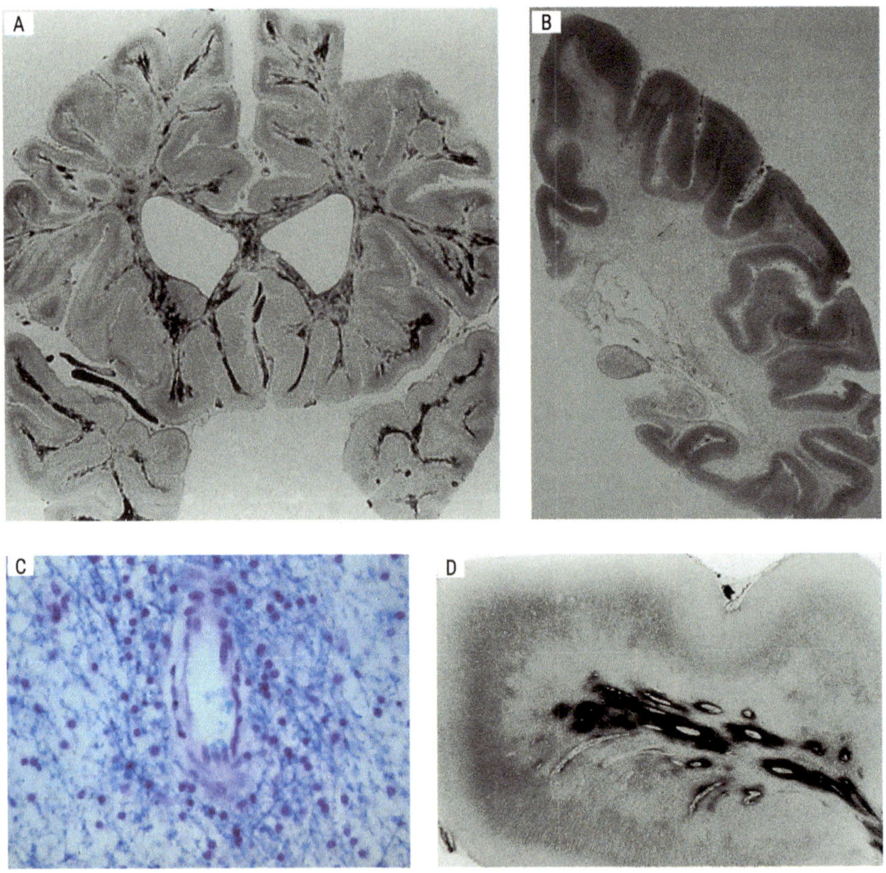

FIGURE 10.17 Pelizaeus–Merzbacher disease: (**A**) typical infantile form of Pelizaeus–Merzbacher tigroid leukodystrophy (Loyez) (courtesy of Professor Jean Lapresle); (**B**) massive congenital form of Seitelberger disease/NBIA2A (Loyez); (**C, D**) microscopic appearance with relative preservation of the myelin around blood vessels (**C**, Luxol fast blue–cresyl violet; **D**, Loyez).

severe symptoms in infancy. This leukodystrophy, although sharing clinical features, is an autosomal recessive disorder caused by mutations in the *AIMP1* gene located on chromosome 4q24.

10.10.3. Congenital Disorders of Glycosylation

Congenital disorders of glycosylation (CDG) are a recently identified and rapidly expanding group of hereditary, largely autosomal recessive, mono- or multi-organ disorders in young children caused by defects in protein glycosylation (i.e., developmental defects). Mutations in approximately 250 glycosylation-related genes produce a broad heterogeneous clinical and morphological spectrum of conditions, individually labeled by the gene affected and the suffix CDG (e.g., PMM2-CDG). There are two main subgroups of diseases, one associated with N-glycosylation (of asparagine groups) and the other related to O-glycosylation (often of Ser or Thr hydroxyl groups) that is located in the cytosol–endoplasmic reticulum–Golgi apparatus region. The former may, in different forms, affect the brain, foremost the cerebellum, well documented by MRI, rarely in individual case reports by neuropathological examination. The CNS structures are marked by loss of neurons in the cerebral cortex and more often in the cerebellar cortex with depletion of Purkinje and granule cells, aberrant neurons in the cortex and dendritic pathology, and "asteroid bodies." Reports on the latter group of O-glycosylation deficiencies may entail developmental defects in brain and eye (known as Walker–Warburg and muscle–eye–brain diseases) and skeletal muscle (resulting in congenital muscular dystrophies). The myopathology is marked by immunohistochemical sarcolemmal deficiency of α-dystroglycan and is described in Chapter 12. Abnormal values of transferrin in the serum and genetic analyses may be the clue to further diagnostic steps arriving at a final CDG diagnosis.

11

Congenital Malformations and Perinatal Diseases

HOMA ADLE-BIASSETTE, BRIAN HARDING, AND JEFFREY A. GOLDEN

11.1. GENERAL CONSIDERATIONS

Congenital anomalies are deviations from normal form or structure, present at birth. *Malformations* are developmental failures due to a primary disruption of normal embryologic development, which can be genetic or environmental in origin or, most commonly, multifactorial as a result of complex interactions between genes and the environment. In contrast, a *disruption* represents the perturbation or abrogation of the normal developmental process; examples of this include a vascular accident resulting in porencephaly or hydranencephaly or the well-known consequences of in utero infection (e.g., with cytomegalovirus [CMV]). These also can be environmental, genetic, or multifactorial. Finally, *deformations* exist when external forces alter but do not disrupt normal development. An example of this is the nongenetic arthrogryposis that frequently accompanies oligohydramnios. Once again, deformations can occur on a genetic, environmental, or multifactorial basis. Understanding the underlying pathogenesis for any congenital anomaly of the central nervous system (CNS) is of importance for genetic counseling of parents and siblings of affected infants.

The neuropathological diagnosis of CNS diseases and malformations in fetuses and newborns should take into account the family history, maternal diseases and risk factors (including environmental factors and teratogens), pregnancy history, fetal conditions, imaging, placental examination, autopsy findings in fetus or infant, postnatal clinical history, karyotype, and when necessary genetic investigations. The distinction between malformations and disruptions is important for pathogenesis and genetic counseling.

During the past decade, significant progress has been made in understanding the molecular/genetic basis of many congenital anomalies, and with that has come a greater appreciation for the complexity of brain development. For example, neural tube closure defects (e.g., myelomeningocele and anencephaly) have largely eluded molecular characterization. However, extensive and ongoing studies have clearly implicated a multifactorial pathogenesis for these disorders involving the planar cell polarity signaling pathway, along with adequate maternal nutrition, folate intake in particular.

Another example of this complexity has come through the greater elucidation of the pathogenesis of holoprosencephaly (HPE). This complex malformation can arise in the setting of a mutation in a single gene, in the presence of multiple genetic alterations, due to gross chromosomal alterations (e.g., trisomy 13), or on a multifactorial basis. Further confusing the evaluation, a mutation in a known causative gene for HPE, such as *SHH*, does not always correlate with this specific brain anomaly and can be seen in individuals with a normal brain, even in the same family with an individual with the same mutation but exhibiting HPE, further supporting the complex genetic, or multifactorial, basis of most congenital anomalies.

A clear understanding of normal brain development is critical for the evaluation of congenital anomalies, as the effect of an exogenous factor on the brain is dependent on the timing of the exposure. For example, exposure of the fetus to alcohol in the first trimester can result in microcephaly and other disorders, whereas exposure in the second or third trimester can result in a normal brain structure but potential functional perturbation.

11.2. CONGENITAL MALFORMATIONS

11.2.1. CNS manifestations of chromosomal change

Cytogenetic studies should be considered if there is evidence of any of the following: congenital malformation, intrauterine growth restriction, hydrops, ambiguous genitalia, or dysmorphic features. A wide range of craniofacial, morphologic, and functional abnormalities of the CNS are found in patients with chromosomal defects.

11.2.2. Neurulation failure

The transformation of the neural plate into the neural tube begins around the end of the third gestational week and is complete by the end of the fourth gestational week. Failure of this process results in neural tube defects (NTDs) involving closure. NTDs are the most frequent CNS malformations, with an incidence of 1 or 2 per 1,000 live births, although there is wide geographic variability; for example, the incidences in Ireland and Punjab, India, are reported to reach 8 per 1,000 live births. As mentioned above, NTDs are widely believed to result from a complex interaction between genetics and environmental influences because the risk of recurrence among couples who have had an affected offspring is increased over that for the general population. Nongenetic risk factors include certain maternal disease states, poorly controlled maternal diabetes mellitus, hyperthermia, and teratogens such as anticonvulsants. Preconception multivitamin and folate supplementation reduces the recurrence risk for women with one affected child and appears to reduce the overall risk in all women. Successful screening programs using a panel of maternal serum markers along with a follow-up ultrasound or magnetic resonance imaging (MRI) examination for positive cases identify the majority of cases with a high degree of sensitivity and specificity. NTDs may be isolated malformations or found in association with other malformations as part of a syndrome, the latter primarily being occipital encephalocele associated with several Mendelian disorders, such as Meckel–Grüber syndrome (a ciliopathy) and Walker–Warburg syndrome (a congenital disorder of glycosylation).

11.2.2.1. CRANIAL NTDS

Exencephaly and *anencephaly* are characterized by the absence of the calvarium, abnormalities of the skull base, and variable disruption of the intracranial neuroepithelium. The commonly involved sphenoid bone often induces shallow orbits, causing protrusion of the eyes (Fig. 11.1).

Anencephaly is the most common form of cranial NTD. In this condition, there is variable loss (destruction) of the forebrain, diencephalon, and rostral brainstem, which are replaced by an irregular web of neurovascular tissue that includes ependyma-like epithelium and choroid plexus ("area cerebrovasculosa").

Exencephaly (Fig. 11.2) is a very rare related condition in which the cerebral hemispheres, although disorganized and rudimentary, are usually present. Experimental studies suggest the neural tissue, growing outside the confines of the skull

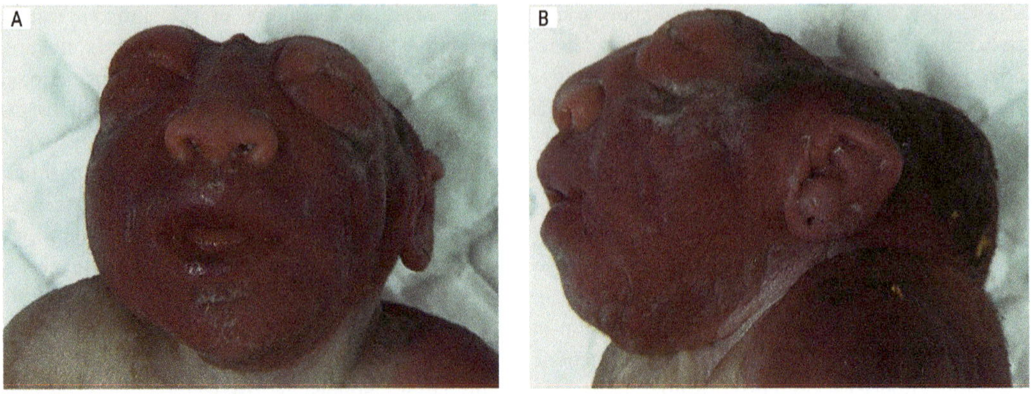

FIGURE 11.1 Anencephaly: (**A**) face and (**B**) profile.

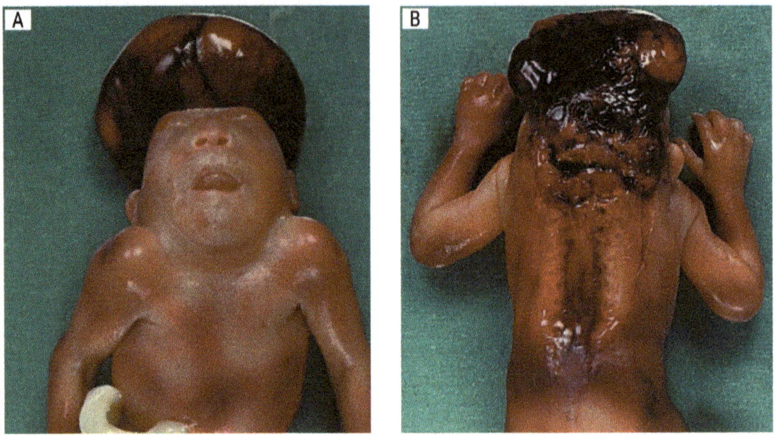

FIGURE 11.2 Exencephaly (**A**) associated with craniorachischisis (**B**).

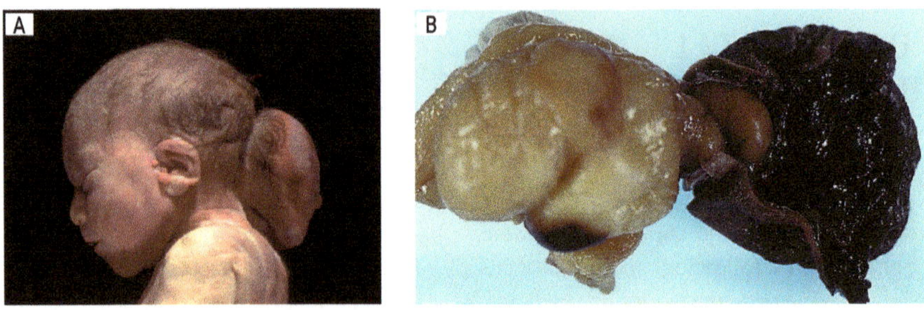

FIGURE 11.3 Occipital meningoencephalocele.

and resulting in the malformation, is protected from the amniotic fluid, likely by the meninges. Destruction of the neural tissue occurs when the neurepithelial tissue is in contact with the amniotic fluid, eventuating in the area cerebrovasculosa. Involvement of the cranial contents along with the upper or entire spinal cord is referred to as craniorachischisis.

Encephalocele (or *meningoencephalocele*) is the herniation of cerebral tissue or meninges (meningocele if involving the meninges only) through a calvarium defect of variable size. In 80% of cases, the bone defect occurs in the occipital region and is associated with skin and hair abnormalities (Fig. 11.3). The neural tissue within the encephalocele is usually disorganized, occasionally showing polymicrogyria and frequently showing evidence of ischemic injury. Occipital encephalocele is an important feature of Meckel–Gruber syndrome, a lethal form of the ciliopathies.

11.2.2.2. SPINAL NTDS

Spinal NTDs (Fig. 11.4) have a complex and often interchangeably used nomenclature. Generic terms such as *spina bifida* have been used to describe all forms, and this has been further subdivided by some to be either open ("aperta") or closed ("occulta").

It is perhaps more accurate to use the descriptive terminology of *spinal* or *vertebral dysraphism* if only the vertebral body is involved but not either the spinal cord or the meninges, *meningocele* when only the meninges are involved with a vertebral anomaly, and *myelomeningocele* when there is involvement of all three: the vertebrae, the meninges, and the spinal cord.

Defining the location in addition to the type is also important, with the lumbosacral region being involved most commonly. *Iniencephaly* is a related disorder in which the cervical posterior vertebral arches are foreshortened and fused, resulting in a fixed extension and shortening of the neck, usually and often associated with abnormalities of the brainstem. Similar to that described for the cranial region, when the defect is open to the amniotic fluid, there is destruction of the neuroepithelium, with resulting neurovascular tissue referred to as area myelovasculosa or medullovasculosa. If covered by meninges but involving the neural placode, the developing spinal cord is variably disorganized but recognizable, although the dorsal aspect will be splayed open. The spinal cord adjacent to the defect, where

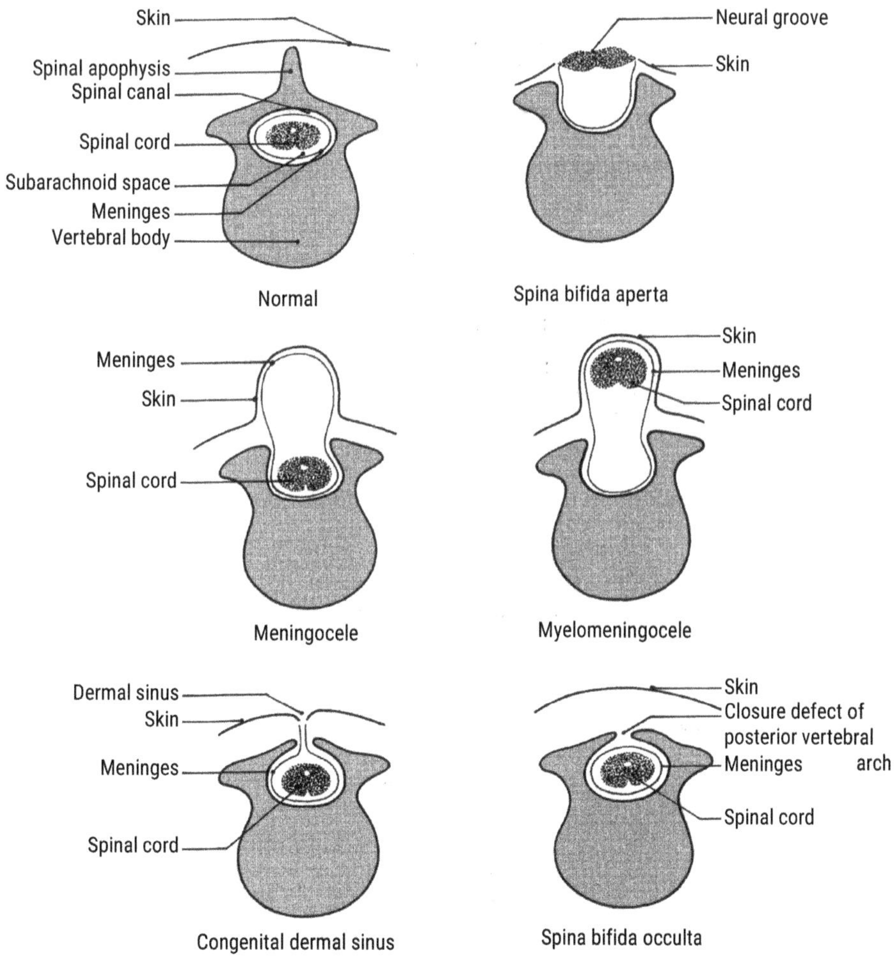

FIGURE 11.4 Spinal neural tube closure defects.

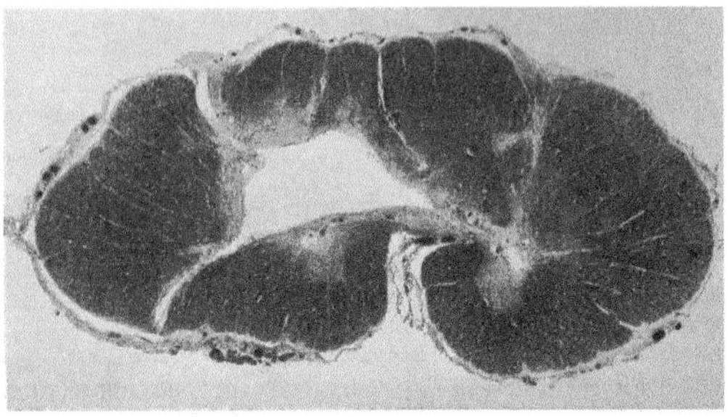

FIGURE 11.5 Syringomyelia, with expansion of the central canal and compression of the posterior horn and column (Loyez stain for myelin).

the neural tube has closed, and in cases in which the neuroepithelium is not involved, may show syringomyelia (Fig. 11.5), hydromyelia (overdistension of the central canal), diplomyelia (duplication of the cord), or diastematomyelia (coexistence of two hemi-cords). A related condition is the presence of a congenital dermal sinus where a communication persists between the skin surface and the subarachnoid space, which can lead to recurrent meningitis.

Lumbosacral meningomyelocele is nearly always associated with a characteristic composite of posterior fossa anomalies. They include a low-set tentorium and small posterior fossa, lengthening of the cerebral peduncles, an "S-shaped" deformation of the medulla oblongata, and cerebellar hypoplasia with downward displacement of the cerebellar vermis through an enlarged foramen magnum (overlying the dorsal surface of the cervical spinal cord) (Fig. 11.6). This complex, called the Chiari type II (or Arnold–Chiari) malformation, is further characterized by hydrocephalus, and sometimes with a polygyria pattern of the cerebral convolutions and subependymal heterotopia. Of considerable interest, recent advancements in the repair of lumbosacral myelomeningocele in utero (fetal surgery) have resulted in the elimination of the cerebral components of the Chiari II malformation in most cases, suggesting some of the changes described in the posterior fossa are due to a secondary deformation, rather than a true malformation.

11.2.3. Disorders of development of the prosencephalon

The most rostral subdivision of the neural tube is known as the prosencephalon. Bilaterally symmetric outgrowths from the prosencephalon give rise to the telencephalic vesicles in the fifth week of gestation. These paired structures will become the cerebral hemispheres and the basal ganglia. The caudal–medial part of the prosencephalon, which remains as a single entity, becomes the diencephalon (future thalamus) and also gives rise to the optic vesicles. The most rostral aspect of the neural tube becomes the lamina terminalis, where the cerebral hemispheres meet as corpus callosum fibers decussate at approximately the 12th week of gestation. The cerebral hemispheres and the olfactory placodes derive from the telencephalic vesicles. In humans, the olfactory vesicles regress at approximately 10 weeks and form the olfactory bulbs, but they persist in many other vertebrates.

11.2.3.1. HOLOPROSENCEPHALY

Failure of the two telencephalic vesicles to grow out from the prosencephalon results in a spectrum of malformations called *holoprosencephalies*, which are associated with ocular and midline facial abnormalities, such as cyclopia, cebocephaly, ethmocephaly (nose with single nostril), facial median cleft due to the absence of the premaxilla, and hypo- or hypertelorism. Recognizing a correlation in severity between brain and craniofacial anomalies, DeMyer famously concluded that the "face predicts the brain."

The HPEs are now recognized as signaling defects from the ventral or dorsal midline. The most common teratogenic association in humans is maternal diabetes mellitus. Most cases of HPE have a recognizable genetic etiology. Approximately 50% of cases have a cytogenetic/chromosomal basis, and 25% are syndromic. The genetic basis is most often attributed to a mutation in one of several pathways essential for normal midline signaling. The four HPE genes of major importance are *SHH*, *SIX3*, *ZIC2*, and *TGIF*. In the cases belonging to the cytogenetic/chromosomal category, trisomy 13 and, much less commonly, trisomy 18 as well as other chromosomal aberrations may be found.

Prenatal ultrasound may detect the malformation as early as the 12th week of gestation; fetal MRI possibly even earlier. The HPE spectrum ranges from complete absence of the prosencephalon to instances in which only a minimal abnormality is observed (e.g., isolated absence of the olfactory bulbs and tracts), with a broad range of transitional forms. Not all of these midline anomalies have the same pathogenesis; for example, absence of the olfactory bulbs and tracks may also be seen as a result

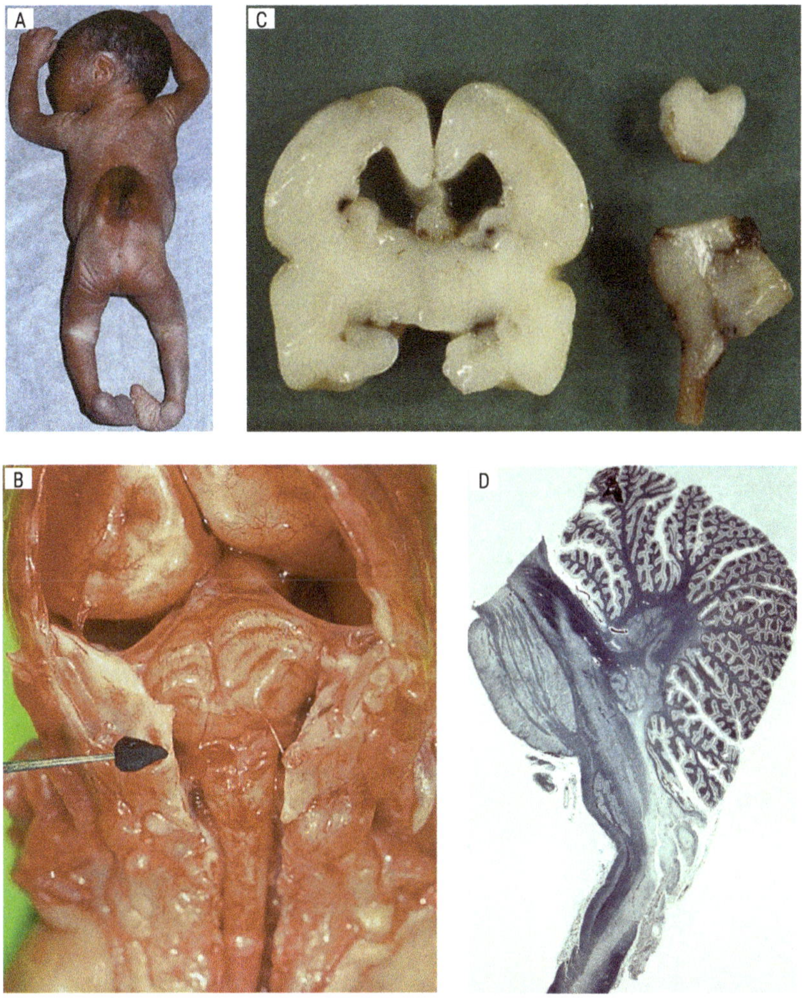

FIGURE 11.6 Arnold–Chiari malformation: (**A**) dorsolumbar meningomyelocele (courtesy of Dr. J. C. Larroche); (**B**) dorsal view of the posterior fossa showing cerebellar engagement and "S-shaped" abnormality of the medulla oblongata (courtesy of Dr. J. C. Larroche); (**C**) coronal section of the cerebral hemispheres and midbrain showing bilateral ventricular dilation; sagittal section of the brainstem and cerebellum showing cerebellar tonsil herniation and S-shaped abnormality of the medulla oblongata; (**D**) sagittal whole-mount section of the brainstem and cerebellum showing cerebellar tonsil herniation and S-shaped abnormality of the medulla oblongata (Loyez stain).

of failed induction or outgrowth. Individuals who are severely affected often die in utero or early childhood. Children with milder forms (semilobar, lobar, or with the middle interhemispheric variant) may survive to adulthood.

- *Aprosencephaly* and the related atelencephaly are extremely rare conditions characterized by a rudimentary prosencephalon and extreme microencephaly.
- *Alobar HPE* (Fig. 11.7) consists of an undivided holospheric cerebrum, or prosencephalic monoventricle, which may open posteriorly into a dorsal sac-like structure. The thalamic and other diencephalic nuclei are most often totally or partly fused, with a narrow or absent third ventricle. The corpus callosum and septum pellucidum are absent. The cerebral convolutions may be aberrant and pachygyric. The olfactory bulbs and hypophysis are usually absent (arrhinencephaly). The brainstem and the cerebellum may also be affected (mesencephalo/rhombencephalosynapsis).

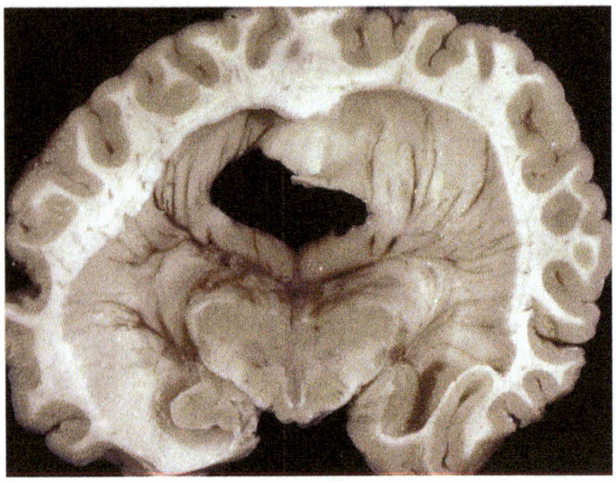

FIGURE 11.7 Alobar holoprosencephaly.

- *Semilobar HPE* is characterized by the presence of an interhemispheric fissure only in the parieto-occipital region, in contrast to cases with continuous cortical gyri bridging over the midline in frontal regions (Fig. 11.8). The prosencephalic monoventricle is frontal, divided posteriorly in two temporal and occipital horns where the cortex is continuous across the midline. There may be no, partial, or complete fusion of the diencephalic structures and the basal ganglia. Again, the olfactory bulbs and tracts are absent.
- *Lobar HPE* is characterized by two well-developed hemispheres connected by an orbital frontal bridge of cortical convolution. The corpus callosum is absent or sometimes hypoplastic, and the septum pellucidum is absent.
- The *middle interhemispheric variant* of HPE is characterized by a variable-size nodule of heterotopic gray matter extending across the dorsal midline and often protruding into or even obliterating the ventricles. The corpus callosum is absent from the regions of heterotopic gray matter, and the cerebral cortex is continuous across the midline. Ventral structures are usually preserved, including the olfactory bulbs and tracts.
- *Arrhinencephaly*, the least severe form of the HPEs, consists of isolated absence of olfactory bulbs and tracts and of the straight sulci along the orbital frontal cortical surface (Fig. 11.9).

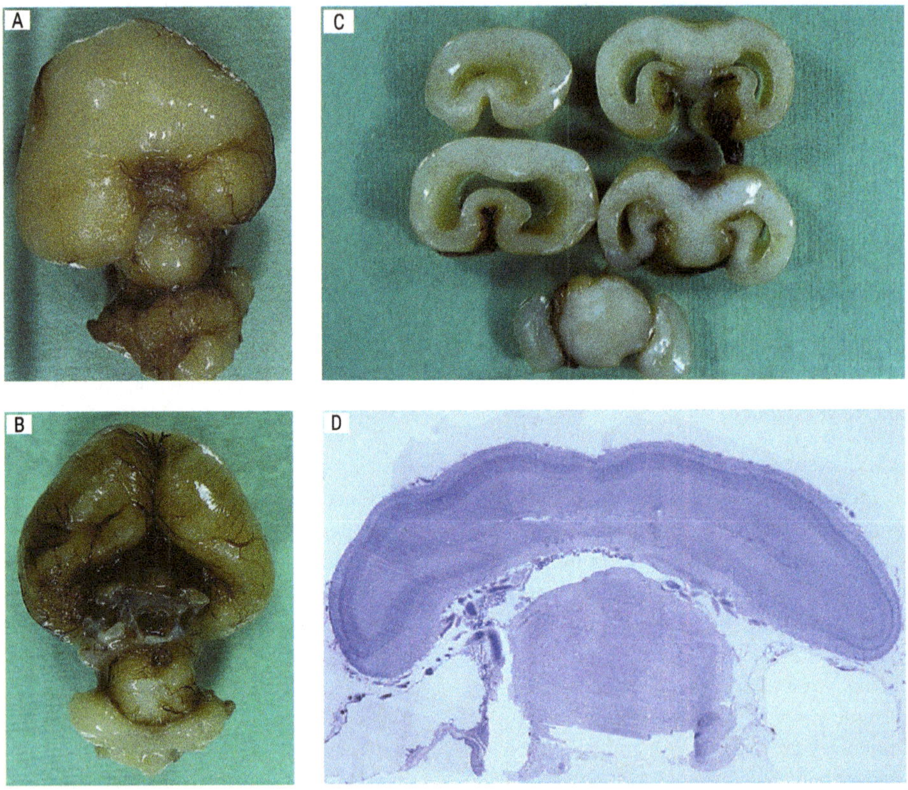

FIGURE 11.8 Semilobar holoprosencephaly: (**A**) basal view; (**B**) dorsal view; (**C**) coronal section; (**D**) microscopic appearance.

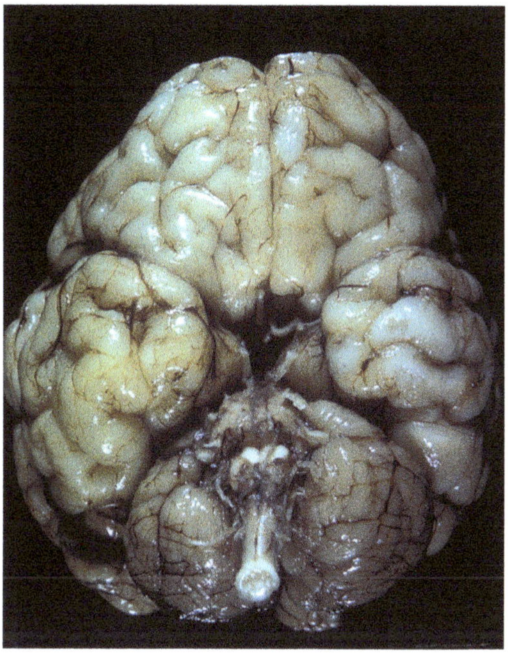

FIGURE 11.9 Arrhinencephaly.

Histologic findings in HPE differ from case to case. Hypoplastic deep nuclei and cytoarchitectonic abnormalities with subependymal heterotopias have been most often observed.

11.2.3.2. OTHER ABNORMALITIES OF MIDLINE STRUCTURES

11.2.3.2.1. Agenesis of the corpus callosum. Agenesis of the corpus callosum (ACC) is a relatively common malformation that may be present in isolation or be associated with other brain or systemic anomalies. The disorder may occur sporadically, as part of chromosome aberration syndrome (e.g., trisomy 18 and 8) or as a metabolic/genetic disease (e.g., L1 syndrome). Familial cases also have been reported. Some cases occur as incidental findings at autopsy in adults with no history of neurologic or developmental abnormalities.

The corpus callosum develops rostrocaudally from the crossing of telencephalic commissural axons between the 10th and 20th weeks of gestation; thus, this abnormality can be seen by prenatal ultrasound examination even in early gestation.

In instances of *complete agenesis*, the medial surfaces of the hemispheres show secondary abnormalities, characterized by an aberrant callosal artery and replacement of the normal cingulate gyrus by perpendicular ("radiating") gyri and sulci. On coronal sections, in addition to the absence of a crossing tract, the corners of the lateral ventricles show a vertical ("batwing" or "staghorn") orientation (Fig. 11.10). The ventricular roof is membranous and may bulge into the interhemispheric fissure. In most cases, the misdirected callosal fibers form an aberrant anteroposterior tract along the dorsal–medial margin of the ventricle and are known as Probst's bundle (Fig. 11.10B).

Partial agenesis of the corpus callosum typically occurs in the posterior portion of the structure; the presence of a normal rostrum, genu, and anterior body of the corpus callosum is variable (Fig. 11.11). The presence of an intact cingulate gyrus occurs only to the extent of the development of the corpus callosum.

Whether total or partial, callosal agenesis may be accompanied by lipomatous tissue, vascular abnormalities, or calcifications along the dorsal midline at the site of the absent callosal fibers. ACC may be sporadic or familial and associated with mutation affecting a single gene or complex chromosomal abnormalities.

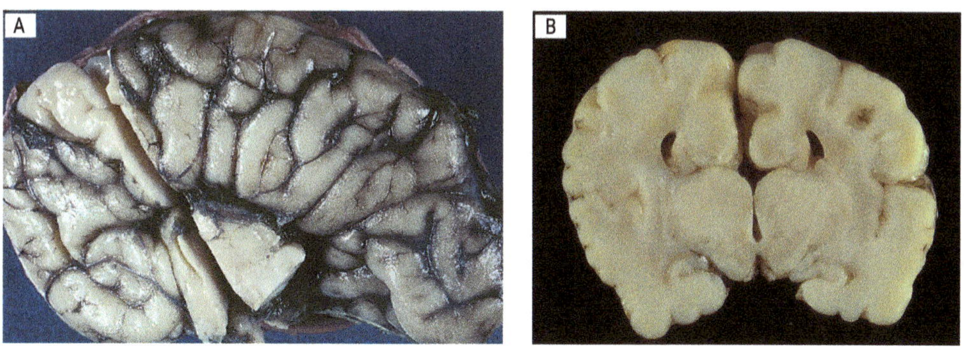

FIGURE 11.10 Agenesis of corpus callosum: (**A**) interhemispheric view; (**B**) coronal section.

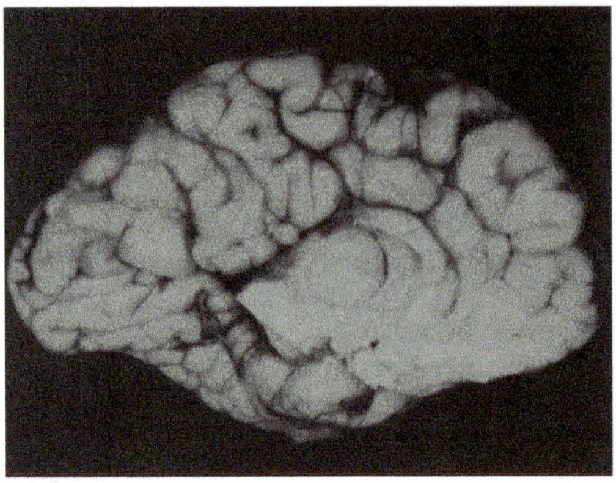

FIGURE 11.11 Partial agenesis of the corpus callosum.

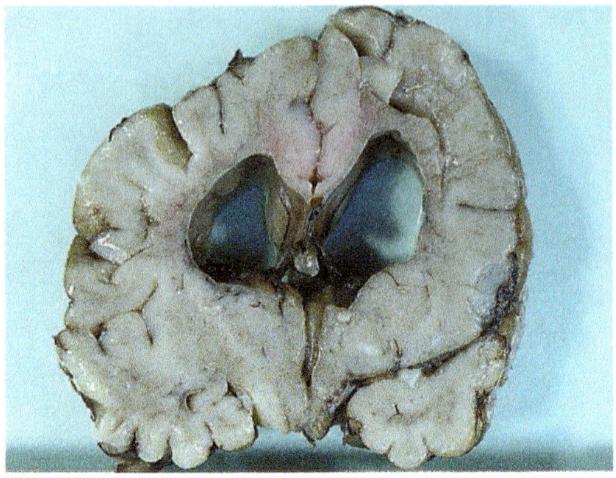

FIGURE 11.13 Septal rupture.

11.2.3.2.2. Anomalies of septum pellucidum. *Cavum septum pelludidum* (rostral) and *cavum septi vergae* (caudal) are seen in fetuses as developmentally normal midline cavities lying between the two leaves of the septum (Fig. 11.12). They tend to become obliterated toward term, but they persist postnatally in a minority of individuals.

Agenesis of the septum pellucidum gives rise to a pseudomonoventricle. True primary agenesis of the septum pellucidum must be distinguished from secondary destruction. Septo-optic dysplasia is characterized by two or more features of the classical triad of (1) optic nerve hypoplasia; (2) pituitary hormone abnormalities; and (3) midline brain defects, including agenesis of the septum pellucidum and/or corpus callosum. Many of these cases are now recognized as a Mendelian disorder related to mutations in one of several genes.

In hydrocephalic brains, the destruction of one or both leaves of the septum may also lead to a similar appearance; however, the retinal dysplasia and hypothalamic/hypophyseal defects are not present in these cases (Fig. 11.13).

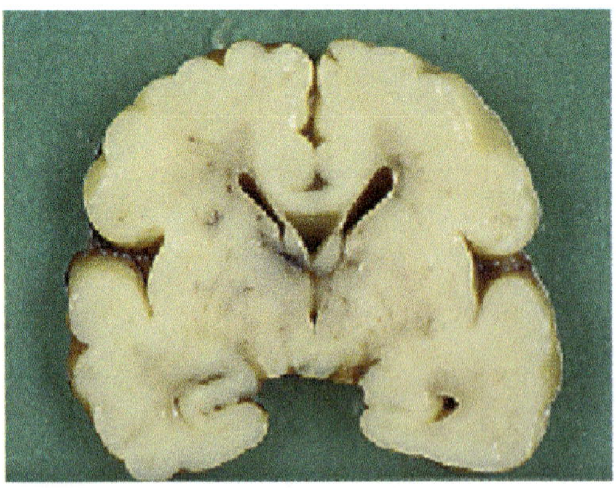

FIGURE 11.12 Cavum septum pellucidum.

11.2.4. Malformations of the cortical plate

Disorders of normal cortical cell genesis, migration, and maturation lead to a spectrum of cytoarchitectonic abnormalities, leading to external gyral abnormalities (agyria/pachygyria or polymicrogyria) or to more subtle lesions, such as the presence of heterotopic neurons in the white matter.

11.2.4.1. DISORDERS OF BRAIN SIZE

Proliferation of neural progenitor cells along the lumen of the neural tube (nascent ventricles) is critical for the generation of normal numbers of neurons in the CNS. Perturbations of this process alone result in reduced numbers of neurons in the brain and subsequently a small brain (i.e., primary microcephaly). Primary microcephaly may have a normal-appearing gyral pattern or a simplified gyral pattern. Although most cases do not have a known etiology, the genetic basis of a subset of cases has been elucidated and in most cases is the result of mutations in centrosomal proteins required for normal cell division of neural progenitors. Other genetic causes include chromosomal anomalies and several monogenic syndromes. Clinical assessment considers secondary microcephaly a progressive condition occurring after birth and attests to white matter developmental abnormalities or to neurodegenerative processes. From the perspective of neuropathological study, secondary microcephaly is seen in the setting of acquired/environmental insults related to infections (e.g., TORCH [toxoplasmosis, other, rubella, cytomegalovirus, or herpes virus] syndrome), vascular ischemic–hemorrhagic lesions, or toxic insults.

Megalencephaly and hemimegalencephaly are developmental abnormalities of brain growth characterized by early onset, often progressive, brain overgrowth affecting both or one cerebral/cerebellar hemisphere. Many cases are caused by constitutional or mosaic mutations resulting in overactivation of the PI3K-AKT-MTOR signaling pathway.

11.2.4.2. NEURONAL HETEROTOPIA

Neuronal heterotopia is defined by the presence of heterotopic neurons in the white matter (Figs. 11.14–11.16).

11.2.4.2.1. Laminar, subcortical band heterotopia. Laminar, subcortical band heterotopia consists of bilateral, often symmetrical, bands of gray matter, of variable thickness, within the centrum semiovale, separated from the normal-looking cortex by a band of white matter composed of numerous small nodules of gray matter, which frequently coalesce into irregular larger nodules (Fig. 11.14A). Histologically, heterotopia reveals well-differentiated, randomly oriented and focally clustered neurons, including pyramidal cells, forming bands or aggregates (Fig. 11.14B). The overlying cortex usually has a normal hexalaminar organization.

The syndrome is most commonly linked to mutations in *DCX* on chromosome Xq22.3-Xq23. The gene encodes a signaling protein, doublecortin (DCX); to date, all cases are in females. Male patients in the same family have lissencephaly; subcortical band heterotopia is rarely observed. However, this condition may also be seen in males and in sporadic cases. At least some of these are associated with a *LIS1* mutation.

11.2.4.2.2. Periventricular nodular heterotopia. Periventricular nodular heterotopia consists of small clusters of neurons adjacent to the ventricle and frequently protruding into the ventricle. Single or several periventricular heterotopias may occasionally be found in an otherwise normal brain. When periventricular nodular heterotopias are numerous, essentially lining the walls of the lateral ventricles, the condition is almost always genetic in origin. In these cases, the heterotopias appear as discrete or confluent, well-defined nodules (2 to >10 mm) beneath the ependymal lining protruding into the ventricle, giving a lumpy appearance to the normally smooth ventricular surface (Fig. 11.16). The trigones and occipital horns of the lateral ventricles are the most commonly affected regions. Histologically, nodules consist of islands of mature cells resembling cortical neurons, sometimes with a concentric arrangement as well as interneurons and glia. Nodular heterotopia may be an isolated finding or complicate other cerebral malformations, such as hydrocephalus, microcephaly, and agenesis of the corpus callosum, cerebellar hypoplasia, polymicrogyria, agyria, pachygyria, and cortical dysplasia.

Periventricular nodular heterotopias represent a failure of migration of immature neuroblasts from

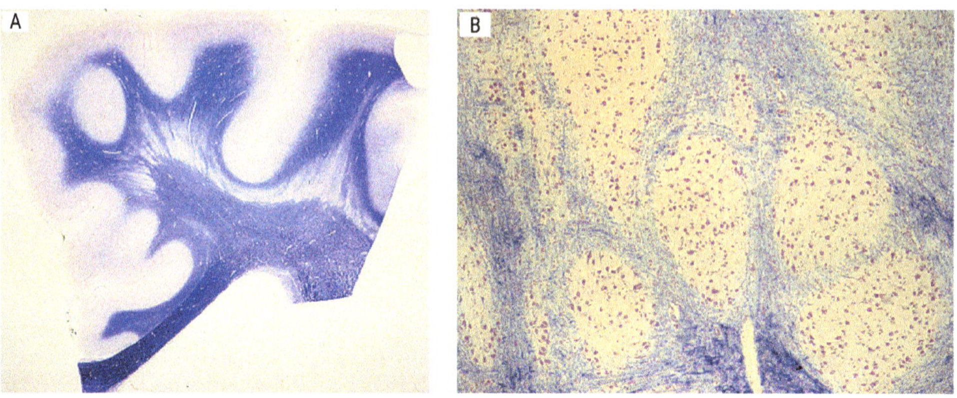

FIGURE 11.14 Laminar subcortical heterotopia: (**A**) heterotopic tissue separated from the normal cortex by a layer of normally myelinated white matter (Luxol fast blue/cresyl violet); (**B**) neurons in the heterotopic gray matter are arranged in irregular aggregates of normal-appearing pyramidal cells (Luxol fast blue).

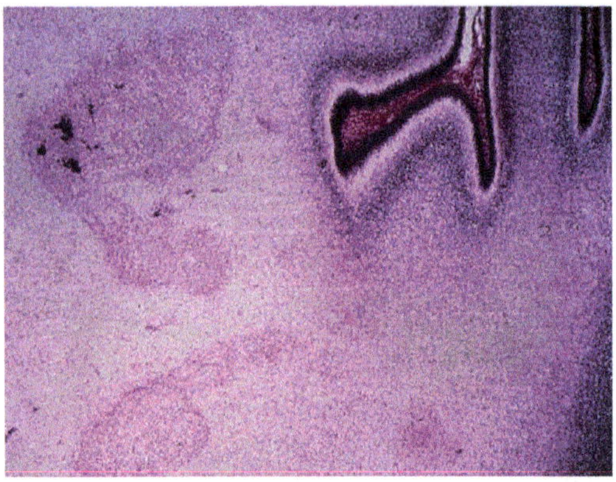

FIGURE 11.15 Cerebellar heterotopia.

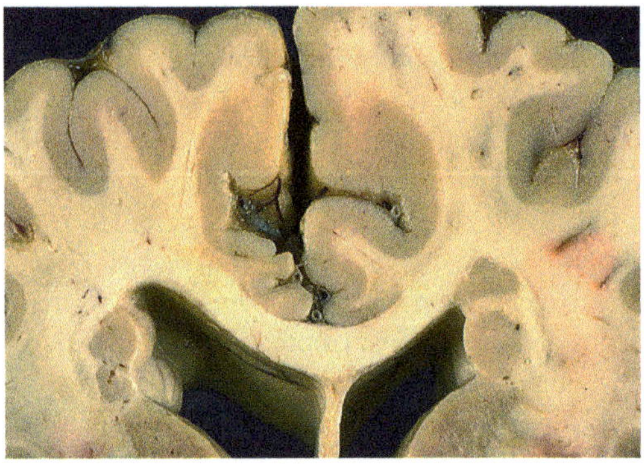

FIGURE 11.16 Subependymal/periventricular heterotopia: section of frontal lobe showing multiple nodules of gray matter next to the caudate nucleus.

the ventricular zone, due, in some cases, to a mutation in the *FilaminA* (*Filamin-1*) gene on the X chromosome. Females, who carry one copy of the mutant gene and one normal copy, have a subset of neuroblasts that are able to migrate normally to the cortex. The random inactivation of the normal allele, then, results in a subpopulation of neurons with the mutant allele that are unable to migrate and thus remain in the ventricular region. Males carrying the mutant gene (i.e., only one X chromosome) have major migrational failure, which most commonly results in prenatal lethality. There are, however, rare occurrences of nodular heterotopia in males who are germline mosaics, a mechanism that is also responsible for phenotypically normal mothers of affected daughters. Additional genes are involved in nodular heterotopia associated with malformations confined to the CNS or with multisystem disorders. Isolated periventricular heterotopia may be found on neuroimaging obtained in patients with intellectual disability and epilepsy or incidentally in normal subjects. The mechanistic relationship of heterotopia to intellectual disability or epilepsy remains uncertain.

11.2.4.3. POLYMICROGYRIA

Polymicrogyria refers to a cortical malformation characterized by an excessive folding and irregular fusion of adjacent gyri with a thin cortical ribbon. The leptomeninges covering the polymicrogyric cortex can be abnormally vascularized and may contain ectopic (i.e., displaced and disorganized) neuroglial tissue (Fig. 11.17).

Polymicrogyria may be seen in several conditions. There are now well-defined Mendelian disorders that include polymicrogyria, some in specific patterns (e.g., perisylvian, bilateral frontal, bilateral frontal–parietal, and others). Polymicrogyria may also be found in patients with complete triploidies. Mutations in at least 50 genes have been associated with polymicrogyria, including the Zellweger syndrome, a primary metabolic disorder, and in patients with congenital disorders of glycosylation. Mutations in fibroblast growth factor receptor gene (*FGFR3*), which give rise to thanatophoric dysplasia, a form of chondrodysplastic dwarfism associated with temporal lobe enlargement and abnormal deep transverse sulci across the temporal surface, are also associated with polymicrogyria. Finally, polymicrogyria may result from disruptions of cerebral cortical development in a narrow window of time from approximately 16 or 17 gestational weeks through approximately 23 or 24 gestational weeks. Examples of these disruptions resulting in polymicrogyria include the margins of porencephaly and hydranencephaly (see Sections 11.3.1.1.1 and 11.3.1.1.2). Congenital CMV infection is also well known to cause polymicrogyria,

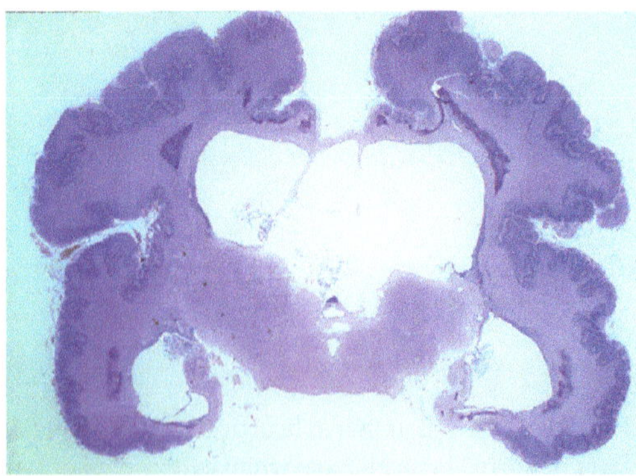

FIGURE 11.17 Polymicrogyria.

likely on a disruptive basis. Thus, the pathogenesis of polymicrogyria is likely to be multifactorial.

On microscopic examination, regions affected by polymicrogyria show variable expression from a chaotic (called *unlayered*) organization of the isocortex to a "four-layer" organization. Both forms can be seen in the same brain, as may occur in thanatophoric dysplasia (Fig. 11.18). *Four-layer polymicrogyria* refers to the description by Bielschowsky in 1915, characterized by a superficial, acellular molecular layer that infolds and fuses to produce a microsulcus; a second cellular layer comprising neuronal types of cells normally belonging to cortical laminae II and III; a third layer devoid of neurons, containing mostly glial cells; and a fourth layer contiguous with normal layer VI of the adjacent cortex (Fig. 11.19). This microscopic appearance, along with the facts that the lesion may be focal and border porencephalic defects, suggests that four-layer polymicrogyria may be a sequela of laminar necrosis of layers IV and V due to early ischemic, toxic, or infectious injury such as in TORCH syndrome (see Section 11.3.1.1.1).

Focal polymicrogyria may also be found in Chiari II malformations and in encephaloceles, as well as in fetal alcohol syndrome.

11.2.4.4. LISSENCEPHALY

The term *lissencephaly* means "smooth brain" and refers to the macroscopic appearance of the brain where external examination shows few or no sulci, although the major fissures (interhemispheric and Sylvian) are preserved intact. The term is used interchangeably with agyria, but when involvement is localized to smaller regions of the brain, the term pachygyria is preferred. Hemilissencephaly (involving only one cerebral hemisphere) may be seen in some children/infants with intractable epilepsy.

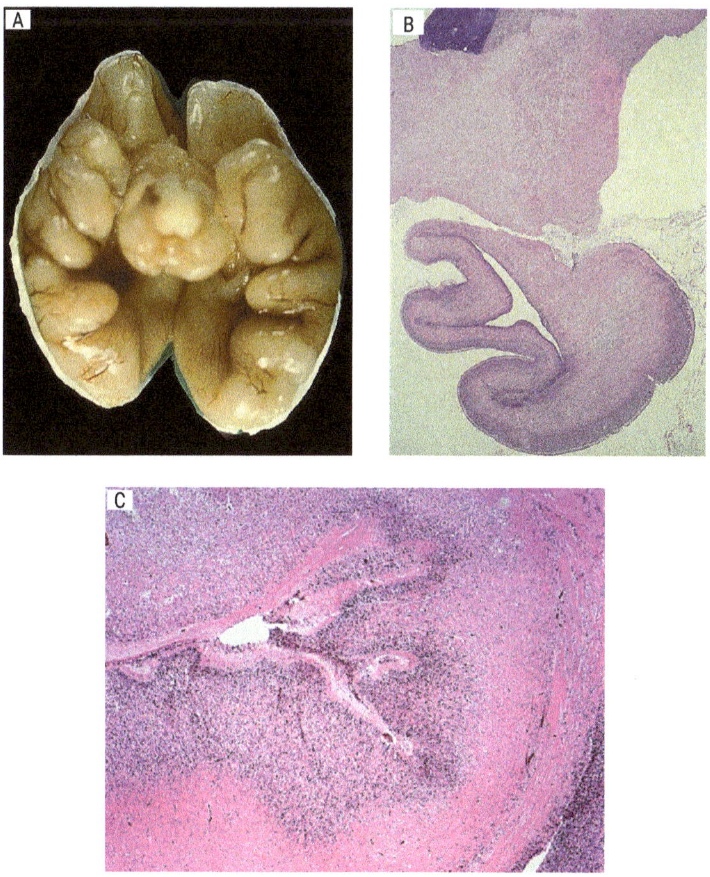

FIGURE 11.18 Thanatophoric dysplasia: (**A**) basal view; (**B**) temporal sulcus; (**C**) cytoarchitectonic abnormalities.

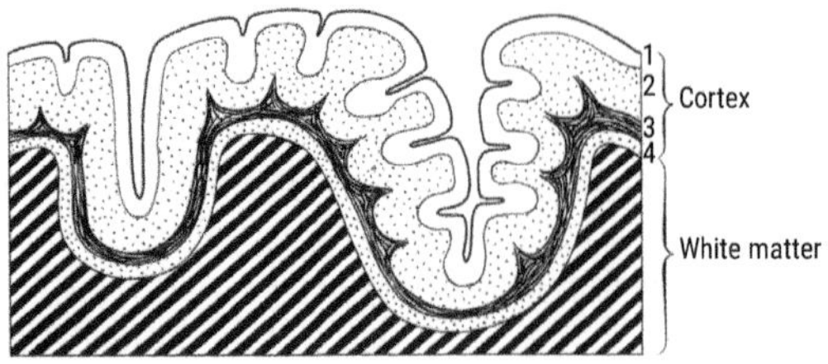

FIGURE 11.19 Cortical changes in polymicrogyria. (After Crome, L., and Stern, J. (1972). *Pathology of mental retardation* (2nd ed.). Baltimore: Williams & Wilkins.)

11.2.4.4.1. Type I lissencephaly. Classic or type I lissencephaly is characterized by a markedly thickened cortex overlying a reduced volume of white matter (Fig. 11.20). Ventricular enlargement is also frequent. These macroscopic features, especially the altered white:gray ratio, can be seen on fetal or postnatal MRI. Histologically, the thickened gray matter displays an abnormal horizontal lamination, with most cases showing a four-layer cortex in an indistinct "inside-out" pattern: The most superficial layer is an acellular molecular layer, followed by a highly cellular zone of large pyramidal neurons; a sparsely cellular layer with numerous myelinated fibers; and a deep, densely cellular layer of disorganized neurons (Fig. 11.21). The adjacent periventricular white matter may contain single or grouped heterotopic neurons. The four-layer pattern is seen with mutations in both *LIS1* and *XLIS* (*DCX*), the most common causes of lissencephaly. Mutations in *ARX* result in a three-layer lissencephaly. A two-layer lissencephaly has been identified, but no specific genetic mutations have been associated. The brains of patients with *TUBA1A* mutations show multiple anomalies, including abnormal white matter bundles and defects of the cortex (e.g., bilateral, often asymmetric, perisylvian polymicrogyria), basal ganglia, hippocampus, brainstem, and cerebellum. The pathologic findings described in cases associated with other lissencephaly genes are more variable. Anomalies of the corpus callosum, inferior olivary nuclei, cerebellum, or corticospinal tracts may be present.

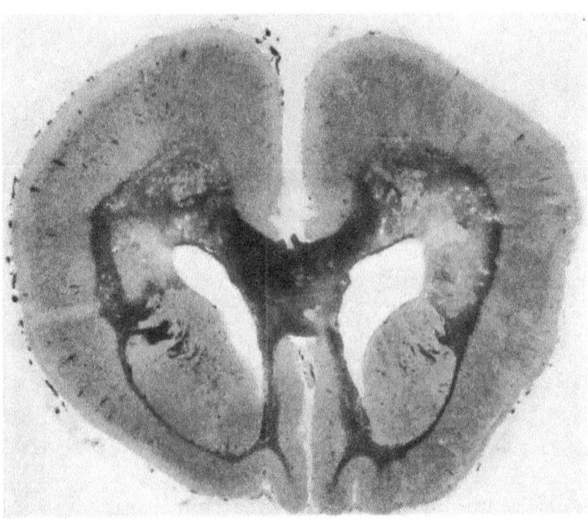

FIGURE 11.20 Agyria/pachygyria (Loyez stain).

Mutations in *LIS1* are the most common cause of lissencephaly. The autosomal dominant Miller–Dieker syndrome includes lissencephaly and characteristic facial features. This syndrome is due to a deletion of the short arm of chromosome 17, involving 17p13, which includes not only *LIS1* but also *14-3-3ε* (also called YWHAE), which functionally interacts with *LIS1* to disrupt cell migration. Isolated mutations in *LIS1* give rise to lissencephaly but without the full Miller–Dieker syndrome.

In X-linked lissencephaly, the gene *XLIS* encodes the protein DCX, also important in normal migration of neuroblasts. *XLIS* mutations in the female result in subcortical band heterotopia, as described previously. Males exhibit four-layer lissencephaly, particularly severe in the frontal lobes.

Other genes also associated with type I lissencephaly include *RELN, ARX, CDK5, NDE1, VLDLR*, tubulin genes (e.g., *TUBA1A* and *TUBG1*), molecular motor genes (e.g., *DYNC1H1* and *KIF2A*), and actin genes (e.g., *ACTB* and *ACTG1*).

11.2.4.4.2. Type II lissencephaly. Type II (LISII) or "cobblestone" lissencephaly (Fig. 11.22A, B) is a distinct cytoarchitectonic disorder characterized by overmigration of numerous clusters of neurons and glial cells into the subarachnoid space associated with disrupted leptomeninges. The obliteration of the subarachnoid space by the infiltration of neural glial tissue impairs cerebrospinal fluid dynamics and often leads to early hydrocephalus, which may be severe and is detectable by ultrasound examination as early as 16 weeks of gestation.

In LISII, there is no recognizable pattern of lamination. Instead, the superficial disorganized band of neurons, glia, and vascular connective tissue (meninges) overlies a band of neurons likely representing the remnant of the cortical plate. These bands are separated by an ill-defined line thought to represent the early embryonic pial surface (Fig. 11.22C). The pathogenesis of this type of lissencephaly is due to the overmigration of neurons and glia through a defective pial–glia limitans. The

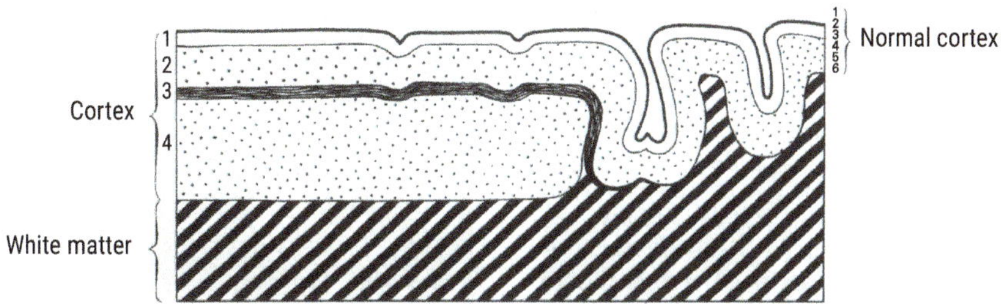

FIGURE 11.21 Cortical changes in agyria/pachygyria. (After Crome, L., and Stern, J. (1972). *Pathology of mental retardation* (2nd ed.). Baltimore: Williams & Wilkins.)

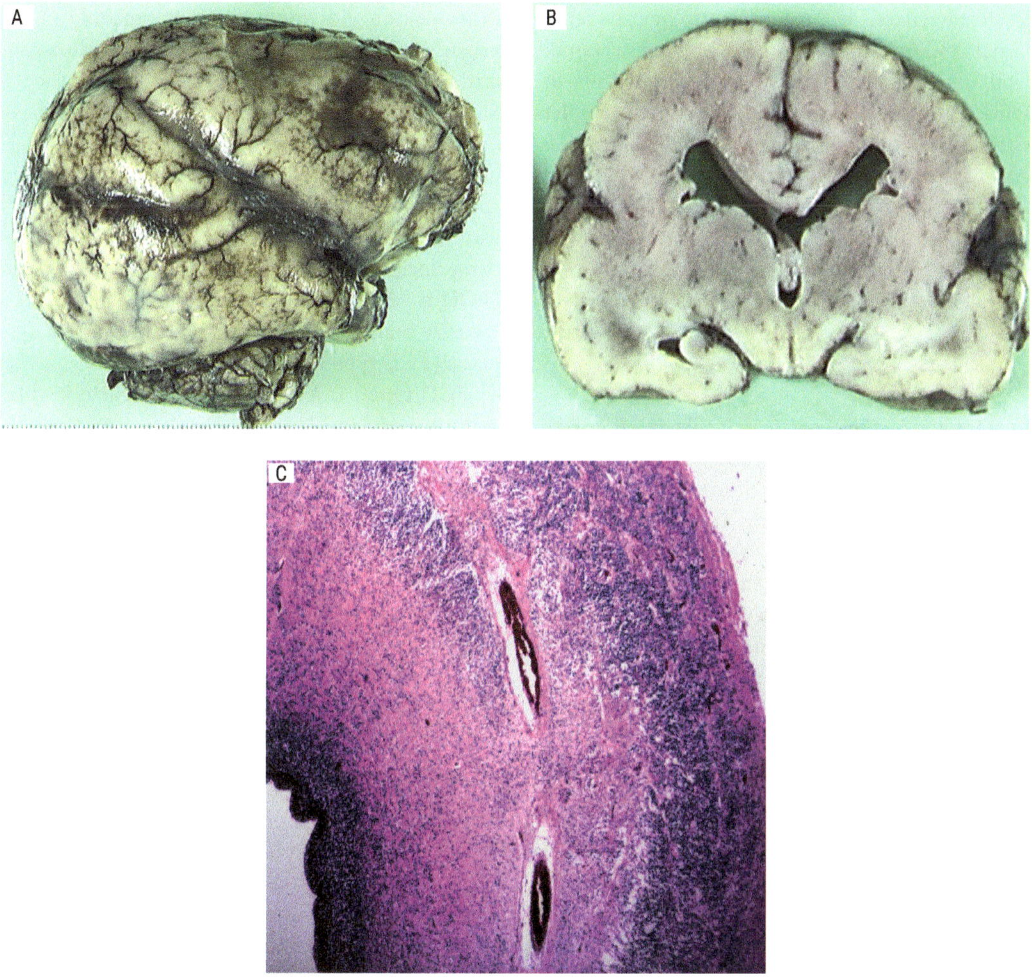

FIGURE 11.22 Type II lissencephaly: external appearance of cerebral hemispheres: cobblestone (**A**); coronal section (**B**) and whole-mount histological preparation (cresyl violet stain) (**C**) showing ventricular enlargement and characteristic cortical malformation with neuroglial ectopia extending into and obliterating the arachnoid space. Arachnoidal vessels are seen at the interface between the ectopic tissue and the residual cortical plate.

underlying molecular defect in all known cases is a disruption in O-glycosylation, primarily affecting dystroglycan. The known genes, including *POMT1, POMT2, POMGNT1, FKTN* (fukutin), *FKRP* (fukutin-related protein), *B3GALNT2, B4GAT1* (B3GNT1), and *LARGE1,* are all glycosyltransferases. Mutations in one of these genes have been found in 32–50% of patients. Newly identified genes have been described. In addition to the cerebral hemisphere defect, involvement of the brainstem and cerebellum is commonly seen.

This class of disorders represents a continuum, with brain, ocular, and muscular involvement, the most severe called Walker–Warburg syndrome, and also including the muscle–eye–brain diseases and Fukuyama muscular and cerebral dystrophy. The Walker–Warburg syndrome (Online Mendelian Inheritance in Man [OMIM] 236670), also known under the HARD±E acronym (hydrocephalus, agyria, retinal dysplasia, encephalocele), is characterized by major neurological deficit, visual and muscular impairment, and a rapidly fatal outcome. Less severe examples within the same spectrum, with subtle eye abnormalities, less significant neurological deficit, and a milder muscular dystrophy, include muscle–eye–brain disease, first described in the Finnish population (OMIM 253280), and Fukuyama muscular and cerebral dystrophy, common in Japan (OMIM 253800).

11.2.4.5. LOCALIZED OR FOCAL MALFORMATIONS

11.2.4.5.1. Focal cortical dysplasia. Focal cortical dysplasia (FCD) is a localized or multifocal, or even multilobar, cortical malformation, frequently found in surgical corticectomy or hemispherectomy specimens removed from patients with intractable epilepsy. The younger the child or infant from whom a specimen originates, the greater the likelihood that it will represent severe FCD. There is much overlap of imaging features between the different types of FCD; however, MRI may be normal. MRI alterations typically associated with FCD type II include increased cortical thickness, a blurring of the gray–white matter junction, a transmantle sign, and/or gyration anomalies.

Macroscopic examination of the resected specimen is often unremarkable, although thickening of the gyri or blurring of the gray–white matter border have been reported. Early neuropathological reports of FCD by Crome and later Taylor described "the congregations of large, bizarre neurones" sometimes in association with "grotesque cells, probably of glial origin" in a brain with cytoarchitectural disorganization in the cerebral cortex of epileptic patients. Since then, a large spectrum of anomalies have been described in the diagnosis of FCD. An international consensus classification system described specific clinicopathological entities in 2011, which was updated recently (Table 11.1). It distinguishes two principal forms of cortical dysplasia in isolation (FCD types I and II) from cases associated with a separate brain lesion distinct from the cortical dysplasia (FCD type III) (Table 11.1).

FCD type I is a malformation characterized by abnormal cortical layering, consisting of a microcolumnar, rather than a horizontal laminar, cortical architecture (FCD type Ia) or, alternately, in defective horizontal lamination with lamina-specific neuronal paucity, but this pattern is much more controversial (FCD type Ib). The combination of the abnormalities seen in both Ia and Ib is designated as FCD type Ic.

Table 11.1 Classification System of Focal Cortical Dysplasia (FCD) Proposed by the International League Against Epilepsy (ILAE)

FCD type I (isolated)	FCD with abundant microcolums (FCD type Ia)	FCD with abnormal tangential cortical lamination (FCD type Ib)	FCD with abnormal vertical and horizontal abnormalities (FCD type Ic)	
FCD type II (isolated)	FCD with dysmorphic neurons (FCD type IIa)		FCD with dysmorphic neurons and balloon cells (FCD type IIb)	
FCD type III (associated with principal lesion)	Cortical dyslamination in the temporal lobe associated with hippocampal sclerosis (FCD type IIIa)	Cortical dyslamination adjacent to brain tumor (FCD type IIIb)	Cortical dyslamination adjacent to vascular malformation (FCD type IIIc)	Cortical lamination abnormalities adjacent to lesion acquired during early life (e.g., from trauma, ischemic injury, encephalitis) (FCD type IIId)

Source: From Najm et al., *Epilepsia*, 2022;63:1899–1919.

The designation FCD type II requires evidence of dysplastic, megalocytic neurons (dysmorphic neurons) mixed with normal neurons (FCD type IIa) without balloon cells. In FCD type IIb, both dysmorphic neurons (Fig. 11.23A) and balloon cells (Fig. 11.23C, D) are present.

Abnormal neurons in areas of FCD show cytoskeletal changes, such as coarse intracytoplasmic fibrillary inclusions, which stain with antibodies to high and medium molecular weight (phosphorylated) neurofilaments, to microtubule-associated protein (MAP), as well as weakly to ubiquitin. Although these inclusions are reminiscent of neurofibrillary tangles seen in Alzheimer disease (and can be readily identified with silver impregnation techniques), they do not stain with antibodies to paired helical filaments (PHFs). As well, ultrastructural examination fails to show PHFs; instead, the cytoplasm contains skeins of interwoven filaments.

In addition, dysplastic cortical cells are positive with antibodies to immature MAPs (MAP1B, 2C); this may reflect an increased plasticity and remodeling of dendrites in these cells. Dysplastic cells also stain with antibodies to the embryonal form of the cell adhesion molecule N-CAM (E-NCAM) and to developmental neurofilaments nestin and internexin, supporting the idea that the phenomenon represents a failure of maturation. Balloon cells in FCD stain with anti-glial fibrillary acidic protein (GFAP), vimentin, GFAP-delta, and nestin antibodies, in keeping with their ultrastructural identity as intermediate cytoplasmic filaments, and αB-crystallin. In addition, some cells contain neuronal markers, and dual labeling has been demonstrated, thus reflecting intermediate glial and neuronal differentiation. The proliferation index of these cells is low.

An extreme form of neuronal migration abnormality is represented by the rare epileptogenic malformation of hemimeganencephaly (HME), in which a malformed cerebral hemisphere is markedly enlarged compared to the more "normal" hemisphere. Neuropathologic findings in resected HME

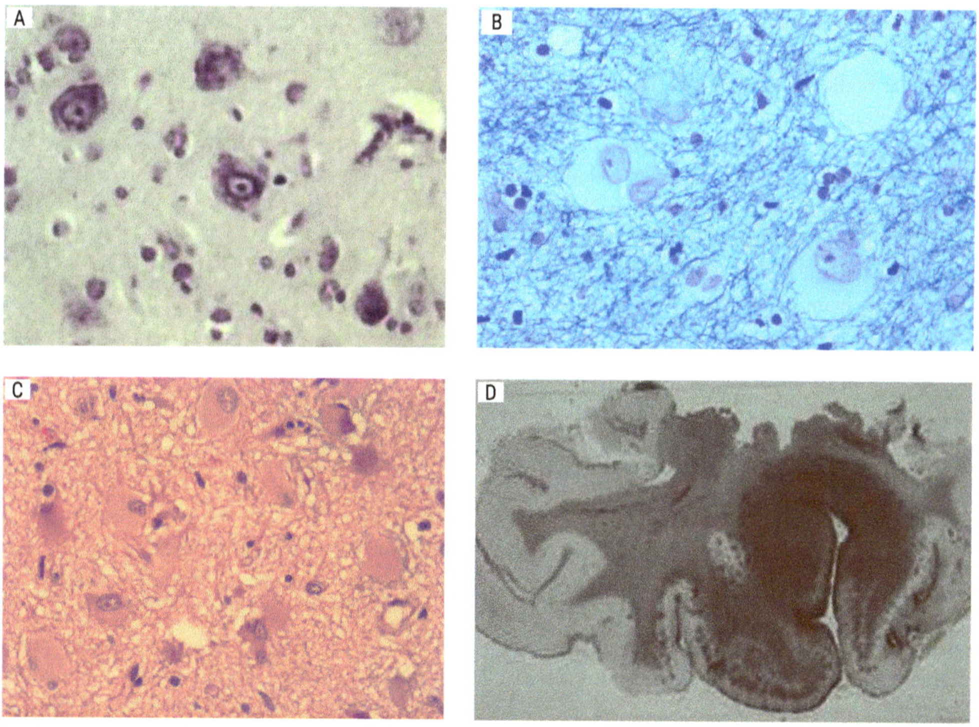

FIGURE 11.23 Focal cortical dysplasia. (**A**) Dysplastic neurons in focal cortical dysplasia. The neurons are enlarged and show thickening of the nuclear membrane. They are abnormally oriented within the isocortex (cresyl violet stain). (**B**) Aggregates of balloon cells in the white matter underlying an area of focal cortical dysplasia (Luxol fast blue/Nissl). (**C**) Balloon cells in the isocortex in a region of focal cortical dysplasia (H&E). (**D**) An area of cortical dysplasia with marked gliosis as seen on GFAP immunostaining.

specimens are extremely variable; some cases show features of severe FCD type II, although many lack the balloon cell change described, despite pronounced neuronal disorganization and abnormal polarity. In others, hemilissencephaly (see Section 11.2.4.4) has been observed.

Most cases of FCD occur sporadically, but rare familial cases are reported. In patients with FCD type II and hemigalencephaly, somatic gain-of-function variants in the mammalian target of rapamycin (mTOR) and its activators (e.g., AKT3, MTOR, PIK3CA, and RHEB), as well as germline, somatic, and two-hit loss-of-function variants in its repressors (DEPDC5, TSC1, and TSC2), are found. Dysmorphic neurons and balloon cells both carry the pathogenic variants activating the mTOR pathway. Consequently, immunostaining of phosphorylated S6 protein, a marker of mTOR pathway activation, highlights the dysplastic cells.

The category FCD type III refers to a disorder of cortical lamination that is associated with a separate brain lesion, usually adjacent to the cortical dysplasia or at any rate affecting the same area/lobe. Four categories are proposed for FCD type III: FCD type IIIa associated with HS, FCD type IIIb associated with tumors, FCD type IIIc associated with vascular malformation, and FCD type IIId associated with another brain lesion acquired during early life.

Additional histological features reported in FCD include subpial layers of myelinated axons, reactive gliosis (Fig. 11.23D), subpial fibrillary ("Chaslin") gliosis (a nonspecific abnormality found in resection specimens from corticectomy for epilepsy, regardless of etiology), loss of axons, and increased numbers of corpora amylacea.

FCD with dysplatic neurons and balloon cells has overlapping features with the cortical tubers associated with tuberous sclerosis (TSC). However, the following characteristics should help distinguish between the two disorders: Patients with FCD show no systemic or cutaneous stigmata of TSC, absence of subependymal lesions or calcifications, and no family history or genetic cause of TSC. Tubers in TSC tend to be multiple and distributed throughout the cerebral hemispheres and are macroscopically recognizable, whereas lesions in FCD are more often solitary. Microscopic examination of tubers shows dysmorphic enlarged neurons and balloon cells with eccentric nuclei and glassy eosinophilic cytoplasm. Gliosis, vascular hyperplasia, and calcifications may be prominent. A peculiar "wheat sheaf" arrangement of astrocytes in the subpial region is typical of tubers. However, differentiation from FCD is not always possible on microscopic examination alone, and genetic analysis can be carried out when there is uncertainty. The two genes (*TSC1* and *TSC2*) in which mutations/deletions occur to cause TSC can be analyzed. Although antibodies to the respective gene products (hamartin and tuberin) are widely available, staining of a suspected tuber or FCD specimen with these reagents is not of value in differentiating the two types of lesions. Several studies have also been able to distinguish these two entities based on the activation of S6 kinase in the mTOR pathway.

11.2.4.5.2. Mild malformations of cortical development. Mild cortical malformations may not be visualized by either imaging or naked eye examination. The spectrum of abnormalities recognized on microscopic examination features blurring of the gray–white matter boundary and increased numbers of heterotopic neurons in the white matter (mild malformations of cortical development [mMCD] type II). These abnormalities can be associated with seizure disorders. Heterotopic neurons in cortical layer 1 (mMCD type I) have not been observed in surgical case series. mMCD (type II) can be characterized on MRI by a hyperintense signal of the white matter with blurring of the gray–white matter junction.

11.2.5. Disorders of hindbrain development

11.2.5.1. MALFORMATIONS OF THE CEREBELLUM

A broad range of anomalies affect the cerebellum, ranging from macroscopic structural defects to subtle abnormalities visible only at microscopic examination. The malformations may affect primarily the vermis, parts of the vermis, the lateral hemispheres, or the vermis and lateral hemispheres.

11.2.5.1.1. Dandy–Walker malformation. The Dandy–Walker malformation (Fig. 11.24) consists of an anteriorly rotated, incompletely formed cerebellum giving rise to a cyst-like dilation of the fourth ventricle (i.e., no true cyst is present). The tentorium is superiorly positioned, thus resulting in a relatively expanded posterior fossa. The vermis may be absent or hypoplastic; when

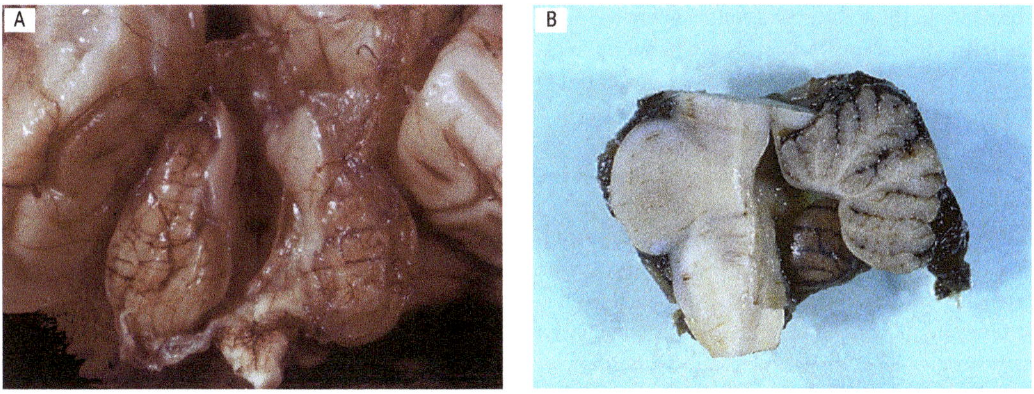

FIGURE 11.24 Dandy–Walker syndrome, with agenesis of the vermis and cystic dilation of the fourth ventricle: (**A**) posterior view; (**B**) sagittal section of brainstem and cerebellum.

hypoplastic, it is primarily the inferior vermis that is affected. Microscopic examination of the inferior vermis and contiguous posterior membrane around the foramen of Magendie demonstrates an atretic cerebellum. The lateral hemispheres of the cerebellum may be normal or show variable degrees of hypoplasia. Malformations of the brainstem and supratentorial structures are sometimes also present in association with the Dandy–Walker malformation and should be investigated by imaging studies inasmuch as the finding of additional anomalies can be associated with a worse prognosis. Many chromosomal anomalies have been associated. The etiology of most, if not all, cases of human Dandy–Walker malformation appears to be genetic in origin. Mutations in *FGF17*, *NID1*, *LAMC1*, and *AP1S2* have been found in patients with the Dandy–Walker malformation. Approximately 20% of patients with Walker–Warburg syndrome are reported to also have a Dandy–Walker malformation, but in addition the cerebellum in these patients shows more severe dysplasia, including loss of folia in the lateral hemispheres.

11.2.5.1.2. Joubert syndrome. Joubert syndrome includes cerebellar vermis hypoplasia along with a deep ventral midline cleft in the pons. The cerebellar peduncles are abnormally elongated, such that when the brainstem is viewed in the horizontal plane, the hindbrain has been described as having a "molar tooth" appearance.

Although originally believed to be a single entity, Joubert syndrome is now recognized as part of a broad range of disorders, which fall into a variety of subtypes depending on whether affected individuals also have other CNS and extra-CNS abnormalities. All of these subtypes are associated with mutations in cilia-related genes; accordingly, Joubert syndrome is now classified as one of the ciliopathies. More than 30 genes have been implicated in this syndrome.

11.2.5.1.3. Chiari malformations. In the late 1800s, Chiari described a series of what he referred to as cerebellar herniation anomalies. In the Chiari II malformation as described above, the cerebellar vermis is displaced below the foramen magnum and overlies the lower medulla and dorsal rostral spinal cord. The Chiari I malformation involves the cerebellar tonsils, as opposed to the vermis, which extend below the foramen magnum (by definition >1.5 cm inferior). While in the setting of increasing intracranial pressure within the posterior fossa, brain herniation can lead to displacement and, ultimately, necrosis of the cerebellar tonsils, modern imaging techniques have shown that displacement of the tonsils can be seen in patients with no symptoms. The displaced tonsils may show dysplasia; syringomyelia, hydromyelia, syringobulbia, or hydrobulbia may coexist. Chiari III malformations are quite rare and represent the herniation or inclusion of posterior fossa elements, mainly the cerebellum, in an occipital encephalocele.

11.2.5.1.4. Rhombencephalosynapsis. In rhombencephalosynapsis, the vermis is replaced by medially situated (fused) cerebellar hemispheres containing the dentate nucleus crossing the midline. The fourth ventricle is obtruded. The malformation may be extended rostrally to the mesencephalon, and in such cases, forking or atresia of the aqueduct with secondary obstructive hydrocephalus is observed. In these cases, the colliculi may be indistinct. Rhombencephalosynapsis can be found in association with HPE but is more commonly found as an isolated defect.

11.2.5.1.5. Posterior fossa arachnoid cyst. Arachnoid cysts may arise in the posterior fossa as they do at other intracranial sites. When in the midline, these true cysts may compress and displace the cerebellar vermis and cause hydrocephalus. It may at times be difficult to distinguish these arachnoid cysts from a Dandy–Walker malformation; however, the presence of a compressed fourth ventricle is more in keeping with a retrocerebellar arachnoid cyst, whereas expansion of the fourth ventricle is the hallmark of Dandy–Walker malformation.

11.2.5.2. ABNORMALITIES OF THE AQUEDUCT OF SYLVIUS

Isolated aqueductal stenosis, in which there is narrowing or forking of the lumen, in the absence of microscopic abnormalities of the aqueduct is rare. A rare form of X-linked recessive hydrocephalus with stenosis of the aqueduct of Sylvius (HSAS) has been reported in males with hydrocephalus, absence or severe hypoplasia of the medullary pyramids, and abducted thumbs. This combination of findings is known as X-linked hydrocephalus or MASA (mental retardation, aphasia, shuffling gait, and adducted thumbs) syndrome, SPG1 (X-linked complicated hereditary spastic paraplegia type 1), and X-linked agenesis of the corpus callosum, and it is associated with mutations in *L1-CAM*.

In cases of atresia of the aqueduct of Sylvius, the aqueduct is abnormally shaped (forking) or may be entirely replaced by a few rosettes. Atresia of the aqueduct may be post-hemorrhagic or found in fetal disruption syndromes, including intrauterine strokes (Fig. 11.25). Occlusion of the aqueduct may occur in the setting of infectious, neoplastic, or hemorrhagic disease and can result in triventricular hydrocephalus. In such cases, a portion of the lumen of the aqueduct may be of normal size (or dilated), but at other sites it may be occluded by necrotic tissue, inflammatory debris, or hemorrhage. The ependymal layer of the aqueduct, as well as elsewhere in the ventricular system, is disrupted and replaced by reactive gliosis and pigment-laden macrophages. At later stages, the aqueduct may be occluded by a glial plug or covered over by a glial septum.

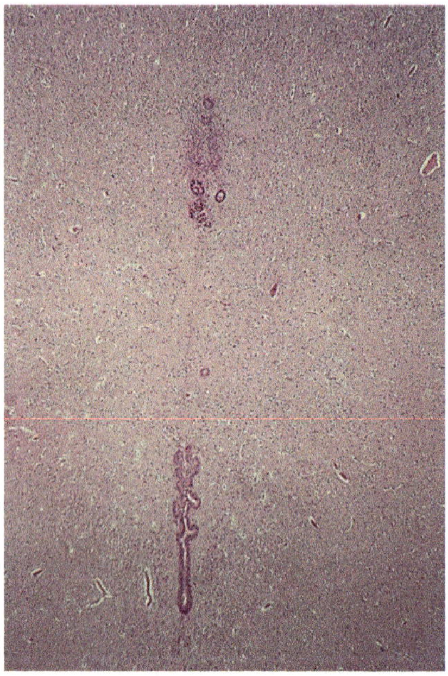

FIGURE 11.25 Aqueductal atresia.

11.3. DISRUPTIONS OF DEVELOPING BRAIN

The foregoing sections have considered primarily abnormalities of development related to genetic or environmental influences on early organogenesis. Disruptions often affect both gray (i.e., cortical and deep nuclear elements) and white matter at the same time, manifested clinically as "hypoxic–ischemic encephalopathy." However, their distinct neuropathologic patterns are discussed separately. Disruptive lesions are reported in association with a variety of situations causing altered in utero hemodynamics, including trauma, gas intoxication, drug abuse, and twin gestations.

11.3.1. Lesions of developing gray matter

Exogenous processes disrupting the normal sequence of neuronal migration and cortical differentiation (encephaloclastic processes) usually act after midgestation. They lead to a spectrum of cortical abnormalities, ranging from disturbed cytoarchitecture, often at the margins of cysts (porencephaly), to loss of cortical plate segments ("basket brain") and complete absence of supratentorial brain tissue (hydranencephaly). Lesser degrees of insult may have effects on selective neuronal populations.

Finally, disruptions of germinal matrix and deep nuclei of the diencephalon and brainstem have distinctive features. The vast majority of disruptions have in common some element(s) of decreased perfusion (ischemia) and low oxygen tension (hypoxia), phenomena that tend to occur together (hence the commonly used term *hypoxia–ischemia*).

11.3.1.1. ENCEPHALOCLASTIC LESIONS OF DEVELOPING NEOCORTEX

11.3.1.1.1. Porencephaly. *Porencephaly* refers to any defect extending from the brain surface toward the ventricle. Most usually, these are in the region of the Sylvian fissure (Fig. 11.26). They may be bilateral, sometimes denominated "schizencephaly." The margins are smooth and have abnormal gyral architecture, either polymicrogyria or gyri radiating outwardly from the lips of the defect. The polymicrogyria found at the margins in some cases is thought to be due to incomplete ischemia in the tissue lying near the defect.

Porencephalies lack significant glial scarring. These features are consistent with an intrauterine insult occurring after neuroblast migration and prior to gyration. The basal ganglia, cerebellum, and brainstem are not affected, although the thalamus and descending white matter tracts may be secondarily atrophic. Clinical manifestations are related to the area of involvement and may include hemiparesis, blindness, and seizures.

11.3.1.1.2. Hydranencephaly. Hydranence phaly ("bubble brain") refers to the residua of intrauterine massive hemispheric necrosis. Various insults, including trauma, attempted abortion, TORCH infection, and household gas intoxication, have been correlated with hydranencephaly, although most antecedent events are unknown. The extent of destruction dictates the clinical picture, which typically includes spasticity, severe seizures, and vegetative signs; mortality in infancy is high. Because the areas involved are often in the distribution of the carotid arteries, the inferior temporal and occipital lobes tend to be preserved, with polymicrogyria at the interface. The basal ganglia are variably affected, but the thalamus and descending tracts are always atrophic. Head enlargement develops in longer surviving infants as a result of scarring of the aqueduct leading to hydrocephalus. Hydranencephaly has been reported in a familial form due to a distinctive proliferative vasculopathy (Fowler hydrancephaly or Fowler's syndorme) caused by deletions and mutations in the *FLVCR2* gene.

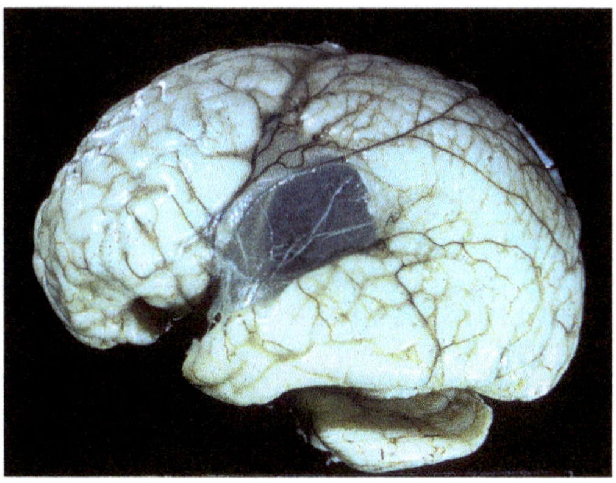

FIGURE 11.26 Porencephaly.

11.3.1.1.3. Basket brain. Basket brain is considered intermediate between porencephaly and hydranencephaly. The cingulate gyri and medial hemispheric structures are preserved (corresponding to the "handle" of the basket), while the lateral parietal and frontal lobes are cystic bilaterally.

11.3.1.1.4. Multicystic encephalomalacia. Multicystic encephalomalacia (also known as multicystic leukoencephalopathy) differs from porencephaly and hydranencephaly by the occurrence of innumerable cysts separated by glial septa, involving the cortex and white matter in all lobes (Fig. 11.27). Microscopic evidence of resolved infarction and hemorrhage, including macrophages and hemosiderin, can be seen accompanying the marked gliosis and suggests an insult in the perinatal period (i.e., late gestation to early infancy). As with porencephaly and hydranencephaly, associated events have included maternal suicide attempts, infection, and parturition-related complications such as cord prolapse. In surviving infants, severe cognitive and motor deficits along with epilepsy are common.

11.3.1.1.5. Ischemic strokes. Perinatal ischemic strokes, usually arising in the territory of the middle cerebral artery, can be seen often in the setting of congenital heart disease, for example, or other conditions requiring extracorporeal membrane oxygenation. These strokes are similar to those occurring in adults in terms of their histologic evolution.

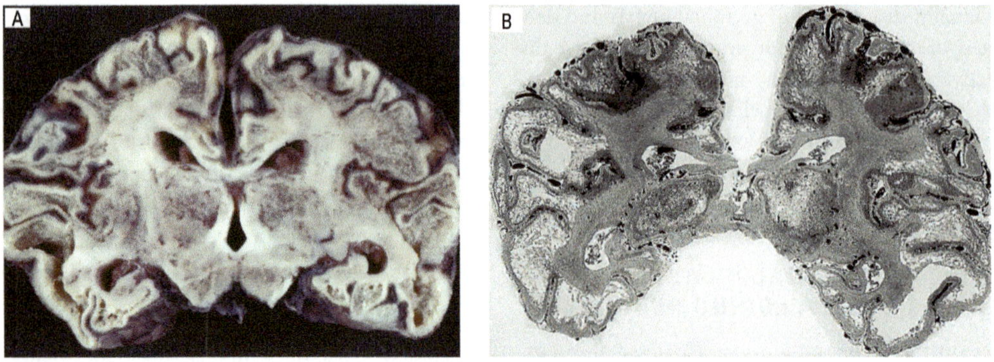

FIGURE 11.27 Multicystic encephalomalacia in a case of neonatal carbon monoxide poisoning: (**A**) gross appearance; (**B**) Loyez stain.

11.3.1.1.6. Selective neuronal necrosis. The premature infant has a somewhat different profile of neuronal vulnerability to hypoxia–ischemia than that of the full-term baby, believed to be due to variations in patterns of cerebral blood flow. For example, the parasagittal regions, which are the border zones between anterior and middle cerebral artery territories, are especially susceptible to hypoxia–ischemia. Injury in these areas gives rise to basket brain or lesser degrees of porencephaly, as described previously. The depths of sulci are end-arterial regions so that neurons there are susceptible to hypoxia–ischemia, leading to ulegyria, a mushroom-like appearance of sulcal atrophy with preservation of gyral crests (Fig. 11.28). For unclear reasons, neurons within the deeper cortical layers are more prone to injury than are neurons in upper layers, giving rise to laminar necrosis, a layer of destruction within the cortical ribbon. The pattern of vulnerability depends on the developmental stage; for example, Sommer's sector of the hippocampus is vulnerable in the term baby, whereas the subiculum is susceptible in the premature. Coexistence of neuronal necrosis in predictable patterns, as in pontosubicular necrosis, may be seen and may be highly associated with white matter necrosis (discussed in Section 11.3.2).

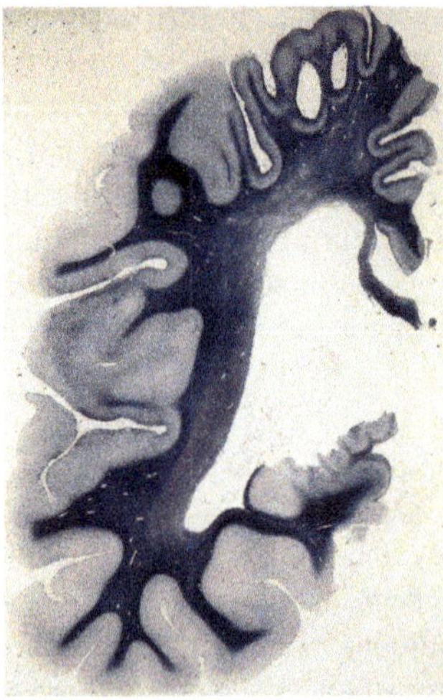

FIGURE 11.28 Ulegyria: Loyez stain showing atrophy of sulci with relative preservation of gyral crests.

11.3.1.2. ENCEPHALOCLASTIC LESIONS OF DEVELOPING BASAL GANGLIA AND THALAMUS

In both term and premature infants, thalamic and basal ganglionic neurons may undergo necrosis, resulting in mineralization (or ferrugination) of individual cells. In babies surviving a year or more, damage to the thalamus and basal ganglia may lead to disturbed architecture known as *status marmoratus* (or "état marbré"), in which aberrant myelination of disoriented axons and glial processes leads to a marbled gross appearance.

Clinical features accompanying status marmoratus classically include static (nonprogressive) bilateral choreoathetosis, motor and intellectual retardation, spastic diplegia, and sometimes epilepsy; the inexact term *cerebral palsy* has been applied to these symptoms in many such affected individuals.

11.3.1.3. LESIONS OF THE GANGLIONIC EMINENCE (GERMINAL MATRIX)

The periventricular gray matter in utero is composed of immature cells (neural progenitors, neuroblasts, and glial progenitors), proliferation and migration of which peak between the 18th and 26th gestational weeks. Because the vessels of this region are remodeling actively during this time and therefore have incompletely formed basal lamina and loosely interdigitated glial end feet, they are particularly vulnerable to any alterations in hemodynamics.

Periventricular hemorrhages are a common lesion in prematurely delivered infants who typically have respiratory compromise and are hemodynamically labile. Large periventricular hemorrhages can result in extensive destruction of precursor cells as well as adjacent mature structures, such as the caudate and internal capsule, and can interrupt the overlying ventricular (ependymal) surface, leading to intraventricular hemorrhage and hydrocephalus. Individual cases vary from small hemorrhages limited to the germinal matrix (Grade I) to those with intraventricular extension, ventricular enlargement, and intraparenchymal hemorrhage (Grade IV). In surviving infants, macrophages resorb the hemorrhage, resulting in periventricular cysts. Hemosiderosis, gliosis, and rosette-like remnants of ependymal cells may remain. In noncavitating healed lesions, mineralization of cell bodies and processes may persist as markers of injury.

Hemorrhages of the choroid plexus, although not ganglionic eminence lesions, are mentioned here because they can have the same sequelae (i.e., hydrocephalus) as intraventricular hemorrhages arising from the germinal matrix.

Coexistence of deep (germinal matrix) and surface (cortical plate) disruptions is common in the porencephalies described previously. Likewise, some forms of perisylvian polymicrogyria are thought to reflect a combination of disruption of the local glia limitans and cortical plate together with interruption of precursor migration leading to complex cortical dysplasia and deep gray matter heterotopia.

11.3.2. Lesions of developing white matter

In the human, white matter development lags behind gray matter development, such that the vulnerable period for the former is the final trimester through the first year of life—that is, the period of myelinogenesis.

The major cerebral white matter lesion in the perinatal period is diffuse white matter injury (DWMI), encompassing the previously used terms *periventricular leukomalacia* (PVL), defined as focal white matter necrosis, as well as diffuse cerebral white matter gliosis (DWMG), with which PVL is virtually always associated; these two patterns represent points along a spectrum of severity, rather than separate pathologic entities. DWMI frequently accompanies gray matter lesions comprising the "encephalopathy of prematurity."

Diffuse white matter injury generally arises in the sick premature infant with immature lungs, respiratory distress syndrome, and hemodynamic instability. In these critically ill preterm infants with multiple metabolic derangements, it is difficult to distinguish specific clinical signs secondary to white matter injury. However, lower limb weakness may occur in the first weeks of life in infants with cystic PVL documented by neuroimaging. In term infants, DWMI typically arises in the setting of severe cardiopulmonary dysfunction. The long-term consequences of cystic PVL include spastic diplegia or quadriplegia ("cerebral palsy"), intellectual disability, learning deficits, and seizures.

On MRI, cystic cavities may be obvious, along with evidence of delayed or permanently deficient myelination as determined by signal characteristics. In children followed by MRI over time, early cavitations may be replaced by glial scars with adjacent white matter hypomyelination and hydrocephalus ex vacuo, suggesting a capacity for remodeling in some lesions.

11.3.2.1. NEUROPATHOLOGIC FINDINGS

11.3.2.1.1. Macroscopy. In severe PVL forms, the necrotic changes occur mainly, but not exclusively, in the periventricular regions within 15 mm of the ventricular wall, with a predilection for sites anterior to the frontal horn; lateral corners of the lateral ventricles at the level of the foramen of Monro; and lateral regions of the trigone and occipital horn, including the optic radiations. Typically, they measure 2–6 mm in diameter. The acute foci (i.e., coagulation necrosis) may not be identifiable grossly. Organizing foci are identified as chalky "white spots" due to the presence of lipid-laden macrophages. Cavitation occurs within a few weeks, and eventually the cysts may collapse to form a solid glial scar. In severe damage, periventricular cavitation remains (Fig. 11.29). In some instances, widespread necrosis and cavitation of the white matter occur. Severe or long-standing damage is characterized by an overall reduction in the cerebral white matter, thinning of the

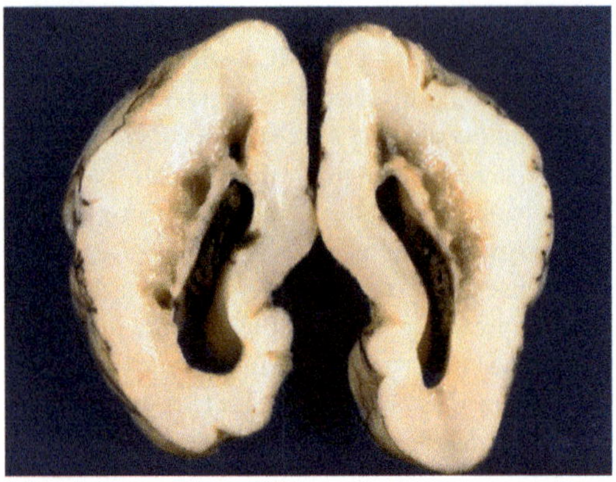

FIGURE 11.29 Periventricular leukomalacia.

corpus callosum, and ventriculomegaly. The volume loss also likely represents the consequences of diffuse injury of the white matter surrounding the necroses.

In cases of early or mild DWMI lacking any focal necroses (DWMG), there are no specific gross findings. In severe cases, DWMG may be appreciable as duskiness of the white matter, accompanied by pallor of the overlying cortex ("white ribbon effect"), and may result in decreased overall volume of the cerebral white matter, thinning of the corpus callosum, and ventriculomegaly of varying degree.

11.3.2.1.2. Histopathologic findings. In DWMI (with or without necrosis), the predominant feature is reactive ("hypertrophic") astrocytes, defined morphologically in hematoxylin and eosin--stained sections by pale vesicular nuclei and eosinophilic, irregular, hyaline cytoplasm. They are usually smaller than the conspicuous reactive astrocytes seen in the adult brain and are present throughout the periventricular, central, and even intragyral white matter. The cell body stains positively for GFAP. Reactive astrocytes may occur in association with amphophilic globules and acutely damaged glia, as well as microscopic mineralization. DWMI is also accompanied by microgliosis.

White matter necroses undergo a stereotyped evolution histologically, beginning with changes within 24 hours of the insult. This process is characterized by hypereosinophilia; nuclear pyknosis; and acutely necrotic, swollen axons (spheroids), which stain immunocytochemically for β-amyloid precursor protein. Within a week, the necrotic foci become organized, with infiltrating macrophages in the center and reactive astrocytes at the margin. Cavitation with the development of periventricular cysts occurs within a few weeks. In some instances, the cysts collapse and focal glial scars form, typically with lipid-laden macrophages and mineralized axons. The accompanying gliosis/microgliosis preferentially involves the deep, as compared to the intragyral, white matter.

The long-term consequences of DWMI include delayed myelination, thought to reflect adverse effects on the developing oligodendrocytes (OLs) in the deep white matter. Myelination delay is noted as pallor of staining on Luxol fast blue, or complete absence of staining in dense glial scars, with mineralization, even many years after the insult.

Perinatal white matter damage typically coexists with a variety of other CNS lesions, including germinal matrix hemorrhage, thalamic infarcts or gliosis, and hippocampal and brainstem gliosis; occasionally, widespread cortical injury is also present.

11.3.2.2. PATHOGENESIS

Diffuse white matter injury involves immature cerebral white matter in the fetal period and early infancy when it is populated predominantly by pre-OLs and active myelin sheath synthesis has not begun. The peak age occurrence of PVL between 24 and 32 weeks, before mature myelin basic protein+ OLs arise, coupled with the long-term outcome of delayed myelination, suggests that pre-OLs, particularly in the diffusely gliotic white matter, are the main target of the insult. Multiple factors contribute to this age-dependent vulnerability and reflect these cells' sensitivity to excitotoxicity, damage from reactive oxygen species (ROS) and reactive nitrogen species (RNS), and cytokine toxicity/inflammation.

Immature cerebral white matter is especially vulnerable to ischemia due to the presence of vascular end zones in combination with the propensity for sick premature infants to exhibit a pressure-passive circulation reflecting disturbed cerebral autoregulation. The major causes of DWMI are (1) cerebral ischemia/reperfusion in the critically ill premature infant with impaired regulation of cerebral blood flow and (2) maternal or fetal infection that is postulated to trigger an inflammatory response in the fetal brain. These two insults are not mutually exclusive, and each may potentiate the other. According to the multiple-hit hypothesis, maternal and/or fetal infection/inflammation can act as predisposing factors, making the brain more susceptible to a second stress (sensitization process), such as hypoxic–ischemic or excitotoxic insults.

In cystic PVL, one may consider the focal necrosis as the central core of tissue damage (i.e., an infarct), resulting from the most severe ischemic insult in the arterial end zones, and the surrounding diffuse gliosis (or whole lesion in DWMG) as the "penumbra" in the surrounding tissue (where the blood flow reduction is less severe), with the capacity to recover on restoration of perfusion. In DWMG, the initial acute stage of injury to the targeted pre-OLs evolves into the subacute and chronic stages, characterized by an inflammatory response with activated astrocytes and microglia and subsequent production and release of cytokines. The final stage includes recovery and repair, with potential reinitiation of myelination by repopulated developing OLs that mature to myelin-producing OLs in the absence of additional cerebral ischemia/reperfusion, weeks or months following the perinatal insult.

Regarding specific cellular mechanisms of damage in DWMI (with or without necroses), oligodendrocytes and oligodendroglial progenitors are exquisitely vulnerable to oxidative stress and inflammation. Cerebral ischemia leads to oxygen and glucose depletion with energy ("pump") failure in all parenchymal cells in the cerebral white matter, including pre-OLs, astrocytes, and axons traversing it, thereby triggering excitotoxic and nonexcitotoxic mechanisms of injury and cell death.

Reperfusion is hazardous because there may be an increase in oxygen in excess of consumption, resulting in the formation of ROS. Production of excessive RNS is also suggested by the presence of nitrotyrosin in developing OLs. Both ROS and RNS are postulated to preferentially injure pre-OLs, leading to their loss, subsequent decreased mature myelin basic protein (MBP+) OLs, and delayed myelination in long-term survivors.

In addition to these "nonexcitotoxic" mechanisms of cell injury following oxygen deprivation that are shared by virtually all systemic cells, during the period of risk for PVL, developing OLs are also susceptible to excitotoxicity (i.e., cell injury induced by excessive levels of the excitatory amino acid neurotransmitter glutamate).

Finally, upregulation of cytokines in response to both hypoxia–ischemia and infection may exert cytokine toxicity to the vulnerable fetal cerebral white matter.

12

Pathology of Skeletal Muscle

TERESINHA EVANGELISTA, ANTHONY A. AMATO, BASIL T. DARRAS, AND UMBERTO De GIROLAMI

12.1. GENERAL CONSIDERATIONS

Neuromuscular pathology must always be evaluated in a multidisciplinary context. The integration of clinical features (age of onset, pattern of muscle involvement, disease course, family history, concurrent medical problems, and medications), electrophysiological studies (electromyography [EMG] and nerve conduction velocity studies), laboratory results (creatine kinase [CK] levels, the presence of a monoclonal gammopathy), and radiologic muscle imaging allows for the formulation of the most probable clinical diagnostic hypotheses preceding the biopsy.

The objective of the biopsy is then to confirm, extend, or perhaps disprove these initial hypotheses. Determining the need for a muscle biopsy and ensuring its performance and interpretation are best accomplished by a collaborative effort between the referring physician and the neuropathologist.

12.2. BIOPSY OF SKELETAL MUSCLE

To obtain the best result possible from a muscle biopsy, some important aspects must be considered: the site of the biopsy (choice of the muscle to be sampled), the protocol chosen to process the tissue, and the histopathologic methods utilized to examine it. The surgical procedure may be an open muscle biopsy, or the tissue may be sampled through a muscle biopsy needle. The choice of one or the other method varies depending on the local expertise. The quantity of muscle tissue obtained by a needle biopsy is smaller than that usually available from an open incision, and that difference should be considered in the procedure chosen by the physician who requests the biopsy.

12.2.1. Site of the biopsy

The diagnostic yield of a muscle biopsy is higher if obtained from a moderately affected muscle. Biopsy of clinically severely involved muscles should be avoided because it may only reveal nondiagnostic end-stage changes. Thus, if access to muscle imaging (magnetic resonance imaging [MRI], computed tomography, or ultrasound) is unavailable, the chosen muscle to be biopsied should have a Medical Research Council grade of about 4/5. When the clinical deficit is only mild muscle weakness (e.g., only in the hip girdle musculature, that is not typically biopsied), an EMG can help select the muscle for the procedure. The EMG should be performed on one side of the body and the biopsy on the contralateral limb. Sites of prior EMG needle examination, injections, or previous trauma should not be chosen because there may be focal necrosis or inflammation, leading to misleading information.

12.2.2. Techniques

12.2.2.1. TISSUE PREPARATION

Muscle biopsies are performed in a wide range of circumstances, from cases with a systemic disease that may manifest with neuromuscular deficit (e.g., vasculitis) to primary neuromuscular disorders. The choice of the initial techniques is often made considering the patient's clinical picture. However, many laboratories have a set panel of techniques they routinely use as a starting point.

Careful handling of the muscle samples at all stages is mandatory to avoid artifacts and obtain the maximum information from the biopsy. During the procedure, cauterization should not be used for hemostasis; the muscle should not be infiltrated with the anesthetic; and it should be processed immediately, particularly the frozen segments, to avoid degradation of enzymatic activity.

The following protocol is recommended: collection of one or two segments frozen in isopentane cooled in liquid nitrogen for cryostat sections, one fragment frozen in liquid nitrogen for molecular and biochemical studies, one fragment fixed in formalin for paraffin-embedded sections, and one smaller fragment fixed in glutaraldehyde to be embedded in plastic for electron microscopy. Where expertise is available, a specimen can be submitted for cell culture, allowing for research studies.

The study of the muscle biopsy includes the evaluation of paraffin and cryostat cross sections (and often longitudinal sections) stained with a battery of standard stains and often analysis of plastic-embedded sections to be further evaluated by electron microscopy as necessary. Histological stains routinely employed on frozen sections include hematoxylin and eosin (H&E), the modified Gomori trichrome (GT), periodic acid–Schiff (PAS), and oil red O (ORO). Histochemical reactions ordinarily employed include nicotinamide adenine dinucleotide–hydrogenated/reduced (NADH), succinate dehydrogenase (SDH), cytochrome *c* oxidase (COX) and/or COX/SDH, and adenosine triphosphatase (ATPase) at acid and alkaline pHs. Other specific histochemical stains are used in selected cases. Paraffin sections are particularly useful to assess the status of vessels, infectious/inflammatory changes, and the presence of neoplastic infiltrates. The study can be complemented with immunocytochemistry for specific proteins or immunologic markers and Congo red stain for assessment of amyloid deposits. Electron microscopy is utilized for the demonstration of specific ultrastructural abnormalities.

12.2.2.2. HISTOLOGICAL STAINS

12.2.2.2.1. Hematoxylin and eosin and modified Gomori Trichrome. H&E staining reveals the overall structure of the muscle and demonstrates abnormalities in fiber size and integrity, inflammatory infiltrates, and connective tissue. GT allows for evaluation of the distribution of the connective and adipose tissue; the mitochondria appear as fine red dots. Furthermore, abnormal accumulations of mitochondria such as in ragged red fibers, and red inclusions such as nemaline rods or other protein aggregates, can be demonstrated.

12.2.2.2.2. Periodic acid–Schiff technique and oil red O. PAS demonstrates the glycogen content of the muscle fibers. When there is an accumulation of PAS-positive material, the specificity for glycogen can be evaluated by digestion with α-amylase. If the material is resistant to digestion with α-amylase, that indicates the presence of polyglucosan. The content of intracytoplasmic lipids is revealed with ORO stain, where lipids appear as small orange-red droplets; they are more abundant in type 1 fibers. Under normal instances, the content in intracytoplasmic lipids and glycogen can be affected by diet and exercise.

12.2.2.3. MUSCLE ENZYME HISTOCHEMISTRY

Assessment of muscle pathology also relies on enzymatic reactions aimed at detecting endogenous enzymatic activities of muscle fibers. Selected methods convert soluble substrates into insoluble precipitates to demonstrate enzyme activity, such as myosin ATPase, COX, lysosomal enzymes, and the glycolytic pathway enzymes. These methods require frozen, unfixed tissue sections in which the native enzymatic activities are preserved and are used to differentiate fiber types or detect subcellular abnormalities.

12.2.2.3.1. Analyzing the different fiber types. By convention, muscle fibers can be of two types, type 1 and 2. Type 2 fibers may be further subdivided into 2A, 2B, and 2C (Table 12.1).

- One of the defining characteristics of type 1 or slow-twitch muscle fibers and type 2 fast-twitch fibers is that the two myosin ATPase isoforms have a different optimal pH. Advantage is taken of this difference by preincubating tissue at pH 4.3 or 9.4, respectively, and as a result, the histochemical reaction selectively demonstrates type 1 or type 2 fibers. The ATPase activity of type 1 fibers is weak at alkaline pH (9.4) but strong at pH 4.3; thus, type 1 fibers appear pale at pH 9.4 and dark at pH 4.3, and the reverse is true of type 2 fibers. This distinction can be further refined by carrying out the ATPase reaction at pH 4.63, which permits differentiation of type 2A, type 2B, and type 2C fibers (Fig. 12.1). A small percentage of fibers appear dark (i.e., strongly reactive at both acid and basic pH), and these are designated 2C fibers. They are interpreted as fetal/regenerating fibers because this lack of pH sensitivity appears to be a normal feature of fibers expressing a different myosin isoform that may be re-expressed in pathological conditions during regeneration.
- Type 1 fibers are rich in oxidative enzymes and stain strongly by NADH tetrazolium reductase (NADH-TR) and SDH, whereas type 2 fibers stain relatively weakly. One caveat in this fiber type differentiation is that there is an apparent "concentration" of organelles in atrophic fibers and a tendency for all small atrophic fibers to stain darkly with oxidative (some may be type 2C "pathologic" fibers) reactions.

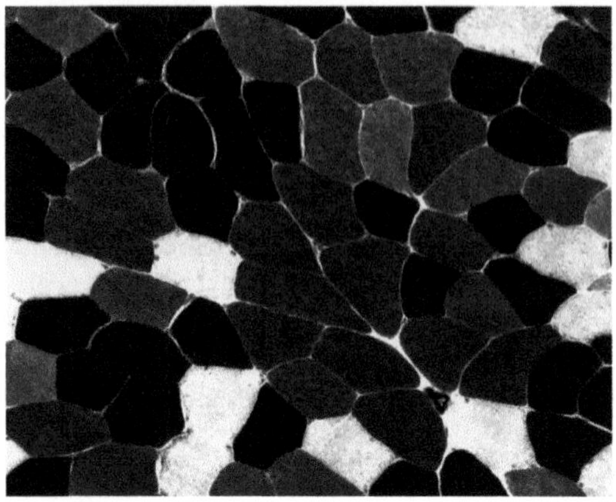

FIGURE 12.1 Frozen section of normal muscle with ATPase reaction at pH 4.63: mosaic pattern of the different fiber types. Darkest fibers are type 1 and lighter fibers are type 2 of differing subtype (ATPase, pH 4.63).

12.2.2.3.2. Demonstrating subcellular phenomena. The acid phosphatase reaction reveals increased lysosomal activity. Mitochondria are reactive to NADH-TR, SDH, and COX; SDH and COX are more specific for mitochondria because the T-tubule system and other membranous organelles are also reactive to NADH-TR.

12.2.2.3.3. Detecting or specifying certain structural abnormalities. NADH-TR reveals structural anomalies or alterations in the distribution of mitochondria and myofibrils, such as target fibers, cores, lobulated fibers, or "moth-eaten" fibers.

Table 12.1 Enzyme Histochemical Characteristics of the Different Types of Muscle Fibers

	TYPE 1	TYPE 2A	TYPE 2B	TYPE 2C
ATPase 9.4	+	+ + +	+ + +	+++
ATPase 4.6	+ + +	–	++	+++
ATPase 4.3	+ + +	–	–	++
SDH	+++	++	+	++
NADH-TR	+ + +	+ +	+	+++

12.2.2.3.4. Demonstrating specific enzymatic defects. Myophosphorylase deficiency can be identified in McArdle disease. Focal COX deficiency affecting individual fibers is observed in most cases of mitochondrial myopathy and selected fibers in inclusion body myositis (IBM) and in the elderly. Combining COX and SDH reactions in the same section may help detection of COX deficiency by showing blue fibers corresponding to COX-negative, SDH-positive fibers among brown double-positive fibers.

12.2.2.4. IMMUNOHISTOCHEMISTRY

Immunohistochemistry (IHC) is a valuable tool for studying muscle biopsies because it allows for the study and localization of selected proteins. Depending on the antibody, frozen or paraffin sections can be used for IHC. For genetic myopathies, Western blot analysis complements IHC studies.

12.2.2.4.1. Identifying the different fiber types. Immunohistochemistry for fast myosin expressed in type 2 fibers, α-actinin expressed in type 1 fibers, or an antibody to slow myosin are excellent means for fiber typing on paraffin sections and are practical alternatives when frozen tissue is not available.

In normal muscle, most fibers express either slow or fast myosin heavy chain; this is equivalent to the ATPases with type 1 and 2 fibers. In pathological muscle, fibers co-expressing the two isoforms of myosin heavy chain are common. Another indicator of disease or immaturity is the expression of developmental (embryonic and fetal) myosin in muscle fibers. These myosins are highly expressed in the neonatal period, and the number of fibers with developmental myosin gradually decreases from birth until approximately age 12 months. Their presence after age 2 years is abnormal.

12.2.2.4.2. Demonstrating muscle regeneration. The neural cell adhesion molecule (NCAM) isoform CD56/Leu19 is a marker of human satellite cells. Satellite cells are mononucleated muscle precursor cells that normally reside between the basal lamina and the cell membrane of muscle fibers. They account for more than 10% of myonuclei in young people and approximately 2% or 3% in adults. Postnatal muscle growth and regeneration result from activation, proliferation, and fusion of satellite cells into muscle fibers. Increased expression of NCAM, neuron-specific enolase, or neonatal myosin reactivity by muscle fibers is useful to assess muscle regeneration following injury or reinnervation.

12.2.2.4.3. Detecting structural protein deficits in muscular dystrophies. See Section 12.6.1.

12.2.2.4.4. Identifying specific immunopathological reactions in inflammatory myopathies. See Section 12.9.

12.2.2.4.5. Detecting abnormal accumulations of proteins. Immunohistochemistry can be used to detect abnormal accumulations of proteins such as actin, myosin, or proteins that interact with the Z line in the case of myofibrillar myopathies.

12.2.3. Normal appearance on frozen section

Much information is gained from the initial histological examination of the overall architecture of the muscle biopsy. In cross section, muscle fibers are polygonal in shape, with little intervening space between them and relatively uniform size. In infants and very young children, muscle fibers have a round shape and only take the polygonal cross-sectional shape at approximately ages 3–6 years.

Neuromuscular spindles (Fig. 12.2) are rounded structures (approximately 50–100 μm in diameter)

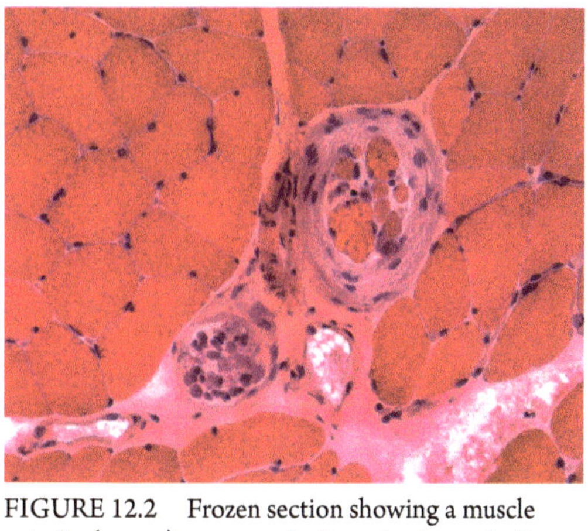

FIGURE 12.2 Frozen section showing a muscle spindle (center) composed of intrafusal muscle fibers surrounded by a capsule of connective tissue. Presence of an intramuscular myelinated nerve (lower left center) (H&E).

containing round intrafusal muscle fibers and myelinated nerve terminals, enclosed by a connective tissue capsule.

The nuclei of muscle fibers are predominantly located in a subsarcolemmal position; however, in samples without neuromuscular disease, as many as 3–5% of fibers have internally located nuclei. Endomysial connective tissue consists typically of thin, delicate septa between the fibers and around the capillary network. The perifascicular connective tissue, or perimysium, contains small arteries, arterioles, veins, and nerve twigs. The epimysium, situated around the fascicles, contains neurovascular bundles and adipocytes. A motor unit (i.e., a single motor neuron and its innervated myocytes) contains muscle fibers of a single histochemical type. Normally, the muscle fibers belonging to a given motor unit are not adjacent but are spatially dispersed in a muscle fascicle over a distance of several millimeters. With the histoenzymatic reactions that allow differentiating the fiber types, the muscle appears as a mosaic (checkerboard) of the two fiber types (Fig. 12.1). Adjacent fibers may be of the same histochemical type but are not necessarily part of the same motor unit. In the adult, the number of type 1, 2A, and 2B fibers is roughly comparable in the muscles that are usually studied (i.e., type 1, 30–40%; type 2A, 20–30%; type 2B, 40–50%; type 2C, 1% or 2%), with some differences between specific muscles. The fiber diameter and the percentage of each fiber type vary not only according to the muscle studied but also according to gender, age (Table 12.2), metabolic status, and physical activity, making it necessary to evaluate the results in comparison to normative data of matched controls.

Nevertheless, variability in fiber diameter within a muscle is not a function of age, and the distribution of fiber types across a biopsy is not age-dependent (i.e., excessive variation in fiber diameter, or fiber type grouping, is abnormal even in infants). There may be normally increased variability in fiber size and shape near tendinous insertions (sites that should be avoided in biopsy) and certain muscles, such as the extraocular muscle, diaphragm, and paraspinal muscles, but fiber type grouping is never a normal phenomenon.

12.3. BASIC PATHOLOGIC CHANGES

12.3.1. Artifacts

Before considering the spectrum of pathologic change in muscle fibers, one must be cognizant of the histologic artifacts that may occur and avoid interpreting these as significant alterations. Foremost of these is "freeze artifact," or the formation of spaces in the muscle fiber due to the presence of ice crystals, which is the result of inadequate or slow freezing of the muscle tissue (Fig. 12.3). Other common artifacts include shrinkage of the fibers when the sample is not frozen promptly and dries out, the vacuolization of the muscle fibers when in contact with too much saline solution or exposed to local anesthetic, or loss of enzymatic activity secondary to cautery for hemostasis during the biopsy procedure. Tissue fixed in formaldehyde destined for paraffin embedding and not appropriately stretched with a muscle biopsy clamp, or other devices serving the same purpose, can become distorted during fixation and is often not properly oriented. Paraffin sections, under these circumstances, commonly show contraction artifacts that preclude detailed morphological analysis of muscle fibers.

Table 12.2 Mean Diameters of Muscle Fibers According to Age

AGE	DIAMETER (MM)
Newborn	12
1 year	16
10 years	40
Adult female	30–70
Adult male	40–80

Source: After Brooke and Engel, 1969.

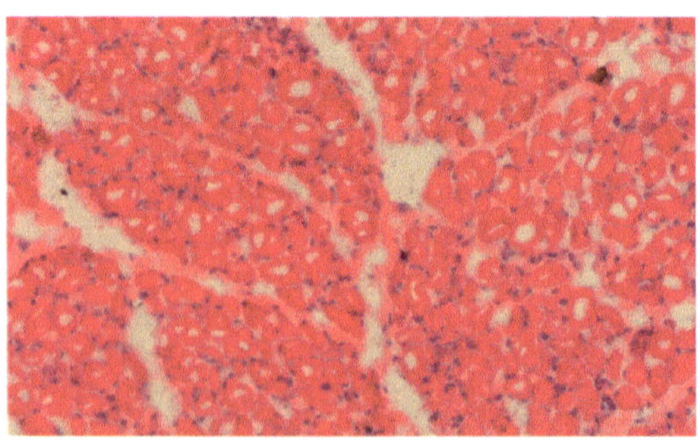

FIGURE 12.3 Frozen section showing a common freezing artifact: intracellular ice crystals (H&E).

12.3.2. Pathologic changes

12.3.2.1. VARIATIONS IN SIZE AND SHAPE

The initial parameters evaluated are muscle fiber size (diameter) and shape uniformity. The fibers should be relatively uniform in size. The mean fiber diameter increases up to ages 12–15 years. If a considerable population of small or larger fibers is present, the condition is described as "excess variation in fiber size." The presence of small, angulated fibers, which are smaller than normal fibers and have a roughly triangular shape, is never normal. "Hypercontracted fibers" (see Section 12.6.1.1.1) are characterized by a round cross-sectional contour in a background of smaller normal polygonal fibers and demonstrating sarcoplasmic hyperchromasia. They can occur in biopsies without definite evidence of neuromuscular disease but are particularly frequent in muscular dystrophies. As mentioned previously, more rounded fibers are normal in fetuses and infants; they assume a polygonal shape in later childhood and adolescence.

12.3.2.2. HYPERTROPHY AND ATROPHY

Hypertrophy consists of an increase in the size of the muscle fibers, often associated with loss of the usual polygonal outline. Some observers have reported that physiological hypertrophy of type 2 fibers may be seen in athletes. In pathological skeletal muscle, hypertrophic fibers are a compensatory change, and they are often accompanied by structural changes such as internalized nuclei and split fibers.

Fiber splitting refers to the phenomenon of longitudinal clefts of the muscle fiber (Fig. 12.4B) and is not present in normal muscle except sometimes at the myotendinous junction.

Atrophic fibers may be rounded in myopathic processes. Angulated fibers are seen in various stages of a neurogenic process in adults. In the latter stages of neurogenic atrophy, the atrophic fibers form "nuclear bags"—that is, clusters of sarcolemmal nuclei within shrunken muscle cells largely devoid of myofibrillar material (see Section 12.4.1.1). In the late stage of a severe myopathic or neurogenic process, the muscle can be severely damaged and is referred to as "end-stage muscle." It is largely replaced by fibro-adipose and connective tissue with few remaining atrophic fibers, and it is often impossible to infer the etiologic basis of the initial insult.

- It is important to determine the distribution of the atrophic fibers; they may occur randomly or be grouped in clusters. Fascicular or group atrophy, a hallmark of denervation, consists of aggregates of atrophic fibers that occupy part of a fascicle. This process differs from perifascicular atrophy, as seen in dermatomyositis (DM), in which atrophic fibers tend to be located at the perimeter of fascicles. Randomly scattered atrophic fibers are less characteristic of a specific pathologic process; when they involve both fiber types, they may represent early stages of denervation.
- Atrophy may select a particular fiber type. Type 1 atrophy (Fig. 12.5), perhaps due to developmental arrest, is usually seen in myotonic dystrophy type 1 and childhood congenital myopathies. The latter may present as a congenital fiber-type

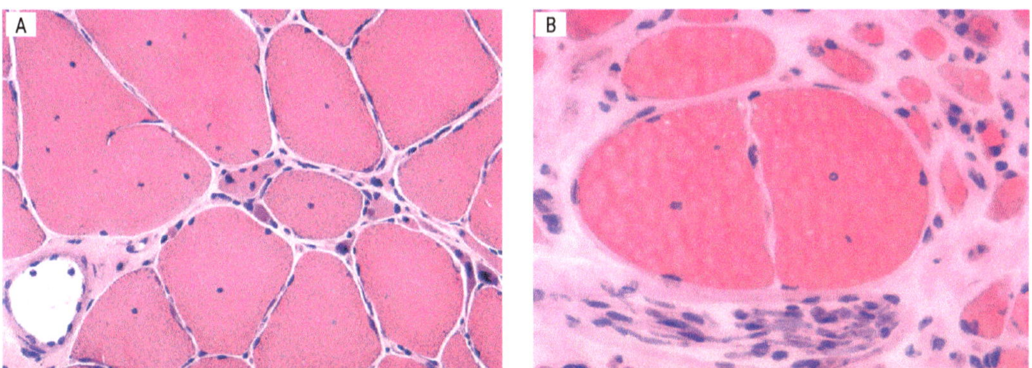

FIGURE 12.4 Variation in size and shape of the muscle fibers: (**A**) small, angulated atrophic fibers contrasting with hypertrophic fibers with internalized nuclei (H&E); (**B**) hypertrophic, split muscle fiber with internalized nuclei in muscular dystrophy (H&E).

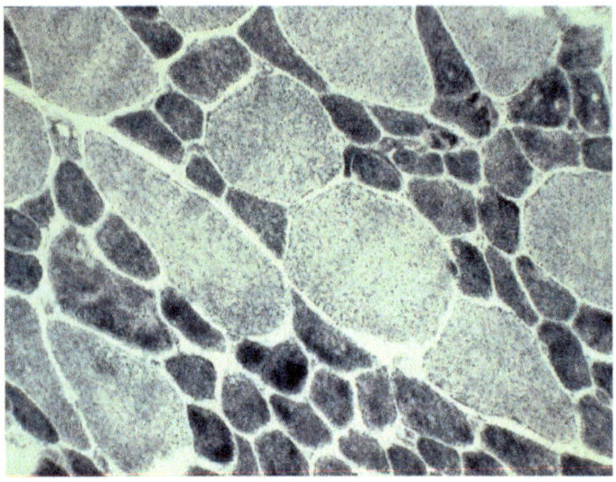

FIGURE 12.5 Type 1 predominance and type 1 atrophy in a case of congenital myopathy (NADH-TR).

disproportion (CFTD). Type 2 atrophy is frequent (mainly involves type 2B fibers) and is seen in a variety of acquired conditions, including immobilization/disuse, myasthenia gravis (MG), chronic debilitating disorders, chronic steroid treatment, and other conditions.

12.3.2.3. PREDOMINANCE OR DEFICIENCY OF A FIBER TYPE

The percentage of type 1 and type 2 fibers depends on the muscle biopsied. For the most frequently biopsied muscles (deltoid, quadriceps, biceps, and gastrocnemius), an abnormal fiber type predominance is considered when the proportion of fibers exceeds 55% of type 1 or 80% of type 2 fibers. Cases of "central hypotonia" often show aberrations of fiber type distribution in the absence of overt denervation. Type 2B deficiency, sometimes total, or the presence of type 2C fibers may be seen in certain myopathic processes. Type 2A deficiency is associated with mutations in the gene *MYH2*. In many neuromuscular diseases, there is a tendency to shift toward type 1 fiber predominance.

12.3.2.4. NUCLEAR ANOMALIES

Inward or central displacement of the nuclei, "internalized nuclei," is considered abnormal when present in more than 3–5% of the fibers (Fig. 12.4). The biological basis of this phenomenon is not clear; it is probably a marker of fibers that have degenerated or are in the process of regeneration. Muscle nuclei may be internalized in hypertrophic fibers, possibly representing an early stage in the process of fiber splitting. In certain diseases, notably myotubular myopathy, nuclei are in the center of the fiber on cross section and, on longitudinal sections, can be seen to aggregate closer together and line up in chains; these are referred to as nuclear chains (Fig. 12.6A). Multiple internalized nuclei also are seen typically in myotonic dystrophies.

12.3.2.5. STRUCTURAL ANOMALIES OF MUSCLE FIBERS

12.3.2.5.1. Split fibers. Split fibers are a common feature of diseased muscle and often associated with hypertrophic fibers. In cross section, splitting is manifest as a fissure extending from the surface of a muscle fiber. This fissure may be branched or contain a capillary (Fig. 12.4).

12.3.2.5.2. Necrosis. Fiber necrosis or degeneration (terms used interchangeably, albeit perhaps imprecisely) is characteristic of dystrophic,

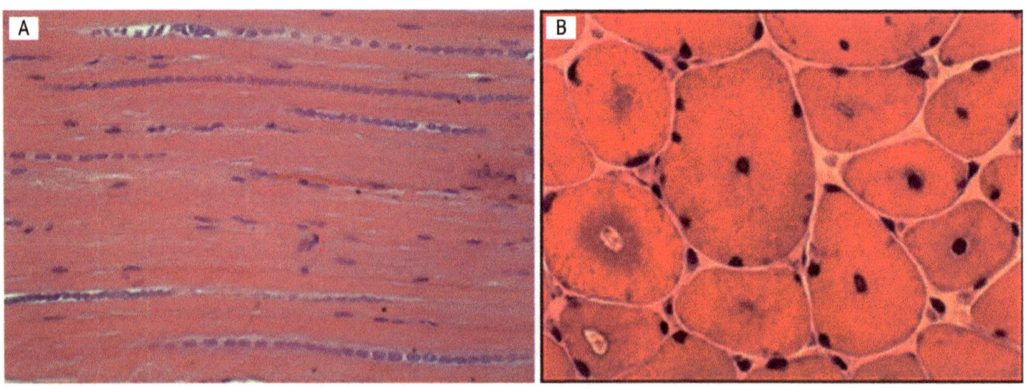

FIGURE 12.6 Centronuclear myopathy: (**A**) nuclear chains in the longitudinal plane (H&E); (**B**) centrally-placed nuclei and central clear channels (H&E).

inflammatory, or toxic myopathic processes that result in destruction of segments along the length of the muscle fiber. Conversely, necrosis is not the primary process in denervation, although it may occur in the late stages of neurogenic atrophy. In H&E preparations, necrotic fibers show a homogenization and glassy appearance of the cytoplasm and poor staining. In longitudinal sections, there is pallor and loss of cross-striations. Over time, the damaged fibers become vacuolated and eventually are invaded by macrophages (Fig. 12.7A). Admixtures of macrophages, T lymphocytes (predominantly T8), and regenerating myoblasts may be seen within the injured muscle fiber tube. This stage progresses to migration of inflammatory cells toward the adjacent blood vessels. In some conditions, muscle fiber necrosis is segmental, best seen in longitudinal sections (Fig. 12.7B).

12.3.2.5.3. Basophilic fibers. Basophilic fibers correspond to regenerating muscle fibers, rich in RNA. The fibers have a basophilic cytoplasm on H&E, may be either faintly striated or nonstriated, and possess larger than normal vesicular nuclei with prominent nucleoli. Regenerating muscle fibers express NCAM/CD56 by IHC. Regeneration may result in complete restitution of the muscle fiber or leave sequelae such as variation in the shape and size of fibers and internalized nuclei.

12.3.2.5.4. Target fibers. Target fibers may be detected with H&E or trichome stains (see Section 12.4.1.3) but are better demonstrated with NADH-TR and are mostly seen in type 1 fibers. They are composed of three concentric zones: a central pale zone, which lacks oxidative enzyme activity; a dark, annular intermediate zone, which is rich in oxidative enzymes; and a normal peripheral zone. They are often found in denervation. A "targetoid" fiber is one in which the darker intermediate zone is absent and is less specific.

12.3.2.5.5. Moth-eaten and lobulated fibers. The moth-eaten and lobulated fibers are recognized

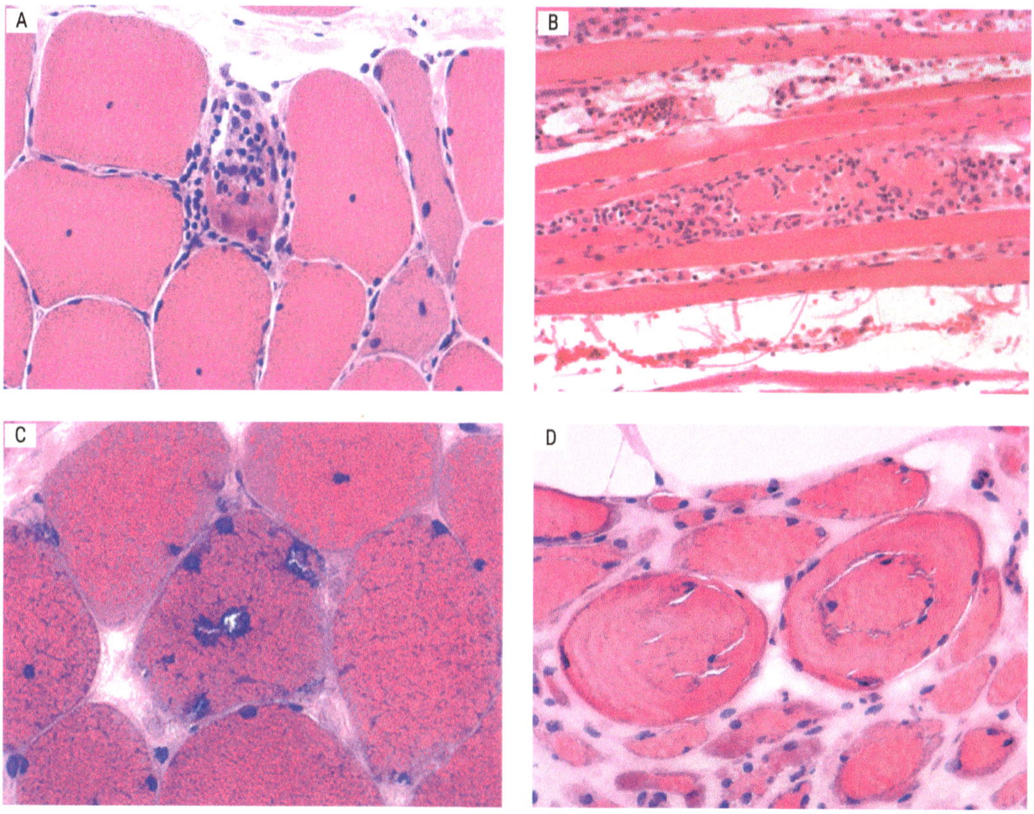

FIGURE 12.7 Structural anomalies of muscle fibers: (**A**) necrotic fiber is invaded by inflammatory cells (H&E); (**B**) central myocyte necrosis on a paraffin longitudinal section (H&E); (**C**) rimmed vacuoles (H&E); (**D**) whorled fibers or "coiled fiber" with central disorganization of the myofilaments (H&E).

in oxidative enzyme preparations. Moth-eaten fibers exhibit ill-defined zones of enzyme loss, resulting in a disorganized aspect of the intermyofibrillar network. They are not specific and are seen in a wide range of conditions, including inflammatory myopathies, fibromyalgia, malignant hyperthermia, and denervation. They must be distinguished from the focal oxidative enzyme loss observed at the site of desmin or other protein aggregates in myofibrillar myopathies.

Lobulated or trabeculated fibers are also best appreciated on NADH-TR. Individual fibers have a lobulated appearance such that there are many small zones of enzyme loss encircled by darker zones within fibers. Certain dystrophies are associated with many lobulated fibers (e.g., calpain-3–related limb-girdle muscular dystrophy [LGMDR1]), but this is a nonspecific myopathic feature. They also may be observed in paraspinal muscle biopsies in patients with axial myopathies (neck extensor myopathy, bent spine syndrome), facioscapulohumeral muscular dystrophy (FSHD), and other dystrophies.

12.3.2.5.6. Cytoplasmic and nuclear inclusions. A variety of cytoplasmic inclusions composed of different types of proteins may be detected. They may be specific or not. They are best seen on the GT staining and mainly include the following:

- Cytoplasmic bodies composed of a homogeneous central region that stains red or dark on GT and an outer zone of radially oriented filaments (Fig. 12.8A).
- Rods characteristic of congenital rod (nemaline) myopathy, which may also be observed in adult acquired myopathies with possible dysimmune origin. Rods are best seen with GT, where they stain red. In areas of accumulation of rods, there is a lack of oxidative and ATPase activity (Fig. 12.8B).
- Cytoplasmic protein accumulations in myofibrillar myopathies that include granular cytoplasmic aggregates with irregular shapes, hyaline inclusions classified as spheroid bodies, and cytoplasmic bodies. They may contain not only the intermediate filament desmin but also αB-crystallin and myotilin.
- Eosinophilic refringent protein aggregates and congophilic inclusions that may be observed in inclusion body myopathy.
- Intranuclear inclusions may be seen in IBM and oculopharyngeal muscular dystrophy.

12.3.2.5.7. Ring fibers and lateral sarcoplasmic masses. Striated annulets (*ringbinden* or ring fibers) are formed by myofibrils that are normal in structure but abnormally arranged so they are perpendicular to the muscle fiber axis, forming a ring on the cross section. Lateral sarcoplasmic masses are delicately granulated nonstriated clear areas that are filled with oxidative enzymes and are situated between the sarcolemmal membrane and a central myofibrillary zone of normal appearance. These two abnormalities may be seen in myotonic dystrophy type 1 and other dystrophies and myotonic disorders.

12.3.2.5.8. Vacuoles. Clear spaces of variable size with the cytoplasm of the muscle fiber are

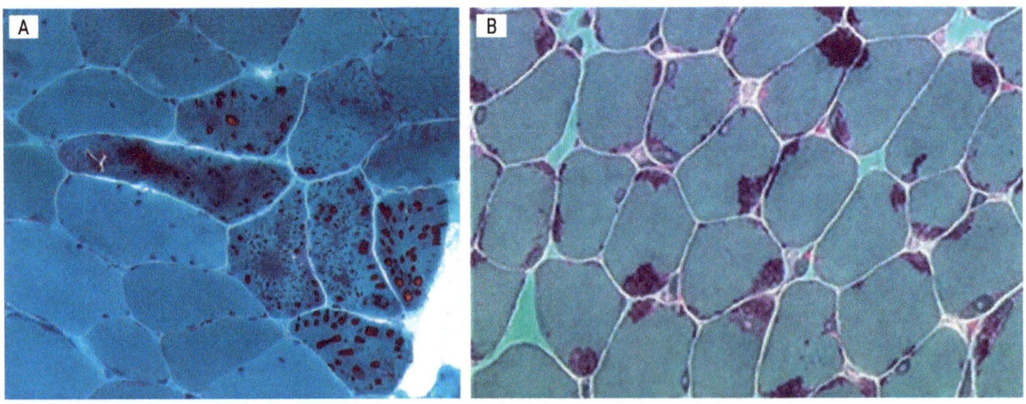

FIGURE 12.8 Cytoplasmic inclusions in cross section of skeletal muscle: (**A**) cytoplasmic bodies (GT); (**B**) aggregates of rods/nemaline bodies at the periphery of myocytes (GT).

visible with H&E, modified GT, and other stains. They have variable pathological significance best determined with the aid of a battery of special stains, but sometimes only after electron microscopy. They occur in the following conditions:

- Non-lysosomal storage diseases (e.g., glycogen in McArdle disease, lipids in carnitine deficiency).
- Lysosomal storage diseases, which are recognized by the acid phosphatase reaction and by identification of the stored material (e.g., glycogen in Pompe disease, autofluorescent lipopigment in ceroid lipofuscinosis).
- Autophagic vacuoles with lysosomal hyperactivity, revealed by the acid phosphatase reaction (e.g., chloroquine myopathy).
- Rimmed vacuoles (Fig. 12.7C), as seen in IBM, where their outer border is granular and basophilic on H&E and reddish with the modified GT stain. By electron microscopy, they are seen to consist of membranous debris and intermediate filaments.
- Vacuoles produced by dilation of the internal membrane systems, as in periodic paralysis, and microvacuoles produced by dilation of the T transverse tubular system and seen amid healthy regions of the sarcoplasm next to recent zones of segmental necrosis. Accumulation of sarcotubular material may be identified at the ultrastructural level in sarcotubular myopathy.
- Vacuoles resulting from the disappearance of myofibrillar material with prominent myosin lysis, as in DM and critical-illness myopathy, in which the content may have a reticulated honeycomb appearance.

12.3.2.5.9. "Ragged red" fibers. Subsarcolemmal or intermyofibrillar abnormal accumulations of mitochondria are the hallmarks of mitochondrial myopathies. They appear reddish with GT (see Section 12.6.4.1) (Fig. 12.9A), hence the name, and bluish with H&E. These aggregates

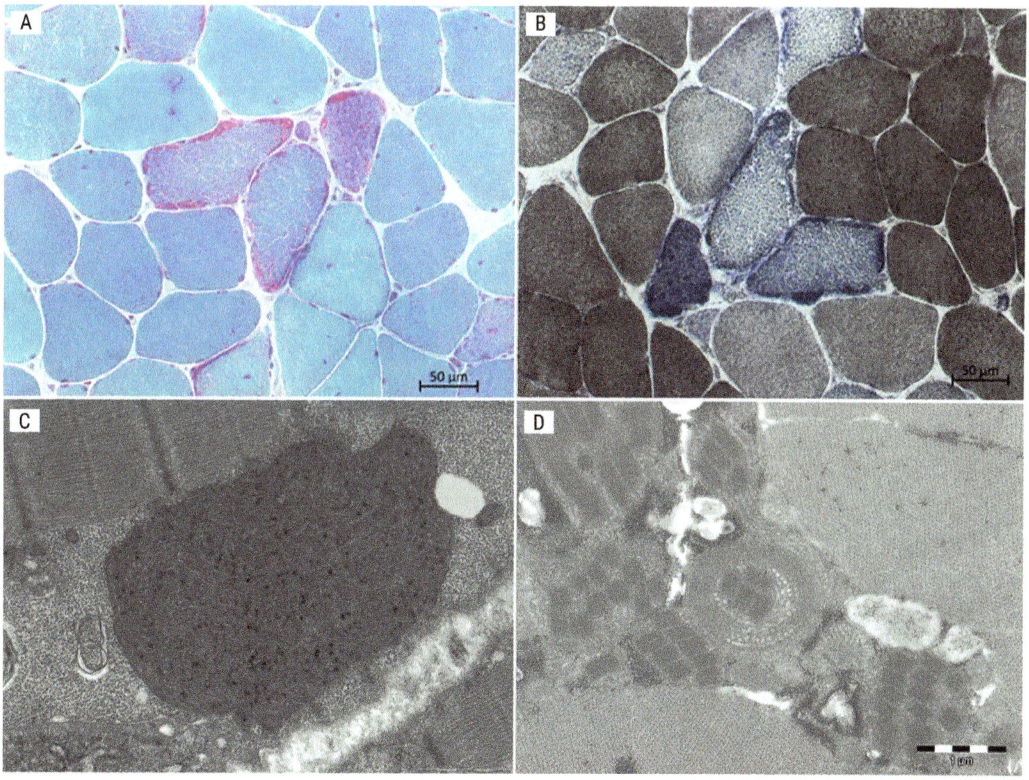

FIGURE 12.9 Mitochondrial myopathy: (**A**) Ragged red fibers have granular staining of mitochondria, with red subsarcolemmal aggregates creating a "ragged" perimeter (GT); (**B**) increased number of mitochondria are evident on histochemical stains that identify mitochondrial enzymes (SDH); (**C**) enlarged mitochondrion with abnormal arrangement of cristae (electron microscopy [EM]); (**D**) multiple enlarged mitochondria with paracrystalline cristae (EM).

contain oxidative enzymes, and therefore stain strongly with the NADH-TR and SDH reactions. Ragged red fibers that are SDH-positive but are COX-negative may harbor an underlying mutation in the mitochondrial DNA (mtDNA) or in nuclear genes that encode mitochondrial respiratory chain subunits; they show subsarcolemmal aggregates on NADH or SDH histochemistry (Fig. 12.9B). Ultrastructurally, they are associated with the accumulation of abnormal mitochondria, including both enlarged mitochondria and those with concentric or paracrystalline cristae (Fig. 12.9C, D). Increased glycogen and lipids may also be seen. Scattered ragged red fibers may also occur in muscle biopsies in the elderly in other clinical settings.

12.3.2.5.10. Tubular aggregates. Tubular aggregates are well-circumscribed zones that are usually subsarcolemmal, located mainly in type 2 fibers, and stain blue with H&E and red with GT (Fig. 12.10). They are strongly reactive with NADH-TR and COX, but they are SDH-negative. By electron microscopy, they are composed of aggregates of dilated T-tubules arranged in a *pipe-organ* pattern. They are often encountered in hyperkalemic paralysis and represent the principal histopathologic abnormality in the myalgia/cramps syndrome associated with tubular aggregate myopathy. They can also be seen in some cases of the congenital myasthenic syndrome, and they may occur in other disorders.

12.3.2.5.11. Reducing bodies. Reducing bodies are basophilic cytoplasmic structures on H&E, stain red with GT, and may be misinterpreted as cytoplasmic bodies. They can be identified with the menadione nitroblue tetrazolium stain as dark inclusions.

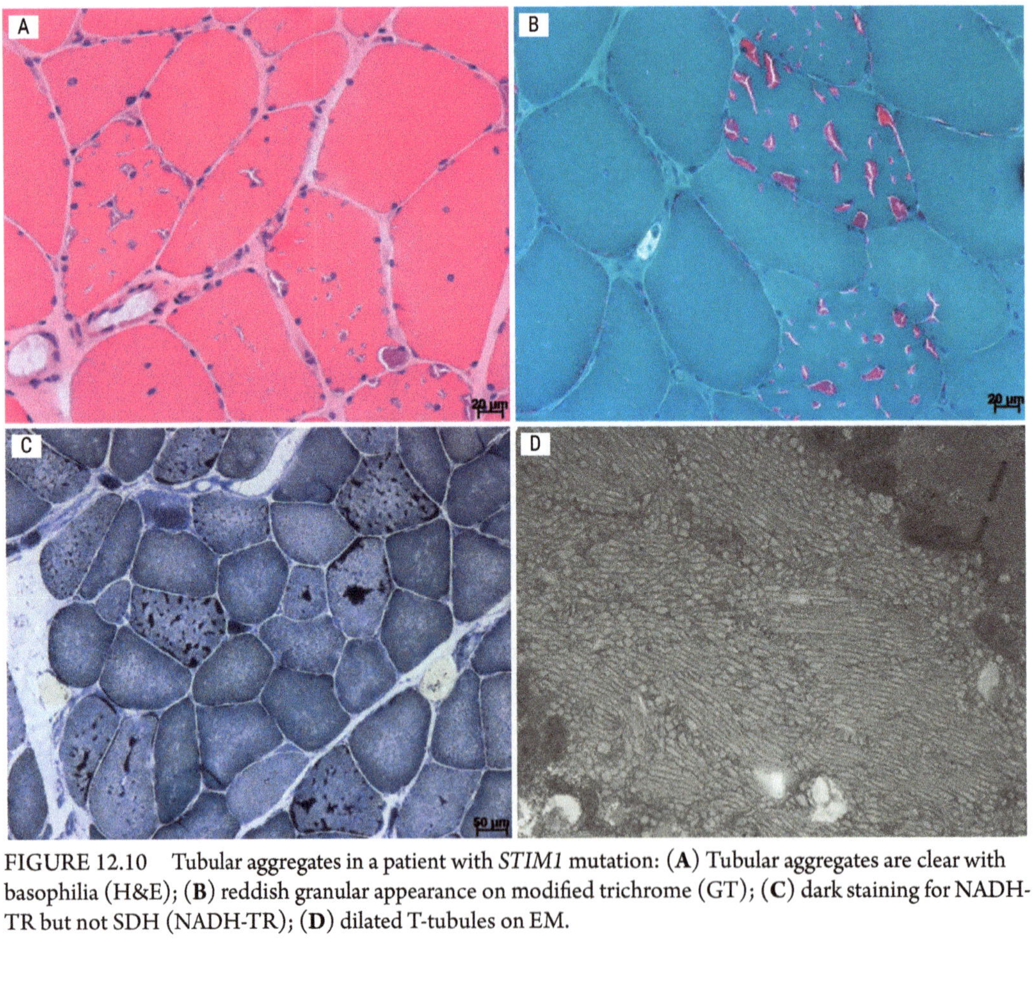

FIGURE 12.10 Tubular aggregates in a patient with *STIM1* mutation: (**A**) Tubular aggregates are clear with basophilia (H&E); (**B**) reddish granular appearance on modified trichrome (GT); (**C**) dark staining for NADH-TR but not SDH (NADH-TR); (**D**) dilated T-tubules on EM.

12.3.3. Interstitial changes

Changes seen in the supporting connective tissue may have diagnostic significance and help establish the etiology of the process (e.g., sarcoidosis, amyloidosis). Increased endomysial connective tissue or "endomysial fibrosis" is typical of certain types of muscular dystrophy. In end-stage muscle of whatever cause, there is infiltration and replacement of muscle by connective and adipose tissue.

Inflammatory cellular infiltrates may be seen in a variety of conditions: to some extent in muscular dystrophies such as dystrophinopathies, dystroglycanopathies, dysferlinopathies, and FSHD and in some cases of calpainopathy or γ-sarcoglycanopathy, in which eosinophils may be conspicuously present; in rhabdomyolysis (in the setting of a toxic or metabolic myopathy) in relation to myonecrosis; and in idiopathic inflammatory myopathies, such as DM, anti-synthetase syndromes, immune-mediated necrotizing myopathies, inclusion body myositis, and overlap myositis. The topography and the cellular composition of the inflammatory infiltrate are important clues to establish an etiologic basis.

12.4. NEUROGENIC ATROPHY

Two broad diagnostic categories of muscle disease are recognizable on muscle biopsy: neurogenic muscle disease and myopathic muscle disease (Table 12.3). These major subdivisions denote fundamental differences in the pathogenesis of the muscle disorder: (1) Diseases characterized by *denervation* (Fig. 12.11) are neurogenic disorders and result in muscle atrophy due to loss of innervation; and (2) diseases characterized by injury to the myocyte are *myopathies*, and the primary insult involves constituents of the muscle fiber itself, resulting in functional and structural abnormalities and potential degeneration of the myocyte.

In denervation, the site of injury may be the innervating motor neuron cell body in the spinal cord (or brainstem), the axon in the anterior root, peripheral nerve, the intramuscular terminal nerve twigs, or rarely the motor end plate. Microscopic examination of the muscle alone ordinarily cannot determine the precise locus; correlative clinical and neurophysiologic data are requisites to make that determination.

12.4.1. General features

12.4.1.1. DENERVATION ATROPHY

Denervation of skeletal muscle fibers results in a progressive reduction in the size of the fiber and loss of contractile proteins with preservation of the integrity of the cell membrane, intracellular organelles, and myocyte nuclei, which may facilitate fiber size restoration with reinnervation. An early detectable change is a reduction in the caliber of the cell and an alteration in its cross-sectional contour, which loses its polygonal shape and becomes less rounded ("angulated"). The small, angulated fibers are scattered throughout the fascicle and affect both type 1 and type 2 fiber types as assessed by ATPase reactions or fast myosin immunocytochemistry. Affected fibers are uniformly darker on

Table 12.3 Characteristic Myopathic and Neurogenic Processes: Differential Histological Features

MYOPATHIC PROCESSES	NEUROGENIC PROCESSES
Considerable variation in the fiber size	Groups of atrophic fibers
Rounded fibers	Angular fibers
Increase in the number of nuclei	Pseudo multiplication of the nuclei due to cytoplasmic atrophy
Internalized nuclei	Internalized nuclei not a feature
Necrotic and basophilic fibers	Rare, if any, necrotic or basophilic fibers
Cytoplasmic alterations in contractile proteins	Target fibers
Conspicuous interstitial fibrosis	Minimal interstitial fibrosis
Inflammatory cellular infiltrates	Rare inflammatory cellular infiltrates

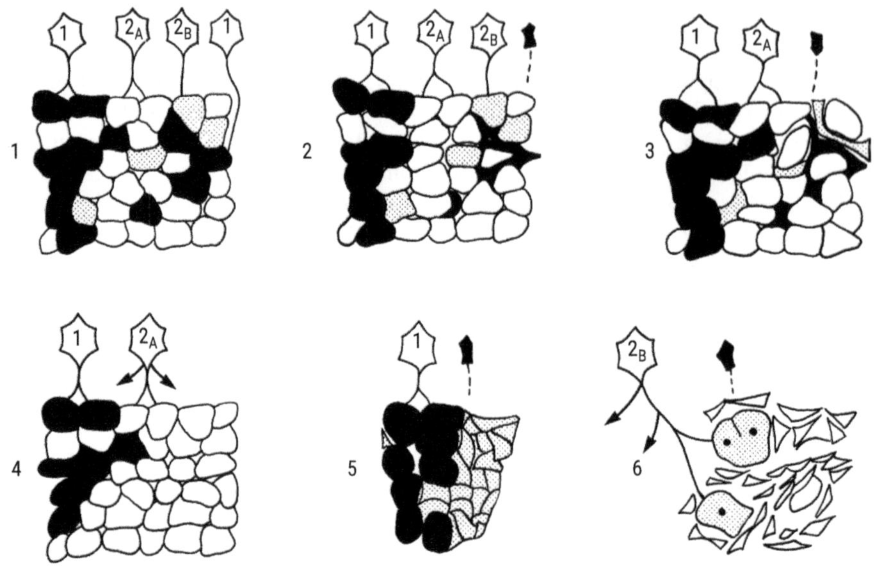

FIGURE 12.11 Mechanisms of denervation. (1) Normal muscle with checkerboard distribution of motor units. (2) Scattered fiber atrophy due to loss of a single type 1 motor neuron or axon (angular atrophic fibers). (3) Scattered fiber atrophy due to multiple motor unit damage. (4) Type grouping secondary to reinnervation leading to "giant" type 2A motor unit. (5) Group atrophy secondary to atrophy of "giant" motor unit. (6) Pseudomyopathic changes in chronic denervation.

oxidative enzyme staining. As the denervation process progresses, the atrophic fibers may be grouped in small nests and, later, in larger patches. The chronic denervation leads to myocytes with clusters of muscle fiber nuclei and little contractile apparatus, sometimes referred to as *nuclear knots* or *bags* (Fig. 12.12C).

12.4.1.2. GROUPING OF FIBERS OF THE SAME HISTOCHEMICAL TYPE (TYPE GROUPING)

The denervated muscle fibers may recover normal, or near normal, size when reinnervated by collateral sprouting from unaffected motor axons. Because the histochemical fiber type is determined by the innervating motor neuron, the fiber type may change with reinnervation. When the sprouting axons go on to reinnervate atrophic fibers near unaffected fibers of the same motor unit, this results in patches of contiguous fibers of the same enzyme histochemical type. Repeated cycles of this process result in the progressive pathological enlargement of motor units, composed of a single fiber type, and, gradually, the formation of giant motor units (recognized with neurophysiological methods). As a result, there is progressive disappearance of the normal checkerboard pattern. The development of patches of contiguous fibers of the same histochemical type, involving both fiber types, is called *fiber type grouping* and is virtually pathognomonic of denervation/reinnervation (Fig. 12.12A).

As the disease progresses, when the newly innervating axon that had incorporated the atrophic fibers in its motor unit also becomes damaged, there is atrophy of the muscle fibers that were grouped together, a phenomenon termed *group atrophy*. The phenomenon is apparent in H&E (Fig. 12.12D) and histochemical preparations. Pseudo-grouping may occur in myopathies when multiple fiber splits are present.

The definitive number of contiguous fibers required to be certain that one is dealing with genuine type grouping is debatable. The presence of fibers of a given fiber type, surrounded by nearest neighbors all of the same fiber type, so-called enclosed fibers, may be used as a rough guide, particularly when the phenomenon is observed in both fiber types. If one fiber type is predominant in a given muscle, enclosed fibers of that type will inevitably be found and, therefore, not indicative of pathologic type grouping.

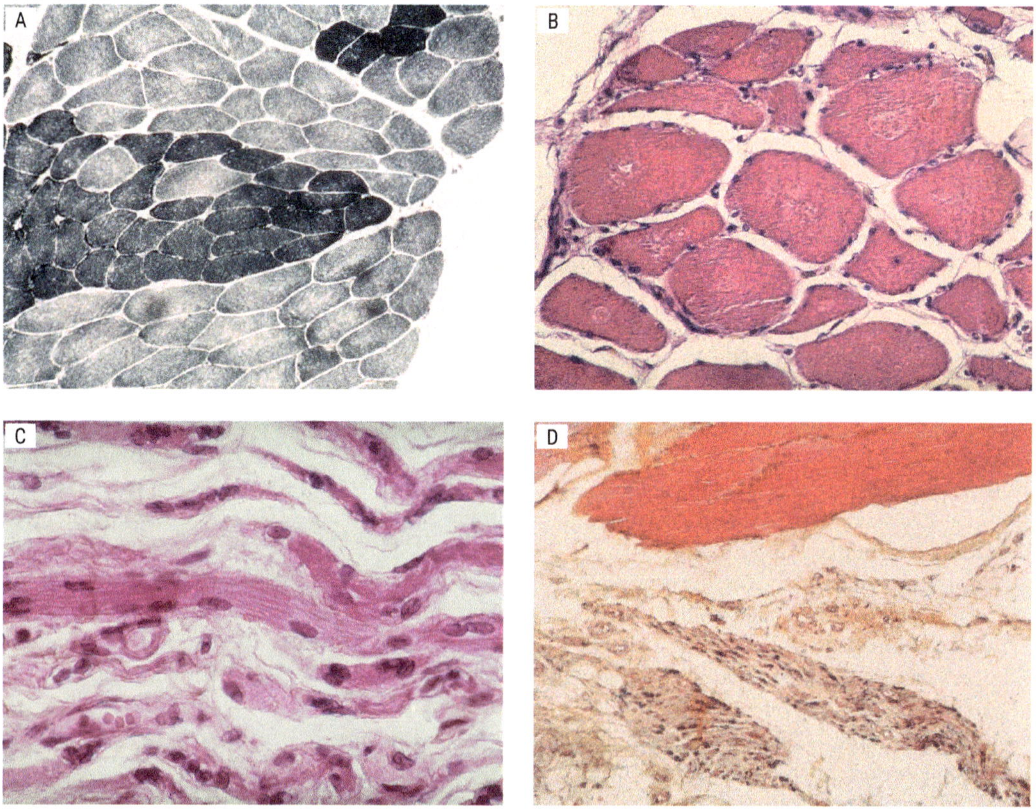

FIGURE 12.12 Neurogenic atrophy; morphological appearances: (**A**) fiber type grouping (NADH-TR); (**B**) angular atrophy and target fibers (H&E); (**C**) atrophic fibers forming nuclear bags (i.e., clusters of nuclei within muscle cells largely devoid of myofibrillar material) (H&E); (**D**) group atrophy (H&E).

12.4.1.3. TARGET FIBERS

Target fibers are commonly seen in denervation. They are best visualized in oxidative enzyme preparations such as NADH-TR, but they may also be suspected in paraffin sections stained with H&E (Fig. 12.12B) and especially with Masson's trichrome.

12.4.2. Neurogenic atrophy in infants

In infantile spinal muscular atrophy type 1 (SMA1; Werdnig–Hoffmann disease), muscle biopsy demonstrates numerous hypotrophic type 1 and type 2 fibers with rounded (not angulated) outlines. This form of atrophy is associated with groups of hypertrophic fibers, predominantly of type 1 (Fig. 12.13). There may be relatively little capacity to reinnervate denervated muscle fibers in these patients, and as a result, fiber type grouping is seldom seen.

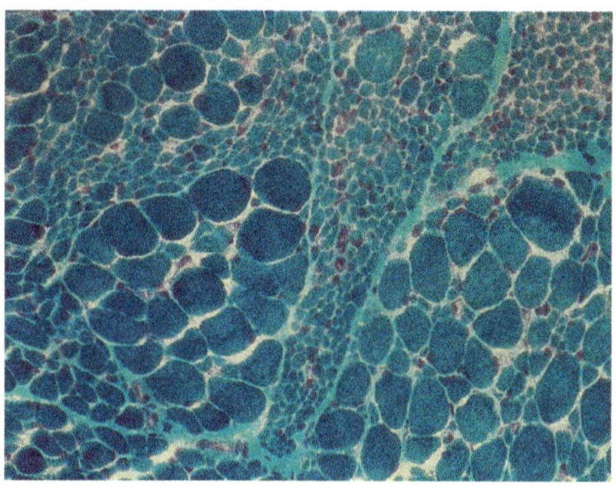

FIGURE 12.13 Neurogenic atrophy in an infant with Werdnig–Hoffmann disease (SMA1). Numerous hypotrophic fibers with rounded outlines are associated with groups of hypertrophic fibers (GT). In the juvenile form, Kugelberg–Welander disease or SMA3, more typical findings of denervation are the rule; in the intermediate form, SMA2, the findings are similar to those for SMA1.

12.4.3. Acute and chronic neurogenic processes

The histologic findings described give some sense of the tempo of the process, implicating the stage of the disease:

- The hallmark of acute denervation is the presence of random atrophy of angulated muscle fibers.
- With time, the denervated atrophic fibers may be reinnervated and regain their former size, but ATPase histochemistry will reveal fiber type grouping, which implies a further evolution of the process.
- In the late stages of the disease, the neuron responsible for reinnervated fibers may become affected, resulting in group atrophy.
- In slowly evolving denervation, or prolonged chronic denervation, in addition to typically neurogenic changes, muscle fiber hypertrophy, with excessive numbers of central nuclei, split fibers, and interstitial fibrosis, "pseudomyopathic" changes may be found, including scattered perivascular mononuclear cellular infiltrates of necrotic fibers.

12.5. NEUROMUSCULAR TRANSMISSION DEFECTS

These diseases present clinically with a myasthenic syndrome characterized by weakness and fatigability, which may be generalized or be more noticeable in the extraocular and eyelid muscles. The basic mechanism of injury is the dysfunction of the neuromuscular junction, resulting in impaired neuromuscular transmission. The diseases may be separated into acquired, autoimmune myasthenic syndromes, including MG and Lambert–Eaton syndrome, and congenital myasthenic syndromes (CMSs). In infants, botulism may enter in the differential diagnosis.

12.5.1. Myasthenia gravis

Myasthenia gravis is due to an antibody-mediated autoimmune response to nicotinic acetylcholine receptors (AChRs) or, less often, to muscle-specific tyrosine kinase (MuSK) and to low-density lipoprotein-related protein 4 (LRP4) localized on the postsynaptic neuromuscular junction complex. MG may be associated with other autoimmune disorders. Thymus hyperplasia is found in 70% of patients with MG, and thymoma is found in 10%.

The diagnosis is often evident by clinical examination combined with (1) electrophysiological studies showing the characteristic decremental response to repetitive nerve stimulation; (2) pharmacological tests, particularly the pyridostigmine test; and (3) detection of antibodies in serum. Muscle biopsy is generally not necessary, but it may be performed in seronegative cases to eliminate other diseases with a similar clinical presentation, such as mitochondrial cytopathies. Lymphocytic infiltrates, patchy major histocompatibility complex (MHC) class I immunostaining of muscle fibers, mild type 2 atrophy, and membrane attack complex (MAC; C5b9 complement fraction) deposits in the postsynaptic membrane may be observed. Ultrastructural study of the neuromuscular junction shows widening of the synaptic cleft, simplification of the postsynaptic apparatus with atrophy, and flattening of the postsynaptic folds.

12.5.2. Lambert–Eaton syndrome

Lambert–Eaton syndrome is also an acquired autoimmune disorder that typically presents as a paraneoplastic syndrome in association with small cell carcinoma of the lung. Patients develop antibodies against voltage-gated calcium channels on the presynaptic nerve terminal in neuromuscular junctions (see Chapter 9). Muscle biopsy is not useful to establish the diagnosis.

12.5.3. Congenital myasthenic syndromes

The CMSs represent a heterogeneous group of disorders due to genetic abnormalities of the proteins of the neuromuscular junction. Given the large number of these proteins, increasing numbers of new genes will likely be discovered in the future.

These conditions affect mainly children but may also occur in adults. Clinical and electrophysiological symptoms may be those of myasthenia, but serologic tests for anti-AChR, anti-MuSK, and anti-LRP4 antibodies are negative.

According to the site of the defect, one may separate presynaptic CMS, synaptic CMS, or postsynaptic CMS. Table 12.4 lists selected affected genes described thus far.

Table 12.4 Genes Associated with Congenital Myasthenic Syndromes

LOCATION	GENE	INHERITANCE	CHARACTERISTICS
Presynaptic	*CHAT*	AR	
	SLC5A7	AR	
	SLC18A3	AR	
	VAMP1	AR	
	SYT2	AR, AD	
	PREPL	AR	
	MYO9A	AR	
	SLC25A1	AR	Subtle mitochondrial changes
	UNC13A	AR	
Synaptic	*COLQ*	AR	
	COL13A1	AR	
	AGRN	AR	
Postsynaptic	*CHRNA1*	AR, AD	AChR deficiency (AR)
	CHRNB1	AR, AD	Slow-channel CMS (AD)
	CHRND	AR, AD	Fast-channel CMS (AR)
	CHRNE	AR, AD	
	RAPSN	AR	
	DOK7	AR	
	LRP4	AR	
	MUSK	AR	
	PLEC	AR	
	SCN4A	AR	
		AR	
Pre- and postsynaptic CMS; glycosylation defects	*ALG2*		Presence of tubular aggregates
	ALG14		*GFPT1* mutations may have autophagic vacuoles.
		AR	
	DPAGT1		
	GFPT1		
	GMPPB		

AD, autosomal dominant; AR, autosomal recessive; CMS, congenital myasthenic syndrome.

The diagnosis of CMS is usually based on the clinical features, EMG studies, and molecular results (CMS gene panel) rather than histology. A muscle biopsy studied by the traditional histologic and histochemical stains is usually normal or shows minimal nonspecific changes, such as fiber size variability, type 2 fiber atrophy, and type 1 fiber predominance. An exception is CMS caused by mutations in *GFPT1*, *DPAGT1*, *ALG2*, and *ALG14*, which are associated with a limb-girdle syndrome and may show tubular aggregates on muscle biopsy.

12.6. DISEASES OF SKELETAL MUSCLE

The diseases affecting primarily the skeletal muscle may be acquired or genetically determined. The latter may be classified into five main categories: (1) muscular dystrophies, which are clinically progressive myopathies and pathologically characterized by conspicuous degeneration, regeneration, and variability of fiber size (myotonic dystrophies, although fundamentally a separate category, are considered with the muscular dystrophies); (2) congenital myopathies, in which clinical manifestations typically become apparent early in life, with a nonprogressive or very slowly progressive course and can show distinctive muscle biopsy alterations allowing a specific morphological diagnosis; (3) metabolic myopathies, including glycogen, lipid storage, and mitochondrial cytopathies; (4) myofibrillar myopathies and rimmed vacuolar myopathies; and (5) ion channel disorders. Classifications that include specific molecular abnormalities have largely replaced prior categories. Mutations may involve the genes encoding skeletal muscle structural proteins or, less often, enzymes. Importantly, involvement of a single gene may result in different phenotypes and clinical presentations.

12.6.1. Muscular dystrophies

The muscular dystrophies are a group of genetically determined myopathies characterized clinically by chronic and progressive weakness and often markedly elevated serum creatine kinase. The past few decades have witnessed a revolution in the understanding of genetic and molecular basis of muscular dystrophies.

Central to our understanding of this broad group of disorders is the recognition of the associated mutations in genes that encode functionally related cytoskeletal proteins of the muscle fiber. These can be proteins or glycoproteins that link cytoskeletal actin and the extracellular matrix (Fig. 12.14), including transmembrane and membrane-associated proteins (dystrophin, sarcoglycans, dystroglycans, caveolin-3, α_5- and α_7-integrins, and dysferlin). Also recognized are mutations in genes encoding (1) extracellular matrix components (merosin/laminin 2, collagen VI); (2) intracellular proteases (calpain-3); (3) cytoplasmic proteins associated with organelles and the sarcomere (titin, telethonin, myotilin, and fukutin and related enzymes); and (4) nuclear membrane proteins (lamin A/C, emerin) (Fig. 12.15). It seems likely that this complex of cytoskeletal proteins stabilizes the muscle fiber plasma membrane (the sarcolemma) against the mechanical stress of repeated cycles of contraction and relaxation. Proteins such as dystrophin and dysferlin are involved in restoring sarcolemmal integrity. It has been speculated that some members of the complex are involved in signal transduction, although what these signals are remains unknown.

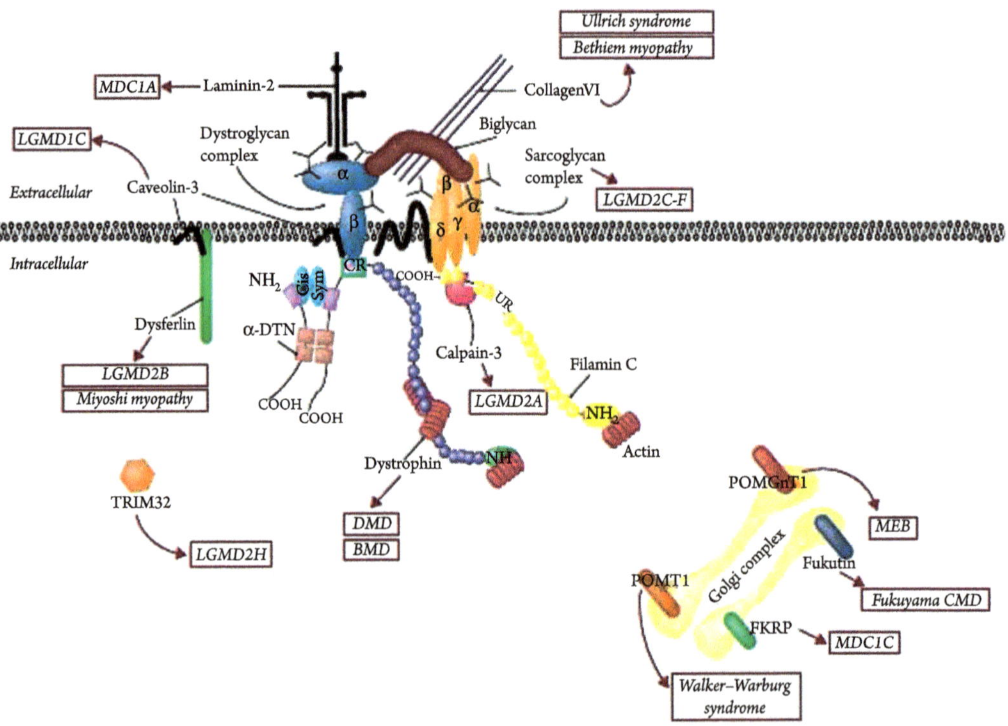

FIGURE 12.14 Diagram of cytoskeletal proteins involved in the pathogenesis of muscular dystrophies. (Modified from Dalkilic and Kunkel, 2003.)

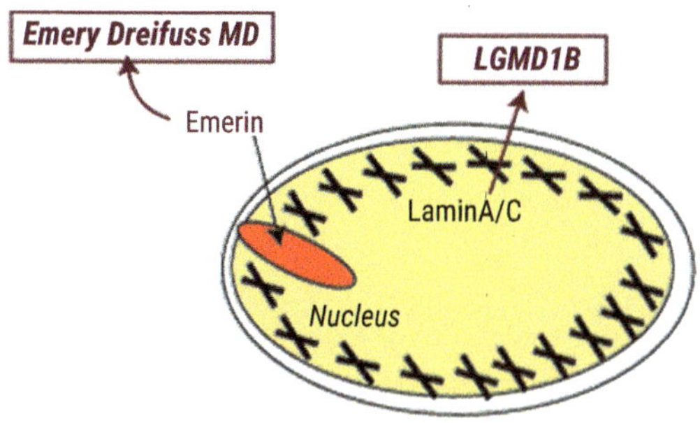

FIGURE 12.15 Diagram of the nuclear proteins involved in the pathogenesis of muscular dystrophies. (Modified from Dalkilic and Kunkel, 2003.)

The current and evolving classification schemes of the muscular dystrophies reflect progress in the understanding of the genetic and molecular biology of the diseases while taking into account the collected body of knowledge regarding the mode of genetic transmission (i.e., X-linked, autosomal dominant/recessive) and the clinical aspects of the disease.

12.6.1.1. X-LINKED MUSCULAR DYSTROPHIES

12.6.1.1.1. Duchenne muscular dystrophy. Duchenne muscular dystrophy (DMD) is the paradigmatic muscular dystrophy and the foundation for many of the recent advances in the understanding of these diseases. The affected gene is the *DMD* gene, the largest gene in the human genome, spanning 2700 kb and encoding the 427-kDa cytoskeletal protein dystrophin. Located on the X-chromosome, DMD is inherited as X-linked recessive (i.e., affecting males and transmitted by females). However, approximately one-third of DMD cases result from spontaneous mutations. Females are carriers and generally asymptomatic. Manifesting carriers reflect skewed inactivation of the X chromosome carrying the intact copy of the *DMD* gene.

The myopathy is of early onset in the muscles of the pelvic limb girdle. The muscles present a pseudohypertrophic appearance most evident in the calves but occurring elsewhere. CK is characteristically markedly increased into the range of greater than 10,000 IU. Dystrophin is also expressed in cardiac muscle and brain, so cardiac dysfunction and cognitive impairment may occur. The course is rapid, leading to death in young adulthood. The life expectancy of Duchenne patients has increased in the past few decades due to better management of cardiac and respiratory complications, such that patients may now survive into their late 20s or 30s.

The appearance of the muscle biopsy differs greatly depending on the patient's age at the time of biopsy. Biopsies performed in the first 2 years of life when the patient is asymptomatic may already show pathologic changes.

Muscle biopsy taken of the moderately affected boy in late childhood shows striking variation in fiber size, with smaller than normal fibers admixed with rounded hypertrophic fibers (Fig. 12.16A, B), increased internalized nuclei, fibers with opaque sarcoplasm (so-called hypercontracted fibers), regenerating fibers with basophilic cytoplasm (Fig. 12.16B), myophagocytosis, and scattered chronic inflammatory infiltrates (Fig. 12.16A). There is also a marked increase in endomysial connective tissue (Fig. 12.16C). As the diseases progresses, there a reduction in the number of muscle fibers and gradual infiltration by adipose and connective tissue. Enzymatic staining methods (i.e., ATPase reactions) show poor fiber differentiation.

Typically, at approximately age 2 years, the biopsy will show rounded fibers. At this early stage of the disease, there may be small numbers of degenerating and regenerating fibers. Endomysial fibrosis is subtle, if present, and fatty infiltration of the endomysium is not seen. When the biopsy is performed at the end of the age spectrum or autopsy, it will show abnormalities largely consisting of adipose tissue and abundant fibrosis with only scattered surviving muscle fibers (Fig. 12.16E). In the later stages of the disease, with extensive loss of muscle, the CK is often lower than at any time in the antecedent years due to the severe reduction in muscle mass.

The absence of dystrophin from muscle, demonstrated by IHC or Western blot, is the defining feature of this disorder, and the diagnosis should be confirmed by genetic analysis. Three antibodies directed toward the rod (DYS1), C-terminal (DYS2), and N-terminal (DYS3) domains of dystrophin should be used for IHC demonstration of an absence of dystrophin.

- Immunocytochemistry with the three antibodies shows that the normal subsarcolemmal distribution of dystrophin is lost in DMD, contrasting with the normal expression of spectrin control. In DMD, a few positive fibers, called *revertant fibers*, may be detected with

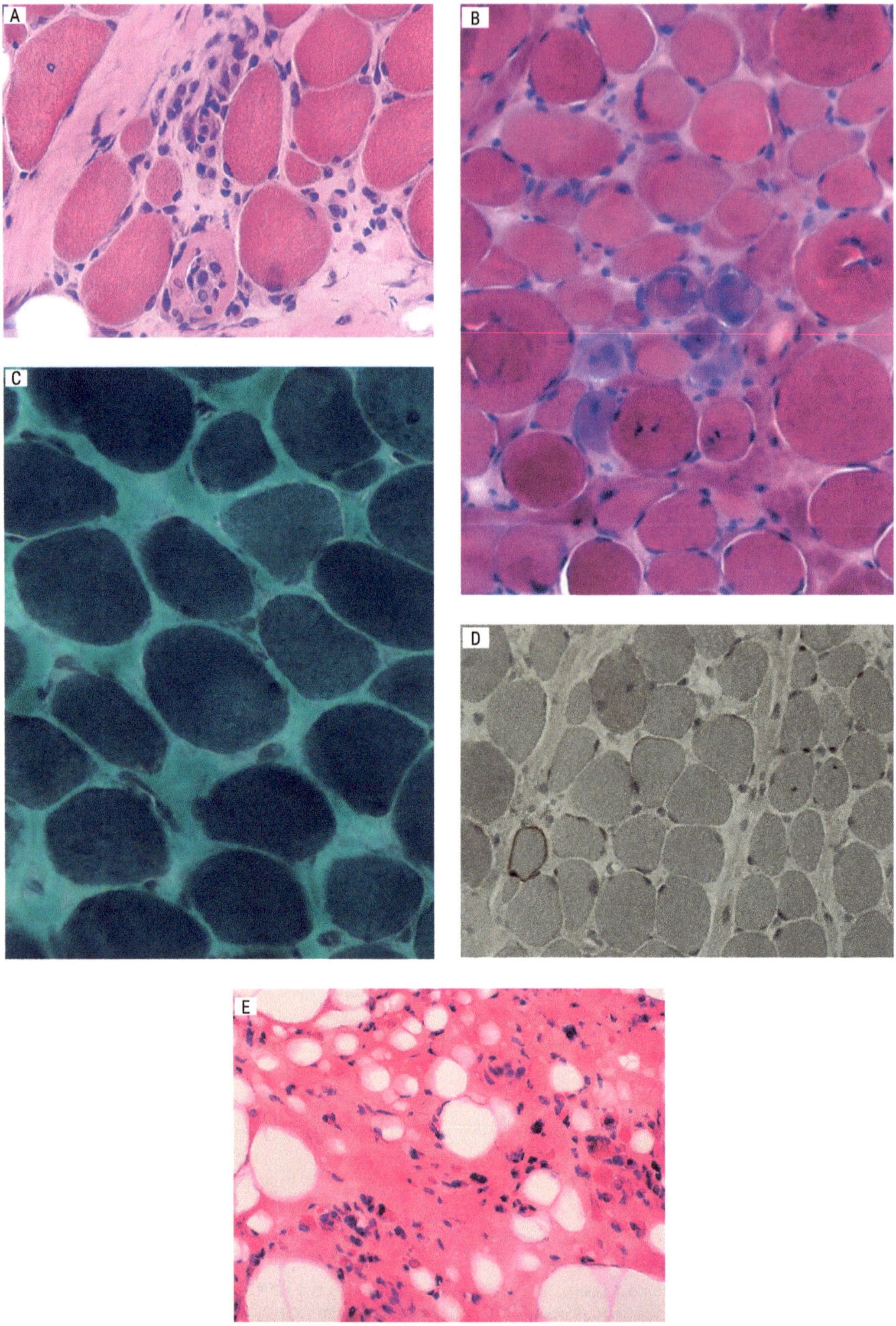

FIGURE 12.16 Duchenne muscular dystrophy (DMD): (**A**) necrotic fibers with myophagocytosis, variation in fiber size, with atrophic fibers mixed with hypertrophic fibers and internalized nuclei (H&E); (**B**) a focus of small basophilic fibers surrounded by rounded "hypercontracted fibers" (H&E); (**C**) increased endomysial connective tissue (GT); (**D**) absence of expression of dystrophin at immunocytochemistry using an antibody to the C-terminus except for one "revertant fiber"; (**E**) morphological appearance of the muscle at a late stage of the disease, with only scattered surviving muscle fibers within fibrosis and infiltration of adipocytes (H&E).

specific mutations. Occasionally, weak expression may be found with monoclonal antibodies to the N-terminus or the rod domain but never with antibodies to the C-terminus (Fig. 12.16D), allowing distinction with Becker dystrophy (see Section 12.6.1.1.2). Female carriers show a mosaic of dystrophin-positive and -negative fibers.
- Western blotting on muscle homogenate tissue identifies a marked decrease of dystrophin (the usual threshold is less than 5%).
- Genetic testing is now the gold standard to identify mutations in the *DMD* gene and to establish the diagnosis. The genetic information can also be used for carrier identification and prenatal diagnosis in subsequent pregnancies.

12.6.1.1.2. Becker muscular dystrophy. Whereas DMD occurs in patients with a nearly total loss of dystrophin, Becker muscular dystrophy (BMD) results from mutations associated with the retention of some dystrophin, albeit abnormal either in amount (underexpression) or in molecular size (either truncated protein or, in rare instances, larger than normal dystrophin, which does not function normally).

Clinically, this type of myopathy can be similar to DMD, but its hallmark is its wide variation in clinical course—that is, onset occurs later, the disease course extends later in life, and there is broader variability in severity. Individuals with severe forms of BMD may not fare much better than patients with DMD, whereas patients with mild forms of the disease may be capable of ambulation for a longer period in life. Patients with the mildest forms of BMD, identified only by molecular testing, may have only myalgias and/or an elevated serum CK, but they are at risk of developing a cardiomyopathy.

In keeping with this clinical and molecular finding, the appearance of the muscle biopsy is variable; in some patients, the extent of involvement is comparable to what is seen in DMD, whereas others show much less severe findings. Dystrophin immunochemistry in patients with BMD is characterized by irregular labeling intensity between fibers and in the same fiber. It is essential to use antibodies to different regions of the dystrophin molecule to avoid false-negative results. Using a triad of dystrophin antibodies may be informative in BMD, but the diagnosis rests on demonstrating the causative mutation.

Most mutations of the dystrophin gene result in deletions of one or more exons, and they are found in approximately 65–75% of DMD patients and 65–70% of BMD patients. DMD gene duplications are also detected in approximately 11–13% of affected individuals. Duplication of exon 2 is the most common duplication in the *DMD* gene (6.3–9.8% of all duplications).

The mutations in patients without detectable deletions or duplications are single nucleotide variants, microdeletions or insertions in the coding sequence, or splice site variants. Patients with clinical phenotypes suggestive of DMD or BMD but without a clear X-linked pattern of inheritance may have defects in other genes, including those encoding the dystrophin-associated glycoproteins.

There is no clear correlation between the size of dystrophin gene deletions and the severity and progression of the DMD/BMD phenotype. The molecular basis of DMD (more severe) versus that of BMD (less severe) is related, at least in part, to whether the amino acid translational reading frame is disrupted or preserved by the deletion mutations ("reading frame" rule).

Exceptions to the reading frame rule as a predictor of phenotype occur in approximately 8% of DMD cases and up to 34% of BMD cases. These exceptions may occur because of mutations in critical domains, exon skipping events, posttranslational mechanisms, and other factors. Thus, affected males and their families should be informed that phenotype prediction may not be accurate when based on the reading frame rule. Some regions of the dystrophin protein are more critical to function than others. Deletions in the regions coding for the amino-terminal or carboxy-terminal domains of dystrophin often result in more severe phenotypes than mutations affecting the rod domain. However, exceptions occur. Very large deletions or deletions in protein-binding domains (e.g., cysteine-rich domain), even if in-frame, can result in a severe phenotype. Out-of-frame deletions of exons 3–7 or exon 45 can result in BMD, DMD, or an intermediate phenotype. Exon-skipping events or activation of new cryptic translational start sites may create situations in which apparently out-of-frame deletions behave as in-frame deletions or vice versa.

12.6.1.1.3. X-linked Emery–Dreifuss muscular dystrophy and similar phenotypes. Emery–Dreifuss muscular dystrophy (EDMD) is the less common X-linked muscular dystrophy. Prominent features that distinguish the disease clinically from DMD are the later age of onset, prominent contractures, and the type of cardiac involvement. The early muscle contractures characteristically involve elbows, Achilles tendons, neck extensors, and scapulohumeroperoneal muscles. Disturbances in cardiac conduction can be lethal by the fifth decade. Female carriers rarely express the disease but are at higher risk of developing cardiac abnormalities.

In the various forms of EDMD, the changes observed on muscle biopsy are comparable, though not distinctive. These include a dystrophic pattern with fiber size variability, a tendency to atrophy of type 1 fibers, and considerable endomysial fibrosis. The number of fibers with internalized nuclei varies from scarce to abundant. Muscle fiber necrosis/regeneration is infrequent.

In X-linked EDMD with mutations in *EMD*, the immunocytochemistry for emerin shows an absence of labeling of all the nuclei. In female carriers of the disease, the immunocytochemistry reveals that the antibody does not label some nuclei. Emerin is a 34-kDa nuclear envelope transmembrane protein that supports the nuclear membrane (Fig. 12.15); it is expressed in all cells. Absent immunocytochemical expression of emerin can be assessed in muscle as in other tissues, such as skin.

When considering an Emery–Dreifuss phenotype, in addition to the X-linked EDMD with mutations in *EMD*, there are at least five genetically distinct forms of EDMD, both X-linked and autosomal dominant and in most cases associated with mutations in genes that code for nuclear envelope proteins. Emerin mutations are the most common cause of X-linked EDMD, although mutations in *FHL1* may also be associated with a similar phenotype, which is also X-linked. Mutations in *FHL1* are also the cause of X-linked scapuloperoneal myopathy/dystrophy.

Mutations in lamin A/C are the most common cause of autosomal dominant EDMD (also known in the former LGMD classification as LGMD1B; it has been excluded from the new LGMD classification). Mutations in this gene are also a common cause of hereditary cardiomyopathy. Nonmuscular phenotypes of laminopathies, such as lipodystrophy, may also occur. Autosomal dominant EDMD can occur less commonly with mutations involving SYNE1, which codes for nesprin 1, SYNE2 for nesprin 2, and the transmembrane protein 43 (TMEM43) gene. The distinction between the different forms of the Emery–Dreifuss phenotype frequently requires genetic analysis and histopathology, and the forms can vary in phenotype and pattern of inheritance (Table 12.5).

12.6.1.1.4. X-linked myopathy with excessive autophagy. The rare condition of X-linked myopathy with excessive autophagy (XMEA) manifests as progressive proximal muscle weakness, usually of childhood onset, with increased CK levels. There is neither cardiac nor intellectual involvement. It is due to mutations in the *VMA21* gene at Xq28, required for lysosomal proton pump function and resulting in increased lysosomal pH. There is a decrease in lysosomal degradative ability (autophagy) with subsequent accumulation of undigested autophagosomal material. Muscle biopsy shows increased acid phosphatase activity and intracytoplasmic giant (2–10 μm) autophagic vacuoles encircling sections of cytoplasm. The vacuoles represent internalized sarcolemma (i.e., they have membrane components including dystrophin, sarcoglycan, spectrin, and merosin). The phagosomes with undigested material

Table 12.5 Genes Associated with Emery–Dreifuss Muscular Dystrophy Phenotype

CHROMOSOME	PHENOTYPE OMIM NO.	INHERITANCE	PROTEIN	GENE
Xq26.3	300696	XLR	Four-and-a-half LIM domains protein 1	*FHL1*
Xq28	310300	XLR	Emerin	*EMD*
6q25.2	612998	AD	Nesprin 1	*SYNE1*
1q22	181350	AD	Lamin A/C	*LMNA*
14q23.2	612999	AD	Nesprin 2	*SYNE2*
3p25.1	614302	AD	Transmembrane protein 43	*TMEM43*

AD, autosomal dominant; XLR, X-linked recessive.

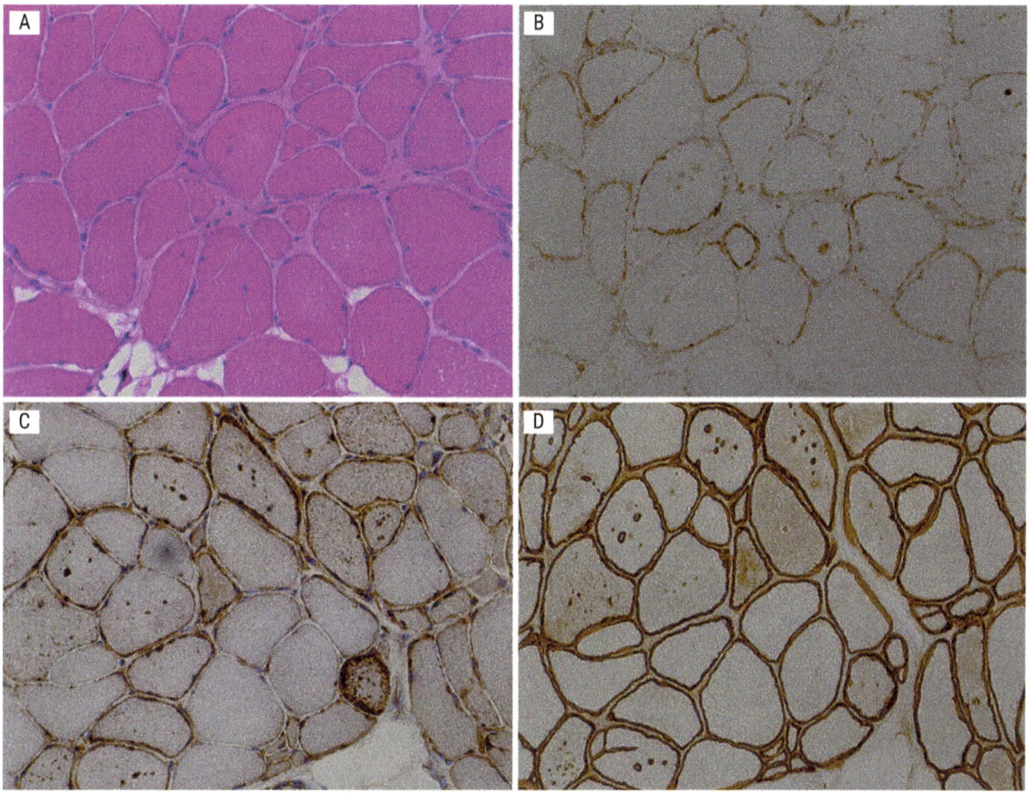

FIGURE 12.17 XMEA: (**A**) vacuoles within myocytes, fiber size variability, fiber splitting, and increased connective tissue (H&E); (**B**) complement complex C5b-9 in the sarcolemma of multiple fibers (C5b-9 IHC); (**C**) expression of autophagocytic protein in vacuoles and sarcolemma (LC3 IHC); (**D**) dystrophin within the phagosome membranes, in addition to the sarcolemma (dystrophin IHC).

tend to migrate to the myofiber surface, fuse with the sarcolemma, and extrude their contents, forming a field of extracellular debris around the fiber. Calcifications, deposition of the C5b-9 complement MAC, and expression of MHC class I antigen can also occur (Fig. 12.17).

12.6.1.2. AUTOSOMAL DYSTROPHIES

12.6.1.2.1. Limb-girdle muscular dystrophies. The LGMDs form a heterogeneous group of myopathies of autosomal recessive or, less commonly, autosomal dominant inheritance (Table 12.6). LGMDs have clinical and myopathological features overlapping with those of DMD or BMD, although they are clinically and histopathologically more variable. In referral-based clinical populations, fukutin-related protein (FKRP) deficiency (LGMD2I/LGMDR9), calpainopathy (LGMD2A/LGMDR1), and, to a lesser extent, dysferlinopathy (LGMD2B/LGMDR2) appear to be the most common LGMDs.

Onset of LGMDs is most often in the second or third decade of life but may range from childhood to late adulthood. Patients usually present with weakness of the pelvic/hip girdle muscles and shoulder girdle muscles. There may be scapular winging, calf hypertrophy, or calf atrophy, depending on the subtype of LGMD. In addition, some forms of LGMD are associated with early cardiac (see below) or respiratory muscle involvement. The CK value may range from the upper limit of normal to several hundred times normal.

Muscle biopsies of slightly affected muscles show mild irregularities in fiber size and some increase in the number of fibers with internalized nuclei. Weaker muscles demonstrate a higher degree of muscle degeneration along with progressive rounding of fibers, increasing variation in fiber diameter, internalized nuclei, muscle fiber degeneration and regeneration, increase in endomysial and perimysial connective tissue (fibrosis), and fatty replacement. Mild inflammatory infiltrates may be seen. Inflammation may be misleading for idiopathic inflammatory myopathy in dysferlin and anoctamin 5 deficiencies and eosinophilic myositis in calpain and γ-sarcoglycan deficiencies. Hypertrophic fibers subsequently show splitting and various other cytoplasmic changes that include whorled fibers, motheaten fibers, and lobulated fibers.

Molecular genetics revolutionized the understanding of these diseases. The older classification of LGMDs was based on their pattern of inheritance (autosomal dominant and recessive) and chromosomal locus or linkage. The nomenclature would assign the prefix LGMD followed by 1 (autosomal dominant) or 2 (autosomal recessive), followed by a letter (A, B, C, etc.) in sequential order of their identification. Since 2018, a consensus classification of LGMDs has been established; the new classification assigns the letters D and R for dominant and recessive, respectively, and is followed by a number in sequential order of the discovery of the affected protein (e.g., LGMD 2B is now LGMD R2 dysferlin-related) (Table 12.6).

Cardiac involvement is common in LGMD R4 (β-sarcoglycan-related) and LGMD R9 (FKRP-related). It is rare in LGMD D1 (DNAJB6-related), LGMD R1 (calpain-3–related), and LGMD R3 (α-sarcoglycan–related). In LGMD R3, the heart is spared presumably because ε-sarcoglycan replaces α-sarcoglycan in the myocardium. Dilated cardiomyopathy and cardiac conduction system abnormalities are the most common types of cardiac involvement. Intellect is usually normal, although intellectual disability is a feature of LGMD R11 (POMT1-related) and has been reported in LGMD R14 (POMT2-related).

For many LGMDs, particularly the recessive forms, the mutated gene and abnormal or absent protein have been identified. For most of the LGMD-associated proteins, specific antibodies are commercially available, allowing immunocytochemical diagnosis of a number of these conditions.

Sarcoglycans have a sarcolemmal distribution identical to that of dystrophin and are absent in the homozygous forms. Sarcoglycans and dystroglycans form a complex of dystrophin-associated proteins, which means that their expression may be altered secondary to the loss of one of the other proteins of the complex. Loss of one sarcoglycan may produce variable secondary loss of other sarcoglycans, although they do not have a similar secondary effect on either dystrophin or dystroglycans. Thus, confirmation of a specific defect by molecular genetics remains mandatory.

12.6.1.2.2. Distal myopathies/muscular dystrophies. The distal myopathies/muscular dystrophies (Table 12.7) are a heterogeneous group of disorders clinically notable for preferential early involvement of distal muscles, in contrast to proximal weakness as occurs in most other myopathies. The mode of inheritance is autosomal dominant or recessive. The clinical course is usually slowly progressive so that patients may not recognize their illness until reaching their late 40s or 50s. Myotonic dystrophy type 1 (DM1) and FSHD are discussed separately from this subgroup, even though prominent distal muscle weakness can be a feature of these diseases.

Muscle biopsy findings in distal myopathies vary from characteristic findings to nonspecific changes. Notable abnormalities include dystrophic changes with amyloid deposition in the endomysium and surrounding small vessels (e.g., dysferlin and ANO-5–related myopathies); rimmed vacuoles (e.g., GNE-related myopathy, hereditary inclusion body myopathies/multisystem proteinopathies, and myofibrillar myopathies), protein aggregates (e.g., myofibrillar myopathies) and fiber type disproportion (e.g., congenital myopathies), central nuclei (*DYN2* mutations), nemaline rods (*NEB* mutations), hyaline bodies (*MYH7* mutations), and reducing bodies (*FHL1* mutations).

Muscle IHC helps identify deficient structural proteins in recessive dystrophies (e.g., LGMD R2 dysferlin-related) or abnormal protein accumulation in myofibrillar myopathies (e.g., DES-related myopathy). Characteristics of the principal distal myopathies are summarized in Table 12.7.

Many distal myopathies are allelic to LGMDs:

- Dysferlin mutations cause Miyoshi myopathy type 1 as well as LGMD2B/LGMDR2. Dysferlin is involved in sarcolemmal repair. As a result, dysferlinopathies are associated with high CK levels. Miyoshi myopathy prominently affects calves at the onset. Muscle biopsy exhibits necrotic fibers but no vacuolar changes. IHC demonstrates reduced dysferlin on the sarcolemma of muscle fibers. In addition, sarcolemmal deposition of C5b9 complement fraction and inflammation are commonly found. Amyloid deposits around blood vessels and muscle fibers may rarely be seen (Fig 12.18). Lack of dysferlin is easily assessed by IHC. *ANO-5* mutations can also cause a Miyoshi myopathy phenotype (MM3) or a limb-girdle

Table 12.6 Classifications of Limb-Girdle Muscle Dystrophies

OLD CLASSIFICATION	NEW CLASSIFICATION (2018)	GENE	REASON FOR EXCLUSION
Autosomal Dominant			
LGMD 1A	Excluded, MFM	*MYOT*	Distal weakness
LGMD 1B	Excluded, EDMD	*LMNA*	Emery–Dreifuss phenotype
LGMD 1C	Excluded, rippling muscle disease	*CAV 3*	Mainly rippling muscles and myalgia
LGMD 1D	LGMD D1 DNAJB6-related	*DNAJB6*	
LGMD 1E	Excluded, MFM	*DES*	Primarily false linkage; distal weakness
LGMD 1F	LGMD D2 TNPO3-related	*TNPO3*	
LGMD 1G	LGMD D3 HNRNPDL-related	*HNRNPDL*	
LGMD 1H	Excluded	?	False linkage
LGMD 1I	LGMD D4 calpain-3–related	*CAPN*	
Autosomal Recessive			
LGMD 2A	LGMD R1 calpain-3–related	*CAPN*	
LGMD 2B	LGMD R2 dysferlin-related	*DYSF*	
LGMD 2C	LGMD R3 γ-sarcoglycan–related	*SGCG*	
LGMD 2D	LGMD R4 α-sarcoglycan–related	*SGCA*	
LGMD 2E	LGMD R5 β-sarcoglycan–related	*SGCB*	
LGMD 2F	LGMD R6 δ-sarcoglycan–related	*SGCB*	
LGMD 2G	LGMD R7 telethonin-related	*TCAP*	
LGMD 2H	LGMD R8 TRIM32-related	*TRIM32*	
LGMD 2I	LGMD R9 FKRP-related	*FKRP*	
LGMD 2J	LGMD R10 titin-related	*TTN*	
LGMD 2K	LGMD R11 POMT1-related	*POMT1*	
LGMD 2L	LGMD R12 anoctanin 5–related	*ANO 5*	
LGMD 2M	LGMD R13 fukutin-related	*FKTN*	
LGMD 2N	LGMD R14 POMT2-related	*POMT2*	
LGMD 2O	LGMD R15 POMGnT1-related	*POMGnT1*	
LGMD 2P	LGMD R16 α-dystroglycan–related	*DAG1*	
LGMD 2Q	LGMD R17 plectin-related	*PLEC*	
LGMD 2R	Excluded; MFM	*DES*	Distal weakness
LGMD 2S	LGMD R18 TRAPPC11-related	*TRAPPC11*	
LGMD 2T	LGMD R19 GMPPB-related	*GMPPB*	
LGMD 2U	LGMD R20 ISPD-related	*ISPD*	
LGMD 2V	Excluded, POMPE disease	GAA	Glycogen storage disease
LGMD 2W	Excluded, PINCH-2–related myopathy	PINCH-2	Reported in one family
LGMD 2X	Excluded, BVES-related myopathy	BVES	Reported in one family
LGMD 2Y	Excluded, TOR1AIP1-related myopathy	TOR1AIP1	Reported in one family
LGMD 2Z	LGMD R21 POGLUT1-related	*POGLUT1*	
New Entities			
Bethlem myopathy recessive	LGMD R22 collagen VI–related	*COL6A1, COL6A2, COL6A3*	

(*continued*)

Table 12.6 Continued

OLD CLASSIFICATION	NEW CLASSIFICATION (2018)	GENE	REASON FOR EXCLUSION
Bethlem myopathy dominant	LGMD D5 collagen VI–related	*COL6A1, COL6A2, COL6A3*	
Laminin α_2-related muscular dystrophy	LGMD R23 laminin α_2-related	*LAMA2*	
POMGNT2-related muscular dystrophy	LGMD R24 POMGNT2-related	*POMGNT2*	

EDMD, Emery–Dreifuss muscular dystrophy; MFM, Myofibrillar myopathy.

Table 12.7 Classification and Characteristics of the Principal Distal Myopathies

TYPE	GENE/PROTEIN	INHERITANCE	CHARACTERISTIC FEATURES AND MUSCLE BIOPSY (MB) FINDINGS
Miyoshi myopathy type 1 or dysferlinopathy Allelic with LGMD R2	*DYSF* Dysferlin	AR	Onset: young adulthood. Calf involvement at onset; increased CK levels MB: myopathic or dystrophic changes; amyloid deposition
GNE myopathy (hereditary inclusion body myopathy type 1)	*GNE* UDP-*N*-acetylglucosamine 2-epimerase/*N*-acetylmannosamine kinase	AR	Onset: early adulthood. Bilateral foot drop; prominent tibial anterior involvement; quadriceps sparing; CK moderately elevated (<5× normal) MB: myopathic; rimmed vacuoles
Miyoshi myopathy type 3 Allelic with LGMD R12	*ANO5* Anoctamin 5	AR	Onset: early adulthood. Atrophy of posterior compartment of the forelegs; increased CK levels MB: myopathic or dystrophic changes; amyloid deposition
Distal Myopathy	*ADSS1* ADSSL1	AR	Onset: adolescence. Slow progression; facial muscle weakness common MB: myopathic; rimmed vacuoles; rods; increased lipid droplets
	KLHL9 Kelch-like homologue 9	AR	Childhood–adolescence onset. Dystrophy or nonspecific myopathy
Markesbery–Griggs myopathy (myofibrillar myopathy)	*LDB3* ZASP	AD	Late onset. Bilateral anterior foreleg weakness and foot drop; cardiomyopathy; CK levels normal or mildly elevated MB: myofibrillar myopathy; desmin inclusions; RV

Table 12.7 Continued

TYPE	GENE/PROTEIN	INHERITANCE	CHARACTERISTIC FEATURES AND MUSCLE BIOPSY (MB) FINDINGS
Scapuloperoneal myopathy FHL1 associated; allelic with reducing body myopathy, EDMD	*FHL1* Four and a half LIM domains 1	X-linked	Onset: 20–58 years. Distal lower limbs; CK: ↑ 1.5× to 10× MB: myopathic, focal; desmin inclusions; myofibrillar myopathy; reducing bodies
Myotilinopathy; myofibrillar myopathy	*MYOT* Myotilin	AD	Late onset. Slowly progressive; distal or proximal and distal weakness; TA contractures; cardiomyopathy; CK levels mildly elevated MB: myofibrillar myopathy; phagocytic vacuoles
Myofibrillar myopathy, αB-crystalline–related	*CRYAB* αB-crystalline	AD	Adult onset. Distal > proximal; respiratory involvement; cataracts; velopharyngeal muscle weakness; CK mildly elevated MB: myofibrillar myopathy; desmin aggregates
Myofibrillar myopathy, desmin-related	*DES* Desmin	AD or AR	Onset second to third decades. Lower limbs distal muscle weakness; may have facial and bulbar weakness Cardiomyopathy; respiratory involvement; CK mildly elevated MB: myofibrillar myopathy; desmin aggregates; vacuoles
Williams distal myopathy	*FLNC* Filamin C	AD	Early adult onset. Sparing of the anterior tibial compartment; distal upper and lower limbs; CK levels normal or mildly elevated MB: variation in fiber size; type 1 fiber predominance; no vacuoles; myofibrillar myopathy pathology
Laing distal myopathy (allelic with congenital myopathies; scapuloperoneal myopathy; cardiomyopathy hypertrophic and dilated)	*MYH7* Myosin heavy chain β	AD	Childhood onset. Selective weakness of foot extensors and great toe extensors; paraspinal, neck, and facial muscle involvement may occur; cardiomyopathy; CK levels normal or mildly elevated MB: nonspecific myopathic (outside the congenital myopathies)
Welander distal myopathy (allelic with ALS-FTD)	*TIA1* TIA 1 protein	AD or AR	Late adult onset. Distal upper limbs weakness, affecting wrist and finger extensors at onset; CK levels normal or mildly elevated MB: myopathic with RVs

(continued)

Table 12.7 Continued

TYPE	GENE/PROTEIN	INHERITANCE	CHARACTERISTIC FEATURES AND MUSCLE BIOPSY (MB) FINDINGS
Finnish (tibial; Udd)	*TTN* Titin	AD	Adult onset. Anterior lower legs; CK levels normal or mildly elevated MB: myopathic with RV
HMERF	*TTN* Titin	AD	Adult onset. Distal lower limbs weakness with foot drop; early respiratory insufficiency; CK levels normal or mildly elevated MB: myofibrillar myopathy; cytoplasmic bodies; RV
Distal myopathy with vocal cord involvement (allelic with ALS)	*MATR3* Matrin-3	AD	Onset: 35–57 years. Progressive foot drop; dysphagia/dysarthria and pharyngeal weakness; CK normal to ↑ 8× MB: myopathic with RV
VCP disease Multisystem proteinopathy 1	*VCP* Valosin containing protein	AD	Onset: 20–40 years. Legs; proximal and distal weakness; ± Paget disease of the bone and FTD; CK mildly elevated MB: inclusion bodies; RV
Myopathy with Paget disease with or without FTD Multisystem proteinopathy 2	*HNRNPA2B1* heterogeneous nuclear ribonucleoprotein A2/B1	AD	Onset: early adulthood. Distal weakness > lower limbs; scapular weakness; CK elevated MB: inclusion bodies; RV
Myopathy with Paget disease without FTD Multisystem proteinopathy 3 Allelic with ALS	*HNRNPA1* Heterogeneous nuclear ribonucleoprotein A1	AD	Onset: 32–45 years. Distal; legs and hands; CK elevated MB: inclusion bodies; RV
Distal dystrophy with rimmed vacuoles Allelic with LGMD D1	*DNAJB6* DnaJ homolog subfamily B member 6	AD	Onset: 10–50 years; Upper and lower limbs distal weakness; CK normal, or slightly elevated MB: dystrophic; RV; myofibrillar disintegration; tubulofilamentous inclusions DNAJB6 and TDP43-immunoreactive; RV
Distal myopathy with caveolin-3 deficiency Allelic with rippling muscle disease	*CAV3* Caveolin-3	AD	Onset: adulthood. Distal muscle weakness particularly affecting the hands; calf hypertrophy; pes cavus; increased serum CK MB: internal nuclei; absence of caveolin-3 staining
Distal myopathy with dynamin 2 deficiency	*DNM* Dynamin 2	AD	Allelic to form of dominant deficiency; intermediate CMT Centronuclear myopathy

Table 12.7 Continued

TYPE	GENE/PROTEIN	INHERITANCE	CHARACTERISTIC FEATURES AND MUSCLE BIOPSY (MB) FINDINGS
Distal myopathy with nebulin deficiency	*NEB* Nebulin	AR	Childhood onset Nemaline myopathy (small and scares in distal phenotype
	ACTA 1 α-Actin-1	AD	Early onset: childhood–adolescence Myofibrillar pathology Nemaline myopathy
Neuromyopathy	*HSPB8* Small heat shock protein 22-kDa protein 8	AD	Myofibrillar myopathy pathology
	HSPB1 Heat-shock 27-kDa protein 1	AD	Autophagy; misfolded protein degradation

AD, autosomal dominant; AR, autosomal recessive; ALS, amyotrophic lateral sclerosis; CK, creatine kinase; EDMD, Emery–Dreifuss muscular dystrophy; FTD, frontoemporal dementia; RV, rimmed vacuoles.

pattern of weakness (LGMD2L/LGMDR12) and also may have amyloid deposition around blood vessels.

- Udd (or Finnish) tibial muscular dystrophy caused by mutations in titin (*TTN*) prominently affects the tibialis anterior muscles, leading to progressive foot drop in mid- or late adulthood.
- Markesbery–Griggs myopathy manifests similar to Udd myopathy but is associated with mutations in Z-band–associated protein (ZASP).

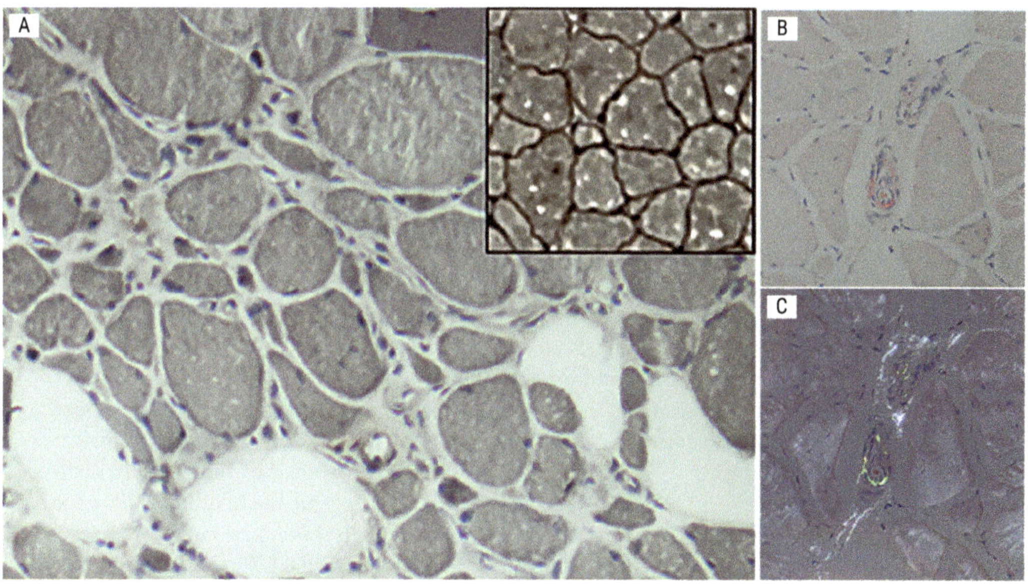

FIGURE 12.18 Dysferlinopathy: (**A**) complete loss of dysferlin expression compared to normal sarcolemmal expression (inset; dysferlin IHC); (**B**) amyloid deposits may be seen around small endomysial blood vessels (Congo red); (**C**) amyloid is birefringent green under polarized light (Congo red).

Distal myopathies may also be allelic to congenital myopathies:

- Early onset Laing distal myopathy is due to mutation in the myosin heavy chain 7 gene (*MYH7*).
- Later onset distal myopathies are also caused by mutations in nebulin and dynamin 2.

Distal myopathies with rimmed vacuoles form a distinct group: The best-characterized form is GNE myopathy (previously referred to as Nonaka distal myopathy or autosomal recessive hereditary inclusion body myopathy type 1). The myopathy is caused by mutations in the *GNE* gene that encodes for UDP-*N*-acetylglucosamine-2-epimerase/*N*-acetylmannosamine kinase enzyme. It is an autosomal recessive myopathy associated with progressive anterior tibial weakness with relative sparing of the quadriceps. Muscle biopsy shows myopathic changes, rimmed vacuoles, and protein agglomerates similar to those observed in sporadic IBM (sIBM), but inflammation is usually absent.

12.6.1.2.3. Congenital muscular dystrophies. Congenital muscular dystrophy (CMD) is within the differential diagnosis of the hypotonic infant. CMDs are usually caused by molecular defects altering structural relationships between muscle fibers and the extracellular matrix. Muscle biopsies of CMD are comparable between the different types within this group, showing increased endomysial connective and adipose tissue and variability in fiber size with a rounded rather than polygonal shape. Degenerating and regenerating fibers and chronic inflammatory cell infiltrates ae also seen. IHC is an important tool for diagnosis. These diseases may be subdivided into three main categories: (1) merosin (laminin α_2) negative, (2) merosin positive, and (3) CMDs associated with central nervous system (CNS) structural or functional abnormalities, including principally Walker–Warburg syndrome (WWS), muscle–eye–brain disease (MEB), and Fukuyama CMD. The last two categories are genetically heterogeneous (Table 12.8).

Merosin-negative CMD or MDC1A: This form is typically associated with contractures; CK elevation to more than 10 times normal; diffuse MRI changes in the cerebral white matter; and dystrophic features on muscle biopsy with increased endomysial connective and adipose tissue, variability in fiber size, and fibers that take a round shape. Degenerating and regenerating fibers may be seen, and inflammatory infiltrates, although rare, can be extended in some cases. Merosin immunocytochemistry shows an absence of the normal expression of the α_2 subunit of laminin (merosin encoded by the *LAMA2* gene) in the basement membrane. A partial merosin-deficient state may have a milder clinical course than a total absence of the protein.

Merosin-positive CMD: Merosin-positive CMD comprises a heterogeneous group of patients with dystrophic muscle biopsies in the neonatal period and apparently normal immunolabeling for merosin. However, the term *classic merosin-positive CMD* has become obsolete as molecular genetic studies characterize distinct disorders. Patients with CMD with mutations in selenoprotein N gene (*SELENON*; old nomenclature, *SEPN1*) typically present with rigid spine syndrome, scoliosis, and respiratory insufficiency. Muscle biopsy may show multi-minicores on oxidative stains. Another example is CMD with mutation of the α_7 integrin gene (*ITGA7*).

Secondary α-dystroglycanopathies: α-Dystroglycan–related dystrophies constitute a third class of CMD associated with brain and often eye malformations. CK levels are often high. In this category are MDC1B, a CMD with partial merosin deficiency with locus in 1q42; MDC1C, caused by mutations in *FKRP*; MDC1D, related to mutations of the *LARGE1* gene; Fukuyama congenital muscular dystrophy (FCMD), which is caused by mutation in *FKTN* and involves predominantly Japanese patients; MEB disease, typically caused by mutations in *O*-mannose β-1,2-*N*-acetylglucosaminyltransferase (*POMGNT1*); and WWS, in which there is genetic heterogeneity with mutations having been demonstrated in the *O*-mannosyltransferase 1 (*POMT1*) gene, the *O*-mannosyltransferase 2 (*POMT2*) gene, the fukutin *FKTN* gene, and the *FKRP* gene. Less common mutations are found in *ISPD*, *GTDC2*, *B3GALNT2*, *B3GNT1*, *TMEM5*, *GMPPB*, *SGK196*, and the dolichyl-phosphate mannosyltransferase subunit genes (*DPM1*, *DPM2*, and *DPM3*).

Table 12.8 Classification of Congenital Muscular Dystrophies: Clinical, Biochemical, and Genetic Characteristics

BIOCHEMICAL DEFECT	GENE	DISEASE PHENOTYPE(S)
Extracellular matrix proteins	*LAMA2*	Primary merosin deficiency (MDC1A)
	COL6A1	Ullrich CMD
	COL6A2	
	COL6A3	Ullrich CMD
Basal membrane proteins	*ITGA7*	Integrin α_7-related CMD
	ITGA9	Integrin α_9-related CMD
Primary dystroglycanopathy	*DAG1*	LGMD with early onset and intellectual disability, normal brain MRI
Secondary dystroglycanopathies	*POMT1*	WWS, MEB, CMD with cerebellar involvement, CMD with intellectual disability and microcephaly
	POMGnT1	WWS, MEB, CMD with cerebellar involvement
	POMT2	WWS, MEB, CMD with cerebellar involvement, CMD with intellectual disability and microcephaly, CMD without intellectual disability
	FKRP	WWS, MEB, CMD with cerebellar involvement, CMD with intellectual disability and microcephaly, CMD with no intellectual disability and normal brain MRI
	FCMD	Fukuyama CMD, WWS, CMD without intellectual disability
	LARGE	WWS, MEB, white matter changes, CMD with intellectual disability
	DPM2/DPM3	CMD with intellectual disability and severe epilepsy
	ISPD	WWS, LGMD, polycystic kidneys
	GTDC2	WWS
	B3GALNT2	MEB, WWS, CMD with intellectual disability, epilepsy
	GMPPB	CMD with intellectual disability and severe epilepsy, MEB, LGMD, isolated CK elevation
	SGK196/POMK	MEB, WWS, LGMD
Endoplasmic reticulum protein	*SEPN1*	CMD with spinal rigidity (RSMD1)
Nuclear envelope proteins	*SYNE1* (*nesprin 1*)	CMD with adducted thumbs
	LMNA	Congenital laminopathy
Mitochondrial membrane protein	*CHKB*	Mitochondrial CMD (CMDmt)

Note: Classification based on combined clinical, genetic, and pathological data. This table does not list all 18 genes involved in the pathogenesis of α-dystroglycanopathies.

CK, creatine kinase; CMD, congenital muscular dystrophy; CMDmt, CMD with mitochondrial structural abnormalities; LGMD, limb-girdle muscular dystrophy; MDC, muscular dystrophy congenital; MEB, muscle–eye–brain disease; MRI, magnetic resonance imaging; RSMD1, rigid spine muscular dystrophy 1; WWS, Walker–Warburg syndrome.

A primary mutation in α-dystroglycan also has been reported. In these diseases, α-dystroglycan immunostaining is usually weaker than in controls.

Collagenopathies: This fourth group of CMDs includes Ullrich and Bethlem myopathies. Both disorders share a uniform combination of contractures in proximal joints, including rigid spine, with distal laxity. CK levels are normal or subnormal. In older infants and children, other typical features include prominent calcanei, keratosis pilaris, and hypertrophic scars (keloids). Subsequent motor development is severely delayed, and walking independently occurs in the minority. Ullrich myopathy is a relatively severe disorder with onset in young infants and children. Bethlem myopathy is a milder, usually autosomal dominant disease, with onset in the first or second decade. Both conditions are connected to mutations in the three genes that encode collagen 6, an extracellular matrix protein: *COL6A1*, *COL6A2*, and *COL6A3* (Table 12.8). Ullrich CMD is caused by either autosomal recessive or dominant mutations in any one of these three genes. However, demonstration of collagen 6 deficiency by IHC requires concurrent double labeling or very high-resolution electron microscopy at a level capable of assessing collagen microfibrils.

12.6.1.2.4. Facioscapulohumeral muscular dystrophy. The classical form of FSHD usually begins in adolescence and is typically slowly progressive. It predominantly involves the face, perihumeral musculature, and the scapular girdle with the notable exception of the deltoid muscle. Peroneal involvement is frequent.

Muscle biopsies reveal nonspecific dystrophic features along with whorled fibers, moth-eaten fibers, and, especially, lobulated fibers (well seen with the NADH-TR reaction in the shape of irregularities in the intermyofibrillar network); and a myositis-like appearance due to the presence of inflammatory mononuclear infiltrates. Considerable histological differences are seen from one muscle to the next. Endomysial fibrosis, of variable intensity, is frequent.

The FSHD myopathy is inherited in an autosomal dominant pattern, but penetrance can be quite variable. Approximately 97% of cases (so-called FSHD1) are associated with deletions of tandem 3.3-kb D4Z4 repeats at 4q35. The deletion reduces the number of repeats to EcoRI/BlnI fragments of less than 35 kb in most patients. The number of D4Z4 repeat units in the general population varies from 11 to 100. In most patients with FSHD1, one D4Z4 allele is contracted (1–10 repeats) and the other D4Z4 allele has the normal number (11–100) of repeat units. Within these repeats lies the *DUX4* gene, which normally is not expressed. In FSHD1, the deletion in the setting of a specific haplotype (4qA) results in hypomethylation of the region and toxic expression of the *DUX4* gene.

Approximately 5% of patients with FSHD have an identical clinical phenotype without the classic deletions in D4Z4 (FSHD2). Mutations in different genes have been described; however, it is important to acknowledge that for the disease to manifest, the patient still needs to have the haplotype 4qA and hypomethylation of the region that leads to the permissive overexpression of the *DUX4* gene. FSHD2 is caused more frequently by mutations in *SMCHD1* and rarely in the *DNMT3B* and *LRIF1* genes. In both FSHD1 and FSHD2, the permissive haplotype introduces a polyadenylation signal that results in an aberrant, toxic *DUX4* transcript. The SMCHD1 protein is an epigenetic modifier that directly binds to the D4Z4 repeat to maintain a repressed chromatin state in somatic cells via methylation; its reduced activity in FSHD2 patients leads to hypomethylation of the D4Z4 repeat array and thus the derepression of DUX4 transcription. Mutations that result in lower levels of the SMCHD1 protein lead to chromatin relaxation of D4Z4, independent of the number of repeats. The *SMCHD1* gene also may act as a modifier of disease severity in families with FSHD1, in which a combination of an larger FSHD1 D4Z4 repeat array of 9 or 10 units and a mutation in *SMCHD1* causes a more severe phenotype and high levels of *DUX4*.

12.6.1.2.5. Oculopharyngeal muscular dystrophy. Oculopharyngeal muscular dystrophy (OPMD) is uncommon, usually autosomal dominant, and characterized by the late-life appearance of external ophthalmoplegia with severe dysphagia. Discrete limb-girdle involvement may be present. Muscle biopsy demonstrates rare "rimmed vacuoles," intranuclear inclusions, and occasionally type 1 fiber predominance. Necrotic fibers are not typical. Ultrastructural studies show intranuclear tubulofilamentous inclusions measuring 8 nm in diameter, not found in the cytoplasm.

OPMD is caused by a GCN trinucleotide repeat expansion (where "N" represents any A, C, G, or T nucleotide) in the first exon of polyadenylate binding protein nuclear 1 gene (*PABPN 1*; previously called *PABP2*). Although immunocytochemistry shows PABPN 1 to be present in the intranuclear inclusions, the confirmatory diagnostic study is the identification of the expanded GCN repeat. The normal *PABPN 1* gene contains 10 repeats. In OPMD, autosomal dominant inheritance occurs with expanded alleles that range from 12 to 17 repeats. Autosomal recessive inheritance has been reported also with alleles that have 11 repeats.

12.6.1.3. MYOTONIC DYSTROPHY AND NONDYSTROPHIC MYOTONIAS

The pathogenesis of myotonia disorders, including dystrophic myotonias (DMs), is complex. and the disorders are heterogeneous. Myotonic dystrophies have been classified among muscular dystrophies for historical reasons. Muscle biopsy is not usually needed to diagnose these conditions because the changes in muscle structure are mostly mild and nonspecific (fiber size variability and internalized nuclei). Muscle biopsy may be helpful to exclude other conditions.

12.6.1.3.1. Dystrophic myotonias *12.6.1.3.1.1. Myotonic dystrophy type 1 (DM1 or Steinert disease).* Myotonic dystrophy type 1 affects individuals at all ages. It is a multisystem disorder that includes characteristic facial involvement, distal limb amyotrophy and weakness, myotonia, and systemic manifestations. The last include frontoparietal baldness, posterior cataracts, endocrine disturbances dominated by hyperinsulinism, thyroid dysfunction, diabetes mellitus, calcium dysregulation, genital hypoplasia, CNS manifestations, and cardiac involvement. Neonatal myotonic dystrophy affects children who have inherited the genetic anomaly from their mother and is manifest by severe hypotonia with facial, oropharyngeal, and respiratory involvement.

Muscle biopsy abnormalities vary greatly in different patient populations and different muscles. Characteristic anomalies include selective atrophy of type 1 fibers and multiple internalized nuclei in many individual muscle fibers. Atrophic fibers may cluster as nuclear bags or occur randomly as angular fibers. In longitudinal sections, internalized nuclei are arranged in chains at various depths of the sarcoplasm. The presence of striated annulets (*ringbinden*) and sarcoplasmic masses is common. Endomysial fibrosis and evidence of degeneration and regeneration are seen to some extent.

Myotonic dystrophy is a "trinucleotide repeat disorder," an unstable heritable expansion of a CTG repeat in the 3′ untranslated region of the "DM protein kinase" gene (*DMPK*) on chromosome 19. Normal individuals have 5–34 CTG repeats at this locus, whereas individuals with classic DM1 have repeats in the hundreds to thousands. In DM1, the expansion of a normal allele (<35 repeats) into the abnormal range is rare.

- Individuals with a CTG repeat size between 35 and 49, designated premutation status or mutable normal, are asymptomatic.
- A mutation of 50 to approximately 150 CTG repeats can manifest as a phenotype characterized by mild myotonia, weakness, or cataracts.
- Repeats in the range of 50 to 1,000 are seen in individuals with the classic DM1 phenotype

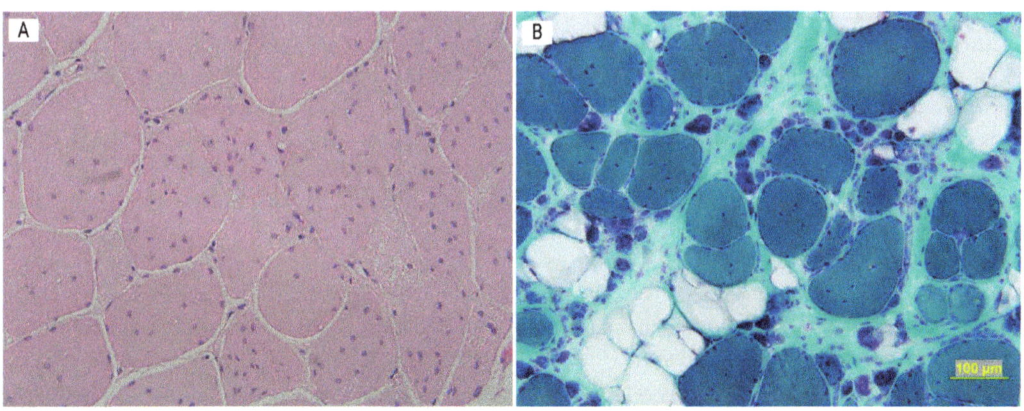

FIGURE 12.19 Myotonic dystrophy type 2. (**A**) Muscle fibers often contain 10 or more internalized nuclei in cross section (H&E). (**B**) Atrophic fibers with nuclear clumps or bags may be frequent (GT).

(onset between ages 10 and 30 years) characterized by muscle wasting and weakness, myotonia, cataracts, frontal balding, and cardiac conduction defects. Average lifespan is reduced.
- With CTG repeat lengths greater than 1,000 (up to 6,500), DM1 may manifest at birth with infantile hypotonia, respiratory dysfunction, and the emergence of intellectual disability; congenital DM1 has also been observed with CTG repeat lengths between 730 and 1,000. There is a tendency for the number of repeats to increase in successive generations, with earlier onset of symptoms, a genetic mechanism known as "anticipation."

12.6.1.3.1.2. Myotonic dystrophy type 2 (DM2 or PROMM). Another dystrophic myotonia (DM2), also called *PROMM* (proximal myotonic myopathy), is caused by a DNA expansion mutation consisting of a CCTG repeat in intron 1 of the *ZNF9* gene located at chromosome 3q13.3-q24. Myotonia may be less prominent than in DM1. Muscle biopsy shows variable atrophy of type 2 fibers. Internalized nuclei with formation of nuclear clumps are also seen. Unlike DM1, ring fibers are not common in DM2.

The DNA expansions in DM1 and DM2 lead to a toxic gain of function of the mutant messenger RNA (mRNA). In both disorders, the mutant RNA appears to form intranuclear inclusions composed of aberrant RNA, with repeats that are detectable by fluorescent in situ hybridization. These RNA inclusions sequester RNA-binding proteins that are essential for proper splicing of a variety of other pre-mRNAs. This results in abnormal transcription of multiple proteins in a variety of tissues/organ systems and explains the systemic manifestations associated with DM1 and DM2.

Although muscle biopsies are usually not performed in DM1, they are not infrequently performed in patients with DM2 because the diagnosis is often not expected. This is because patients with DM2 do not always have significant clinical myotonia or myotonic discharges on electromyography. Biopsy is indicated for nonspecific proximal weakness, elevated CK, or muscle pain. In the appropriate clinical setting, muscle biopsy may suggest the diagnosis in DM2 with findings of markedly increased internalized nuclei in individual muscle fibers (Fig. 12.19), thereby leading to diagnosis by molecular testing.

12.6.1.3.2. Nondystrophic hereditary myotonias. The nondystrophic hereditary myotonias include myotonia congenita (MC) and paramyotonia congenita (PMC) (Table 12.9). Autosomal dominant MC, also known as Thomsen disease, is associated with prominent myotonia and generalized muscular hypertrophy presenting in childhood. The autosomal recessive variant is known as Becker disease (not to be confused with BMD) and is more frequently associated with proximal weakness in addition to myotonia. PMC is inherited in an autosomal dominant fashion and typically presents in early childhood. Unlike the myotonic dystrophies and MC, in which muscle stiffness (myotonia) improves with repetitive activity, the myotonia paradoxically worsens with repetitive activity in PMC. In addition, some patients with PMC have periodic paralysis and develop fixed weakness.

Serum CK levels are usually mildly elevated in MC and PMC, and EMG reveals myotonic discharges. Muscle biopsies may demonstrate nonspecific myopathic features but are not diagnostically useful. MC is caused by mutations in the chloride channel (CLCN1), whereas PMC is caused by mutations in the muscle sodium channel α subunit 4 (SCNA4).

12.6.1.3.3. Related disorders (periodic paralyses). Related classes of disease are hyperkalemic periodic paralysis and hypokalemic periodic paralysis. The former may exhibit myotonia because it is often allelic with PMC. Both are dominantly inherited. Both may have mutations in a sodium channel subunit, but hypokalemic periodic paralysis is more often associated with a mutation in a calcium channel. Both diseases show gradually increasing vacuolations, which ultrastructurally are expansions of the T-tubule system and sarcoplasmic reticulum. Tubular aggregates may be seen and are related to the sarcoplasmic reticulum.

There are also rare myopathies characterized by cramps and prominent tubular aggregates. The proximal myopathies with tubular aggregates described to date are autosomal dominant and associated with mutations in *STIM1*, *ORAI1*, and *CASQ1* (Fig. 12.10). Furthermore, *GDPAGT1*, *GFPT1*, and *ALG2* mutations are associated with congenital myasthenia and may have tubular aggregates on biopsy.

At the light microscopic level, tubular aggregates are red with the modified GT stain and are reactive with NADH, so the distinction from ragged red fibers and mitochondrial myopathy is important. The tubular aggregates do not exhibit cytochrome oxidase or SDH activity, which are specific for mitochondria,

Table 12.9 Genetic, Clinical, and Pathologic Characteristic of Muscle Ion Channel Diseases

DISEASE	GENE	GENE PRODUCT AND FUNCTIONAL CHANGE	SYMPTOMS	PATHOLOGY
Myotonia congenita (Becker)	*CLCN1*	Chloride channel 1 Loss of function	AR; childhood onset; transient weakness	Muscle fiber hypertrophy
Myotonia congenita (Thomsen)	Same as above	Chloride channel 1 Gain of function	AD; second decade	Mild fiber hypertrophy at onset; myofibrillar disarray loss of 2B fibers
Potassium-aggravated myotonia	*SCN4A*	Sodium channel α subunit Gain of function	AD; variable onset; no weakness	T-tubule dilatation (electron microscopy)
Paramyotonia congenita	*SCN4A*	Sodium channel α subunit Gain of function	AD; childhood onset; cold-induced stiffness; weak	Mild nonspecific changes; occasional tubular aggregates
Hypokalemic periodic paralysis type 1	*CACNL1A3*	Calcium channel	AD; second decade onset Episodic weakness triggered by carbohydrates or exercise	Tubular aggregates, debris filled T-tubule dilatation (electron microscopy) Vacuoles
Hypokalemic periodic paralysis type 2	*SCN4A*	Sodium channel α subunit Loss of function	No myotonia; improved by potassium	Tubular aggregates, debris filled T-tubule dilatation (electron microscopy) Vacuoles
Hyperkalemic periodic paralysis	*SCN4A*	Sodium channel α subunit Loss of function	AD; childhood onset Episodic weakness, triggered by rest after exercise; no paramyotonia	Similar to above
Malignant hyperthermia (King–Denborough) (Barnes)	*RYR1* *CACNA1S* *SCN4A*	Ryanodine receptor Calcium channel Sodium channel α subunit	Lethal hyperthermia in response to inhalation anesthetics; no weakness	Can be associated with central core myopathy
Hyperkalemic or hypokalemic periodic paralysis (Andersen–Tawil syndrome)	*KCNJ2*	Potassium channel Loss of function Dominant negative	AD Cardiac arrhythmias Episodic weakness triggered by K+ or exercise	Tubular aggregates

AD, autosomal dominant; AR, autosomal recessive.

Table 12.10 Tubular aggregates myopathies

NAME	GENE	CHARACTERISTICS	MUSCLE BIOPSY
TAM 1	*STIM1*	Extraocular movements limitation CK high	Type 2 fiber atrophy Tubular aggregates in type 1 and 2 fibers
TAM 2	*ORAI1*	Congenital miosis CK high	Tubular aggregates in type 1 fibers
TAM	*CASQ1*	Onset: 4th to 6th decades Myalgias, cramps, fatigue, exercise intolerance CK may be very high	Vacuolar myopathy with tubular aggregates Vacuoles usually clear, and in type 2B fibers they are surrounded by desmin

CK, creatine kinase; TAM, tubular aggregate myopathy.

and tubular aggregates ultrastructurally are not confused with mitochondria (Table 12.10).

12.6.2. Congenital myopathies

Congenital myopathies are a heterogeneous group of myopathies characterized by the presence of structural changes in the muscle fibers. They usually manifest in the neonatal period or early infancy with hypotonia and muscle weakness, and affected individuals have a slow or nonprogressive course.

In general, the clinical course of patients with "congenital myopathies" differs from those with muscular dystrophies in that the tempo of the disease is either nonprogressive or very slowly progressive. Nevertheless, this distinction is imprecise. In some patients, the disease becomes manifest in utero with fetal akinesia or as neonatal hypotonia, whereas other cases are first detected in the neonatal period or later due to delayed motor development or muscle weakness of variable distribution. Associated skeletal dysmorphism is frequently observed, reflecting the early, and even prenatal, muscular dysfunction. CK levels in serum are usually only slightly elevated or normal. The mode of inheritance differs among the congenital myopathies. Next-generation sequencing techniques have allowed the identification of affected genes and mutations.

The classification of congenital myopathies is regularly updated as new genetic information is discovered, but the following is a current understanding:

1. Nemaline myopathy (subtypes: rod, core–rod, cap, and zebra body myopathy)
2. Core myopathy (subtypes: central core and multi-minicore myopathy)
3. Centronuclear myopathy (subtypes: myotubular myopathy and autosomal centronuclear myopathy)
4. Congenital fiber-type disproportion
5. Congenital myopathy with protein accumulation

The muscle biopsy changes most frequently found in congenital myopathies are (1) type 1 atrophy/hypotrophy or marked predominance/uniformity of type 1 fibers; and (2) internalized nuclei, characteristically associated with centronuclear or myotubular myopathies but may also be prominent in RYR1-related myopathies. Fibrosis, necrosis, and regeneration are less common than in other genetically determined myopathies.

12.6.2.1. NEMALINE MYOPATHIES

Nemaline myopathies are a heterogeneous group of disorders with muscle biopsy findings characterized by the presence of intracytoplasmic rods or *nemaline bodies* that are visible by light microscopy (reddish on modified GT, most often within hypotrophic type 1 fibers) (Fig. 12.20; see also Fig. 12.8B). By electron microscopy, they are seen as electron-dense structures, measuring 1–3 μm in length and 0.3 μm in diameter; anchoring thin (actin) filaments; they are close to, or in continuity with, Z disks. Nemaline rods can also be found within nuclei, most frequently in association with mutation in *ACTA1*, but can also be found in cases with mutations in *CFL2* and *MYPN*. In affected younger children, rods may not be as conspicuous in muscle biopsies, due in part to the small size of the fibers in this age group; electron microscopy helps increase the diagnostic yield in this

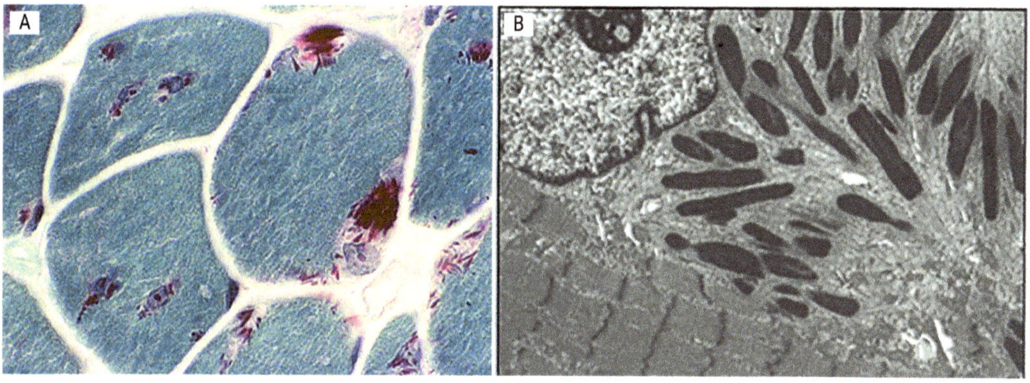

FIGURE 12.20 Nemaline myopathy: (**A**) intracytoplasmic rods that appear reddish and bacilliform on GT; (**B**) ultrastructure of nemaline rods of Z-band density (EM).

age group. Rods are composed mainly of α-actinin, actin, and other Z-band filaments. The number of affected fibers is highly variable and is not correlated with the clinical severity of the disease. Type 1 fibers often predominate. Both dominant and recessive forms and variants with infantile (most severe), childhood (most common), and adult onset have been described. Muscle weakness typically involves proximal, facial, bulbar, and respiratory muscles.

Nemaline myopathies are associated with variants in more than 13 genes of thin filament–associated molecules, including sarcomeric actin (ACTA1), tropomyosin (TPM2 and -3), troponin T (TNNT types 1 and 3), nebulin (NEB), and cofilin (CFL2). Core–rod myopathy (*RYR1* mutations), cap–rod myopathy, and zebra body myopathy (*ACTA1* mutations) are variants of nemaline myopathy and should be considered part of the nemaline myopathies (Table 12.11).

Table 12.11 Nemaline myopathies

GENE	INHERITANCE	PROTEIN	CHARACTERISTICS AND PHENOTYPE OMIM NO.
ACTA1	AD (AR)	Sarcomeric α-actin	May show intranuclear rods, clumped filaments, cores, or fiber-type disproportion; 161800
NEB	AR	Nebulin	Nemaline myopathy with NEB mutations is allelic to one form of arthrogryposis multiplex congenita; 256030
TPM3	AD (AR)	α-Tropomyosin-3	Genetic heterogeneity and variable clinical severity; 609284. Mutations in TPM3 are also responsible by CAP myopathy
TPM2	AD	β-Tropomyosin-2	Mutations in TPM2 are also responsible by CAP myopathy; 609285
TNNT1	AR	Slow troponin or troponin T1	Also called Amish nemaline myopathy (ANM); children with ANM had tremors evident at birth or within a few days of birth; 605355
TNNT3	AR	Fast troponin	Allelic with arthrogryposis, distal, type 2B2
CFL2	AR	Cofilin 2	Very early onset; 610687
KBTBD13	AD	Kelch repeat and BTB domain-containing protein 13	Nemaline rods, cores devoid of oxidative enzyme activity; 609273
KLHL40	AR	Kelch-like protein 40	Very severe, onset in utero; 615348
KLHL41	AR	Kelch-like protein 41	615731
LMOD3	AR	Leiomodin 3	Very severe, onset in utero; 616165

AD, autosomal dominant; AR, autosomal recessive.

Nemaline rods may also occur as a secondary phenomenon in other myopathies (dystrophic, inflammatory, and mitochondrial), and even as an acquired response to tenotomy, neoplasia, and weightlessness. Acquired cases of nemaline myopathy in adulthood, referred to as sporadic late-onset nemaline myopathy (SLONM), are quite rare, thought to be autoimmune, and associated with HIV or monoclonal gammopathy of uncertain significance. Clinically, patients manifest progressive proximal and axial muscle weakness.

12.6.2.2. CONGENITAL MYOPATHIES WITH CENTRAL NUCLEI

The centronuclear and myotubular myopathies are characterized by the presence of a centrally placed nucleus in most fibers (Fig. 12.21); at least three forms are recognized. The term myotubular myopathy is reserved for the X-linked infantile disorder, and the term centronuclear myopathy (CNM) is used for both the autosomal recessive and autosomal dominant forms. Mutations in *MTM1* are associated with myotubular myopathy, and *DNM2*, *BIN1*, *MTMR14*, *RYR1*, *TTN*, *SPEG*, and *CCDC78* have been associated with CNMs.

Myotubular myopathy is a severe X-linked infantile congenital myopathy caused by mutations in *MTM1*, which encodes the protein *myotubularin*, a tyrosine phosphatase. Muscle fibers are uniformly abnormally small and have a central nucleus (or central clear core) giving an "immature" myotube appearance to the fibers, similar to a fetal stage of development (myotubular stage). Female carriers of myotubular myopathy and patients with milder cases of myotubular myopathy may show "necklace fibers" (Fig. 12.22).

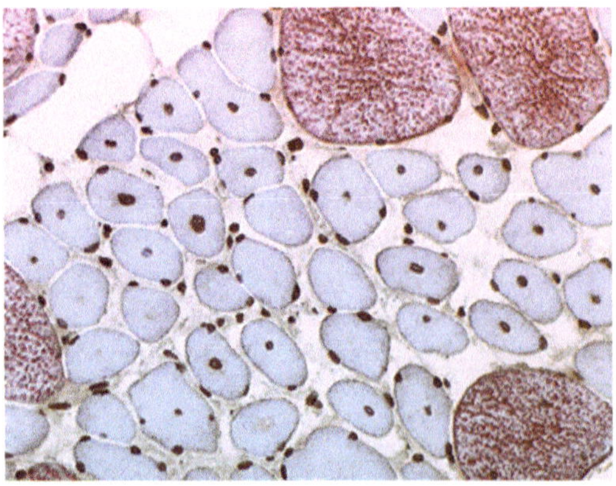

FIGURE 12.21 Adult centronuclear myopathy showing many fibers with central nuclei as well as increased endomysial connective tissue (GT).

The autosomal dominant milder childhood or adulthood forms are mostly due to mutations in *DNM2*. A characteristic feature is the presence of fibers with sarcoplasmic strands radiating from the center like the spokes on a wheel and best observed with PAS and NADH-TR.

Recessive mutations in *BIN1*, which encodes for amphiphysin, are a rare cause of CNM. A prominent feature in these biopsies is the presence of multiple, clustered, central nuclei that may form nuclear chains down the length of fibers and often have a surrounding zone of enhanced oxidative enzyme staining.

Other less frequent forms of CNMs are the autosomal recessive mutations in *SPEG* that cause a severe congenital-onset CNM with dilated cardiomyopathy. On immunoblot and immunofluorescence, there is a marked reduction or absence of SPEG protein. Recessive mutations in *RYR1* have also been associated with a CNM. There are often fewer central nuclei than in other forms of CNMs.

12.6.2.3. CORE MYOPATHIES

Core myopathies are a clinically, pathologically, and genetically heterogeneous group of diseases that include central core disease (CCD), multiminicore disease (MmD), dusty core disease, multi-structured core disease, and core–rod myopathy (Table 12.12). Other myopathies with cores and focal disorganization of the intermyofibrillar network are associated with mutations in *TTN* (autosomal recessive [AR], autosomal dominant [AD]). *DHPR* (AD, AR), *PYROX1* (AR), *UNC45B* (AR), and *SRPK3* (X-linked). These congenital myopathies are characterized by the presence of cytoplasmic areas of myofibrillar disorganization (cores/mini-cores) lacking mitochondrial and oxidative enzyme activity and localized centrally or at the periphery of muscle fibers.

Classical CCD is the most frequent and well-recognized subtype of core myopathy. The gene associated with this subtype is usually *RYR1* (AD); however, some other cases have been described involving mutations in *MYH7* (AD). The *RYR1* gene encodes for the ryanodine receptor, which is involved in calcium homeostasis.

Cores appear as well-delineated amorphous areas on H&E and GT and are devoid of oxidative enzyme activity. In longitudinal sections, they

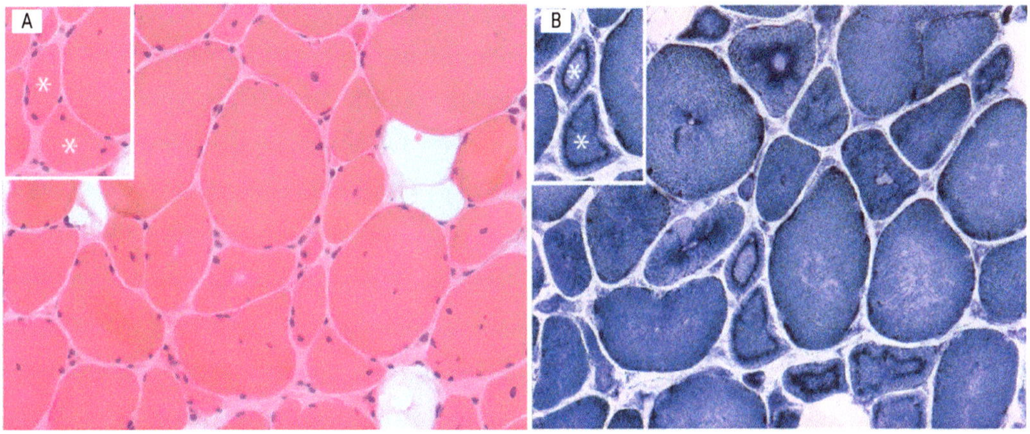

FIGURE 12.22 Necklace fibers: (**A**) atrophic angulated with a faint basophilic layer at the perimeter (H&E); (**B**) oxidative enzyme histochemistry highlights the peripheral "necklace" (NADH). (Necklace fibers duplicated in inset [*asterisks*].)

can extend almost along the full length of the fiber and can have a rim of PAS positivity. In transverse sections, the cores can be central or eccentric, and single or multiple. Cores are most frequently seen within type 1 fibers (Fig. 12.23). They involve predominantly type 1 fibers, and biopsies are sometimes described as "uniform type 1." The central core resembles that seen in target fibers in reinnervation, but the latter (target fibers) involves both muscle fiber types. A few isolated, angular, atrophic fibers may also be seen.

On electron microscopy, cores are devoid of mitochondria, and the sarcoplasmic reticulum and T-tubule networks may be reduced. The areas of myofibrillar disruption have sharply demarcated borders and can vary from poorly aligned sarcomeres and slight irregularity of the Z lines (structured cores) (Fig. 12.23C) to marked disruption and disarray of the sarcomeres (unstructured cores) with Z-line streaming (Fig. 12.23B). Unstructured cores lack myosin ATPase staining. Immunohistochemically, cores show accumulation of several myofibrillar proteins, including desmin, myotilin, αB-crystallin, filamin-C, and heat shock proteins.

CCD may be associated with an increased incidence of the potentially fatal malignant hyperthermia reaction in response to certain general anesthetics. Other phenotypes associated with *RYR1* mutations are a late-onset axial myopathy (bent spine syndrome), recurrent myoglobinuria, and hyper-CK-emia with or without myalgia.

Multi-minicores in MmD are characterized on electron microscopy by multiple small areas of Z-line streaming and loss of mitochondria running over a few sarcomeres. In the oxidative stains, multi-minicores present as multiple areas without enzymatic activity or with an uneven staining that creates an appearance similar to moth-eaten fibers. The genes most frequently mutated are *SELENON* (AR) and *RYR1* (AR). Multi-minicores can be observed in both type 1 and type 2 fibers, although they are more often seen in type 1 fibers. SELENON-related myopathy is clinically characterized by axial myopathy with scoliosis and respiratory failure.

In dominant forms of MYH2-related myopathy, the multi-minicores are present in type 2A fibers, as *MYH2* encodes for myosin heavy chain 2, which is expressed in type 2A fibers. Recessive forms lack type 2A fibers, but there are no true multi-minicores.

MYH7-related myopathies show variable phenotypes. Mutations in *MYH7* encoding the slow skeletal muscle fiber myosin heavy chain may show aspects of CCD; may show hyaline bodies on muscle biopsy; may be associated with Laing distal myopathy, MmD, or deposits of myosin heavy chain beneath the sarcolemma; or may be associated with cardiomyopathy.

Dusty core disease is associated with recessive mutations in *RYR1*. Dusty cores are large irregular areas of myofibrillar disorganization with variable diameter and length that frequently cover the entire diameter of the fiber. GT stain shows reddish-purple granular material, and there is an uneven oxidative staining and negligent ATPase activity. Unlike cores, dusty cores are not well delimited and are not round/ovoid in shape.

Table 12.12 Clinicopathological Features of Core Myopathies

GENE (INHERITANCE)	CCD	MMD	DUCD	CORE ROD MYOPATHY	SYMPTOMS
RYR1 (AR/AD)	+ (AD)	+	+ (AR)	+	External ophthalmoplegia, bulbar involvement, scoliosis, hip dislocation, malignant hyperthermia
SELENON (AR)		+ (both fiber types)			Axial myopathy with scoliosis, respiratory failure, spinal rigidity
MYH2 (AR)		+			Facial weakness and dysmorphism, proximal weakness, scoliosis, ophthalmoplegia
MYH7 (AD)	+	+ (hyaline bodies)			Weakness of great toe/ankle dorsiflexors, neck flexor, finger extensor, facial weakness
TTN (AR)		+ like[a] (multiple internal nuclei)			Neonatal hypotonia, facial muscle weakness, dilated cardiomyopathy
CCDC78 (AD)	+[b]				Neonatal hypotonia, distal weakness, excessive fatigue, myalgias, cognitive involvement
UNC45B (AR)	+[b] 1FP/unstructured cores, eccentric cores				Axial and proximal weakness, delayed motor milestones, calf hypertrophy
ACTN2 (AD)	+ Multistructured core disease [c]				Distal weakness, ophthalmoplegia, ptosis, cardiac abnormalities, respiratory involvement
MEGF10 (AR)		+ Eosinophilic aggregates			Axial, facial, and proximal weakness; scoliosis; respiratory problems; contractures; nasal speech
NEB (AR)				+	Generalized hypotonia, bilateral foot drop
ACTA1 (AD)	+ Unstructured cores				Proximal or generalized muscle weakness, delayed motor milestones, facial weakness
KBTBD13 (AD)				+	Proximal and neck weakness

CFL2 (AR)	+ Nemaline bodies, minicores	Floppy infant, respiratory distress
TRIP4 (AR)	+ Multi-minicores, nemaline rods, cytoplasmic bodies, caps, rimmed fibers	Axial and proximal weakness, rigid spine, dysmorphic facies, cutaneous involvement, respiratory failure, dilated cardiomyopathy
TNNT1 (AR)	+ Multi-minicores in type 1 fibers, nemaline rods in type 1 fibers	Proximal weakness, scoliosis, congenital hip luxation, rhabdomyolysis, rigid spine, respiratory involvement

[a]Marked loss of thin filamentary material; electron microscopy: focal disorganizations, loss of filamentary material, M-line dissolution with almost preserved Z-line over one or two sarcomeres.
[b]Atypical cores.
[c]Well-delimited subsarcolemmal structured cores.
CCD, central core disease; DuCD, dusty core disease; MmD, multi-minicore disease.

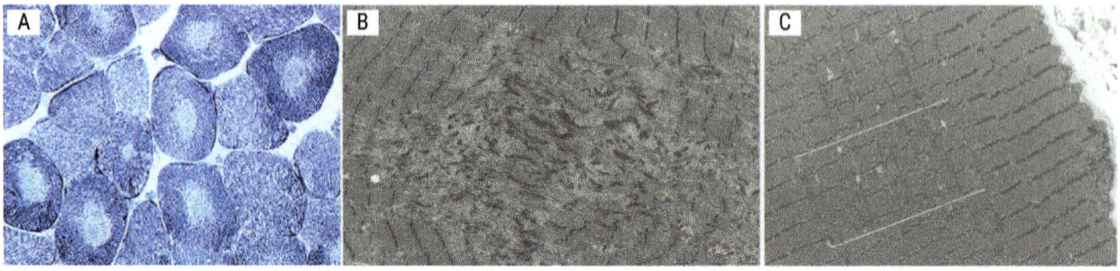

FIGURE 12.23 Central core disease. (**A**) Central cores are devoid of oxidative enzyme activity in type 1 fibers (NADH-TR). (**B**) Cores are devoid of mitochondria, the sarcoplasmic reticulum and T-tubule networks may be reduced, and there is myofibrillar disruption of the sarcomeres in unstructured cores (EM). (**C**) Misaligned sarcomeres with irregularity of the Z bands in structured cores (EM).

12.6.2.4. OTHER TYPES OF CONGENITAL MYOPATHIES

Regarding other types of congenital myopathies, cap myopathy is characterized by the presence of cap-like structures, which are sharply demarcated structures of disorganized, thin filaments at the periphery of muscle fibers. As with nemaline myopathy, the genes associated with cap myopathy (*TPM2*, *TPM3*, and *ACTA1*) encode components of the sarcomeric thin filaments.

Other types of congenital myopathies seen rarely in clinical practice include reducing body myopathy (mutation of the *FHL1* gene), hyaline body myopathy (mutation of the myosin heavy chain 7 gene *MYH7*), congenital myopathies with severe cardiomyopathy (mutations of *MYBPC3* and titin), fingerprint inclusion myopathy, and zebra body myopathy.

12.6.2.4.1. Congenital Fiber-Type Disproportion. Congenital fiber-type disproportion (CFTD) myopathy was originally identified because of the distinctive histologic appearance of small, excessively numerous type 1 fibers (fiber-type disproportion) and a benign prognosis (Fig. 12.5). However, this abnormality may be seen in other congenital myopathies and in DM1. The nosology of this condition remains uncertain. The likelihood is that these cases represent a heterogeneous collection of disorders (e.g., related to mutation of *ACTA1* or *SELENON*) with a common morphologic appearance.

12.6.3. Myofibrillar myopathies

Myofibrillar myopathies are a group of myopathies with common morphologic features characterized by pathological protein aggregates and degenerative changes of myofibrils. Some cases are likely to be identical to what has been described as "desmin myopathy," "cytoplasmic body myopathy," "spheroid body myopathy," or "protein storage myopathies." The mode of inheritance is autosomal dominant or recessive. The disease is clinically manifest by progressive muscle weakness, which often involves or begins in distal muscles, but limb-girdle or scapuloperoneal distributions can also occur. Cardiomyopathy and peripheral neuropathy are frequently observed. Myofibrillar myopathies are characterized on muscle biopsy by a distinct pattern of focal myofibrillar dissolution associated with disintegration of the Z disk, accumulation of myofibrillar degradation products, ectopic expression of multiple proteins, and sometimes congophilic material. In trichrome-stained sections, an admixture of dark blue or blue-red amorphous, granular, or hyaline deposits that vary in shape and size is seen in the abnormal fibers. The hyaline structures are typically devoid of oxidative enzyme activity. In some myofibrillar myopathies, rimmed vacuoles may be present. Immune staining demonstrates accumulation of desmin and other proteins. To date, all myofibrillar myopathy mutations have been traced to Z-disk–associated proteins, namely desmin, αB-crystallin, myotilin, ZASP, filamin C, and Bag3 (Table 12.13).

12.6.4. Metabolic myopathies

12.6.4.1. MITOCHONDRIAL MYOPATHIES

Primary mitochondrial disorders constitute a group of systemic diseases due to mitochondrial enzyme deficits and with a wide range of clinical manifestations (see Chapter 10). Mitochondrial myopathy may be an organ-specific manifestation

Table 12.13 Myofibrillar Myopathies

PROTEIN	GENE	PROTEIN CLASS	EXPRESSION
Desmin	*DES*	Intermediate filament	Skeletal, cardiac, smooth muscle
αB-crystalline	*CRYAB*	Small heat shock protein	Skeletal, cardiac, lens, kidney, lung
Myotilin	*MYOT*	Sarcomere protein	Skeletal, cardiac
Protein Cypher	*ZASP*	Sarcomere protein	Skeletal, cardiac
BAG3	*BAG3*	BAG family	Skeletal, cardiac, smooth muscle
Filamin C	*FLNC*	Filamin family	Skeletal, cardiac
FHL1	*FHL1*	FHL family	Skeletal, cardiac
Titin	*TTN*	Third filament system	Skeletal, cardiac
Plectin	*PLEC*	Intermediate filament	Skeletal, skin
DNAJB6	*DNAJB6*	DNAJ family	Skeletal, brain
α-Actin	*ACTA1*	Thin filament	Skeletal, cardiac
HSPB8	*HSPB8*	Small heat shock protein	Skeletal, cardiac, placenta

of what is more appropriately referred to as a mitochondrial cytopathy. Mitochondrial cytopathies may result from mutations of either mtDNA or, more commonly, nuclear DNA. mtDNA is a 16.5-kb DNA encoding for 22 transfer RNA (tRNA), 2 ribosomal RNA, and 13 mRNA for respiratory chain proteins. The other 67 polypeptides implicated in the mitochondrial respiratory chain are encoded by the nuclear DNA. Many cases appear to be sporadic, but autosomal (dominant or recessive) Mendelian transmission and especially non-Mendelian maternal transmission by the mitochondrial genome are sometimes present. So-called maternal inheritance is only a feature of mutations of mtDNA.

There is a wide range of clinical manifestations, including ptosis, external ophthalmoplegia, heart conduction block, short stature, deafness, diabetes, and epilepsy. Diagnostic features include an elevated lactate:pyruvate ratio in blood and cerebrospinal fluid and muscle biopsy findings. Confirmation requires biochemical and genetic testing.

Muscle biopsy shows increases numbers and abnormalities of mitochondria in muscle fibers. By light microscopy, these are well demonstrated with the modified GT stain, as ragged red fibers (Fig. 12.9A), although this finding is neither specific nor invariable. The number of ragged red fibers is highly variable within a biopsy sample and from one muscle to another. The abnormal accumulations are seen with NADH histochemistry, although SDH and COX are more specific for mitochondria. Histoenzymatic demonstration of COX (complex IV of the mitochondrial respiratory chain) deficiency is extremely useful for assessing mitochondrial dysfunction. In most patients with mtDNA mutations, a COX reaction shows a pattern of reactivity in which selected, randomly distributed fibers are devoid of COX reactivity. Associated altered glycogen and lipid metabolism is manifest with abnormal aggregates of intramuscular lipids or glycogen. Electron microscopy may show mitochondria with structural abnormalities, such as cristae that are concentrically arranged, are honeycombed, or contain paracrystalline inclusions or large osmophilic amorphous granules (Fig. 12.9C, D). Other abnormalities, such as variability in mitochondrial size, shape, and number, are useful adjuncts.

Molecular studies of the mitochondrial genetic material and biochemical studies of the mitochondrial electron transport chain enzymes can be performed on either muscle biopsy samples or lymphocytes. Clinicopathological correlations are complemented by the fact that the same biochemical deficit may be responsible for a highly variable clinical picture. Conversely, identical clinical manifestations may be caused by different enzyme abnormalities.

While a general biochemical classification continues to evolve, several distinct clinical syndromes are well-characterized (Table 12.14).

12.6.4.2. LIPID MYOPATHIES

Lipids are one of the sources of energy for the muscle, and its metabolism occurs in the mitochondria. Lipids are stored in the muscle as lipid droplets lacking a membrane, and they are demonstrable

Table 12.14 Selected Mitochondrial Myopathic Syndromes

SYNDROME	GENETICS	CLINICAL FEATURES	PATHOLOGY
Kearns–Sayre	Single large mtDNA deletion	PEO	Variation in muscle fiber size
	Most common mutation type (80%)	Pigmentary degeneration of retina	Ragged red fibers common
	Identical in Pearson syndrome and PEO	Heart block; mitochondrial myopathy	COX^+ and COX^-
		Weakness: proximal, symmetric	
		Multiple CNS deficits	
MELAS Mitochondrial Encephalomyopathy	mtDNA point mutations	Encephalopathy, seizures, hemiplegia Pigmentary retinopathy	Ragged red fibers, COX^+ Basal ganglia calcification
Lactic acidosis		Myopathy; exercise intolerance	Cerebral focal necrosis
Stroke		Proximal symmetric weakness	
MERRF Myoclonic	mtDNA point mutations	Late adolescence onset; myoclonus	Ragged red fibers, COX^-
Epilepsy Ragged red fibers		Polyneuropathy; myopathy Hearing loss; optic atrophy	

Note: Acquired mitochondrial myopathy may occur in patients treated with azidothymidine (AZT), an antiviral nucleoside analogue interfering with mtDNA replication.

MELAS, *m*itochondrial myopathy, *e*ncephalopathy, *l*actic *a*cidosis, and *s*troke-like episodes; MERRF, *m*yoclonus *e*pilepsy with *r*agged *r*ed *f*ibers; PEO, progressive external ophthalmoplegia.

with ORO or Sudan Black stains (Fig. 12.24A, B). In some lipid myopathies (carnitine deficiency, lipin-1 deficiency, and multiple acyl-CoA deficiency), the number and size of these droplets increase, and there may be secondary mitochondrial changes. In certain cases, such as in carnitine palmityl transferase II deficiency, the content in lipids is not increased, and in other conditions the lipid content varies with the

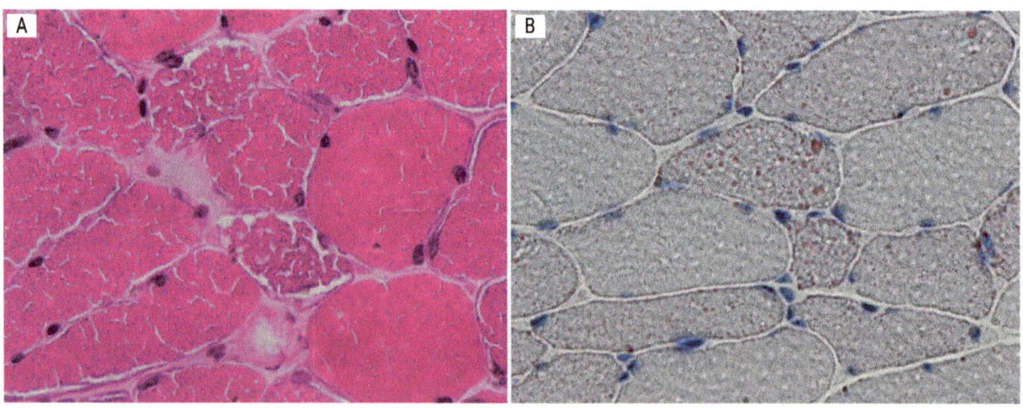

FIGURE 12.24 Multiple acyl-CoA dehydrogenase deficiency (MADD). (**A**) Many fibers with microvacuoles are present (H&E). (**B**) Myocyte content of lipid is increased (ORO).

course of the disease. Clinically, lipid myopathies can be divided into those with fixed weakness and those with exercise intolerance, cramps, and myoglobinuria.

12.6.4.2.1. Carnitine deficiency. Three forms of carnitine deficiency are recognized:

- Muscle carnitine deficiency causes limb-girdle myopathy presenting in the second decade of life. Muscle biopsy reveals vacuolar myopathy. Lipid storage is evident as droplets that can be stained with Sudan Black or ORO. This storage occurs in type 1 fibers and is accompanied by mitochondrial abnormalities. Muscle carnitine levels are low, but serum levels are normal.
- Systemic carnitine deficiency may become clinically apparent early in life manifesting as acute metabolic episodes, in the course of which the myopathy may be detected as a secondary phenomenon.
- Secondary partial carnitine deficiency may be associated with cachexia, liver pathology, chronic hemodialysis, or another form of myopathy, especially mitochondrial myopathy. Carnitine deficiency, and the consequent lipid storage myopathy, may also be drug induced, secondary to valproate anticonvulsant therapy.

12.6.4.2.2. Carnitine palmitoyl transferase II deficiency. Carnitine palmityl transferase II deficiency is manifested from early childhood by episodes of cramps with myoglobinuria, occurring after prolonged effort. Hyperlipidemia may be present. Between these episodes of rhabdomyolysis, muscle biopsy is usually normal. Lipid storage, which is detected in less than one-third of the cases, is less evident than in carnitine deficiency. The enzyme deficit may be demonstrated in the skeletal muscle, leukocytes, and cultured fibroblasts.

12.6.4.2.3. Multiple acyl-CoA-dehydrogenase deficiency. Multiple acyl-CoA-dehydrogenase deficiency (MADD), also known as glutaric aciduria type II, may present with recurrent episodes of exercise-induced myoglobinuria later in childhood or adult life with proximal or distal weakness. The findings on muscle biopsy are indistinguishable from those of primary carnitine deficiency. Serum and urine acylcarnitine analysis profile reveals increased concentrations of all chain lengths, but mainly medium- and long-chain acylcarnitine. The plasma-free carnitine level may be normal or slightly decreased. MADD is caused by mutations in genes that encode for electron transfer flavoprotein ETFA or ETFB or ETF dehydrogenase (ETF-QO). Patients respond successfully to riboflavin treatment.

12.6.4.2.4. Neutral lipid storage disease. Neutral lipid storage disease is recognized as two distinct autosomal recessive forms: (1) neutral lipid storage disease with myopathy (NLSDM); and (2) neutral lipid storage disease with ichthyosis (NLSDI), also called Chanarin–Dorfman syndrome. Both forms can cause progressive proximal or distal weakness as well as cardiomyopathy. Muscle biopsy shows accumulation of lipid (triglycerides rather that fatty acids) and the presence of rimmed vacuoles. Lipid droplets can be seen in the leukocytes (Jordan anomaly). NLSDM is caused by mutations in the *PNPLA2* gene that encodes adipose triglyceride lipase (ATGL), which catalyzes the initial step in triglyceride hydrolysis. NLSDI is caused by mutations in the gene that encodes the coactivator of ATGL. It is an autosomal recessive disease characterized by progressive muscle weakness with high CK levels and occasional cardiomyopathy and cognitive impairment. The onset extends from childhood to early adulthood.

12.6.4.2.5. Lipin-1 deficiency. Lipin-1 deficiency is an autosomal recessive condition and a common cause of rhabdomyolysis in children. It is due to mutations in the gene *LPIN1*. Lipin-1 is a muscle-specific phosphatidic acid phosphatase that catalyzes the conversion of phosphatidic acid to diacylglycerol; thus, it is an important enzyme in the pathway of triglyceride and phospholipid biosynthesis. Lipin-1 also acts as a transcriptional protein that regulates cellular lipid metabolism, including genes involved in fatty acid oxidation and mitochondrial biosynthesis.

The episodes of rhabdomyolysis are triggered by fever, exercise, fasting. or anesthesia. Between attacks, muscle strength is usually normal. CK levels can be very high (20,000–450,000 units/L), but carnitine levels, acylcarnitine profile, urine organic acids, and fatty acid oxidation studies are normal. Muscle biopsy may show an increase in lipid droplets and occasional mitochondrial changes with a diffuse reduction in COX staining.

12.6.4.3. GLYCOGENOSES

In glycogenoses, aggregates of glycogen accumulate within the muscle fiber and are demonstrable in sections stained with PAS; the findings are confirmed with ultrastructural and biochemical studies. The identification of the site of glycogen accumulation in the muscle is important: mainly lysosomal (i.e., type II or Pompe disease) or cytoplasmic (types III–V and VII). A further distinction is the presence of abnormal fibrillary glycogen (polyglucosan) in type IV and phosphofructokinase deficiency.

12.6.4.3.1. Pompe disease (type II, acid maltase deficiency) and Danon disease. Acid maltase deficiency can present in early infancy (classic infantile Pompe) to late adult life. It is caused by homozygous or compound heterozygous mutations in the *GAA* gene, which encodes acid α-1,4-glucosidase, also known as acid maltase. The classic infantile form presents with hypotonia and cardiomyopathy and is usually fatal within 2 years due to cardiopulmonary failure. Late-onset acid maltase is frequently associated with a limb-girdle pattern of weakness (thus it can be mistaken for DMD, BMD, or one of the LGMDs). Respiratory muscles are also frequently involved and may be more severely affected than the limb muscles.

Muscle biopsies in Pompe disease reveal a vacuolar myopathy (Fig. 12.25A). The vacuoles involve a highly variable proportion of muscle fibers, usually of type 1. They may be small and scant and readily stain with acid phosphatase due to the lysosomal origin of the vacuoles. PAS stain shows positive inclusions (Fig. 12.25B) that are digested by amylase. Electron microscopy (Fig. 12.25C) demonstrates excess granular glycogen within membrane-bound lysosomes and extending beyond the lysosomes into the cytosol. Biopsies in late-onset cases may be relatively normal, show nonspecific myopathic features, or even show neurogenic atrophy (probably due to abnormal accumulation of glycogen that also occurs in anterior horn cells). The diagnosis can be confirmed by biochemical assay and/or by genetic testing of the *GAA* gene; enzyme replacement therapy is now available for treatment.

Danon disease, an X-linked vacuolar myopathy associated with mutation and deficiency of lysosome-associated membrane protein 2 (*LAMP-2*), has an onset in childhood or young adulthood

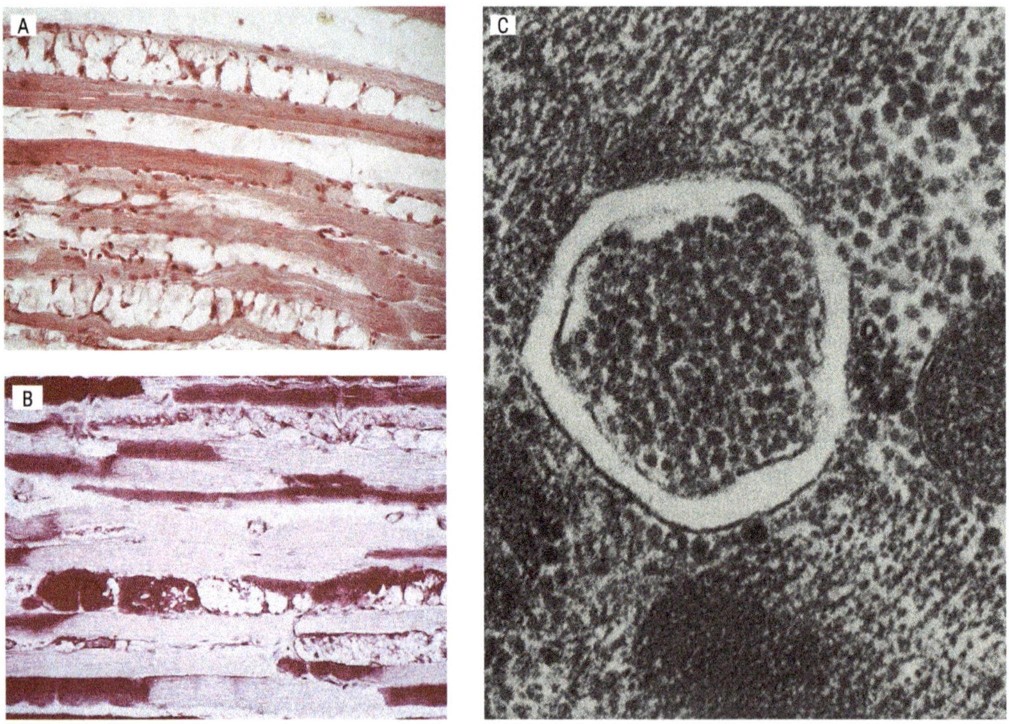

FIGURE 12.25 Pompe disease: (**A**) large clear vacuoles (H&E); (**B**) vacuoles are stained with PAS; (**C**) vacuoles are membrane-bound, indicating lysosomal storage (EM). (Courtesy Pr. M. Baudrimont.)

affects skeletal muscle and the heart. Patients may present with limb-girdle weakness or cardiac signs; there may be associated mild mental retardation. CK levels are elevated. Muscle biopsy shows variability of fiber size and the presence of membrane-bound autophagic vacuoles that are PAS positive and stain with acid phosphatase. IHC shows sarcolemmal proteins in the membranes around the vacuoles (so-called autophagic vacuoles with sarcolemmal features) and an absence of LAMP-2 protein.

12.6.4.3.2. Forbes disease (type III, deficit of the debranching enzyme amylo-1,6 glucosidase). Characterized by the accumulation of dextrin, Forbes disease (type III, deficit of the debranching enzyme amylo-1,6 glucosidase) is usually evidenced in childhood by non0myopathic manifestations.

12.6.4.3.3. McArdle disease (type V, myophosphorylase deficiency). McArdle disease (type V, myophosphorylase deficiency) is caused by homozygous or compound heterozygous mutation in the *PYGM* gene, which encodes muscle glycogen phosphorylase. It is usually recognized in the adult because of painful cramps, which are sometimes associated with myoglobinuria and occur during short and intense bouts of physical exertion. The cramp, which is electrically silent, is followed by a "second-wind" phenomenon that is characteristic as the effort is being made. The curve of hyperlactic acidemia, normally obtained in effort, is flat. Muscle biopsy inconstantly shows subsarcolemmal vacuoles with PAS-positive contents. The diagnosis can sometimes be made with enzyme histochemistry demonstrating absence of phosphorylase activity; however, it is best confirmed by biochemical assay of muscle myophosphorylase activity and/or genetic testing of the *PGYM* gene.

12.6.4.3.4. Tarui disease (type VII, phosphofructokinase deficiency). The clinical picture of Tarui disease (type VII, phosphofructokinase [PFK] deficiency) is similar to that of McArdle disease and is associated with moderate hemolytic anemia. The disorder is caused by mutations in the *PFKM* gene, which encodes the M (muscle) isoform of PFK. Phosphorylase activity is normal. The diagnosis is made either on the basis of enzyme histochemistry or biochemically and confirmed by detection of mutations in the *PFKM* gene.

12.6.4.3.5. Other rare glycogenosis. Among these, a group of disorders characterized by the accumulation of glucose polymers (polyglucosan bodies) is recognized that includes type IV glycogenosis, Lafora disease, and polyglucosan myopathy (see Chapter 10). The accumulated material is PAS positive but resistant to diastase.

12.6.4.4. ENDOCRINE MYOPATHIES

Although muscle weakness is often observed in various endocrine disorders, the corresponding histological changes usually show little specificity.

12.6.4.4.1. Steroid myopathy. Steroid myopathy is seen mostly in Cushing disease or as a result of prolonged corticosteroid therapy. An acute form may occur in status asthmaticus when treatment with curare and high doses of hydrocortisone is necessary. Steroid myopathy is manifest by type 2 muscle atrophy, especially of type 2B. Lipid or glycogen storage, as well as vacuolar myopathy, may also be seen.

12.6.4.4.2. Thyroid myopathy. In hyperthyroidism, the muscle biopsy is ordinarily unremarkable. The muscle biopsies of patients with thyrotoxic periodic paralysis, seen mainly in Japan, show the picture of vacuolar myopathy. In hypothyroidism, abnormalities in the muscle biopsy are more frequent; these include myopathic changes, type 2 fiber atrophy, glycogen storage, and basophilic accumulations in the connective tissue.

12.6.4.5. MYALGIA/CRAMP SYNDROMES

A large number of well-recognized muscle disorders may be manifest primarily as painful myopathies, which present or are accentuated by physical exertion and may be accompanied by cramps. These include some of the glycogenoses, lipidoses, and toxic and endocrine myopathies. In practice, the muscle biopsy in these predominantly myalgic syndromes is often disappointing and shows only nonspecific changes, such as moderate atrophy of type 2 fibers. Such is often the case in rheumatic fibromyalgia. The entity *myopathy with tubular aggregates* is characterized by painful intolerance on muscular exertion and presents in adulthood; tubular aggregates are found in type 2 fibers. The term *myoadenylate deaminase deficiency* is included here for completeness because it is sometimes raised in differential diagnosis, although its distinct nosologic status is tenuous. Deficiency of this enzyme is common in the general asymptomatic population or may be seen in well-characterized myopathies, such as polymyositis (PM), muscular dystrophy, or denervation.

12.6.4.6. MALIGNANT HYPERTHERMIA

Malignant hyperthermia, transmitted as an autosomal disease, is manifested in the course of general anesthesia with halothane or succinylcholine as a severe general syndrome that includes hyperpyrexia and rhabdomyolysis. As mentioned previously, it is sometimes associated with a well-defined myopathy, such as CCD or a myotonic syndrome. In most cases, muscle biopsy performed during the latent phase either is normal or shows only minor nonspecific abnormalities.

12.7. TOXIC MYOPATHIES

In the wide variety of drug-related and chemical toxic myopathies (Box 12.1), both the clinical manifestations and histological appearances are highly variable. The picture may be that of a rhabdomyolysis, a subacute necrotizing myopathy, a hypokalemic myopathy, or a painless proximal myopathy, or it may show various functional manifestations, such as a myalgia/cramp syndrome or myotonia, both of which may be induced by lipid-lowering drugs. Among these medications, "statins," which block the cholesterol synthesis pathway in the liver by inhibiting HMG-CoA reductase (HMGCR) activity, may induce an immune-mediated myopathy, called necrotizing autoimmune myopathy (NAM; see Section 12.9.2.3), associated with anti-HMGCR autoantibodies.

Patients with chloroquine neuromyopathy come to medical attention with a characteristic picture of progressive proximal muscle weakness. Muscle biopsy shows a vacuolar myopathy: The vacuoles often predominate in type 1 fibers, are partially filled by PAS-positive material, and are strongly reactive for acid phosphatase, indicating a lysosomal origin (autophagic vacuoles). Electron microscopy of muscle and nerve shows the presence of membranous whorls, myelin figures, and curvilinear inclusions, the latter persisting many years after cessation of treatment.

Box 12.1 Conditions Associated with Toxic Myopathies

Rhabdomyolysis
Statins
Alcohol
Heroin
Amphetamines
Methadone
Barbiturates
Amphotericin B
Carbon monoxide

Subacute necrotizing myopathies
Statins
Alcohol
Clofibrate
ε-Aminocaproic acid
Emetine
Azidothymidine (AZT)

Hypokalemic myopathy
Diuretics
Laxatives
Licorice

Inflammatory myopathy
Statins (anti-HMGCR myositis)
D-Penicillamine
Cimetidine
Procainamide

Vacuolar myopathy with lysosomal hyperactivity
Chloroquine
Hydroxychloroquine
Amiodarone
Colchicine
Perhexiline maleate

Type 2 fiber atrophy
Corticosteroids

12.8. RHABDOMYOLYSIS

Patients with rhabdomyolysis develop necrosis of muscle fibers, with subsequent regeneration. The inflammatory reaction is often minimal. Rhabdomyolysis may follow a traumatic or ischemic cause, such as crushing, excessive exercise, or compression within an anatomical compartment, particularly in the setting of acute intoxication, generally due to alcohol or psychotropic drugs. It may also be found in conjunction with a metabolic or pseudo-metabolic myopathy (e.g., glycogenosis of the McArdle or Tarui type; deficiency of carnitine palmitoyltransferase; malignant hyperpyrexia; some muscular dystrophies such as dystrophinopathies; or potassium, phosphorus, or magnesium deficiency), a hemoglobinopathy (e.g., sickle cell disease), or an inflammatory muscle disease (e.g., viral myositis).

12.9. INFLAMMATORY MYOPATHIES

Inflammatory myopathies are a group of disorders characterized histopathologically by variable degrees of inflammation, usually associated with destruction of muscle fibers. Patients may be divided into two groups depending on whether the causative agent is a known infectious agent or whether the inflammatory process is believed to be an autoimmune phenomenon.

12.9.1. Inflammatory myopathies caused by microorganisms

12.9.1.1. VIRAL MYOSITIS

The most frequent causes of *acute viral myositis* are (1) influenza virus, which may cause acute benign myositis or severe rhabdomyolysis; and (2) enterovirus, which may be responsible for Bornholm disease or epidemic myalgia (coxsackie B).

In the setting of *HIV infection*, patients who develop muscle involvement can be subdivided into four groups:

- HIV-associated myopathy, which may be the presenting manifestation of the infection and is similar to seronegative PM. HIV antigens may be detected in endomysial and perivascular macrophages, and muscle fibers strongly express MHC class I molecules.
- Azidothymidine (AZT) myopathy is a toxic mitochondrial myopathy frequently associated with an inflammatory component. This condition is associated with myalgia that improve rapidly after AZT withdrawal. Muscle biopsy typically shows AZT fibers (ragged red fibers with marked shrinkage of myofibrils) and COX-negative fibers.
- Muscle involvement linked to immunodeficiency, including pyomyositis, toxoplasmic PM, and primary muscle lymphoma.
- Several other conditions, including HIV-cachectic myopathy, acquired nemaline myopathy, and recurrent myoglobinuria.

12.9.1.2. BACTERIAL MYOSITIS

Bacterial myositis may be a complication of a skin injury (muscle abscess or gas gangrene caused by a clostridium) or part of a pyomyositis. The latter condition is seen in severely debilitated patients in intensive care units and also observed in the tropics (tropical pyomyositis). Patients' clinical presentation if that of a spontaneous, acute suppurative infection culminating in the formation of abscesses in one or several skeletal muscle groups. It is caused by strict anaerobes.

12.9.1.3. PARASITIC MYOSITIS

The most frequent parasitic myositis is trichinosis, which is secondary to the ingestion of meat infested with *Trichinella spiralis*. Trichinosis may be diagnosed in muscle biopsy by the identification of encysted larvae (Fig. 12.26).

Toxoplasma cysts may be detected in muscle biopsies of severely immunocompromised patients, reflecting systemic reactivation of the parasite encysted in brain, retina, myocardium, and skeletal muscle (Fig. 12.27).

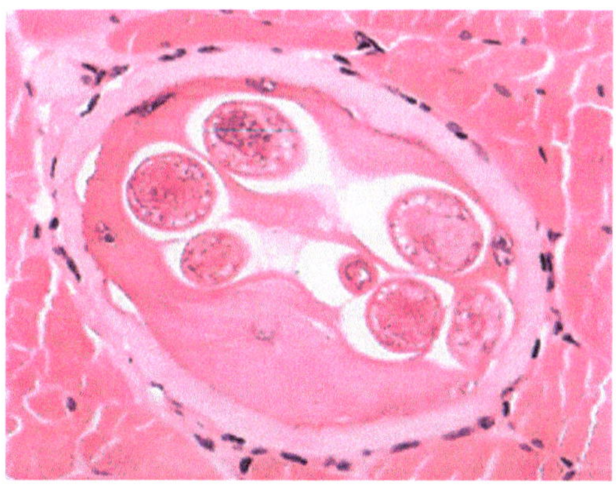

FIGURE 12.26 Muscular trichinosis: encysted larva in a muscle cell.

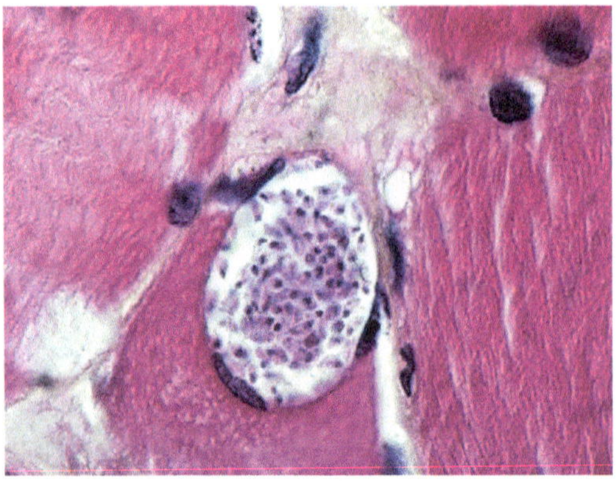

FIGURE 12.27 Muscular toxoplasmosis: toxoplasma cyst in a muscle cell.

12.9.1.4. FUNGAL MYOSITIS

Instances of fungal myositis are most often seen in association with systemic disease.

12.9.2. Idiopathic inflammatory myopathies

The classification of idiopathic inflammatory myopathies has been the subject of extensive recent analysis. Histopathologic characteristics and identification of several myositis-specific autoantibodies have helped identify subsets of inflammatory myopathies with specific clinical and prognostic implications. DM, sIBM, immune-mediated necrotizing myopathy (IMNM) (also known as NAM), antisynthetase syndrome (AS), and overlap myositis are the most common forms. PM is a much less often diagnosed entity because most cases that were previously so designated are now reclassified as IBM, IMNM, or AS.

12.9.2.1. DERMATOMYOSITIS

In DM, proximal muscular weakness, often painful and of acute or subacute onset, is typically associated with cutaneous signs dominated by erythema of the face and the extremities, resulting in a purplish-blue discoloration of the eyelids and periungual hyperemia. Dysphagia, arthralgia, constitutional symptoms, and elevated levels of serum muscle enzymes are frequent. DM may be associated with visceral cancer in adult patients; therefore, when it occurs in adulthood, especially in the elderly, it should be considered as a possible paraneoplastic manifestation and requires investigation for evidence of an occult tumor. In children, it is often accompanied by systemic vasculitis. DM may be difficult or impossible to distinguish from systemic lupus erythematosus (SLE) with muscle involvement.

DM may be associated with different myositis-specific autoantibodies delineating distinct subsets: anti-Mi-2 (classical DM; good response to standard treatment), anti-MDA5 (amyopathic DM or DM with mild myopathy, contrasting with marked extramuscular involvement; severe interstitial lung disease, skin ulcers, and arthritis), anti-TIF-1γ (associated with cancer in adults; classical DM restricted to skin and muscles), anti-NXP2 (associated with cancer in adults, calcinosis, and marked ischemic changes), and anti-SAE (classical DM).

Muscle biopsy is the definitive diagnostic test for DM. Muscle biopsy features of DM are distinctive and reflect primary involvement of the microcirculation with secondary ischemic changes of muscle fibers.

- Inflammatory infiltrates include (1) chronic inflammatory infiltrates (without fibrinoid necrosis) in epimysium/perimysium (Fig. 12.28A), often in perivascular distribution and in perifascicular endomysium; (2) a mixture of mononuclear cells, including $CD4^+$ plasmacytoid dendritic cells, B cells, $CD8^+$ T cells, and macrophages; and (3) no $CD8^+$ lymphocytic invasion of nonnecrotic myofibers.
- Myofiber alterations include (1) progressive reduction in caliber of marginal layers of myofibers (perifascicular atrophy) (Fig. 12.28B) that is preceded by local overexpression of type 1 interferon-inducible proteins, such as myxovirus resistance A (Fig. 12.28C); (2) MHC class I but not MHC class II antigens; (3) myosin lysis and punched-out vacuoles in perifascicular fibers (Fig. 12.28D) or microinfarcts consisting of foci of contiguous necrotic/regenerating fibers; and (4) reduced COX staining of perifascicular muscle fibers.
- Microvascular changes include (1) capillary deposition of the complement C5b-9 membranolytic MAC (Fig. 12.28E), (2) destruction of endothelial cells (free basement membranes) with focal loss of capillaries predominating in perifascicular areas (Fig. 12.28F), and (3) endothelial hyperplasia with

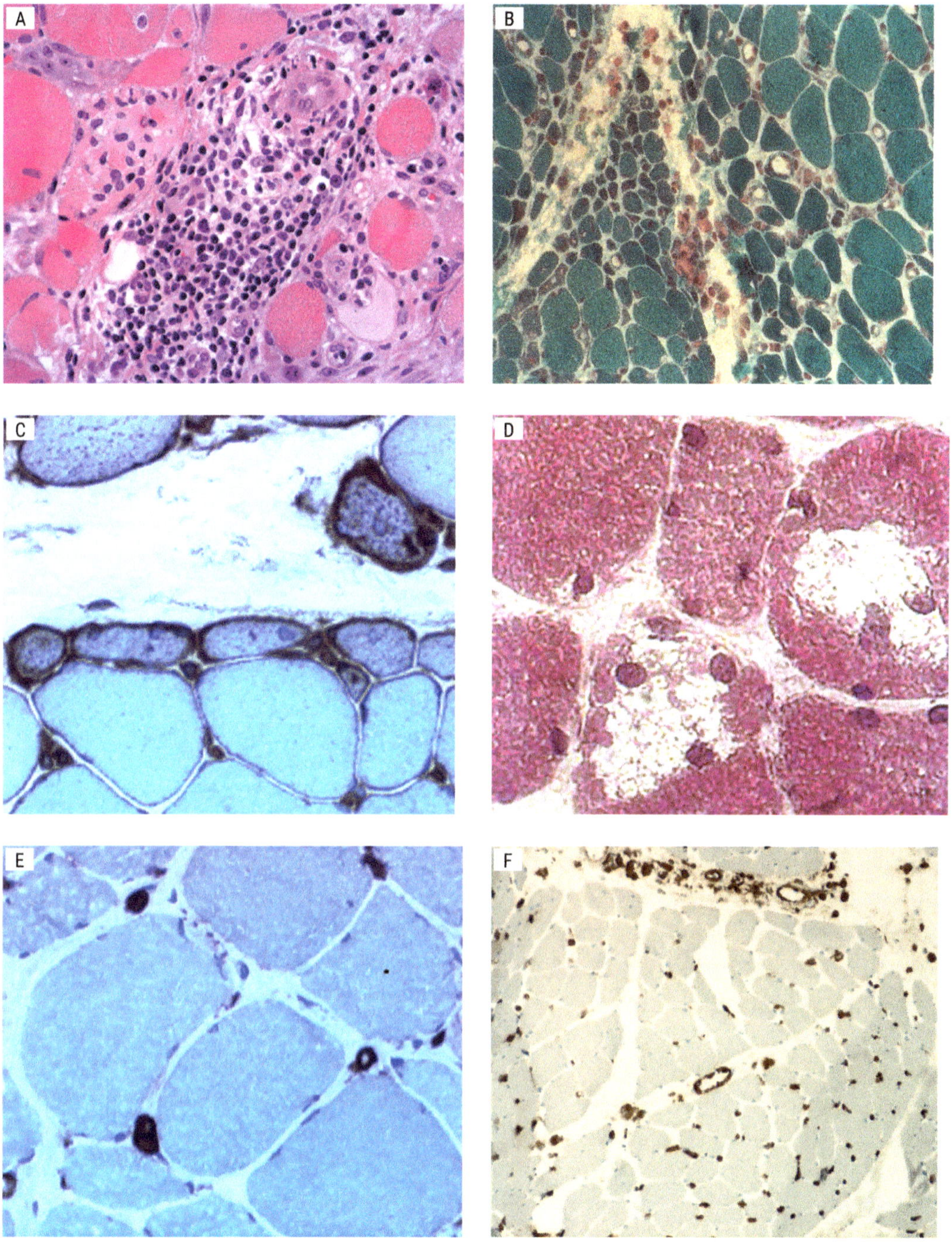

FIGURE 12.28 Dermatomyositis: (**A**) perivascular inflammatory infiltrate in perimysium (H&E); (**B**) perifascicular atrophy (GT); (**C**) expression of type 1 interferon inducible, myxovirus resistance A (MXA) on the sarcolemma of muscle fibers with preferential early involvement of perifascicular fibers (MXA IHC); (**D**) ischemic "punched-out" lesion due to focal myosin loss (H&E); (**E**) complement C5b-9 fraction (membrane attack complex) in muscle capillaries (C5b-9 IHC); (**F**) immunohistochemical evidence of focal loss of CD31-positive capillaries (CD31 IHC).

tubuloreticular inclusions (which are known to be inducible by type 1 interferons).

12.9.2.2. POLYMYOSITIS

As previously mentioned, the diagnosis of PM is increasingly rendered less frequently, and many specialists exclude it from the classification of idiopathic inflammatory myopathies. Most cases of "polymyositis" reported in the literature are believed to be instances of patients with inclusion body myositis, IMNM, AS, or other myopathies with inflammation, such as dystrophies. However, older literature defined PM by an inflammatory pattern suggestive of a $CD8^+$ T-cell–mediated and MHC class I–restricted autoimmune process targeting muscle fibers. This pattern is usually associated with other inflammatory myopathies (mainly sIBM but also overlap myositis with anti-synthetase autoantibodies and connective tissue diseases) or retroviral infections (see Section 12.9.1.1). PM as a separate entity is probably extremely rare. The disease is manifest by symmetrical muscle weakness of subacute or chronic onset in adulthood, with, or more often without, myalgia. There are no skin changes. Focal onset may occasionally occur. CK levels are usually increased, and EMG is consistent with myositis. Because PM has no unique clinical features, its diagnosis is one of exclusion. PM should be considered only after careful consideration of other possible diagnoses: early sIBM, overlap myositis, IMNM, nonspecific myositis, and an inflammatory form of a genetic muscular disease (dysferlinopathy, anoctaminopathy, FSHD, and laminopathy).

The characteristic muscle biopsy finding in PM consists of inflammatory infiltrates, mainly composed of $CD8^+$ T cells (Fig. 12.29) found in endomysium.

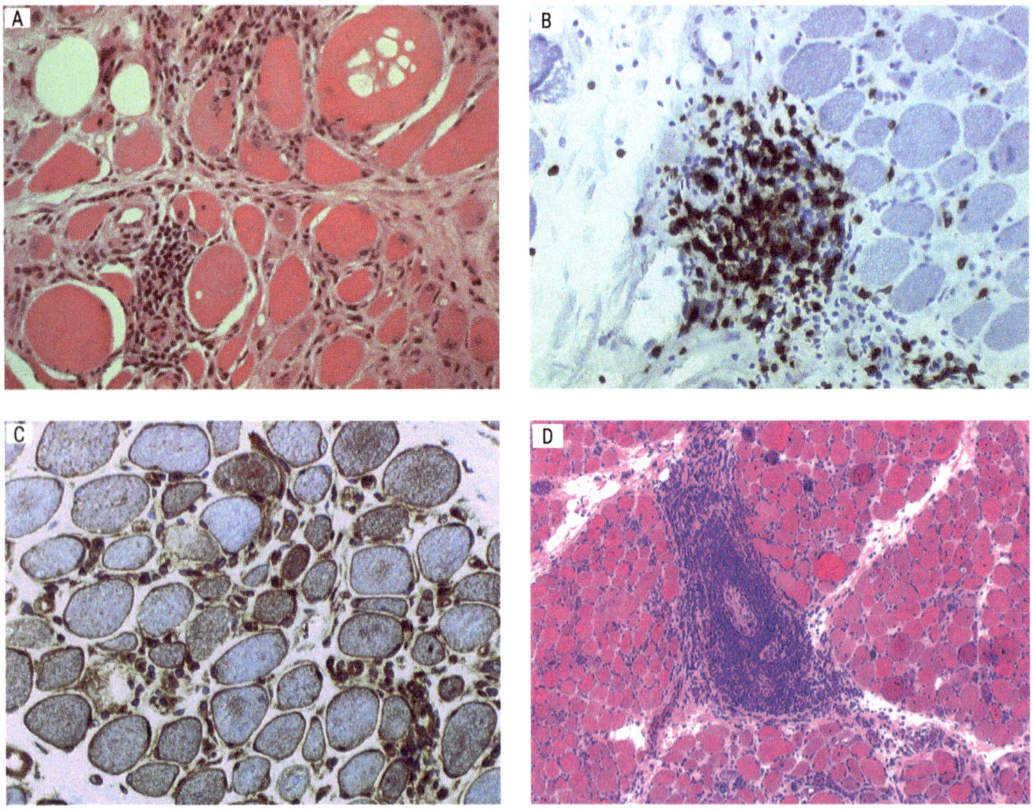

FIGURE 12.29 Polymyositis pattern: (**A**) inflammation in the endomysium surrounding individual muscle fibers, some of which appear invaded by inflammatory cells (H&E); (**B**) predominantly $CD8^+$ cytotoxic lymphocytes within the inflammatory infiltrate (CD8 IHC); (**C**) widespread sarcolemmal expression of MHC class I antigens with occasional sarcoplasmic expression (MHC class I IHC); (**D**) lymphocytic vasculitis in a case of overlap syndrome associated with systemic lupus erythematosus (H&E).

These cells initially surround individual healthy-appearing muscle fibers and then attack and invade them focally, with subsequent macrophage invasion of the damaged segment (Fig. 12.29A). In contrast with DM, there is no associated capillary damage or perifascicular atrophy. Widespread and strong MHC class I overexpression by muscle fibers constitutes a major immunopathologic feature (Fig. 12.29C). The possibility of an association with a connective tissue disease is raised when the disease is associated with perivascular lymphocytic infiltrates (Fig. 12.29D). A PM pattern associated with the presence of rimmed vacuoles or abundant COX-negative muscle fibers is suggestive of sIBM and precludes the diagnosis of PM.

12.9.2.3. IMMUNE-MEDIATED NECROTIZING MYOPATHY

Immune-mediated necrotizing myopathy is an underrecognized form of autoimmune myopathy. Most cases present with acute, proximal-greater-than-distal weakness, with markedly elevated serum CK and myopathic EMG; the clinical presentation in these patients is similar to that of PM. However, muscle biopsies demonstrate scattered necrotic and regenerating fibers with minimal or no inflammatory cell infiltrate (aside from myophagocytosis of necrotic fibers) (Fig. 12.30A). NCAM/CD56 immunostaining usually reveals a larger extent of fiber damage and regeneration than standard

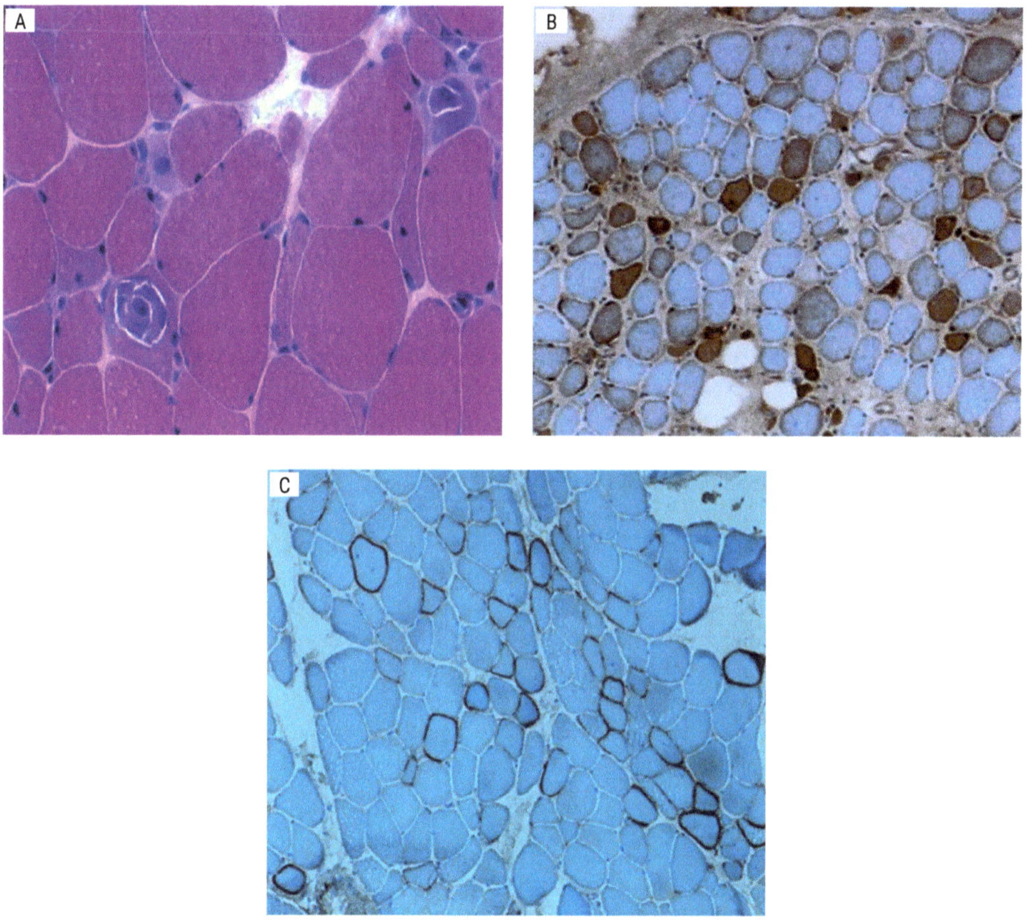

FIGURE 12.30 Immune-mediated necrotizing myopathy: (**A**) several basophilic and necrotic myofibers with myophagocytosis in the absence of endomysial inflammatory infiltrate in a patient with circulating anti-SRP autoantibodies (H&E); (**B**) widespread myofiber regeneration assessed by CD56/NCAM expression in a patient with circulating anti-HMGCR autoantibodies (CD56 IHC); (**C**) widespread sarcolemmal deposition of complement C5b-9 fraction (membrane attack complex) in a patient with anti-HMGCR autoantibodies (C5b-9 IHC).

staining methods (Fig. 12.30B). MHC class I antigen and C5b-9/MAC immunostaining can reveal sarcolemmal deposits on nonnecrotic muscle fibers (Fig. 12.30C). Two myositis-specific autoantibodies are selectively associated with INMN: antibodies directed against signal recognition particle and those directed against HMGCR. The latter may be associated, or not, with exposure to statins. Unlike statin-induced myalgia and increased CK levels without anti-HMGCR antibodies that usually resolve after drug withdrawal, necrotizing myopathy with anti-HMGCR antibodies is a self-autonomous condition that persists after discontinuation of the medication. Anti-HMGCR myopathy is often responsive to monotherapy with intravenous immunoglobulin, but the other subtypes of IMNM are often more difficult to treat and require aggressive immunosuppressive therapy.

12.9.2.4. OVERLAP MYOSITIS AND MYOSITIS WITH ANTI-SYNTHETASE AUTOANTIBODIES

Although there are clinical and histopathological differences between the subsets of myositis, histopathological features may be scarce or nonspecific or sometimes overlap with scleroderma and other connective tissue diseases (e.g., diseases with anti-PmScl, -Ku, -SnRNP, -Ro, and -La antibodies). Another distinct form of myositis is antisynthetase syndrome, which shows anti-tRNA synthetase autoantibodies (ASAs) and is characterized by the combination of inflammatory myopathy, interstitial lung disease, joint involvement, Raynaud phenomenon, and mechanic hands. The most prevalent ASA is anti-Jo-1, but seven other types have been reported (anti-PL7, -PL12, -EJ, -OJ, -KS, -Zo, and -Ha). The anti-Jo-1 syndrome is associated with "immune myopathy with perimysial pathology," which typically includes (1) connective tissue fragmentation with a dramatic increase of alkaline phosphatase activity and abundant infiltration of $CD68^+$ macrophages and dendritic cells in perimysium (Fig. 12.31 A, B); (2) myofiber lesions, including atrophy and necrosis, mostly restricted to perifascicular areas where endomysial infiltrates of auto aggressive $CD8^+$ T cells can be detected (Fig. 12.31 A); (3) myofiber expression of MHC class I antigens, but also, unlike DM, MHC class II (HLA-DR) antigens (Fig. 12.31C), that represents an interferon-γ signature associated with perifascicular $CD8^+$ T-cell infiltrates; and (4) MHC class I and MAC deposition on sarcolemma of perifascicular nonnecrotic fibers (Fig. 12.31D), without capillary deposits. Interestingly, intranuclear inclusions composed of actin filaments have also been reported.

12.9.2.5. INCLUSION BODY MYOSITIS

Inclusion body myositis is a sporadic disease mainly affecting adult males older than age 50 years. Onset is insidious and painless, and it is typically reported as increasing difficulty with everyday tasks requiring proximal or distal limb muscles. Early involvement of quadriceps muscles, remarkable involvement of distal limb muscles (mainly deep finger flexors and foot extensors), and selective and often asymmetrical amyotrophy are typically present. CK levels are normal or slightly elevated. Approximately 40–75% of patients with sIBM have autoantibodies directed against cytosolic 5′-nucleotidase 1A (anti-cN1A), which may also be occasionally detected in Sjögren disease and SLE. EMG shows a mixture of large and small motor unit potentials due to the chronicity of the disease process by the time patients usually come in for evaluations. Progression of IBM is slow and relentless, and patients often do not respond to immunosuppressive treatment. Re-evaluation of muscle biopsy for possible signs of IBM should be performed in patients with presumed PM resistant to steroids.

Typical muscle biopsy findings are required for the histopathological diagnosis of IBM, although findings may not all be present in any given muscle biopsy, perhaps related to sampling error. The characteristic histopathologic picture (Fig. 12.32) consists of the coexistence of a multifocal PM-like inflammatory process composed of $CD8^+$ T cells with a variable number of rimmed vacuoles, the presence of eosinophilic cytoplasmic and even nuclear inclusions, and mitochondrial changes such as ragged red and COX-negative fibers. Myofiber expression of MHC class I and class II molecules is typically present, often restricted to inflammatory areas. Cytoplasmic inclusions may be congophilic, but these are difficult to appreciate (present in only 1% of muscle fibers and only on frozen sections; they are not seen on paraffin sections). Rimmed vacuoles are found in approximately 3% of muscle fibers but may not be easily detected. Cytoplasmic expression of the p62 marker of autophagy is the most sensitive histopathologic biomarker (Fig. 12.32D). On electron microscopy, cytoplasmic and intranuclear

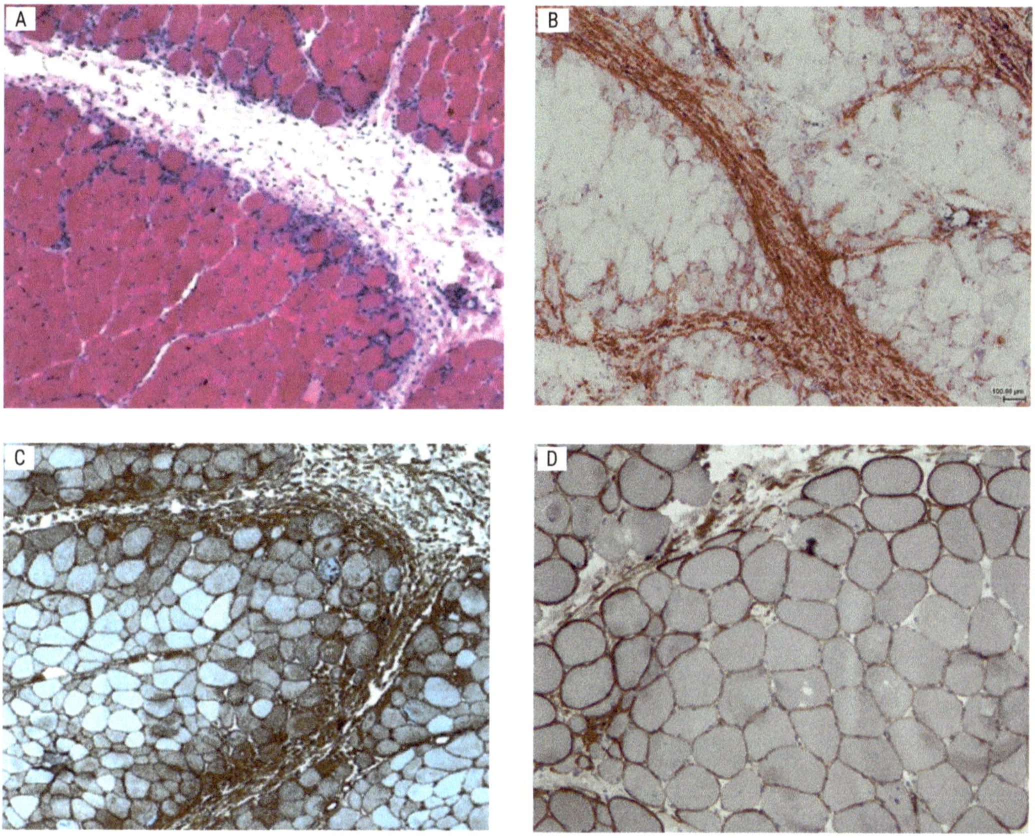

FIGURE 12.31 Myositis with anti-synthetase antibodies (Jo-1): (**A**) breakdown of perimysial connective tissue and perifascicular atrophy, necrosis, and inflammation (H&E); (**B**) dramatic increase of alkaline phosphatase (ALP) activity in perimysium (ALP enzyme activity); (**C**) overexpression of MHC class II antigens predominating in perifascicular areas (MHC class II IHC); (**D**) abundant sarcolemmal deposition of complement C5b-9 fraction (membrane attack complex) predominating on the sarcolemma of perifascicular muscle fibers (C5b-9 IHC).

15- to 21-nm tubulo-filaments can be difficult to find. In muscle biopsies that demonstrate only inflammation but no rimmed vacuoles, which occurs in up to one-third of muscle biopsies, the presence of p62 inclusions and COX-negative fibers is highly suggestive of a diagnosis of IBM as opposed to PM. Of note, rimmed vacuoles are not specific and alone are insufficient to establish the diagnosis of IBM because they can be seen in several forms of muscular dystrophy, particularly the distal myopathies, as previously discussed, and the hereditary inclusion body myopathies.

Regarding hereditary inclusion body myopathy, there is a heterogeneous group of patients with a hereditary myopathy who have muscle biopsy findings similar to those of sIBM, including rimmed vacuoles and immunocytochemical and ultrastructural findings, although the biopsy findings show little or no inflammation. It is really a misnomer. The clinical features, pattern of weakness, and age of onset differ from those of sIBM. Both autosomal dominant and recessive pedigrees are reported. One form, GNE myopathy, is caused by mutation in the *GNE* gene (UDP-*N*-acetylglucosamine 2-epimerase), as previously discussed. Also described is an unusual constellation of autosomal dominant inclusion body myopathy, Paget disease, and premature frontotemporal dementia (IBMPFD). The disease can also be associated with a familial form of motor neuron disease and parkinsonism. Systemic involvement has been termed "multisystem proteinopathies", and these MSPs have a number of genes involved, including mutations in the valosin protein-coding gene.

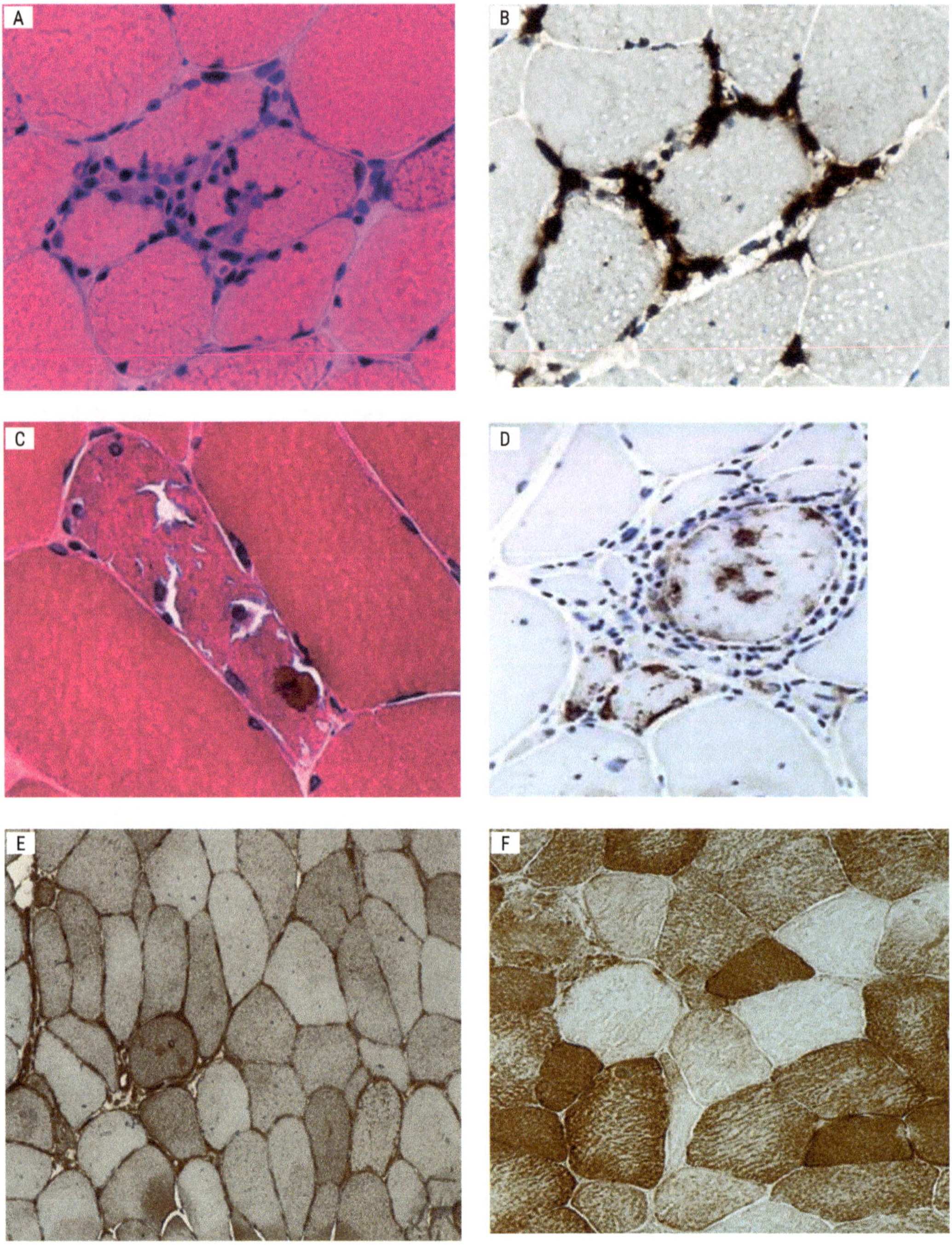

FIGURE 12.32 Sporadic inclusion body myositis (sIBM): (**A**) focal polymyositis-like inflammation consisting of invasion of nonnecrotic myofibers by lymphocytes (H&E); (**B**) focal endomysial CD8⁺ T cells surrounding nonnecrotic myofibers; (**C**) several rimmed vacuoles and one eosinophilic inclusion in an atrophic myofiber (H&E); (**D**) increased autophagy marker associated with the formation of rimmed vacuoles (P62 IHC); (**E**) overexpression of MHC class I antigens (MHC class I IHC); (**F**) COX-negative fibers suggesting mitochondrial dysfunction (COX enzyme activity).

12.9.2.6. SARCOIDOSIS

Interstitial epithelioid and giant cell granulomas may be seen in the muscle of patients with sarcoidosis, particularly at postmortem examination, irrespective of clinical manifestations referable to muscle involvement. A possibly related condition, referred to as *granulomatous polymyositis*, has a similar histologic picture but is not associated with any extramuscular clinical or histological evidence of sarcoidosis.

12.9.2.7. NODULAR FOCAL MYOSITIS

Nodular focal myositis may be seen in various connective tissue diseases but is especially frequent in long-standing rheumatoid arthritis. It is characterized by the interstitial infiltration of lymphocytes and plasma cells, forming compact nodules measuring 1 to 2 mm in diameter, often situated near a small artery or arteriole but without invasion of the vessel wall. There may or may not be changes in the adjacent muscle fibers.

12.9.2.8. EOSINOPHILIC MYOSITIS AND FASCIITIS

Eosinophilic myositis is defined by the presence of inflammatory cellular infiltrates containing eosinophils in muscle and can be associated with necrosis of the muscle fibers. In addition to parasitic diseases of muscle and to systemic vasculitis (especially the Churg–Strauss syndrome), the main causes include hyper-eosinophilic syndrome, which is a rare multisystem disorder in which muscle involvement includes the picture of eosinophilic PM and eosinophilic fasciitis. Rare cases are associated with thymoma or myasthenia gravis.

Eosinophilic fasciitis (or Shulman syndrome) is characterized by a subcutaneous induration that spares the face and fingers and is associated with

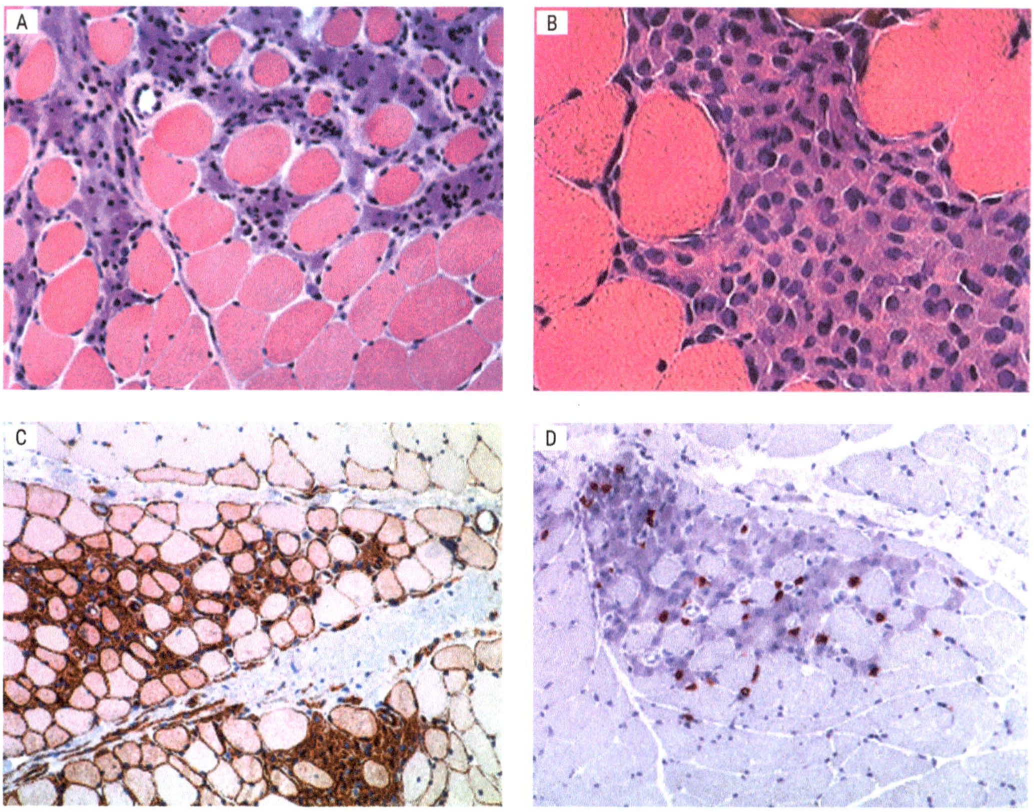

FIGURE 12.33 Macrophagic myofasciitis: (**A**) perifascicular and interstitial infiltration by large macrophages with a basophilic cytoplasm (H&E); (**B**) higher magnification shows the finely granular cytoplasmic content of the macrophages (H&E); (**C**) perifascicular infiltration of the muscle by macrophages (CD68 IHC); (**D**) the presence of T lymphocytes within the infiltrate (T-cell IHC).

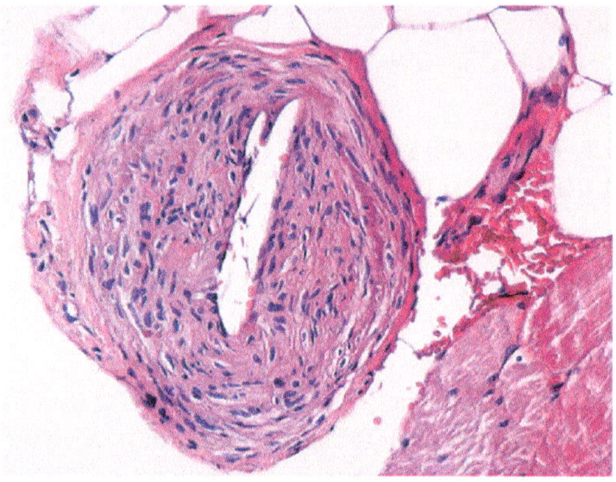

FIGURE 12.35 Paraffin section revels occlusion of a small muscular arteriole by a cholesterol crystal: a cholesterol embolus (H&E).

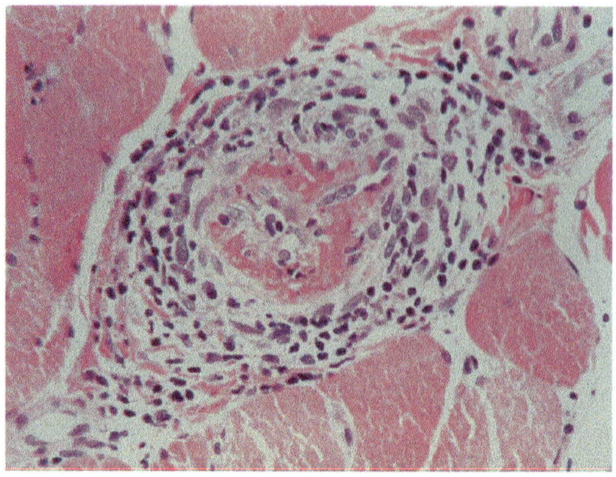

FIGURE 12.34 Polyarteritis nodosa (PAN). Paraffin section reveals transmural inflammation and fibrinoid necrosis of a medium-sized arteriole (H&E).

stiffening of the joints and a raised blood eosinophil count. Inflammatory lesions predominate in the fascia but may extend into the dermis or muscle. In the tissues, eosinophilia is often well circumscribed or absent. The lymphocyte and plasma cell infiltrates are essentially perivascular.

12.9.2.9. MACROPHAGIC MYOFASCIITIS

Macrophagic myofasciitis is a lesion often associated with the site of previous immunizations. It is defined by stereotyped sheets of large macrophages, with a finely granular PAS-positive content, intermingled with lymphocytic infiltrates, in the epi-, peri-, and endomysium without conspicuous muscle fiber damage (Fig. 12.33).

12.9.2.10. LOCALIZED MYOSITIS

Noninfectious myositis localized to a portion of the muscle, to one particular muscle, or to one muscle group essentially includes orbital myositis, sclerosing segmental PM, inflammatory pseudo-tumoral (focal myositis) and proliferative myositis, or recurrent focal myositis. Recurrent focal myositis usually occurs in the lower limbs, but other muscles may be involved; there is focal inflammatory infiltration, necrosis, variation in fiber diameter, and regeneration.

12.9.2.11. VASCULITIS INVOLVING SKELETAL MUSCLE

In the systemic vasculitis (see Chapter 13), combined nerve and muscle biopsy may establish the diagnosis (Fig. 12.34). The lesions in skeletal muscle consist of small inflammatory cellular infiltrates adjacent to the involved blood vessels, nonspecific type 2 atrophy, or evidence of denervation atrophy related to concomitant peripheral nerve involvement. Focal infarction of muscle is sometimes seen involving part of a fascicle. The affected muscle fibers lose their tinctorial affinity, and at their periphery, inflammatory cells may be seen, including acute inflammatory cells.

12.9.2.12. CHOLESTEROL EMBOLI

Within the framework of ischemic myopathies may be included cholesterol emboli, which are often the source of systemic manifestations due to microinfarction of multiple organs. Cholesterol crystals from aortic atheromatous plaques embolize and occlude small arteries (Fig. 12.35), especially those of lower limb muscles, following which they may be surrounded by reactive changes and inflammatory cell infiltrates, including macro phages.

13

Pathology of Peripheral Neuropathy

JEAN-MICHEL VALLAT, DOUGLAS C. ANTHONY, ANTHONY A. AMATO, AND UMBERTO De GIROLAMI

13.1. PERIPHERAL NERVE BIOPSY

13.1.1. Indications for a peripheral nerve biopsy

With advances in clinical, electrophysiology, and molecular diagnostics, the need to perform a nerve biopsy in patients with peripheral neuropathy has decreased. However, the findings derived from nerve biopsy may lead to a change in clinical diagnosis and management in up to 60% of patients with peripheral neuropathy, depending on the expertise of the laboratory handling the biopsy and the selection of patients. The laboratory receiving the biopsy should be capable of performing routine histologic preparations, frozen sections, and plastic embedding, including semithin sections and electron microscopy. In selected cases, teased fiber preparation may be necessary, but this technique requires additional technical and professional expertise. Utilizing these techniques, the highest diagnostic yield is expected in the patient population with focal (or asymmetric) neuropathies, demyelinating neuropathies, or small-fiber neuropathies. The lowest diagnostic yield is in biopsies from patients with chronic, slowly progressive, diffuse, symmetric, axonal sensory polyneuropathies. Because these multiple specialized techniques may be needed to evaluate the patient, the clinical setting and indications for the biopsy and the specific clinical issues to be addressed need to be discussed between the treating physicians and the team evaluating the biopsy.

13.1.2. Site of the biopsy

A peripheral nerve biopsy sample is ordinarily taken from a purely sensory nerve of appropriate caliber to yield meaningful information. In practice, the choice is limited to two nerves in the lower limb: the sural nerve (a branch of the tibial nerve) and the superficial peroneal nerve (a branch of the common peroneal nerve). There is extensive information on the normal fiber composition at these sites, and these nerves in the leg are chosen for biopsy, especially in patients with clinical evidence of distal neuropathy. The superficial peroneal nerve is chosen for biopsy in the setting of foot drop when vasculitis is under consideration and also because the underlying peroneus brevis muscle may be simultaneously sampled with a single surgical incision. The diagnostic yield for vasculitis is increased when both nerve and muscle are biopsied. When there is selective involvement of the limb girdle, a biopsy of the lateral femoral cutaneous nerve is advised; when the neuropathy is restricted to the upper limbs, a sensory superficial branch of the radial nerve of the forearm may be biopsied.

Laboratories equipped with additional expertise are required to perform and analyze skin biopsies, obtained to evaluate small-fiber neuropathies. These biopsies are less invasive than those mentioned above and can also provide information on both myelinated and unmyelinated fibers.

A muscle biopsy may be performed to assess nerve terminals utilizing specialized techniques (e.g., confocal microscopy of fluorescently labeled endplates and scanning and transmission electron microscopy), but nerve endplate studies are not ordinarily required for clinical assessment of peripheral neuropathy.

The sequela of a nerve biopsy is an area of numbness in the distribution of the biopsied sensory nerve. For the sural nerve, the numbness is localized to the heel region. Rare complications of the surgical procedure include allergic reaction to anesthetic agents, operative site infection, and post-biopsy dysesthesias that may last several months.

In disabling neuropathies, nerve biopsy may be considered with somewhat lesser concern because affected individuals may have intense neuropathic sensory symptoms, and the temporary pain and sensory deficits that may be induced by nerve biopsy are not usually perceptible.

13.1.3. Methods

Alerting the laboratory that a nerve biopsy is being performed allows the preparation for the handling that is required. Immediately after removal, the biopsy specimen must be processed using specialized methods so that a number of required studies can be performed. These include routine histologic processing, electron microscopy, and teased-fiber preparations; tissue may also be set aside and frozen for frozen sections and chemical analyses. A critical part of handling a nerve biopsy is maintaining the specimen as a straight segment so that it does not curl up during processing; this can be accomplished using clamps or other methods. The nerve is best analyzed with transverse and longitudinal sections and nerve teasing (depending on the differential diagnostic considerations).

13.1.3.1. ROUTINE HISTOLOGY

Fixation in 10% buffered formalin (3.7% formaldehyde) and paraffin embedding is standard practice and enables the study of abnormalities of connective tissue, including an evaluation of blood vessels, the infiltration of inflammatory cells, and the presence of abnormal deposits such as amyloid. The stains commonly employed on paraffin sections include hematoxylin and eosin (H&E), elastic tissue stains, Masson trichrome, silver impregnation or immunoperoxidase methods for axons, myelin stains, and Congo red stain for amyloid. Paraffin-embedded tissue can also be used for immunohistochemistry should it be necessary to characterize the types of inflammatory cells or to localize specific antigens. Immunofluorescence techniques for the demonstration of immunoglobulins are best performed on frozen sections.

13.1.3.2. PLASTIC EMBEDDING

Plastic embedding following fixation in 2.5% buffered glutaraldehyde allows for semithin (1-μm thick) transverse and longitudinal sections and is the method of choice to examine the structural details of both myelinated and unmyelinated fibers (Fig. 13.1A–C). Semithin, plastic-embedded sections give greater morphologic detail than paraffin-embedded sections because the relative thinness of the section reduces the optical effect of overlapping structures, thereby allowing for a more precise assessment of axonal density, myelin thickness, and subcellular structures. Plastic embedding also is required to proceed to ultrastructural evaluation, when necessary (Fig. 13.1D–F). In some cases, immunoelectron microscopy may be performed to identify specific proteins at the ultrastructural level.

13.1.3.3. TEASED FIBER PREPARATION

The tease fiber technique separates individual myelinated fibers (approximately 1-cm long) after aldehyde fixation and osmication by teasing them apart

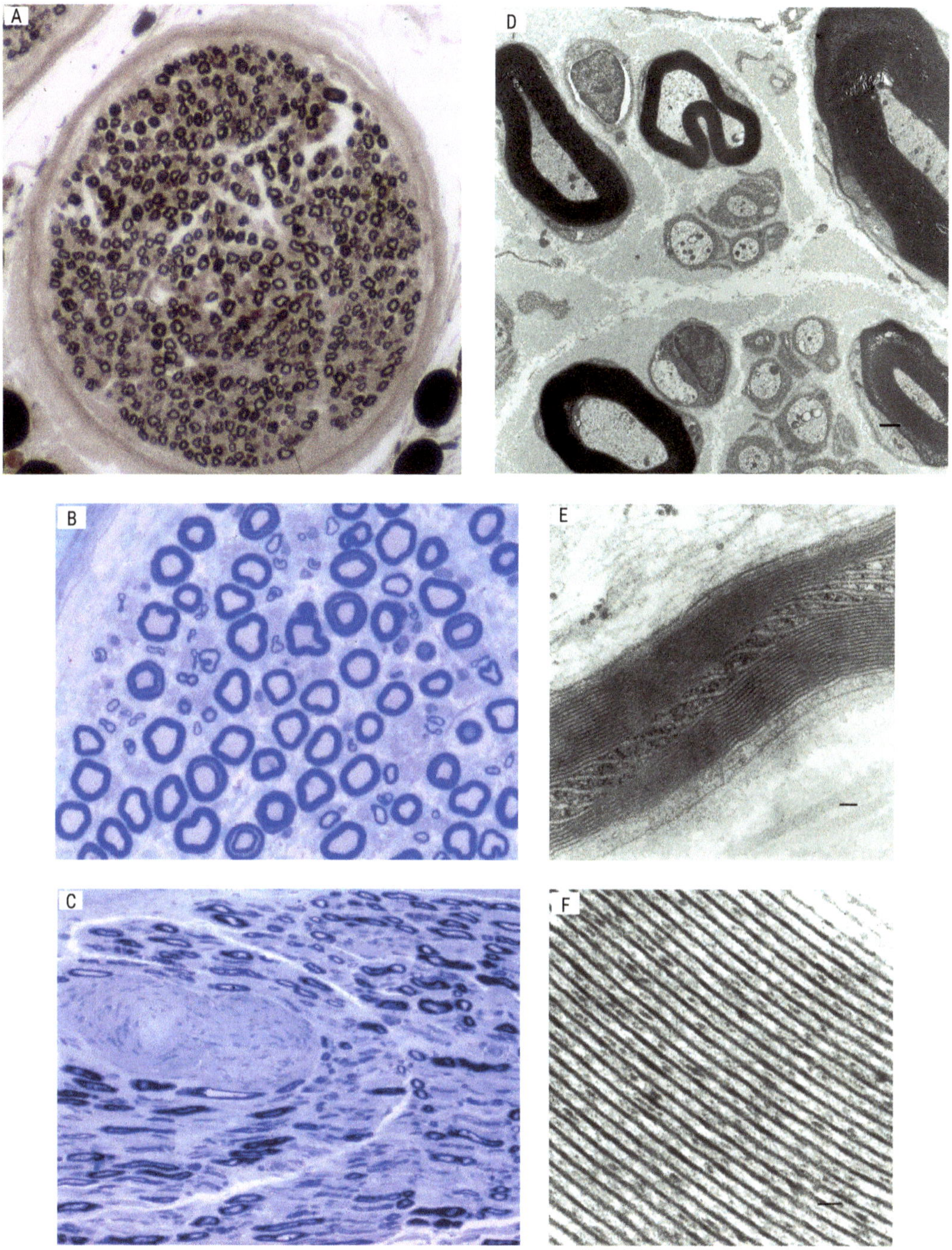

FIGURE 13.1 Normal histologic appearance of peripheral nerve: (**A, B**) semithin transverse sections; (**C**) semithin longitudinal section with Renaut body; (**D**) ultrastructural appearance of myelinated and unmyelinated axons; (**E**) higher magnification showing myelin sheath with Schmidt–Lanterman incisure; (**F**) high-magnification electron micrograph showing periodicity of myelin layers.

with fine needles while visualized with a dissecting microscope. Light microscopic examination of the longitudinally oriented teased fibers shows the site of nodes of Ranvier and is very helpful in discriminating between demyelinating lesions and axonal degeneration. This assessment considers, among other things, the length of the internode and the thickness of myelin sheaths along the long axis of

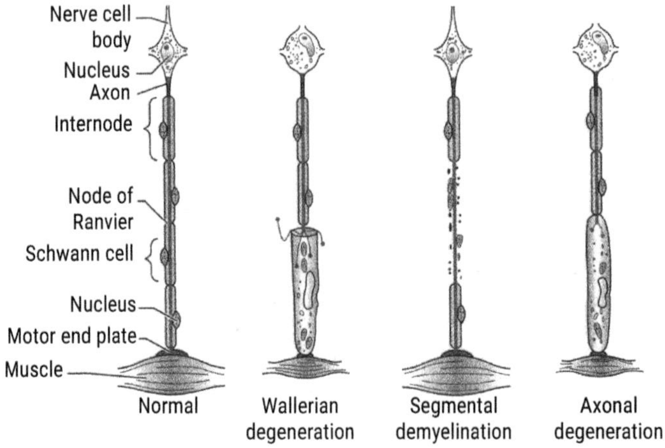

FIGURE 13.2 Diagram showing the primary types of pathologic findings in peripheral neuropathies. Note the distal axon remains intact during segmental demyelination.

the fibers (Fig. 13.2). Because this technique is very time-consuming, it is reserved for selected cases.

13.1.3.4. FROZEN SECTIONS FOR IMMUNOFLUORESCENCE OR CHEMICAL ANALYSIS

Direct immunofluorescence studies can be carried out using specific antibodies to identify abnormal deposits of immunoglobulins in endoneurium or within myelinated fibers. Various markers for inflammatory cells (T lymphocytes, B lymphocytes, and macrophages) as well as amyloid deposits can be used on both frozen and paraffin-embedded sections. Frozen tissue is also useful when testing for metabolic disorders, both because direct chemical analysis of tissue can be performed and because storage materials, which may be removed during routine aldehyde fixation and dehydration, may be detected histochemically in frozen sections.

13.1.3.5. MOLECULAR AND PROTEOMIC ANALYSIS

DNA can be extracted from either paraffin-embedded or frozen tissue, which allows for the molecular classification of archival material. Molecular tests are regularly performed on whole-blood samples during the course of the evaluation of patients suspected of having hereditary forms of peripheral neuropathy. In addition, mass spectrometric proteomic analysis has been used to characterize protein deposits, including the subclassification of amyloid deposits in tissue.

13.1.3.6. QUANTITATIVE AND MORPHOMETRIC ANALYSES

Quantitative and morphometric studies are time-consuming and require a substantial investment in equipment. In routine practice, a trained observer can often give a reliable assessment regarding the density of myelinated fibers, estimate the extent of loss of large or small fibers, and determine the presence and severity of demyelinating or axonal lesions. When morphometric analyses are employed, they can be performed in cross sections or in longitudinal sections.

In the longitudinal plane, morphometric analysis quantifies the internodal distances on single nerve fibers using statistical computer-assisted methods. This is usually represented as a plot of internodal distances against the mean diameter of the fibers for a number of myelinated fibers.

Morphometric analysis of cross sections of the nerve may be carried out either after photography or following whole slide imaging by image analysis. Analysis of myelinated fibers may be performed on either plastic-embedded sections or by electron microscopy; morphometry of unmyelinated fibers requires electron microscopy.

The density of myelinated axons in young adults is 7,000–10,000 fibers/mm^2. The number of fibers decreases progressively with age. The diameter of myelinated fibers ranges from 2 to 12 μm in a bimodal distribution, with peaks at 3–6 and 9–12 μm. There are more small myelinated fibers than large myelinated fibers. The relationships between size of the axon and number of myelin lamellae can only be established with electron microscopic examination and are nearly linear. The "g" ratio is the ratio of axonal diameter to fiber diameter. In most fibers, the g ratio is on the order of 0.5–0.7, and it may be used to evaluate the severity of demyelinating lesions on semithin sections.

Regarding unmyelinated fibers, which can be studied only by electron microscopy, the fiber diameter ranges from 0.2 to 2.5 μm in a unimodal distribution, with a peak at 1.4–1.6 μm. The density of unmyelinated fibers ranges from 20,000 to 35,000/ mm^2. The ratio of unmyelinated fibers to myelinated ones is approximately 4 to 1. Other parameters may also be quantified, such as the thickness of the perineurium and the extent of proliferation of endoneurial connective tissue.

13.2. NORMAL ANATOMY

13.2.1. Connective tissue sheaths of peripheral nerve

The nerve fibers of peripheral nerve trunks are compartmentalized in bundles (fascicles), separated by fibrous connective tissue and adipose tissue: the *epineurium*. Bundles of nerve fibers within each fascicle are surrounded by multiple concentric layers of specialized cells (perineurial cells): the *perineurium*. Individual myelinated and unmyelinated nerve fibers are embedded in a meshwork of delicate connective tissue: the *endoneurium*. The larger vascular bundles that supply the nerve lie within the epineurium. Other components of the endoneurial compartment besides the myelinated and unmyelinated fibers include the Schwann cells that surround myelinated axons, Remak cells around unmyelinated axons, collagen fibers, capillaries, mast cells, fibroblasts, and Renaut bodies. Endoneurial capillaries have tight junctions, forming an effective blood–nerve barrier, analogous to the blood–brain barrier. Renaut bodies (Fig. 13.1C) occur at multiple sites throughout the peripheral nervous system, including at sites of potential entrapment, such as in the median nerve at the wrist and the ulnar nerve at the elbow. Absent in the fetus, they increase in number with age. They are made up of cells showing perineurial differentiation. Their precise function is not known, but a cushioning effect has been speculated.

13.2.2. Axons

The ratio of myelinated to unmyelinated axons and the diameter of the axons vary considerably from nerve to nerve, depending on the number of sensory fibers of various modalities and autonomic fibers plus the number of motor axons within a given nerve. The most extensive body of quantitative data is from the sural nerve, where unmyelinated nerve fibers are approximately four times as numerous as myelinated nerve fibers (Fig. 13.1D). Axonal diameter may be visually estimated across the short axis of the axon or mathematically calculated as the diameter of a circle of equal area to the cross-sectional area of the axon. By convention, the axonal diameter does not include the myelin layers surrounding the axon. The nerve fiber diameter, on the other hand, is the distance across the short axis of the entire fiber (including the myelin layer) and therefore necessarily greater than the axonal diameter.

13.2.2.1. MYELIN SHEATHS

In myelinated fibers, the myelin sheath extends as segments over the length of the axon, beginning just beyond the neuronal cell body and, in motor fibers, ending before the axon terminal. Myelin is produced by Schwann cells, which line up along the axon, with concentric layers of modified plasma membrane. The myelin sheath is not a continuous structure throughout the length of the axon. Instead, one Schwann cell encircles a segment of the axon, with gaps between each Schwann cell along the axonal length. The portion between two adjacent Schwann cells is referred to as a *node of Ranvier*, and the stretch of myelinated axon between one node of Ranvier and the next is referred to as an *internode*. In myelinated axons, the internode represents the segment of an axon myelinated by a single Schwann cell. The length of an internode is fairly constant along a given axon and is greater in larger axons. The Remak cell has a comparable function to the Schwann cell but surrounds multiple unmyelinated axons and does not produce myelin. Each internode of a myelinated axon is supported by a single Schwann cell, whereas several unmyelinated axons are within the purview of one Remak cell. The myelin sheath is made up of very regular concentric lamellae with a 12- to 17-nm periodicity, forming major dense lines separated by electron-lucent zones in which one or two interperiod lines can be observed (Fig. 13.1E, F). Discontinuity in the compaction of the lamellae is seen at the Schmidt–Lanterman incisures (Fig. 13.1E), where the major dense lines open, allowing invaginations of Schwann cell cytoplasm to penetrate between them.

13.2.2.2. MYELINATED AXONS

Myelinated axons vary in diameter between 3 and 12 μm. They are surrounded by a 7- to 8-nm-thick plasma membrane, the axolemma, which communicates directly with the internal mesaxon. The axolemma has the same ultrastructural characteristics as the cytoplasmic membranes of Schwann cells; it is lined by a basal lamina, which passes from one Schwann cell to the next without interruption at the nodes of Ranvier. The axoplasm contains longitudinally oriented mitochondria, smooth endoplasmic reticulum, multivesicular bodies, neurofilaments, and microtubules. Axonal neurofilaments have a mean diameter of 9 to 10 nm, whereas microtubules contain a central lumen and have an external diameter of approximately 25 nm.

13.2.2.3. SCHWANN CELLS

By electron microscopy, Schwann cells can be distinguished from endoneurial fibroblasts by the presence of a basement membrane. Their elongated nuclei are found roughly equidistant from two adjacent nodes of Ranvier. The cytoplasm, between the inner lamella of the myelin sheath and the axon and between the outermost myelin lamella and the cell membrane, is sparse. Located mainly around the nucleus, the cytoplasm contains endoplasmic reticulum, a Golgi apparatus, mitochondria, sometimes a centriole, and complex multilamellar lipid membranous granules (π granules or granules of Reich).

13.2.2.4. NODES OF RANVIER

In myelinated axons, the short (1 μm) nonmyelinated stretch of axon between two adjacent Schwann cells is called the *node of Ranvier*. Within the node, the axon is in direct contact with small, elongated finger-like structures (microvilli) emanating from the cytoplasm of Schwann cells. Between two nodes, the fiber segment corresponding to the myelinated axon is called the internode. At the two ends of the internodes are characteristic regions: the paranodes (just adjacent to the nodes), where the myelin lamellae terminate; and "myelin loops" are apposed to the axon with a gap of 2.5–3 nm and which are attached to the axolemma (septate junctions) by small periodic, dense structures like dots, called the terminal bands. A basal lamina surrounds individual myelinated Schwann cell–axon units and extends through the nodal gap. These structures are embedded in an extracellular matrix-rich material (termed the "cement disk" by Ranvier).

13.2.2.5. UNMYELINATED FIBERS

The axons of unmyelinated fibers have a similar ultrastructural appearance of axoplasm and axolemma as those of myelinated fibers; in comparison, they are, however, smaller in diameter and lack the repetitive layers of myelin lipid membranes. Also, unlike myelinated fibers, multiple unmyelinated axons are usually enclosed by a single Remak cell; they are closely packed and separated from each other by a thin layer of Remak cell cytoplasm.

13.3. GENERAL REACTIONS OF PERIPHERAL NERVE TO DISEASE

The general reaction of peripheral nerve to injury can be separated into two prototypes: those that involve primarily the axon and those that preferentially involve the myelin sheath. Combinations of the two are common.

13.3.1. Primary axonal degeneration

The degeneration of axons may be subclassified based on the cause of the degeneration (Fig. 13.2). By and large, all forms ultimately result in denervation of muscle fibers when the process affects motor axons.

13.3.1.1. TYPES OF AXONAL DEGENERATION

13.3.1.1.1. Wallerian degeneration. Wallerian degeneration is the response of the distal part of an axon to the physical transection or crush of the nerve at some point along its course (Fig. 13.3). In the early stages, the process is characterized morphologically by breakdown of the axon and its myelin sheath at all points distal to the point of transection. A reparative stage begins shortly after transection and consists of proliferation of Schwann cells within the tube formed by the original Schwann cell basal lamina, providing that scaffolding had not been destroyed by the initial injury. In this response, the Schwann cell groups are arranged as a linear tube and constitute a band that may be seen in cross section by electron microscopy,

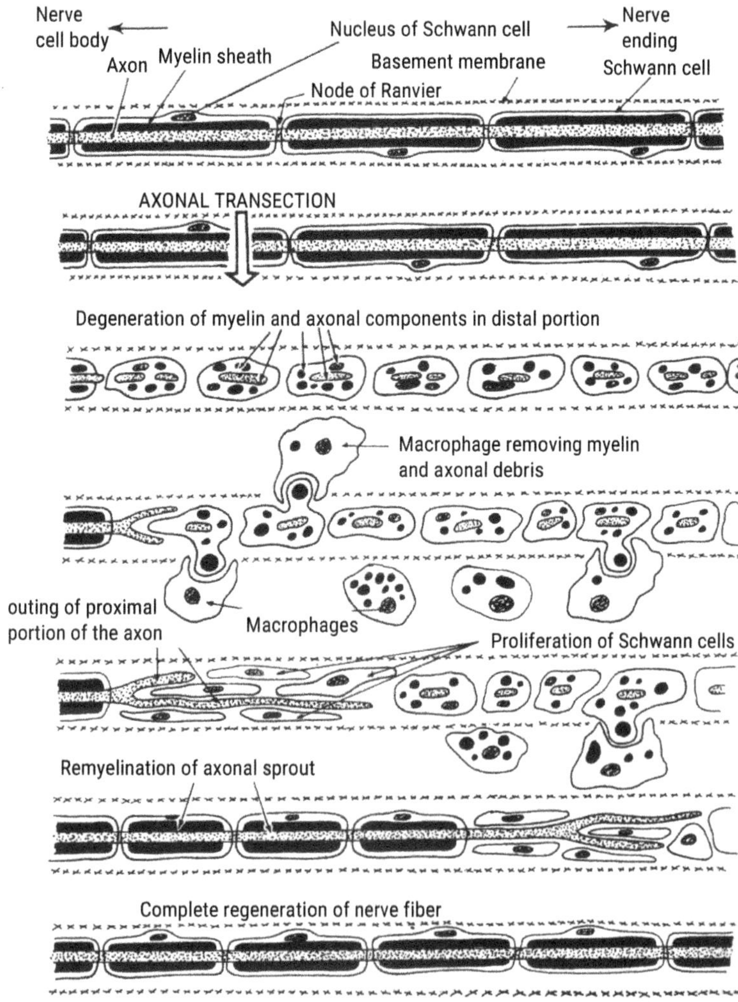

FIGURE 13.3 The main stages of Wallerian degeneration and regeneration of a myelinated fiber. (Redrawn and modified from Bradley, W. G. (1974). *Disorders of peripheral nerves*. Oxford, UK: Blackwell.)

called a band of Büngner. Regeneration occurs from the sprouting of axons from the proximal stump of the sectioned nerve; it begins almost at once after axotomy and progresses relatively slowly (1–3 mm per day). These sprouts, usually two to five per sectioned axon, may enter the bands of Büngner. When this occurs, one may observe the appearance of clusters of small, thinly myelinated groupings of regenerating fibers (see Section 13.3.1.2).

13.3.1.1.2. Progressive distal axonopathy (dying-back neuropathy). The dying-back neuropathy (progressive distal axonopathy) type of axonal injury is characteristic of a group of neuropathies for which the clinical picture is manifest as a fairly symmetrical, subacute or chronic axonal degeneration, first affecting the most distal portions of axons, followed by progressively more proximal degeneration of the axon. The longest and largest axons are usually the first to be involved (size-dependent vulnerability). In the case of sensory fibers, where axons are directed toward the spinal cord or brainstem, the process affects first the most distal portions of the respective sensory ascending fiber tracts; degeneration of the posterior columns, for example, thus starts from the upper end of the spinal cord, especially in the fasciculus gracilis. In the early stages of the disease, nerve conduction studies may show diminished amplitude but preservation of nerve conduction velocity. In later stages of the disease, the conduction velocity is reduced.

The pathogenesis of this distal accentuation of axonal loss is not completely understood. Some investigators have viewed it as a "biochemical transection" whereby there is progressive involvement of more proximal segments of the axon, akin to the morphological manifestations of Wallerian degeneration. There is some evidence to support the concept that the dying-back process is related to abnormalities of fast axonal transport. The neuropathologic picture is characterized by a reduction in the number of myelinated fibers, with evidence of regeneration, including axonal sprouting.

13.3.1.1.3. Neuronopathy. Neuronopathy is a category of axonal neuropathy in which the primary abnormality is thought to be within the neuronal cell body, with a more or less synchronous injury along the entire length of the axon. Because it is the neuronal cell body that degenerates, axonal regeneration is not observed in these cases. The clinical course of the disease of patients with neuronopathies as they affect the peripheral nervous system, comparable to neuronal degenerations in the central nervous system, is characteristically slowly progressive, non-length-dependent, with selective populations of neurons becoming sequentially involved.

Sensory neurons are more often affected than motor neurons in neuronopathic toxic injuries (e.g., pyridoxine intoxication or paraneoplastic neuropathy). The reason for the predilection of sensory systems is not known but postulated to be related to the lack of vascular barrier in dorsal root ganglia, thereby permitting direct access of toxins or paraneoplastic antibodies to the ganglion cells. Preferential involvement of populations of the neurons within dorsal root ganglia is well recognized, as occurs in neuropathies that selectively involve either the small neurons (e.g., Fabry disease) or the large neurons (e.g., sensory paraneoplastic neuropathy, Friedreich ataxia, and abetalipoproteinemia). Another proposed mechanism of cell injury theorizes the uptake of noxious substances in the free sensory terminals, which are devoid of the blood–nerve barrier, thereby allowing access to the perikaryon through retrograde axonal transport ("suicide transport").

13.3.1.1.4. Abnormalities of axonal caliber. Axonal caliber is related to, among other things, the number of neurofilaments and microtubules contained in the axon. In human pathology, axonal atrophy chiefly affects the large fibers, perhaps because they are richest in neurofilaments (caliber-dependent vulnerability). Axonal atrophy is expressed by a loss of the circular outline of the fiber and by a reduction of average axonal diameter. In prolonged insults, secondary demyelination may occur and may be sufficiently severe to mimic a primary chronic demyelinating process. Axonal atrophy has been documented in Charcot–Marie–Tooth (CMT) disease, in uremic neuropathy, in diabetic neuropathy, in neuropathy associated with myeloma, and in various toxic neuropathies. Axonal swelling resulting from focal or multifocal accumulation of neurofilaments and other organelles is characteristic of hereditary neuropathies (e.g., hereditary giant axonal neuropathy [GAN]) (Fig. 13.4A) and of certain toxic neuropathies (e.g., hexane neuropathy) (Fig. 13.4B).

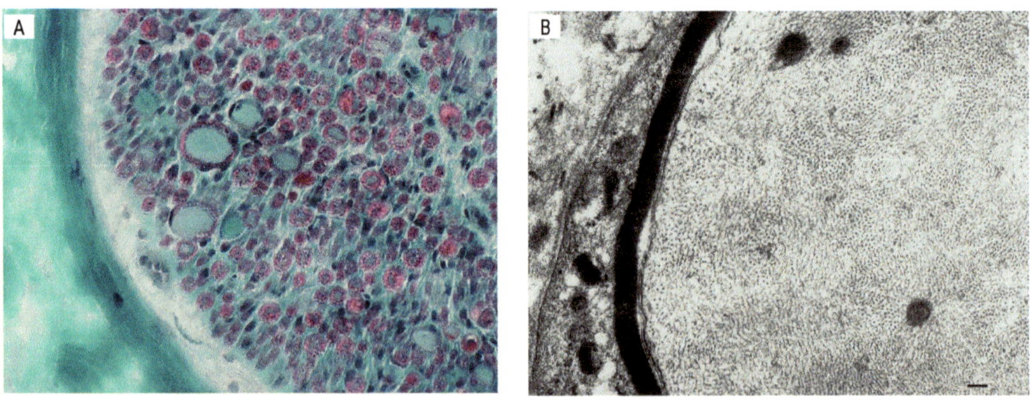

FIGURE 13.4 Axonal swellings on peripheral nerve biopsy: (**A**) light microscopy in a case of hereditary giant axonal neuropathy with multiple distended axons; (**B**) electron microscopy in a case of hexane neuropathy showing accumulation of neurofilaments, distended diameter, and attenuated myelin.

13.3.1.2. MORPHOLOGICAL APPEARANCES OF AXONAL DEGENERATION AND AXONAL REGENERATION IN PERIPHERAL NEUROPATHIES

The histologic appearance of axonal degeneration and axonal regeneration in peripheral neuropathies varies depending on the course of the disease, the interval between biopsy and the onset of the disease, and the site of the nerve sample along the length of the fiber. In the early stages of an axonal neuropathy, axonal degeneration may be seen by light microscopy as *ovoids*, which are axonal fragments surrounded by disintegrating myelin (Fig. 13.5A, D). In cross sections, this form of degeneration is sometimes difficult to distinguish from crush artifact (Fig. 13.5B). The presence of myelin debris and retained cytoplasmic detail in adjacent cells is best appreciated with electron microscopy (Fig. 13.5C). In addition, teasing permits identification of the earliest lesions, which consist of myelin retraction on either side of the node of Ranvier, followed by myelin irregularity and fragmentation in each internodal segment into a row of ovoids. Phagocytosis of degenerating nerve fiber fragments by Schwann cells and by circulating mononuclear phagocytes is seen to better advantage in longitudinal sections, by light or electron microscopy (Fig. 13.5C). Early axonal sprouting may also be seen.

The earliest changes that attend axonal degeneration are best detected by electron microscopy as disruption of the myelin sheath, associated with abnormalities within the axon, including clustering and swelling of organelles. Axonal regeneration is first identifiable by light microscopy when the sprouting axonal extensions are myelinated and form clusters of small, closely packed fibers, which are well seen in semithin cross sections (regeneration fascicles) (Fig. 13.6). Teasing may also demonstrate myelinated axonal sprouts with regularly

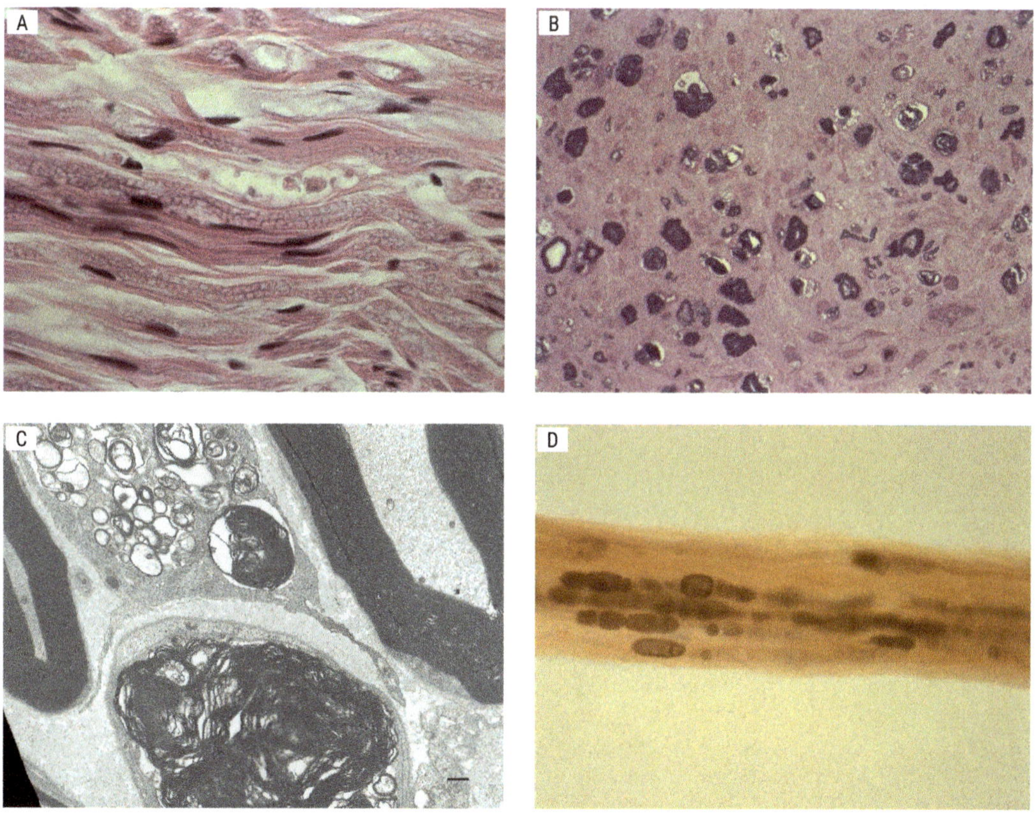

FIGURE 13.5 Acute axonal degeneration showing routine H&E light microscopy (**A**), semithin sections on light microscopy (**B**), at the ultrastructural level by electron microscopy (**C**), and on teased-fiber preparations (**D**). In the longitudinal plane, there are rows of ovoid, lipid-filled vacuoles, whereas in the transverse plane there is a loss of distinction of the axoplasm with myelin debris.

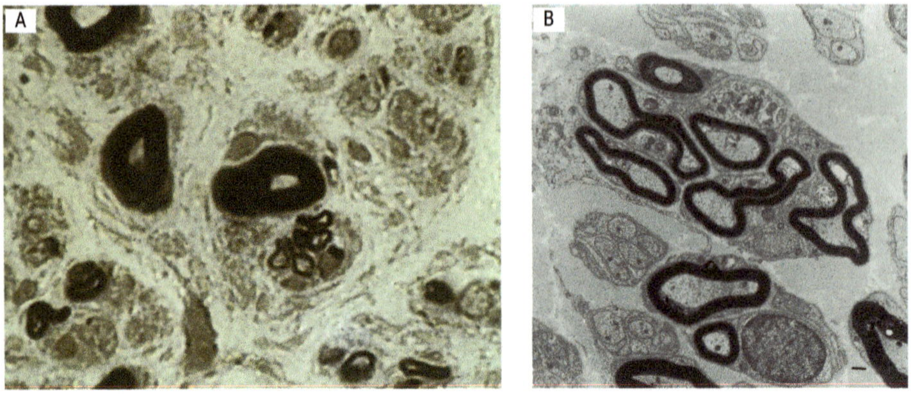

FIGURE 13.6 Clusters of small-caliber, closely packed fibers, typical of "regeneration fascicles," in semithin cross section (**A**) and by electron microscopy (**B**). The band of Büngner is evident only by electron microscopy, where a single basal lamina surrounds the entire group of small axons.

spaced internodes that are too short for the diameter of the fiber.

In the chronic or late stages of axonal degeneration, the principal histologic features include loss of myelinated axons and an increase in endoneurial connective tissue (Fig. 13.7). The presence of regenerating clusters is good presumptive evidence that the underlying pathologic process is due to

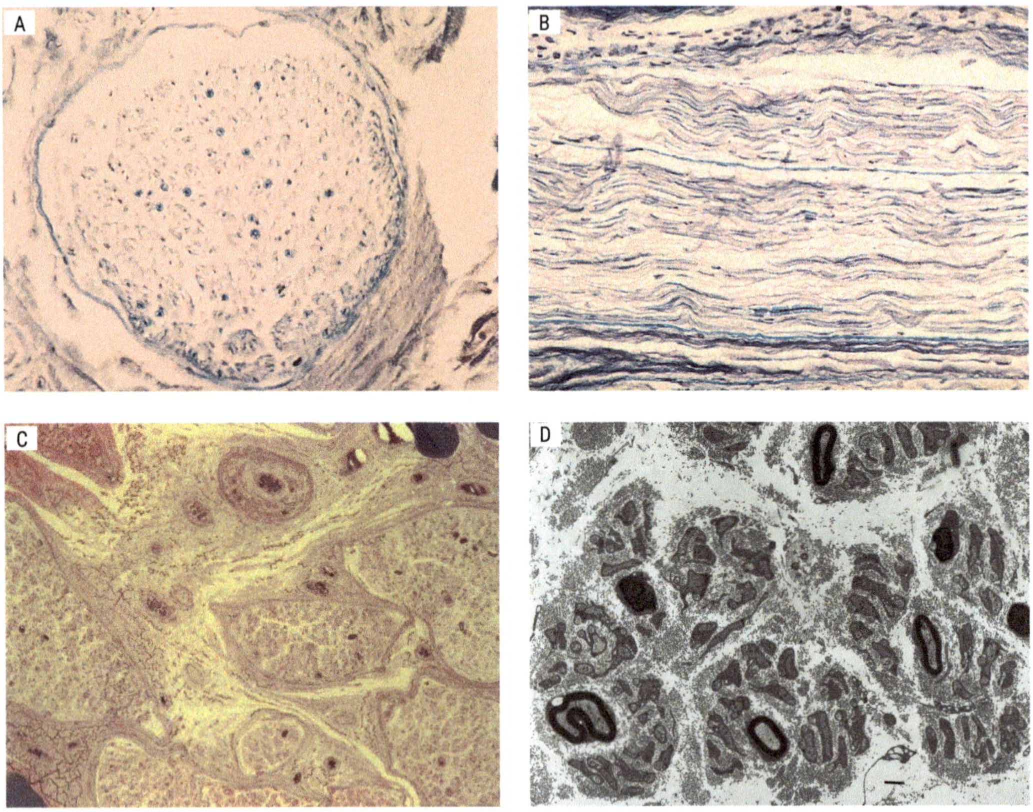

FIGURE 13.7 Severe chronic axonal neuropathy. Axonal loss, resulting from the cumulative effects of chronic axonal degeneration, is seen on transverse (**A**) and longitudinal sections (**B**) (Bodian silver axonal impregnation combined with Luxol fast blue myelin stain in paraffin sections) and on semithin section (**C**). (**D**) Ultrastructural examination shows severe loss of myelinated fibers in a case of autosomal recessive axonal-type Charcot–Marie–Tooth disease.

axonal degeneration. Teased nerve fiber preparations may demonstrate different stages of degeneration and regeneration, which indicate an ongoing process.

13.3.2. Primary segmental demyelination

Primary segmental demyelination is a process whereby the primary site of injury is the myelin sheath. When a motor axon is affected solely by demyelination, denervation atrophy of muscle does not occur as long as the axon remains intact.

13.3.2.1. ACUTE SEGMENTAL DEMYELINATION AND REMYELINATION

Primary involvement of the myelin sheaths or the Schwann cells causes segmental demyelination, with myelin destruction and relative sparing of axons, occurring one internodal segment at a time. This process involves the myelin of individual internodes randomly along the length of fibers, affecting some in sequence while skipping others. The demyelination begins next to the node of Ranvier. Subsequently, Schwann cells and mononuclear phagocytes participate in the phagocytosis of degenerated myelin. Widening of the nodes of Ranvier and denuded stretches of demyelinated internodes affecting most fibers within a nerve interrupt saltatory conduction and, over the course of time, cause reduction in the speed of nerve conduction and conduction blocks. Myelin loss involving only very short segments of the fiber (i.e., less than 15-μm stretches) may be followed by remyelination with Schwann cells and myelin elaboration. When the extent of myelin internodal loss is greater than 15 μm, Schwann cells proliferate and form small, intercalated internodes. In teased-nerve preparations, the characteristic appearance of a fiber that has undergone remyelination after segmental demyelination consists of internodes of unequal size, in which the remyelinated internodes are shorter than normal and have a thinner myelin sheath than that of the adjoining, unaffected internodes (Fig. 13.8). In cross section, remyelinated fibers appear to be hypomyelinated (i.e., the myelin sheaths are disproportionately thin compared to the axon diameter) (Fig. 13.9A).

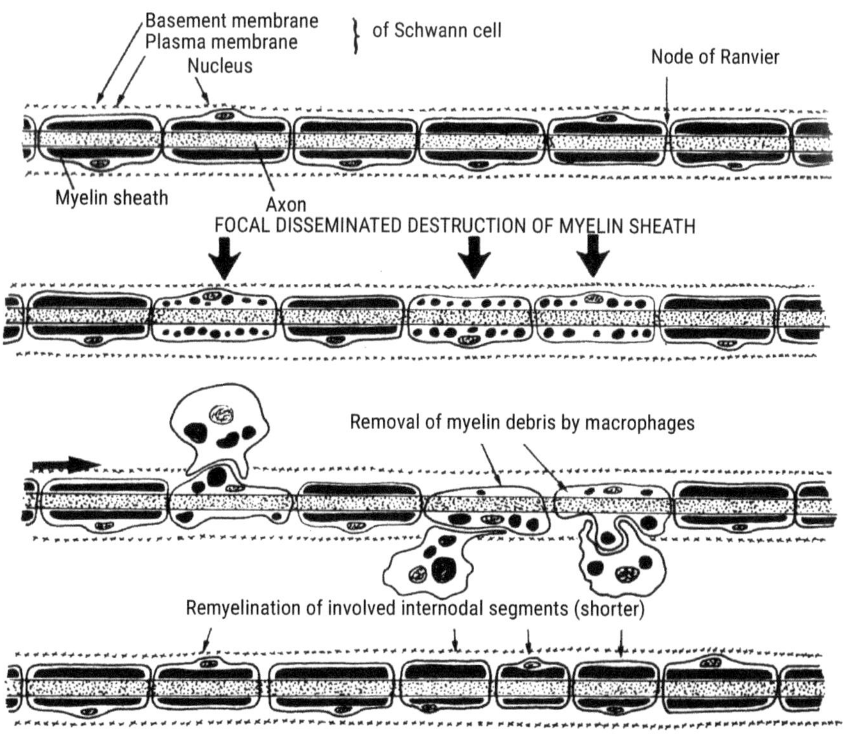

FIGURE 13.8 The main stages of segmental demyelination and remyelination of a myelinated peripheral nerve fiber. (Redrawn and modified from Bradley, W. G. (1974). *Disorders of peripheral nerves*. Oxford, UK: Blackwell.)

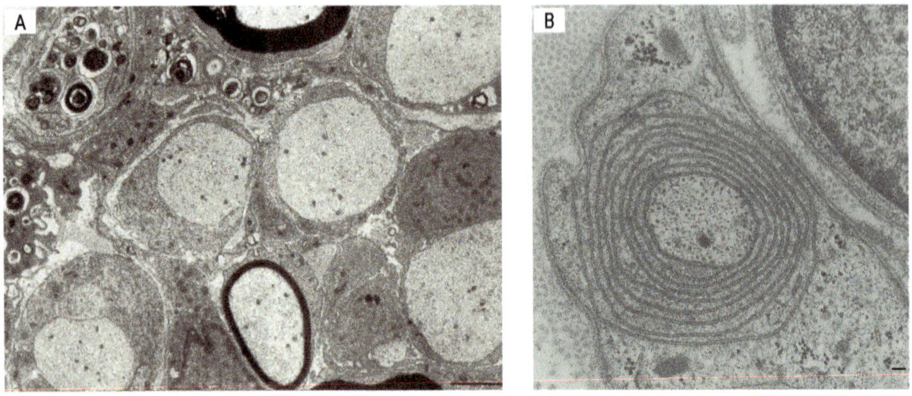

FIGURE 13.9 Ultrastructural appearance of demyelination and remyelination. (**A**) At low magnification, numerous fibers are devoid of myelin (demyelinated) or thinly myelinated, reflecting demyelination and early remyelination. (**B**) Uncompacted myelin is also a feature of the early stages of remyelination.

The concept of "nodopathies" has emerged recently: It has been proposed that structural changes restricted to the nodal or paranodal region may be involved in the pathophysiology of some demyelinating neuropathies, such as anti-ganglioside antibody-mediated neuropathies. These abnormalities of the nodal region may induce axonal degeneration due to alterations of the function of the Na^+/K^+ pump. Thus, the nodal region (Fig. 13.10) has emerged as a hot spot in the field of autoimmune neuropathies.

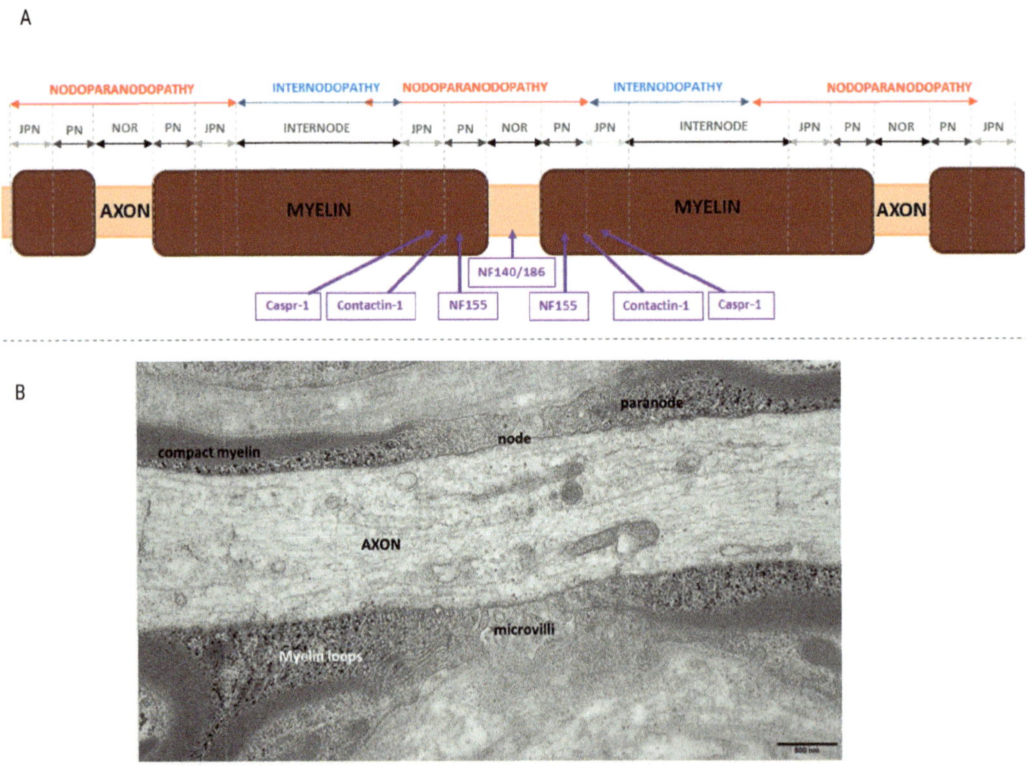

FIGURE 13.10 (**A**) Schematic representation of a nerve myelinated fiber; the regionally restricted expression of some nodo-paranodal proteins (contactin-1, caspr-1, NF155, and NF140/186) are indicated. (Courtesy of Dr. S. Mathis.) (**B**) Electron microscopic longitudinal section of the nodo-paranodal area of a myelinated fiber.

13.3.2.2. OTHER MYELIN LESIONS

During myelination and with remyelination, one may observe incomplete compaction of the outermost myelin lamellae at the ultrastructural level (Fig. 13.9B). In this situation, the spacing between the lamellae is abnormally wide. In pathologic circumstances, this widening of myelin lamellae may stem from abnormalities and genetically determined mutations of certain proteins in compact myelin, such as myelin protein zero. This compaction abnormality may also be observed in neuropathies due to monoclonal gammopathy (often of immunoglobulin M [IgM] type with anti–myelin-associated glycoprotein [MAG] or antiglycolipid activity).

Hypo- or hypermyelination, the presence of abnormally thin or abnormally thick myelin sheaths, respectively, can be seen in genetically determined neuropathies. Hypermyelination is an excess of myelin lamellae relative to the diameter of the axon, often producing redundant, abnormally folded loops of myelin. Focal areas of hypermyelination, referred to as "tomacula," can affect a portion of one internode and are characteristic of certain genetically determined entrapment peripheral neuropathies. In the majority of affected families, the disorder is inherited as an autosomal dominant trait, and individuals have a deletion of the *PMP-22* gene on chromosome 17p11.2. Inheritance of duplication of the *PMP-22* gene leads to CMT type 1A (CMT1A). Patients with hereditary neuropathy with liability to pressure palsies (HNPP) have an underlying demyelinating sensorimotor neuropathy, in addition to a tendency to develop pressure palsies. Tomacula are occasionally seen in conditions other than hereditary pressure-sensitive neuropathy, such as sporadic chronic neuropathy in childhood, neuropathy associated with chronic alcoholism, and benign monoclonal gammopathy. In congenital hypomyelinating neuropathies with onset of symptoms in early childhood, myelin width is considerably thinner than expected normally for the patient's age.

13.3.2.3. SCHWANN CELL PROLIFERATION AND ONION BULB FORMATIONS

Repeated episodes of segmental demyelination and remyelination culminate in Schwann cell abnormalities. Onion bulb formation is a process characterized by an exuberant proliferation of Schwann cells and of basement membrane deposits arranged concentrically around an axon, which may be completely denuded of myelin or may have a thin myelin sheath relative to the diameter of the axon (Fig. 13.11A–C). When the process is severe, the Schwann cell processes form multiple concentric layers (Fig. 13.11C) around a majority of axons and are referred to as *onion bulbs*. There is also an increase of collagen in the endoneurium, which often has a loose, sometimes metachromatic, appearance. The early stages of onion bulb formation may be demonstrable only by electron microscopy (Fig. 13.11D).

13.3.3. Lesions that are both axonal and demyelinating

In chronic peripheral neuropathies, one form of injury predominates at first, but with time, secondary involvement occurs. Thus, a purely axonal or demyelinating chronic neuropathy is seldom encountered. Instead, in a chronic axonopathy, there is a severe depletion of axons and mild degrees of demyelination and remyelination. Conversely, in a chronic demyelinating neuropathy, onion bulb formation may be extensive, and axonal loss is also present to some extent. These pathologic findings correlate with the electrophysiologic studies on the patient. Early stages of an axonal peripheral neuropathy may show decreased amplitude on nerve conduction studies, while the conduction velocity is relatively spared. However, later in axonal neuropathies, the conduction velocity may also be decreased, reflecting an element of secondary demyelination. Similarly, demyelinating neuropathies often show a slowing of conduction velocity as an early finding, and only in later stages when there is substantial axonal loss is there a change in the amplitude on nerve conduction studies. In general, the more severe pathologic abnormality, whether on nerve conduction studies or peripheral nerve biopsy, is usually presumed to be the primary event and may be described as "axonal neuropathy with secondary demyelination," for example.

13.4. INFLAMMATORY POLYNEUROPATHIES

13.4.1. Immunopathologic disorders of unknown cause

13.4.1.1. GUILLAIN–BARRÉ SYNDROME OR ACUTE INFLAMMATORY DEMYELINATING POLYNEUROPATHY

Guillain–Barré syndrome (GBS), the most common form of which is acute inflammatory demyelinating

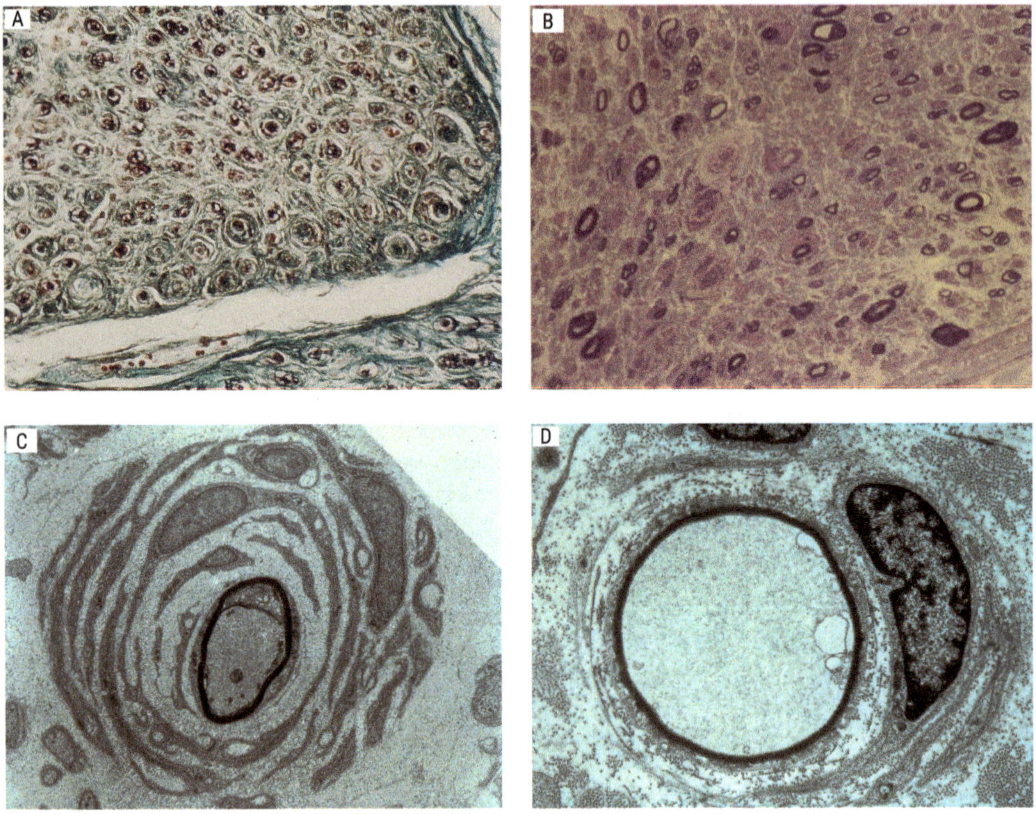

FIGURE 13.11 Onion bulbs: (**A**) microscopic appearance in hypertrophic neuropathy in paraffin-embedded tissue, created by the presence of many onion bulbs. (**B**) Onion bulbs on semithin section, with multiple layers of Schwann cell processes surrounding many of the axons. (**C, D**) Ultrastructural appearance: (**C**) proliferation of Schwann cells and of basement membranes concentrically around an intact axon; (**D**) early stage of onion bulb with a few layers of concentrically arranged Schwann cell processes surrounding a thinly myelinated axon.

polyneuropathy (AIDP), can be the primary manifestation of a neurologic illness or may occur in the setting of systemic disorders, including infections (e.g., by cytomegalovirus, the Epstein–Barr virus, mycoplasma, hepatitis viruses, or HIV), vaccinations, surgery, pregnancy, immunosuppression, and cancer. Immune-mediated myelin damage is believed to be the cause of the peripheral nerve lesions, but precise pathogenesis of the illness is incompletely understood. Nerve biopsy is only rarely needed to establish the diagnosis of GBS, although in rare severe cases with electrically silent nerves, histological examination of biopsy specimens can determine the type and extent of lesions.

In the acute phases of the disease, which is usually demyelinating, lesions typically consist of disseminated segmental demyelination that is accentuated in perivenular locations and are associated with endoneurial edema and mononuclear cellular inflammatory infiltrates. A characteristic feature may be seen by electron microscopy: Macrophages cross the basal lamina and displace the Schwann cell cytoplasm; their processes surround the myelin sheaths and insert themselves between the outer myelin lamellae (Fig. 13.12); the myelin sheaths are thus progressively destroyed so that macrophages are in contact with the axon. Perhaps independent of this process, myelin sheaths undergo vesicular degeneration. Axonal degeneration is also sometimes seen in teased-nerve preparations.

Although the most common form of GBS is a demyelinating condition (AIDP), it appears to be a somewhat heterogeneous electroclinical entity. Neurophysiology and biopsy may identify purely axonal sensorimotor forms of GBS (acute motor–sensory axonal neuropathy) or a subtype of the pure motor form called acute motor axonal neuropathy. Because the process appears

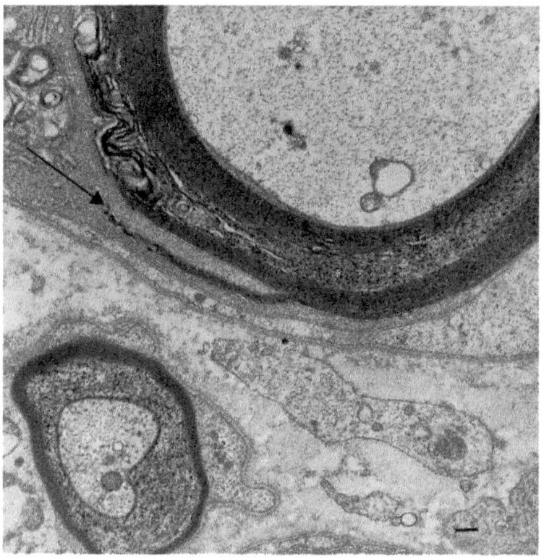

FIGURE 13.12 Guillain–Barré syndrome. A tongue-like macrophage extension inserts itself between the outer myelin lamellae (*arrow*).

first near the node of Ranvier, these axonal autoimmune neuropathies have been described as "nodo-paranodopathies."

Autopsy studies have shown that the inflammatory lesions in GBS tend to predominate in the proximal regions of the peripheral nervous system close to the spinal cord. For this reason, sural nerve biopsies may be less informative. The inflammatory infiltrate in GBS is composed of macrophages and, especially, T lymphocytes in which the CD4:CD8 ratio is identical to that seen in the blood.

13.4.1.2. SUBACUTE OR CHRONIC INFLAMMATORY DEMYELINATING POLYRADICULONEUROPATHY

Subacute or chronic inflammatory demyelinating polyradiculoneuropathy (CIDP) is a demyelinating neuropathy of autoimmune pathogenesis in which the clinical evolution is slower than occurs in patients with GBS. A nerve biopsy can then provide supportive evidence of CIDP in patients with an unusual course or presentation, and when performed, a nerve known to be affected on the basis of clinical or electrophysiological study should be chosen for biopsy. The lesions tend to be most prominent in nerve roots and vary considerably in severity. In sural nerve biopsies, their distribution is typically heterogeneous within a given fascicle and between fascicles; this uneven distribution may be useful in differentiating CIDP from genetic chronic demyelinating processes. Inflammatory infiltrates are usually mild or absent. Light microscopic examination of plastic-embedded sural nerve sections may show demyelination and some loss of myelinated fibers. Some of the remaining axons can be totally devoid of myelin, whereas others are surrounded by a thin sheath of myelin indicative of remyelination.

Teased-fiber preparations may demonstrate segmental demyelination and remyelination. Ongoing demyelination is best seen by electron microscopy. Onion bulb formations may be striking both in plastic sections and by electron microscopy, as the characteristic concentric whorling of Schwann cell cytoplasm with skeins of the basal membrane surrounding normally myelinated or thinly myelinated axons. Regenerating clusters, indicative of concomitant axonal involvement and interpreted as secondary to chronicity, are also seen. There often is also a loss of unmyelinated fibers.

Recently, it has been shown that patients with chronic demyelinating polyneuropathy have IgG4 antibodies to some antigens of the paranodal region, such as Caspr-1, Contactin-1, NFasc155, and NFasc186, as well as other unidentified paranodal proteins. These IgG4 antibodies induce characteristic ultrastructural lesions of the axonal surface at the paranodal region in the absence of macrophage-induced demyelination. These lesions consist of a selective loss of the septate-like junctions. Cell processes may also penetrate into the expanded spaces between the paranodal myelin loops and the axolemma. These antibody-mediated neuropathies were previously subclassified as variants of CIDP but recently have been recategorized as paranodal neuropathies, not CIDP.

13.4.1.3. SARCOIDOSIS

Sarcoidosis is a disease in which a T-lymphocyte–mediated inflammatory process develops in the setting of a response to an unknown antigenic stimulus. The disease has a wide range of clinical and pathological manifestations as it affects the peripheral nervous system. Noncaseating granulomas with giant cells may be seen rarely in nerves, chiefly in the epineurium. Inflammatory infiltrates extend into the endoneurium, following connective tissue septa and blood vessels; a necrotizing vasculitis occurs in some cases. Multifocal heterogeneous axonal loss is the rule; demyelination is rare.

13.4.2. Neuropathies due to infections

13.4.2.1. LEPROSY

The peripheral nervous system is especially vulnerable in leprosy, and the range of manifestations of the disease is wide. The involvement of the peripheral nervous system is typically multifocal, and it may induce mononeuropathies or multiple mononeuropathies while sparing other nerves entirely.

13.4.2.1.1. Multibacillary (lepromatous) leprosy. There is nearly always widespread involvement of cutaneous sensory nerves in lepromatous (multibacillary) leprosy, even in patients without clinical signs of neuropathy, and most cases show morphologic evidence of inflammation with widespread infiltration of the endoneurium, perineurium, and epineurium by numerous macrophages (Fig. 13.13A). The cytoplasm of these macrophages contains *Mycobacterium leprae* (Fig. 13.13B), sometimes in large aggregates called globi. On ultrastructural examination, bacilli predominate in macrophages and Schwann/Remak cells, but they also occur within axons and endothelial cells. Individual bacteria, or groups of bacteria, are surrounded by an electron-lucent halo (Fig. 13.13C).

13.4.2.1.2. Paucibacillary (tuberculoid) leprosy. In the tuberculoid (paucibacillary) form, bacilli are either absent at light microscopic examination or extremely rare. Granulomatous infiltrates predominate and consist of T lymphocytes with some B lymphocytes, plasma cells, Langhans giant cells, and macrophages (Fig. 13.14). In some cases, necrosis may occur, producing abscesses. Marked distortion of the walls of capillaries and small vessels is also found. Axons, Schwann cells, and myelin are lost, and there is fibrosis of the perineurium

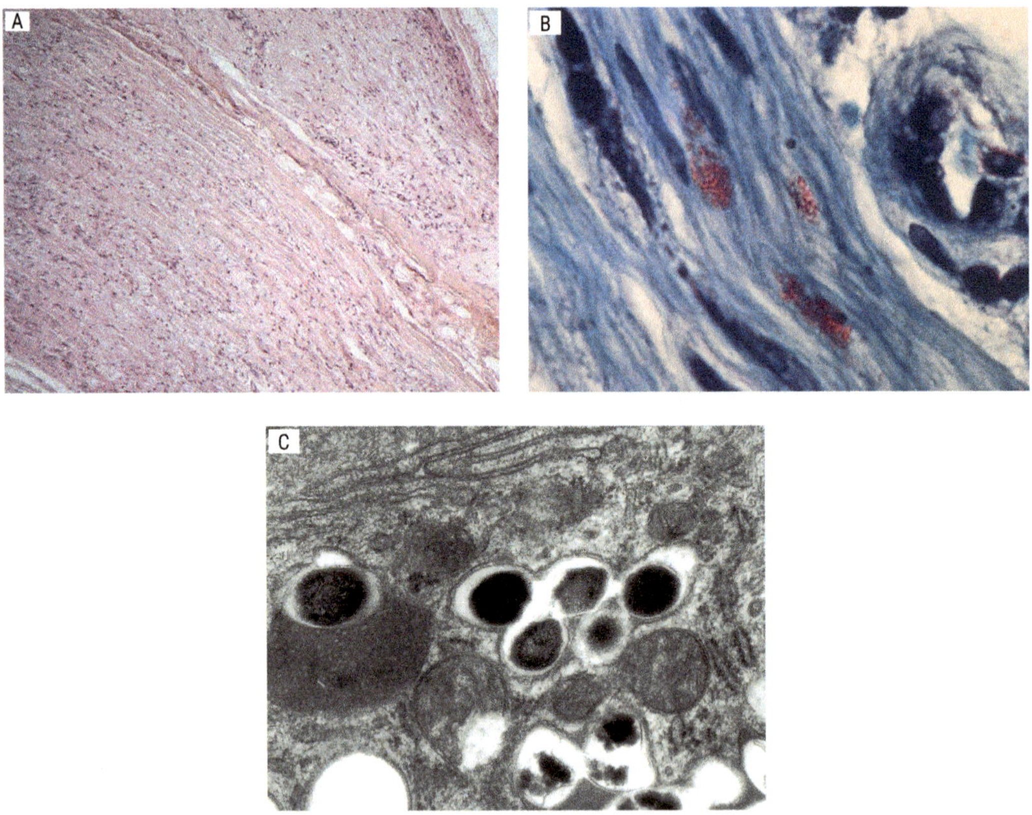

FIGURE 13.13 Multibacillary (lepromatous) leprosy. (**A**) Infiltration of the endoneurium by numerous macrophages. (**B**) The cytoplasm of these macrophages is filled with leprosy bacilli, well demonstrated on Ziehl–Nielsen stain for acid-fast bacilli. (**C**) Ultrastructural examination shows a group of mycobacteria surrounded by an electron-lucent halo.

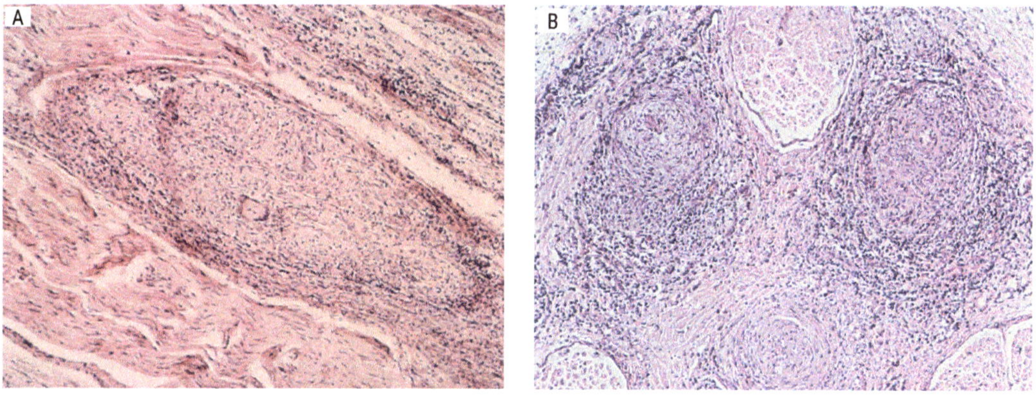

FIGURE 13.14 Paucibacillary (tuberculoid) leprosy. (**A**) Granulomatous inflammatory infiltration of the endoneurium with Langhans-type giant cells. (**B**) On transverse section, note inflammation and fibrosis of the perineurium and endoneurium.

and endoneurium; the nerves adjacent to the foci of granulomatous inflammation undergo nodular thickenings and clinically become abnormally firm.

13.4.2.1.3. Intermediate forms of leprosy. The nerve lesions in patients with intermediate forms of leprosy are characterized by varying amounts of inflammatory infiltrates and acid-fast bacilli. Viable organisms, or more often, organisms in a state of disintegration, can be demonstrated by electron microscopy within the cytoplasm of Schwann cells and macrophages.

13.4.2.2. HIV-ASSOCIATED NEUROPATHY

Different forms of peripheral nerve involvement have been described in patients with HIV infection and can involve small and/or large fibers. Patients with severe neuropathy may develop motor weakness and muscle cramps. Direct viral infection of the nerve is not the cause of the neuropathy. In situ hybridization and immunocytochemical methods have detected viral antigens in mononuclear cells in the endoneurial compartment.

HIV-associated neuropathy may take the form of inflammatory polyradiculoneuropathy (GBS or CIDP), mainly in the early stages of the disease. HIV-related inflammatory polyneuropathy is more frequently observed in patients with cerebrospinal fluid pleocytosis than in patients with GBS or CIDP in the absence of HIV infection.

Distal painful symmetric sensory neuropathies have been described in patients in the late stages of HIV infection and attributed to involvement of the dorsal root ganglia with the destruction of sensory neurons, of uncertain pathogenesis. A necrotizing vasculitis, comparable to that seen in polyarteritis nodosa (PAN), may be observed in HIV-infected individuals who develop multiple polyneuropathy.

A subset of HIV-infected patients have been found to develop persistent CD8 hyperlymphocytosis and a Sjögren-like syndrome associated with multivisceral CD8 T-cell infiltration, known as the *diffuse infiltrative lymphocytosis syndrome*. Nerve biopsy in these cases has shown marked angiocentric CD8 infiltrates without vessel wall necrosis; abundant expression of HIV anti-p24 immunoreactivity in macrophages has been noted.

Some patients with AIDS develop peripheral neuropathy induced by cytomegalovirus, and a particularly dreaded complication is painful meningomyeloradiculitis, which affects the lumbosacral regions. The characteristic viral inclusions are seen on light microscopic examination, highlighted by anti-HIV immunocytochemistry; by electron microscopy, viral particles are present in Schwann cells, macrophages, endothelial cells, and fibroblasts. Iatrogenic axonal painful neuropathy has been associated with several antiretroviral medications used to treat HIV.

13.4.2.3. BORRELIOSIS (LYME DISEASE, TICK-BITE MENINGORADICULONEURITIS)

Acute axonal neuropathy can be seen in peripheral nerve biopsies in the meningoradiculoneuritic or secondary stage of Lyme disease (borreliosis or tick-bite meningoradiculoneuritis). There may also

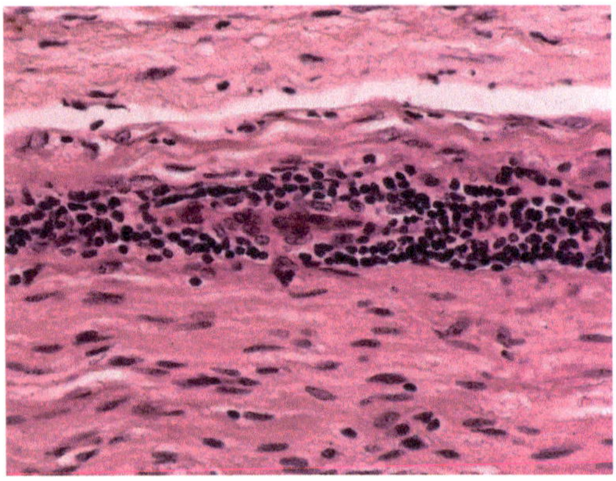

FIGURE 13.15 Lyme disease neuropathy, with perivascular mononuclear cell infiltrate.

be a prominent lymphocytic and plasmacytic reaction around blood vessels in the endoneurium (Fig. 13.15) and epineurium. The inflammatory cell infiltrates have been found to be mainly B lymphocytes. Demyelinating lesions and dissociation of myelin lamellae by inflammatory have not been reported as it has in GBS. Vessel walls are devoid of fibrinoid necrosis or inflammatory infiltrates. *Borrelia burgdorferi* has not been demonstrated in affected nerves.

13.4.3. Vasculitic neuropathies

The *vasculitides* are inflammatory disorders of the vascular system characterized by cellular inflammatory infiltrates involving focal segments of the walls of blood vessels. The presence of fibrinoid necrosis within the vascular wall defines the entity of necrotizing vasculitis. When vasculitis involves the peripheral nervous system, it usually involves the blood vessels of the epineurium. The nerve injury secondary to vascular involvement is characterized by axonal degeneration, which shows variable and focal fascicular localization. Complete cross-sectional infarction of a peripheral nerve is rare. The usual manifestation of the disease is that of partial and segmental loss of nerve fibers, presumably from nerve ischemia caused by damaged vessels at some distance away from the biopsy site being examined. The lesions are typically heterogeneous from one fascicle to the next or within the same fascicle (centrofascicular or eccentric depopulation). The clinical picture most suggestive of vasculitis-induced neuropathy is that of multiple mononeuropathies, sometimes also called "mononeuritis multiplex"; a diffuse polyneuropathy may also be seen.

Two types of vasculitis are most commonly associated with nerve or muscle disease: polyarteritis nodosa (PAN) and anti-neutrophil cytoplasmic antibody (ANCA)–associated vasculitis.

13.4.3.1. POLYARTERITIS NODOSA (SYSTEMIC VASCULITIS AFFECTING MIDDLE-CALIBER ARTERIOLES)

The characteristic lesions of PAN involve the wall of small- and middle-caliber arteries and arterioles (70–200 μm). Systemic vasculitis is characterized by medial fibrinoid necrosis, polymorphonuclear panarterial cellular inflammatory infiltrates, and vascular thrombosis. Lesions of different ages are typical. Hepatitis B virus (HBV) infection is the major known risk factor associated with PAN, although with the prevalence of HBV immunization, the percentage of patients with HBV-associated PAN has decreased considerably. ANCAs are not present in PAN.

Patients with rheumatoid arthritis may have peripheral nerve lesions comparable to those seen in PAN but also involving the microcirculation, and the inflammatory lesions are often rich in plasma cells. Less often, necrotizing panarteritis may occur in other collagen diseases, such as systemic lupus erythematosus or Sjögren syndrome.

13.4.3.2. ANCA-ASSOCIATED VASCULITIDES

The ANCA-associated vasculitides, strongly associated with circulating anti-neutrophil antibodies, include three major entities: granulomatosis with polyangiitis (GPA), eosinophilic granulomatosis with polyangiitis (EGPA; or Churg–Strauss syndrome), and microscopic polyangiitis (MPA). There are specific clinicopathologic features of each of the ANCA-associated vasculitides, in addition to their association with ANCAs. EGPA and MPA have a tendency to involve peripheral nerves.

In patients with EGPA (Churg–Strauss syndrome), involvement of small- to medium-caliber arterioles or venules occurs in individuals with a history of asthma; many of these patients have received prolonged treatment with corticosteroids.

A very high circulating eosinophil count is also seen in these patients. The vascular lesions are similar to those of PAN but differ by the great abundance of eosinophils in the inflammatory infiltrates, by the frequency with which both veins and capillaries are involved, by the less frequent occurrence of fibrinoid necrosis, and by the presence of extravascular granulomas in some cases. The serum is often positive for p-ANCA (most often anti-myeloperoxidase) in Churg–Strauss syndrome, but c-ANCA (most often anti-PR3) is usually negative.

Microscopic polyangiitis is characterized by a vasculitis affecting blood vessels less than 70 μm in diameter and commonly is associated with serum ANCA. Microvasculitis, which affects mainly not only the postcapillary venules but also the arterioles, capillaries, and small veins, is characteristic of hypersensitivity angiitis. It may follow various antigenic exposures, such as a drug, a heterologous protein (Zeek angiitis), an infectious agent such as HBV, or a neoplastic antigen. It may also supervene in the course of a systemic disease. The lesions are usually all the same age. In some cases, various degrees of vessel wall necrosis are associated with cellular infiltrates composed of altered neutrophils. This lesion is typically seen in skin biopsies but may be demonstrable in nerve or muscle biopsies. In other cases, lymphocytic vascular infiltration is present as a nonnecrotizing vasculitis. Lesions of this type are not infrequent in peripheral nerve biopsies in various clinical settings; their pathogenetic role is uncertain. Nevertheless, the presence of sizable numbers of chronic inflammatory cells in the endoneurial or epineurial compartments, angiocentric or otherwise, must be regarded as abnormal, although this finding is not specific for any given disorder. A similar pathologic picture may be seen in collagen vascular diseases (e.g., rheumatoid arthritis, systemic lupus erythematosus, Sjögren disease, or scleroderma) or with carcinoma, especially when muscle lesions of the same type are also present.

GPA is a distinctive necrotizing or nonnecrotizing granulomatous angiitis involving large- and middle-caliber blood vessels. Involvement of lung, kidney, and air sinuses is common, whereas nerve involvement is less so. In addition to the vascular lesions, interstitial granulomatosis is common, and the characteristic lesions may be seen in muscle and nerve biopsies. ANCA is usually positive (PR3; c-ANCA) on serum serology.

13.5. NEUROPATHIES ASSOCIATED WITH HEMATOLOGIC DISEASES AND NEOPLASMS

13.5.1. Paraneoplastic neuropathies

Patients with carcinoma or lymphoma may develop a diffuse peripheral neuropathy in the setting of circulating paraneoplastic immunoglobulins; the disease manifests at the time of diagnosis, before diagnosis, or months, or even years, after the initial diagnosis of neoplasia. In paraneoplastic sensorimotor peripheral neuropathy, axonal lesions involving fibers of all fiber diameter may be observed on nerve biopsy; sometimes, perivascular lymphocytic infiltrations are seen. The pathologic findings of typical CIDP may also occur in these cases.

The paraneoplastic sensory neuropathy originally described by Denny-Brown is characterized by extensive loss of neurons in the spinal sensory ganglia, with secondary degeneration of the respective axons extending from the dorsal spinal nerve roots to the posterior columns of the spinal cord. Lymphocytic infiltration, indicating a prominent inflammatory component of the disorder, has been found in peripheral nerves in some cases, and the presence of anti-Hu antibodies in blood has a high specificity for paraneoplastic sensory neuropathy (see Chapter 9).

13.5.2. Neuropathies associated with malignant lymphomas

Patients with non-Hodgkin malignant lymphomas (NHMLs) may develop a distal sensorimotor peripheral neuropathy. In these cases, malignant B-cell or T-cell proliferation may be demonstrated in nerve biopsies by immunolabeling of the infiltrates. Due to the patchy distribution of the lesions, a negative biopsy does not rule out the existence of lymphomatous infiltrates in the nerve. Instances of widespread polyradiculoneuropathy have also been seen in patients with NHML, often with intravascular lymphomatous infiltrates, described under the term *neurolymphomatosis*.

13.5.3. Monoclonal gammopathies

13.5.3.1. PERIPHERAL NEUROPATHY WITH MONOCLONAL GAMMOPATHY

Peripheral nerve involvement may occur in patients with monoclonal gammopathies induced by one of several different pathogenetic mechanisms. Patients with the osteosclerotic form of myeloma with monoclonal IgG are at increased risk to develop peripheral neuropathy compared to patients with multiple (osteolytic) myeloma. Patients with the POEMS syndrome (polyneuropathy, organomegaly [hepatosplenomegaly, lymphadenopathy], endocrinopathy, M-protein [IgG or IgA of the lambda type in 95% of cases], and skin changes [thickening, hyperpigmentation, hypertrichosis]) also may develop peripheral neuropathy. In some cases, the diagnosis of POEMS may be initially delayed in the absence of the cardinal signs and symptoms. Vascular endothelial growth factor is a useful biomarker for POEMS, with high sensitivity; it has increased the recognition of early stages of disease.

13.5.3.2. MORPHOLOGIC CHANGES IN MONOCLONAL GAMMOPATHY-ASSOCIATED PERIPHERAL NEUROPATHY

13.5.3.2.1. Widening of myelin lamellae. Widening of myelin lamellae is an abnormality demonstrable by election microscopy that consists of 23-nm spacing between the separated leaflets of the intermediate line, which contains an electron-lucent material. The ultrastructural features of the dense lines remain unchanged. These widened lamellae are associated with dilation of the outer mesaxon and are mainly located on the outer part of the sheath (Fig. 13.16). In some fibers, the widening is restricted to the outermost lamellae, and careful examination is required to document it. This finding, indicative of a dysglobulinemia in a patient with peripheral neuropathy of unknown origin, should prompt the search for an IgM monoclonal peak. Widening of myelin lamellae is observed in Waldenström macroglobulinemia and in monoclonal gammopathy of undetermined significance (MGUS), especially with IgM gammopathy (Fig. 13.16A). Rarely with IgA (Fig. 13.16B) or IgG monoclonal gammopathies and polyneuropathy, and even less often in the absence of dysglobulinemia, comparable widening of the myelin lamellae has been described.

An anti-MAG monoclonal IgM has been implicated as causative in MGUS-associated neuropathy, but the diagnosis may require nerve biopsy for confirmation. With direct immunofluorescence and immunoperoxidase techniques, monoclonal IgM deposits may be identified along the myelin sheaths. Approximately 50% of all patients with IgM monoclonal gammopathy and peripheral neuropathy have monoclonal IgM antibodies that bind to MAG. Due to the high incidence of MGUS and of peripheral neuropathy in aging populations, widening of myelin lamellae is helpful in establishing a causative relationship.

13.5.3.2.2. Uncompacted myelin lamellae. The term *uncompacted myelin lamellae* refers to an ultrastructural abnormality of myelin in which the lamellae are separated by an electron-lucent space that is not present in normally compacted myelin (Fig. 13.9B. This uncommon alteration of myelin is encountered in the POEMS syndrome.

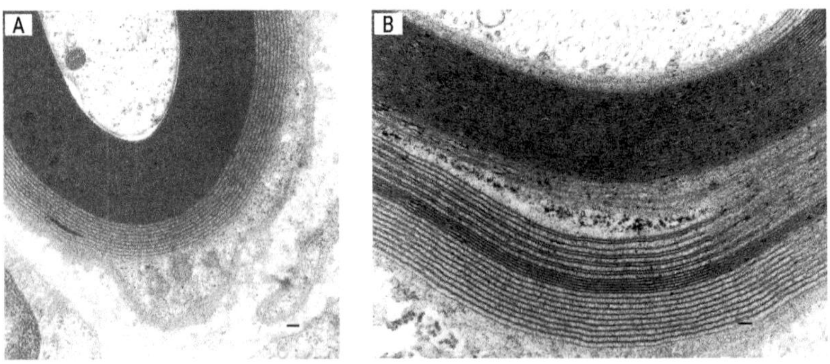

FIGURE 13.16 Widening of peripheral myelin lamellae in a patient with MGUS (**A**) and in IgA monoclonal gammopathy (**B**).

13.5.3.2.3. Endoneurial deposits. Infrequently, *amyloid deposits* have been observed during the clinical course of peripheral neuropathy associated with either multiple myeloma or Waldenström macroglobulinemia. The presence of 7- to 8-nm diameter nonbranching filaments on ultrastructural examination is particularly informative. In these instances, the amyloid is derived from kappa and lambda light chains.

The presence and specificity of *immunoglobulin deposits* can only be established by ultrastructural and immunopathological investigations. Minute deposits may not be detectable on light microscopic examination using any of the current immunopathological techniques. The ultrastructural appearance of these deposits is quite variable, and they may be observed as fingerprints, fibrils, granules, or microtubules or with no defined structure (Fig. 13.17). Such deposits are not specific for any monoclonal dysglobulinemia, and they have been described in MGUS (IgM, IgG, or IgA), myeloma, and Waldenström macroglobulinemia.

13.5.4. Cryoglobulinemias

Cryoglobulins are circulating immunoglobulins that precipitate when cooled to 4°C in the laboratory and redissolve when warmed to body temperature (37°C). Cryoglobulinemias are classified into three distinct categories, depending on the specific immunoglobulin or combination that is present. They can be monoclonal (type 1), as found in paraproteinemia (approximately 25% of cases); mixed, including a monoclonal component (type 2; approximately 25% of cases); or polyclonal (type 3; approximately 50% of cases). Cryoglobulins may be found in patients without underlying disease (essential cryoglobulinemia) or be seen in the context of a specific predisposing disease. The presence of cryoglobulins has been found to be symptomatic in less than one-third of cases.

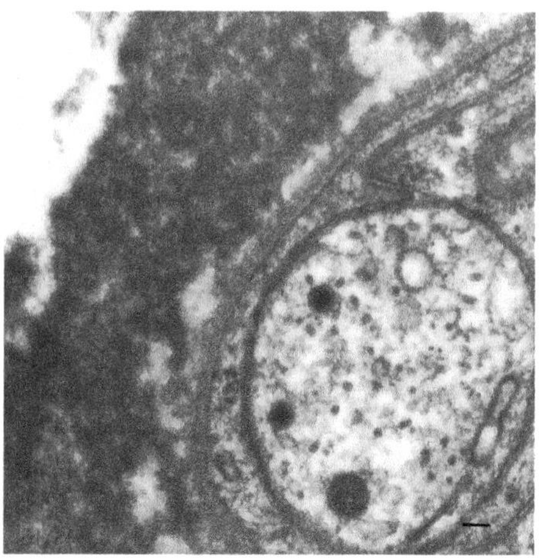

FIGURE 13.17 Myeloma neuropathy: electron-dense endoneurial deposit of IgG.

The clinical manifestations of cryoglobulinemia include purpura; weakness; arthralgia or arthritis; fever; glomerulonephritis; Raynaud phenomenon; and neurologic involvement, which can manifest as peripheral neuropathy, vasculitic encephalopathy, or both. The specific type of cryoglobulinemia needs to be determined; if type 1, antinerve activity (antiglycolipids and anti-MAG) may be present; a few cases have been observed of IgM cryoglobulinemia (type 1) with anti-MAG activity. On both electrophysiological and histological grounds, the neuropathy appears to be demyelinating, just as neuropathies induced by an IgM paraproteinemia with anti-MAG activity. In type 2 or 3 cryoglobulinemia, axonal lesions are often associated with widespread vasculitis affecting medium and small epineurial vessels and, more rarely, endoneurial vessels. In these cases, the presence of axonal lesions in a nerve biopsy requires the careful examination of multiple sections of the nerve segment because deposits or vasculitis tend to be multifocal and nodular. The relationship between vasculitis and circulating cryoglobulins is not clear because globulin deposits in vessel walls have not been observed. A necrotizing vasculitis is observed in approximately 20% of patients infected with hepatitis C virus who have peripheral neuropathy associated with a mixed cryoglobulinemia.

13.5.5. Direct invasion of nerve by neoplasm

In patients with lymphoproliferative neoplasms, nerve invasion is not infrequent at any time during the course of the disease (Fig. 13.18). Patients may or may not be symptomatic, but when so, the peripheral neuropathy is manifest as a painful mononeuropathy or as a polyradiculopathy, and the cerebrospinal fluid may be abnormal. In the typical clinical setting in these patients, peripheral nerve biopsy is rarely necessary, but when indicated by uncertainty in diagnosis, biopsy confirmation may be needed. ^{18}F-FDG positron emission tomography–computed tomography has been shown to be helpful and complementary to nerve biopsy.

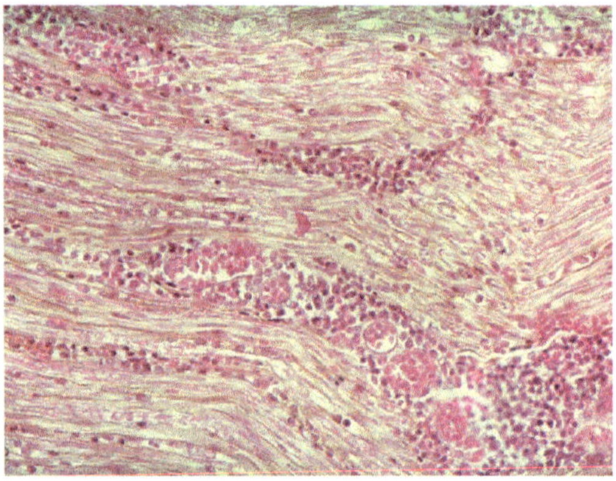

FIGURE 13.18 Infiltration of nerve by neoplastic cells in a case of chronic lymphocytic leukemia.

Primary neoplastic disease of peripheral nerve is beyond the scope of this chapter and is not discussed.

13.6. METABOLIC AND NUTRITIONAL NEUROPATHIES

Functional and structural changes in peripheral nerves develop in response to various metabolic alterations, from either endogenous metabolic disorders or exogenous toxic agents.

13.6.1. Diabetes

The prevalence of peripheral neuropathy in patients with diabetes mellitus depends on the duration of the disease. Up to 50% of diabetic patients develop peripheral neuropathy clinically after 15 years of diabetes, and nearly 100% have nerve conduction abnormalities demonstrable electrophysiologically. Several distinct clinicopathologic forms of diabetic peripheral neuropathy have been recognized. The most common form of diabetic peripheral neuropathy is symmetric neuropathy which involves distal sensory and motor nerves. Another manifestation of diabetic neuropathy is dysfunction of the autonomic nervous system; this is observed in 20–40% of diabetic patients, nearly always in association with distal sensorimotor neuropathy. Some patients, especially elderly adults with a long history of diabetes, develop peripheral neuropathy that manifests as a disorder of a single peripheral or cranial (e.g., oculomotor nerve) nerve (mononeuropathy) or of several individual nerves in an asymmetric distribution (multiple mononeuropathy or mononeuropathy multiplex).

In patients with distal symmetric sensorimotor neuropathy, the predominant pathologic finding is axonal neuropathy. As with other chronic axonal neuropathies, there is often associated segmental demyelination. There is a relative loss of the small myelinated fibers and unmyelinated fibers (Fig. 13.19A), but large fibers are also affected. Endoneurial arterioles show mural thickening, hyalinization, periodic acid–Schiff excess positivity of the thickened vessel wall, and variable reduplication of the basement membrane (Fig. 13.19B). The pathogenesis of the lesions, whether ischemia, metabolic derangement, or another factor or another factor, has not been established.

CIDP may occur in diabetic patients, although whether it occurs randomly or at a higher incidence than expected is still debated; in some atypical cases, nerve biopsy may help confirm the diagnosis and direct immunomodulatory treatment. Autopsy examination in lumbosacral radiculopathy may show

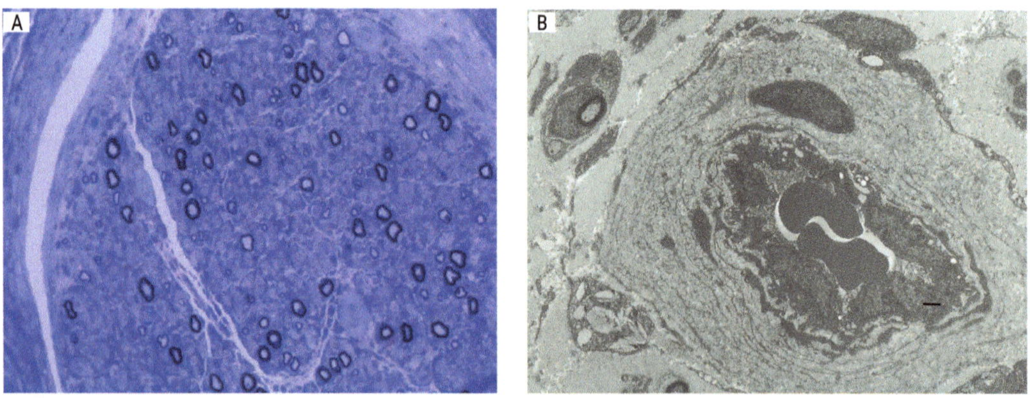

FIGURE 13.19 Diabetic neuropathy: (**A**) loss of myelinated fibers, more severely affecting small myelinated fibers, on semithin section; (**B**) microangiopathy with marked reduplication of the basement membrane.

changes suggestive of ischemic injury and prominent perivascular inflammation without fibrinoid necrosis.

13.6.2. Other metabolic neuropathies

Approximately 65% of patients with renal failure have clinical evidence of peripheral neuropathy before dialysis treatment (uremic neuropathy). The manifestation of the disease is typically a distal, symmetric sensorimotor neuropathy that may be asymptomatic or may be associated with muscle cramps, distal dysesthesias, and diminished deep tendon reflexes. Axonal degeneration is the primary event in these patients. Regeneration and recovery may occur after dialysis treatment.

Peripheral neuropathy can also develop in patients with chronic liver disease, chronic respiratory insufficiency, and thyroid dysfunction. Thiamine deficiency is characterized by axonal neuropathy, a clinical condition termed *neuropathic beriberi*. Axonal neuropathies also occur with deficiencies of vitamins B_{12} (cobalamin) and B_6.

13.7. TOXIC NEUROPATHIES

Peripheral neuropathies can occur after exposure to industrial or environmental chemicals, biological toxins, or therapeutic drugs. Heavy metals, including lead and arsenic, are prominent among the environmental chemicals. In addition, many organic compounds are neurotoxic.

13.7.1. Diphtheria toxin

Peripheral nerve involvement in diphtheria results from the effects of the diphtheria exotoxin, and the initial clinical manifestations are sensory symptoms, including paresthesias and weakness. Early loss of proprioception and vibratory sensation is common. Pathologically, the earliest changes are seen in the sensory ganglia, where the incomplete blood–nerve barrier allows toxin entry. There is selective demyelination of axons that extends into adjacent anterior and posterior roots as well as into mixed sensorimotor nerves.

13.7.2. Accidental and industrial exposures

Toxic peripheral neuropathy has been well documented following exposure to organophosphates and heavy metals, including arsenic, thallium, alkyl mercury, and tri-*ortho*-cresylphosphate.

13.7.2.1. ARSENIC

Arsenic has been known for centuries to be highly toxic, in the context of use with homicidal or suicidal intent. In addition to encephalopathy, mixed sensory and motor neuropathy is a known and disabling consequence of both acute and chronic arsenic intoxication. The characteristic neuropathological feature of this neuropathy is an axonopathy in the most distal parts of the longest nerves. The largest fibers are the most severely affected.

13.7.2.2. LEAD

Lead poisoning in adults occurs most often due to occupational exposure; in children, it usually results from ingestion of dust and fragments of the lead-containing paint that has been extensively used in households. Lead intoxication induces peripheral neuropathy in adults, whereas in children encephalopathy is the more common clinical manifestation. Despite the numerous clinical descriptions of lead-induced polyneuropathy, very little is known about its neuropathologic features in humans; in the few cases described, the lesion is axonal degeneration rather than segmental demyelination.

13.7.2.3. ORGANOPHOSPHORUS COMPOUNDS

The organophosphorus compounds have been extensively used in industry and agriculture as insecticides, modifiers of plastics, petroleum additives, lubricants, antioxidants, and flame retardants. A biological effect of many of them is to phosphorylate acetylcholinesterase (AChE), which leads to irreversible inhibition of the function of this enzyme and, consequently, severe symptoms of excessive cholinergic activity within a day or less of acute exposure to the compound. Death from respiratory paralysis can occur during this acute phase of the intoxication, but if the patient survives this phase, recovery ensues, and there are no delayed effects. Some organophosphorus compounds, however, also induce delayed polyneuropathy that is not due to inhibition of AChE but, rather, correlates with inhibition of another esterase called neurotoxic esterase. The onset of symptoms is delayed from the exposure, and microscopic examination of the peripheral nervous system shows axonal neuropathy with axonal degeneration.

13.7.2.4. HEXANE AND RELATED COMPOUNDS

The six-carbon compounds *n*-hexane and methyl-*n*-butyl ketone, used as industrial solvents, produce striking toxic effects on the peripheral nervous system. The ensuing polyneuropathy, which involves the distal parts of both sensory and motor nerves, is characterized by focal swelling of axons to some two to three times their normal diameter (Fig. 13.4B). The myelin sheaths surrounding these swollen axonal segments are thinned, and myelin is retracted at the nodes of Ranvier, with some segmental demyelination. Electron microscopy of the axonal swellings demonstrates that they contain accumulations of 10-nm neurofilaments, and the axon distal to the swellings undergoes degeneration.

13.7.3. Complications of therapeutic agents

Drug-induced neuropathies with prevailing or notable segmental demyelination include those associated with treatment with amphiphilic cations; these include amiodarone and chloroquine. Amiodarone neuropathy is a subacute polyneuropathy, whereas chloroquine causes a neuromyopathy. Characteristic histopathologic findings may be demonstrated on semithin plastic-embedded sections, showing numerous dense cytoplasmic inclusions in Schwann cells and in endothelial cells. Electron microscopic study may demonstrate polymorphic lysosomal inclusions, some of which have a paracrystalline or multilamellar reticular appearance (Fig. 13.20). The accumulated lipids include gangliosides and phospholipids.

Many other commonly used drugs may cause peripheral neuropathy, which is predominately axonal. These include vincristine, cis-platinum, the nitrofurantoin compounds, metronidazole, isoniazid, disulfiram, almitrine, and pyridoxine.

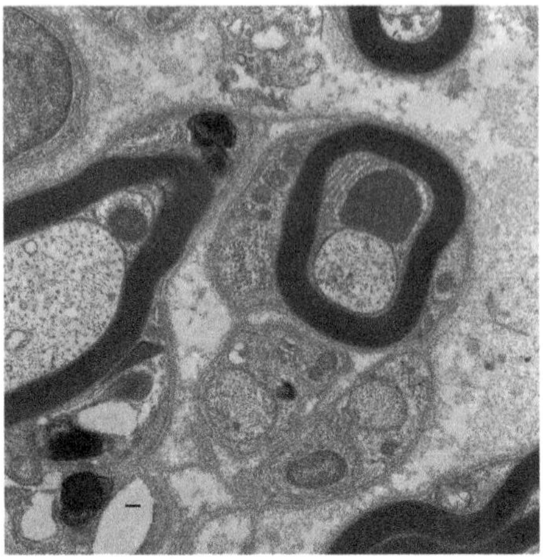

FIGURE 13.20 Amiodarone neuropathy: multiple lipid inclusions in Schwann cells.

13.8. TRAUMATIC NEUROPATHY

Peripheral nerves are commonly injured in the course of trauma, often causing a peripheral mononeuropathy of a limb. Peripheral nerve injury may be a complication of fractures when a sharp fragment of bone lacerates the nerve, avulsions when tension is applied to a peripheral nerve or limb, or compression of a limb when severe or sustained. The most common compression neuropathy results from entrapment of the distal median nerve within the carpal tunnel of the wrist, resulting in carpal tunnel syndrome. Additional compression neuropathies include involvement of the ulnar nerve at the level of the elbow, the peroneal nerve at the level of the knee, and the radial nerve in the upper arm as seen after sleeping with the arm improperly positioned ("Saturday night palsy") or upper arm fractures.

Regeneration of peripheral nerve axons following trauma does occur, albeit slowly. Regrowth may be impaired by discontinuity between the proximal and distal portions of the nerve sheath as well as by the misalignment of individual fascicles. Axons, in the absence of aligned distal segments, may continue to grow, resulting in a mass of tangled axonal processes known as a traumatic neuroma (or amputation neuroma). Within this mass, small bundles of axons appear randomly oriented; each, however, is surrounded by organized layers containing Schwann cells, fibroblasts, and perineurial cells.

13.9. HEREDITARY NEUROPATHIES

Peripheral neuropathy is a clinical manifestation of many hereditary neurologic syndromes where the course of the disease is typically progressive and often disabling. Classification schemes of hereditary diseases affecting the peripheral nervous system are based on whether the disease predominantly affects the motor and sensory modalities (hereditary motor and sensory neuropathies [HMSN]), as well as those predominantly affecting sensory and autonomic modalities (hereditary sensory and autonomic neuropathies [HSAN]). Other hereditary metabolic diseases that may also have symptoms of peripheral neuropathy as an additional component of a broader neurologic and systemic illness are discussed in Chapter 10. Classification of these generalized metabolic disorders is based on the nature of the metabolic defect, such as applies to diseases of lipid metabolism or to mitochondrial disease.

Recent advances in molecular genetics have greatly enhanced the understanding of the hereditary neuropathies. From the clinical perspective, in many cases, knowledge of the mode of inheritance, clinical features, and electrophysiological data may be sufficient to identify the clinicopathologic diagnostic category. However, each clinicopathologic category may be caused by one of several genetic mutations, and currently, screening of the 80 most commonly affected genes is expensive. Also, throughout the years, genetic discoveries have made the classification of hereditary neuropathies more complicated, and new classification systems are emerging.

As technology has improved, targeted testing has been replaced by NGS (next-generation sequencing) panels that may detect many of the most common mutations responsible for the hereditary neuropathies. Genes encoding proteins in the Schwann cell (Fig. 13.21) and neuron are involved in several dynamic processes: myelination, axonal transport, protein aggregation, endosomal sorting, mitochondrial functions, messenger RNA processing/transcription, and channel abnormalities. Mutations in the genes encoding these proteins and the resulting abnormalities of peripheral nerve structure and function are the molecular basis for these hereditary neuropathies. Detailed analysis of clinical phenotypes and sometimes of nerve biopsy

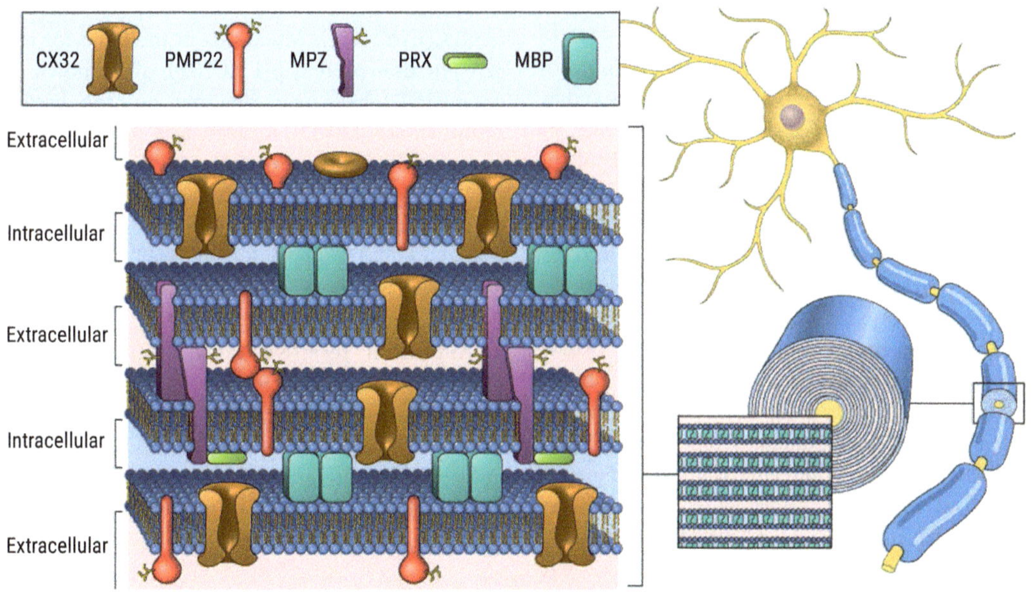

FIGURE 13.21 Diagram of peripheral nerve myelin and proteins affected in hereditary demyelinating neuropathies. Peripheral myelin protein 22 (*PMP22*) is the gene that is duplicated in CMT1A and deleted in HNPP. Myelin protein 0 (*MPZ*) is the gene mutated in CMT1B. Connexin 32 is mutated in the X-linked form of Charcot–Marie–Tooth disease (CMTX), and periaxin (PRX) in CMT3. Myelin basic protein (MBP) is a major component of myelin located in the major dense line of myelin; no hereditary neuropathies involving MBP are known. (Modified from Anthony, D. C., Frosch, M. P., and De Girolami, U. (2010). Peripheral nerve and skeletal muscle. In V. Kumar, A. K. Abbas, N. Fausto, and J. C. Aster (Eds.), *Robbins and Cotran pathologic basis of disease* (8th ed., pp. 1257–1278). Philadelphia: Saunders.)

may be necessary to be certain of the pathogenicity of sequence variants of uncertain significance that are frequently encountered with NGS. Pathologic analysis of the nerve lesions may narrow the search of specific genes when the differential diagnosis is broad.

13.9.1. Hereditary motor and sensory neuropathies

13.9.1.1. CHARCOT-MARIE-TOOTH, DEMYELINATING TYPE

The most common hereditary motor and sensory neuropathy (HMSN) is CMT disease, demyelinating type (CMT1, CMT hypertrophic form, or HMSN I), which usually presents in childhood or early adulthood. Patients may be asymptomatic, but when they come to medical attention, it is often with symptoms/signs that include distal muscle weakness, atrophy of the calf (peroneal muscular atrophy), or secondary orthopedic problems of the foot (e.g., pes cavus). The disorder is autosomal dominant, and although it is slowly progressive, the disability of sensorimotor deficits and associated orthopedic problems are usually limited in severity, and a normal life span is the rule.

In CMT1, a demyelinating neuropathy, both by nerve neurophysiologic conduction velocity and by pathologic criteria, nerve conduction velocities are markedly decreased (often < 30 m/s). Histologic examination shows the consequences of repetitive demyelination and remyelination, with multiple onion bulbs, somewhat more pronounced in distal than in proximal portions of the nerves. The axon is often present in the center of the onion bulb, and the myelin sheath is usually thinner than normal in proportion to the diameter of the axon or absent. In some cases, nearly every axon is surrounded by an onion bulb. The redundant layers of hyperplastic Schwann cells surrounding individual axons may be associated with clinical enlargement of individual peripheral nerves, which are sometimes individually palpable, leading to the term *hypertrophic* neuropathy. Biopsies cut in the longitudinal plane show segmental demyelination. These findings support the view that the pathogenesis of the abnormality is disruption of the maintenance of myelin. In the later stages of the disease, axonal loss also occurs, involving the most distal portions of axons. Autopsy studies of affected individuals have shown degeneration of the posterior columns of the spinal cord.

This clinicopathologic entity is genetically heterogeneous, and subgroups have been identified as CMT types 1A, 1B, 1C, and 1X. In approximately 75% of CMT1 pedigrees (CMT1A), a large region of chromosome 17p11.2-p12 is duplicated, resulting in "segmental trisomy" of the duplicated region. This region includes peripheral myelin protein 22 (*PMP22*), and its expression resulting from the segmental trisomy is thought to be the molecular basis for the disease. A separate genetic locus in some CMT1 families involves myelin protein zero (*MPZ*), located at 1q23.3. This disease has an identical clinical and pathological phenotype with demyelinating lesions and onion bulbs and is classified as CMT1B. Electron microscopic examination may also detect anomalies of myelin compaction that are specific for this subtype of CMT and are related to the fact that MPZ is the main protein of myelin compaction. Some multifocal thickenings of the myelin sheaths may also be encountered. Additional mutations associated with the CMT1 phenotype (autosomal dominant demyelinating HMSN I) include LITAF, EGR2, and NEFL.

Some families with the clinicopathologic phenotype of CMT have a genetic locus on the X chromosome and X-linked inheritance within the family (CMT 1X). Mutations in the gene for the gap junction protein β-1 (*GJB1*), also known as connexin 32, have been identified, and the disease is known as CMT1X. Additional X-linked genetic foci (CMTX) include *PDK3*, *PRPS1*, and foci at Xp22.2 and X126 with unknown gene identification. Several of the proteins involved in autosomal dominant CMT and X-linked CMT are integral membrane proteins of myelin or involved in myelin compaction (Fig. 13.21).

Autosomal recessive cases of demyelinating CMT are much less frequent in Western countries and are identified as CMT type 4. *MTMR2*, *MTMR13* (CMT4B), *SBF2* (CMTSH3TC2), and *frabin* (*FGD4*) mutations (CMT4H) induce severe demyelinating lesions associated with numerous outfoldings of myelin sheaths.

13.9.1.2. CHARCOT-MARIE-TOOTH, AXONAL TYPE

The less common axonal form of autosomal dominant CMT is CMT2; patients develop signs and symptoms similar to those with CMT1, although nerve enlargement is not seen, and clinical manifestations develop comparatively somewhat later in life. This form is recognized electrophysiologically by the demonstration of conduction velocities in the normal range (>38 m/s). Loss of myelinated axons is the predominant finding on nerve biopsy (Fig. 13.7D). Segmental demyelination of internodes is infrequent, and onion bulbs are not present. These findings indicate that the site of primary cellular dysfunction is the axon or neuron.

Also, CMT2 is heterogeneous genetically, and each locus has been identified as a specific subtype. In some dominant families (designated CMT2A), two separate genetic loci have been identified at 1p36.2: CMT2A1 (only one family described) is caused by mutations in the *KIF1B* gene, which encodes a molecular motor of the kinesin superfamily, and CMT2A2 is caused by mutations in the mitofusin 2 (*MFN2*) gene. CMT2A2 represents between 20% and 30% of patients with the axonal form of CMT. In nerve biopsies of CMT2A2 cases, there are distinctive abnormalities of intra-axonal mitochondria, which are demonstrable on longitudinal sections. The mitochondria are abnormally focally aggregated, round instead of tubular, and with irregularities in the external and internal membranes, and they show disruption of the cristae. Many additional, less common, loci have been identified in CMT2 families, namely RAB7 (CMT2B), TRPV4 (CMT2C), GARS (CMT2D), and neurofilament light chain in NEFL (CMT2E). In recessive cases of the axonal form of CMT, several other genes have been identified, including *lamin A/C* (autosomal recessive, LMNA: AR-CMT2B1) and *MED25* (AR-CMT2B2).

13.9.1.3. DEJERINE–SOTTAS DISEASE

Dejerine–Sottas disease (DSD; HMSN III, CMT3) is a progressive demyelinating neuropathy beginning in early childhood, usually before age 2 years, and manifest by delay in developmental milestones, including especially the acquisition of motor skills. Both autosomal recessive and autosomal dominant inheritance have been described. Currently, the validity of the entity is debated by some authors because in clinical practice it may be difficult to differentiate these patients from those with CMT1 or PMP22. Furthermore, MPZ mutations, which are the basis for CMT1B, have been identified in patients with CMT3. The distinction therefore now rests on age of onset in infancy and clinical signs and symptoms.

On physical examination, enlarged peripheral nerves can be detected by inspection and palpation. The deep tendon reflexes are depressed or absent, and nerve conduction velocity is markedly slowed.

On microscopic examination, the size of individual peripheral nerve fascicles is increased, often dramatically, with abundant onion bulb formation as well as segmental demyelination. There is usually evidence of axonal loss, and the remaining axons are often of diminished caliber. These findings are most severe in the distal portions of the peripheral nervous system; however, autopsy studies have shown that similar findings may be present in spinal roots.

Families have been identified with mutations of different genes, but in each pedigree, the mutation has involved genes involved in the formation and maintenance of myelin. The genes identified thus far in DSD include *PMP22*, *MPZ*, early growth response 2 gene (*EGR2*), and periaxin (*PRX*).

Congenital hypomyelinating neuropathy (CHN) is a term that has been used to designate a diffuse symmetrical polyneuropathy that is evident at birth or becomes manifest shortly thereafter. It is characterized pathologically by nearly complete absence of myelin in the presence of normal axons and is closely related clinically to DSD. Patients with this disease are sometimes referred to as having congenital DSD (HMSN III) and sometimes as having CHN (CMT 4E). Mutations thus far have been identified in *EGR2* and *MPZ*.

Due to recent advances in molecular genetics, different mutations of several similar genes have been identified as being at the origin of CMT1, DSD, and CHN; there has not been a clear distinction of one gene associated with one disease. As a result, DSD is considered synonymous with severe early onset CMT1 and within a proposed continuum between CHN and CMT1.

13.9.1.4. TOMACULOUS NEUROPATHY (HNPP)

Tomaculous neuropathy (HNPP) is a disease transmitted as an autosomal dominant disorder and is characterized by recurrent attacks of mononeuropathy, single or multiple. These episodes are characteristically brought on by pressure, such as might affect the ulnar nerve when the elbow rests on a table for an extended period or might occur by traction or stretching. There is generally some recovery (which may require weeks or months), although with repeated attacks some permanent sensory or motor dysfunction may remain.

Examination of peripheral nerve biopsies shows focal enlargements of the myelin sheath either involving entire internodal segments or confined to the paranodal regions (Fig. 13.22A, B). These enlargements create a fusiform enlargement, or sausage-like appearance, in the longitudinal plane referred to as *tomacula* (from the Latin *tomaculum* for "sausage"). Morphometric examinations have shown decreased numbers of large myelinated fibers with relatively normal numbers of smaller myelinated fibers and scattered small onion bulb structures. The tomaculous swellings, when examined by electron microscopy, have been shown to be made up of greatly thickened and abnormally folded myelin sheaths (Fig. 13.22C); axons enclosed by these abnormal myelin structures often appear to be contracted. The disorder is usually caused by deletion of the PMP22 or a whole segment of chromosome 17p11.2 that spans the *PMP22* gene. This is the same region of chromosome 17 that is duplicated in CMT1A.

13.9.1.5. NEUROPATHY ASSOCIATED WITH HEREDITARY ATAXIA

A neuropathy with clinicopathological features closely resembling those in CMT2 is regularly found in the most frequently encountered form of genetically determined progressive ataxia, Friedreich ataxia. This topic is covered in Chapter 8.

13.9.1.6. GIANT AXONAL NEUROPATHY

Giant axonal neuropathy is a disease characterized pathologically by greatly enlarged axons in the central and peripheral nervous systems; the clinical course is that of a gradually progressive sensorimotor neuropathy beginning in early childhood. A pattern of autosomal recessive inheritance occurs in most pedigrees. The disease typically becomes manifest as an awkwardness of gait with a tendency to fall. Increasing motor instability ensues, associated with sensory loss that affects mainly deep sensibility and proprioception, with less involvement of sensations for light touch, pain, and temperature. The disease progresses gradually but relentlessly, and clinical manifestations of dysfunction of the central nervous system become evident in the form of nystagmus, visual impairment with optic atrophy, dysarthria, and intellectual deterioration. Most affected individuals have a distinctive appearance of the hair, variously described as "frizzy" or "kinky."

The characteristic neuropathological feature of this disorder is the presence of greatly enlarged axons, 20–50 μm in diameter (Fig. 13.4A). Overlying the enlarged portion of the axon, the myelin sheath is either markedly thin or absent, and electron

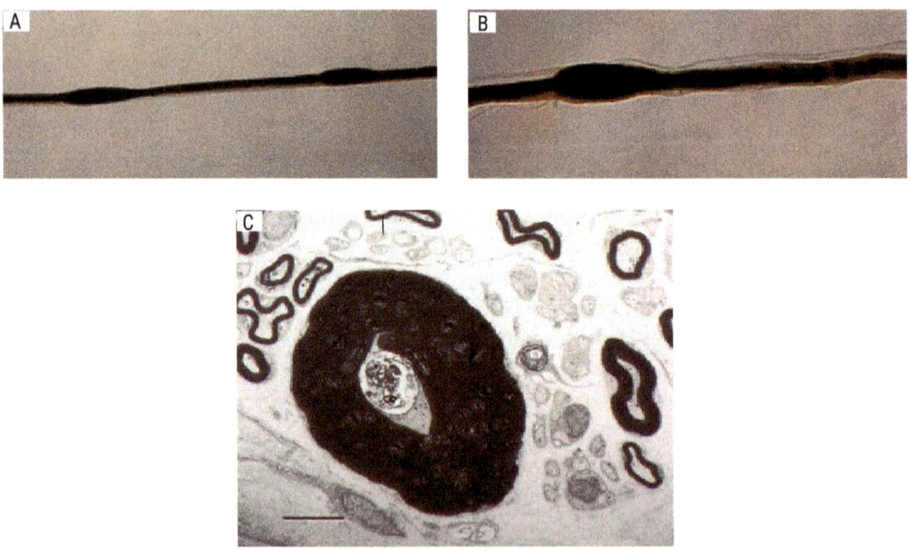

FIGURE 13.22 Tomaculous neuropathy. (**A, B**) Scattered focal swellings of individual myelin sheaths with a sausage-like appearance in the longitudinal plane, seen on teased-fiber preparations. (**C**) By electron microscopy, the swellings are made up of greatly thickened and abnormally folded myelin sheaths.

microscopy shows that the enlarged portions of the axons are filled with masses of densely packed intermediate filaments, 10 nm in diameter, frequently arranged in whorl-like patterns. In addition to the changes in the peripheral nerves, there are striking abnormalities in the central nervous system, including enlarged axons (spheroids) and amorphous masses of glial fibrillary protein in the form of Rosenthal fibers. Aggregates of intermediate filaments also occur in fibroblasts and glia, and the accumulation of aggregates of intermediate filaments occurs in cultures of fibroblasts from patients. The gene responsible for GAN is located on chromosome 16q24.1 and encodes gigaxonin, a member of the E3 ligase family involved in ubiquitination, protein trafficking, and degradation.

13.9.1.7. INFANTILE NEUROAXONAL DYSTROPHY

Schindler disease, or infantile neuroaxonal dystrophy Schindler type, is an autosomal recessive disorder characterized by a relentlessly progressive global deterioration of cerebral function beginning during early infancy after a normal neonatal period and leading to death in childhood. Weakness is profound, associated with hypotonia and muscular wasting, and there is an exaggeration of muscle-stretch reflexes. The typical neuropathological finding is the presence of enlarged axons (spheroids) at all levels of the central nervous system (see Chapter 10) and frequently on nerve biopsies, although they are less frequent than in the brain. The enlarged axons are filled with tubulovesicular or membranous arrays, displacing the cytoplasm and distending the axonal diameter. The disorder is caused by mutations in the *NAGA* gene, encoding *N*-acetyl-α-D-acetylgalactosaminidase, with a deficiency of the encoded protein and enzyme activity.

13.9.2. Hereditary sensory and autonomic neuropathies

The HSANs mainly affect sensation, with relative sparing of motor strength, and are accompanied by varying degrees of autonomic nervous system dysfunction. The most widely accepted classification of these hereditary neuropathies combines them in an overall category of HSANs with several subtypes based on inheritance and the clinical manifestations: HSAN type I (predominantly sensory, autosomal dominant), HSAN type II (predominantly sensory, autosomal recessive), and HSAN type III (predominantly autonomic, autosomal recessive). Other types, including various types of congenital indifference to pain, have also been described.

13.9.2.1. HSAN TYPE I (FAMILIAL ULCEROMUTILATING ACROPATHY OF THEVENARD, DOMINANT)

Type I HSAN is characterized by dominant inheritance and very slow progression. Painless injuries to the feet, with ulcerations of the skin and damage to joints, are typical. Dysfunction of the autonomic nervous system is not prominent. Neuropathologic examination has shown extensive loss of neurons in spinal sensory ganglia, with secondary axonal loss in the posterior roots and posterior columns of the spinal cord and preservation of motor neurons and anterior roots. There also is severe loss of myelinated fibers of all calibers in peripheral nerve. The gene is the *SPTLC1* gene, located on chromosome 9q22, and encodes serine palmitoyltransferase, an important enzyme in sphingolipid biosynthesis.

13.9.2.2. HSAN TYPE II

Autosomal recessive inheritance is the main distinguishing feature of the type II variety of HSAN, and the predominant clinical feature is impairment of pain perception, resulting in painless injuries (insensitivity to pain), often beginning in childhood. Nerve biopsy studies show widespread loss of myelinated fibers of all sizes; unmyelinated fibers are only slightly decreased. A striking vacuolation of the cytoplasm of endoneurial fibroblasts has also been reported. Mutations in the *WNK1* HSAN2 gene and in the *FAM134B* gene have been detected and are subclassified as HSAN 2A and HSAN 2B, respectively.

13.9.2.3. HSAN TYPE III (FAMILIAL DYSAUTONOMIA, RILEY–DAY SYNDROME)

Type III HSAN is a disease characterized by severe autonomic nervous system dysfunction present at birth, as evidenced by absent lacrimation and abnormal reactions to anxiety (lability of blood pressure, salivation, excessive sweating, and erythematous blotching of the skin). The syndrome is inherited as an autosomal recessive trait and tends to occur in children of Ashkenazi-Jewish heritage. Integral components of the syndrome include early appearing lack of pain perception and lack of fungiform papillae in the tongue. Sural nerve biopsy shows a severe decrease in the number of unmyelinated fibers and of large and small myelinated fibers. Teased fibers show some with shortening of the internodal length, but no segmental demyelination or remyelination, and no onion bulb structures. Autopsy studies have reported shrinkage of cell bodies and neuronal loss in dorsal root ganglia, sympathetic ganglia, and the intermediolateral cell column of the spinal cord, suggesting that the primary abnormality is in neurons of the autonomic and spinal sensory ganglia and that the changes seen in peripheral nerve specimens are secondary to the axonal degeneration that results from neuronal death.

The gene for familial dysautonomia is located on chromosome 9q31.3 and encodes an inhibitor of kappa light polypeptide gene enhancer in B cells, a kinase-complex–associated protein, known as *ELP1*. The role of this gene product in the nervous system is not fully understood. More than 99.5% of the alleles in families with the mutation share a common ancestral haplotype, supporting that the ethnic basis of the disease is due to a founder effect.

13.9.2.4. ADDITIONAL TYPES OF HSAN

Some cases of hereditary sensory neuropathy, with or without autonomic dysfunction, have been identified and are recognized rare variants of HSANs. They differ from one another in the details of their clinical expression as well as in the pattern of neuropathological changes, and a number of genetic loci have been identified.

13.9.3. Amyloid neuropathies

Peripheral neuropathy may occur due to deposition of amyloid in peripheral nerve, and there are two major categories of amyloid neuropathies: familial amyloid polyneuropathies and acquired amyloidosis.

13.9.3.1. FAMILIAL AMYLOID POLYNEUROPATHIES

The familial amyloid neuropathies are characterized predominantly by the deposition of amyloid within the peripheral nervous system, with symptoms that may be restricted to those of peripheral neuropathy. Most kindreds exhibit mutations of the transthyretin (TTR) gene, located on chromosome 18q11.2-q12.1. More than 20 forms of mutant TTR have been identified. Rarer forms of hereditary amyloid neuropathy are characterized by the deposition of different amyloid-forming proteins: a variant of apolipoprotein A1 in familial visceral amyloid with polyneuropathy and gelsolin in the Finnish form of familial amyloid polyneuropathy. Clinically, these are sensorimotor and autonomic polyneuropathies with predominant deficiency of temperature and pain sensation, as in the TTR-related familial amyloid neuropathies, but there is corneal clouding in some of these types in addition to the neuropathy.

In all cases, the pathologic amyloid lesions are acellular deposits situated in the endoneurium and in the blood vessel wall, stained by Congo red,

HEREDITARY NEUROPATHIES	CATEGORY	GENES
Sensorimotor (HSMN), types I–IV, and related hereditary sensorimotor neuropathies	CMT1A, AD, onion bulbs	*PMP22* duplication
	CMT1B, AD, onion bulbs	*MPZ*
	CMT1X, X-linked, onion bulbs	*GJB1*
	CMT2, AD, axonal	*KIF1B, MFN2*
	CMT3, DSD, infantile, AR, onion bulbs	*PMP22, MPZ*
	CMT4, AR, onion bulbs	*MTMR2*
	HNPP, AD, tomacula	*PMP22* deletion
	Giant Axonal Neuropathy, AR, giant axons	*GAN*
Sensory and autonomic (HSAN), types I–III (16 genetic types identified)	HSAN I, AD, ulcerating neuropathy, axonal loss	
	HSAN II, AR, axonal loss	*SPTLC1*
	HSAN III, AR, dysautonomia, loss of unmyelinated fibers	*WNK1* *ELB1*
Familial amyloid polyneuropathies	Transthyretin FAP, AD	*TTR*
	Gelsolin FAP, AD, Finnish with corneal clouding	*GSN*

AD, autosomal dominant; AR, autosomal recessive; CMT, Charcot–Marie–Tooth disease; FAP, familial amyloid polyneuropathy; HNPP, hereditary neuropathy with liability to pressure palsies; HSAN, hereditary sensory and autonomic neuropathy; HSMN, hereditary motor and sensory neuropathy.

birefringent by polarized light, and composed of characteristic nonbranching 7-nm fibrils as seen by electron microscopy. Parenchymatous involvement is essentially axonal and typically affects mainly small myelinated and unmyelinated fibers. In the most common form of familial amyloid neuropathy (TTR related), the amyloid fibrils are composed of TTR and can be demonstrated in tissue by immunohistochemistry.

13.9.3.2. ACQUIRED AMYLOID NEUROPATHIES

Acquired amyloidosis may occur in association with B-cell dyscrasias ("primary amyloidosis") or associated with certain inflammatory conditions as reactive systemic amyloidosis ("secondary amyloidosis"). The amyloid in the B-cell dyscrasias is of AL type, composed of fragments of immunoglobulin light chains, most often lambda chains (Fig. 13.23), whereas the amyloid deposits in reactive systemic amyloidosis are of AA type (composed of a fragment of the serum protein, serum amyloid-associated protein). The amyloid deposits, whether familial TTR derived, AL, or AA type, are often discrete and may be demonstrated by immunohistochemistry. They must be distinguished from abnormal globulin deposits that do not have the features of amyloid. AL amyloidosis may also infiltrate the skeletal musculature and the transverse carpal ligament (flexor retinaculum), causing carpal tunnel syndrome. More recent methods allow protein identification of amyloid deposits by mass spectroscopy proteomics from paraffin-embedded tissue.

13.9.4. Porphyria

Polyneuropathy of acute or subacute evolution is characteristic of three varieties of dominantly inherited disorders of heme metabolism: acute intermittent porphyria, variegate porphyria, and hereditary coproporphyria. The polyneuropathy may

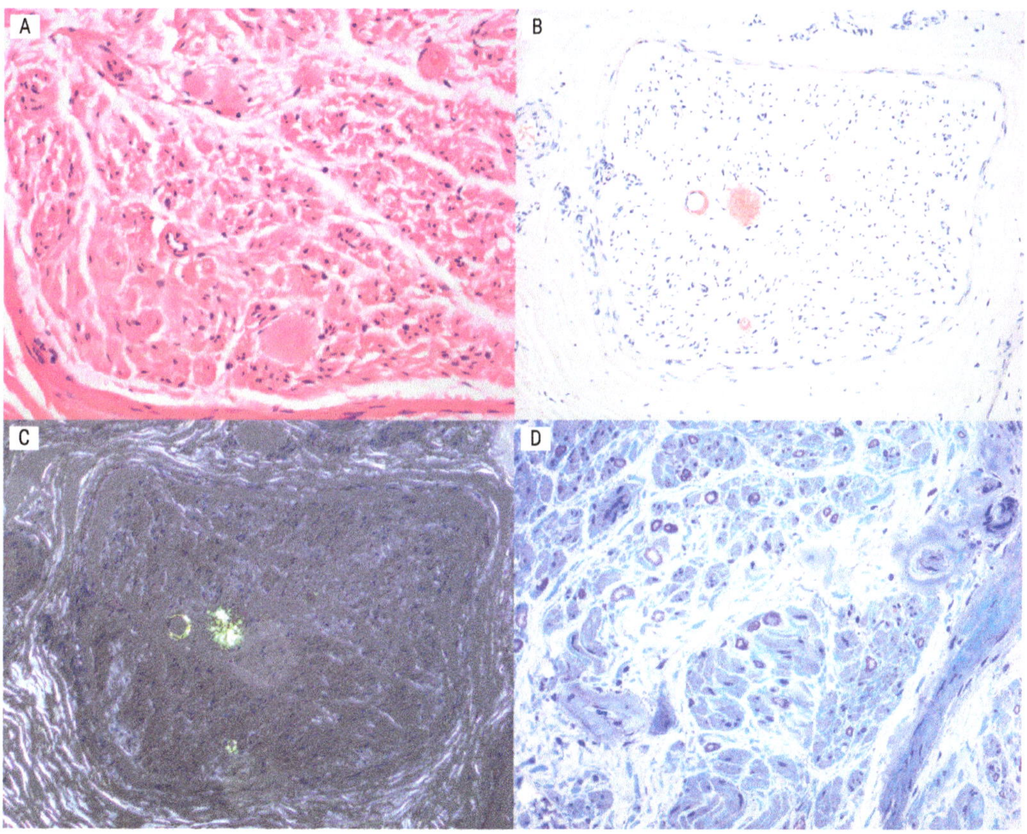

FIGURE 13.23 Interstitial amyloid deposit in peripheral nerve: (**A**) H&E; (**B**) Congo red; (**C**) Congo red under polarized light; (**D**) semithin section stained with toluidine blue with axonal loss particularly affecting small fibers. (Images provided by Alice M. Li, MD, PhD, Harvard Medical School, Brigham and Women's Hospital.)

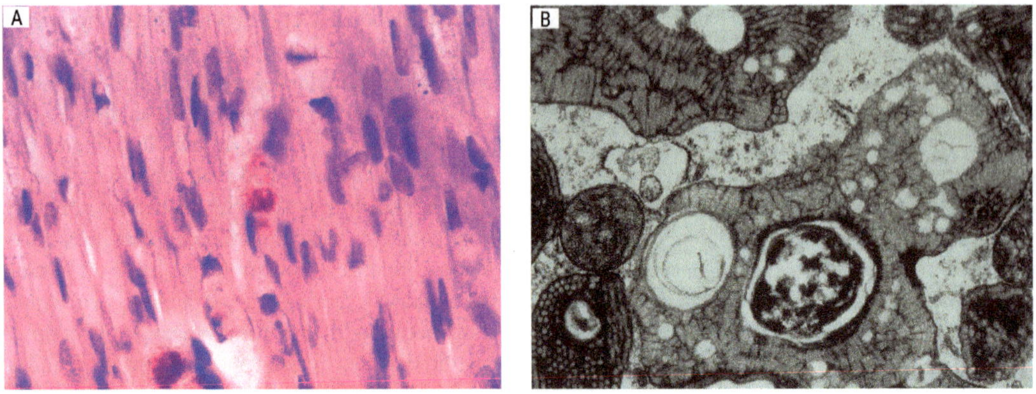

FIGURE 13.24 Metachromatic leukodystrophy. (**A**) The presence of metachromatic material (appearing red on toluidine blue stain) in macrophages in peripheral nerve. (**B**) By electron microscopy, this material has a characteristic "tuffstone" appearance.

be asymmetrical and tends to involve motor fibers more than sensory fibers. The neurologic aspects are the same in all three varieties of porphyria.

The primary axonal neuropathy associated with all forms of porphyria has a distribution that suggests a dying-back axonopathy, an impression confirmed by electrophysiologic observations. Unmyelinated axons are affected, as well as large and small myelinated fibers. In severe cases of long-standing porphyric neuropathy, secondary changes in the spinal cord and sensory ganglia (central chromatolysis; ascending degeneration in the posterior columns) are regularly encountered, as is atrophy of denervated musculature. The relationship of the disorder of heme metabolism to the development of the lesions in the nervous system is still unknown.

13.9.5. Disorders of lipid metabolism

A number of the systemic disorders of lipid metabolism may present with prominent involvement of the peripheral nervous system. In some of these diseases, such as Refsum disease, Bassen–Kornzweig syndrome, or Tangier disease, peripheral nerve involvement may be the presenting sign. For example, Refsum disease, which results from a deficiency of a peroxisomal enzyme, often presents with a demyelinating peripheral neuropathy similar in pathologic features to DSD. In other conditions, particularly in the leukodystrophies (metachromatic leukodystrophy, adrenoleukodystrophy, or Krabbe disease) or in Niemann–Pick disease, involvement of the brain is usually the predominant clinical issue. Other conditions, such as Fabry disease or cerebrotendinous xanthomatosis, present as systemic disorders in which the central and peripheral nervous systems may be involved, among many other organs. In many cases, nerve biopsy may show diagnostic deposits or intracellular inclusions of abnormal lipid (Fig. 13.24; Box 13.1). Most of these diseases may be identified by molecular testing. The neuropathologic aspects of these diseases, including the changes in peripheral nerves, are described in Chapter 10.

Box 13.1 Neuropathies in Disorders of Lipid Metabolism

Lipid Disorders with Prominent Involvement of the Peripheral Nervous System

Refsum disease
Bassen–Kornzweig disease or abetalipoproteinemia
Tangier disease

Lipid Disorders with Predominant Involvement of the Central Nervous System

Metachromatic leukodystrophy
Adrenoleukodystrophy
Krabbe disease
Niemann–Pick disease
Neuronal ceroid lipofuscinosis

Lipid Disorders with Predominant Systemic Involvement

Fabry disease
Cerebrotendinous xanthomatosis

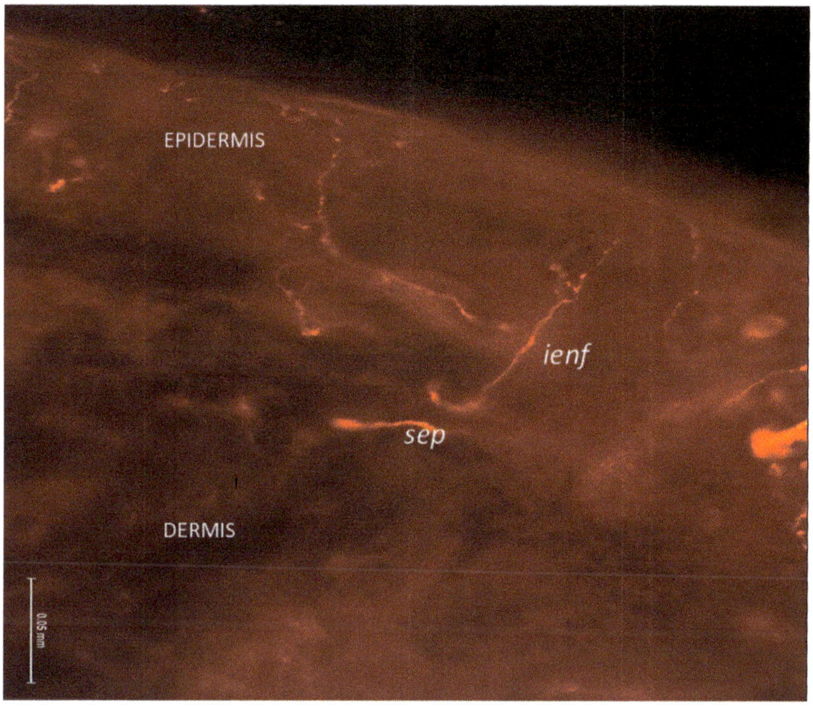

FIGURE 13.25 Skin biopsy; immunofluorescence, anti-PGP 9.5. IENF, intraepidermal nerve fibers; Sep, subepidermal plexus.

13.10. SKIN BIOPSY

Diagnosis of small fiber neuropathy may be clinically challenging due to subtle objective signs and normal nerve conduction studies. Skin biopsy is a less invasive procedure than nerve biopsy, and it allows for quantitation of intraepidermal nerve fiber density utilizing specific immunostaining. Skin samples are obtained using a 3-mm punch, during a sterile procedure with local anesthesia. Routine practice incudes two biopsies, one from a distal site 10 cm above the lateral malleolus (ankle) and a second from a proximal site 20 cm below the anterior superior iliac spine (thigh). Protein gene product 9.5 (PGP 9.5) is expressed in all axons, and anti-PGP immunohistochemistry allows detection and quantitation of axons extending across the dermal–epidermal junction (Fig. 13.25).

The epidermal nerve ending fiber density is compared to normative data obtained on control subjects. When the diagnosis of small fiber neuropathy is raised on the basis of clinical history and physical examination combined with normal nerve conduction studies (which only detect changes in large-diameter nerve fibers), a diagnostic workup is pursued in order to investigate the potential causes of the disorder. Autonomic testing and/or a skin biopsy can be useful to confirm the diagnosis of small fiber neuropathy but does not necessarily define the etiology.

Skin biopsy does not assess large fiber neuropathies because myelinated fibers are not present in the epidermis; they are located in small fascicles only in deeper portions of the dermis.

14

Diseases of the Pituitary Gland

SANDRO SANTAGATA, DAVID MEREDITH, CHIARA VILLA, AND VÂNIA NOSÉ

14.1. GENERAL CONSIDERATIONS

The pituitary, also known as the hypophysis, is a small endocrine gland weighing between 0.5 and 0.8 g, located at the base of the brain, just beneath the hypothalamus. Positioned in a bony cavity called the *sella turcica*, it is surrounded by vital structures including the optic chiasm (superiorly), cranial nerves III–VI (laterally), and the cavernous sinuses and internal carotid arteries (laterally). The floor of the sella turcica forms the roof of the sphenoid sinus; this anatomic relationship enables surgical access via a transsphenoidal approach.

The pituitary consists of an anterior lobe (adenohypophysis) and a posterior lobe (neurohypophysis). The anterior lobe contains six types of specialized hormone-releasing epithelial cells that are organized in clusters referred to as acini, surrounded by sustentacular cells called folliculostellate cells. Hormones produced by the anterior pituitary are stored in secretory granules. Upon release, they exert broad trophic effects, regulating the function of peripheral endocrine organs including the thyroid and adrenal glands. The production and release of these pituitary hormones are regulated by hypothalamic hormones that have stimulatory or inhibitory functions (Table 14.1) and are carried to the anterior pituitary through a portal system of venous blood vessels. The posterior pituitary comprises modified glial cells called pituicytes and axons originating from nerve cells in the supraoptic and paraventricular nuclei of the hypothalamus. These axons traverse the pituitary stalk (infundibulum) to reach the posterior pituitary.

The accurate diagnosis of pituitary pathology requires a comprehensive evaluation that integrates clinical information and laboratory data. Histopathologic examination, including immunohistochemistry, enables accurate classification of the lesions that arise in the sella turcica.

Table 14.1 Major Hypothalamic Hormones and Their Effect on Anterior Pituitary Hormones

HYPOTHALAMIC RELEASING NEUROPEPTIDES	PITUITARY HORMONES/CELL TYPES
Corticotropin-releasing hormone (CRH), released from paraventricular neurons, supraoptic and arcuate nuclei, and limbic system	Proopiomelanocortin (POMC): corticotroph (precursor protein of ACTH and other hormone peptides)
Growth hormone–releasing hormone (GHRH)	Growth hormone (GH): acidophilic/somatotrophs
Gonadotropin-releasing hormone (GnRH), mostly released from preoptic neurons	Luteinizing hormone (LH) and follicle-stimulating hormone (FSH): gonadotrophs
Thyrotropin-releasing hormone (TRH) released from anterior hypothalamic area	Thyroid-stimulating hormone: thyrotrophs
Prolactin-releasing factors (TRH, oxytocin, vasopressin, vasoactive intestinal polypeptide, neuropeptide Y, galanin, substance P, bombesin-like peptides, neurotensin, serotonin, acetylcholine, opiates, and estrogens)	Prolactin (PRL): lactotrophs
Hypothalamic Inhibiting Neuropeptides	
Somatostatin	Inhibits the release of GH, TSH, and PRL
Dopamine	Inhibits the release of PRL

14.2. PITUITARY DEVELOPMENT AND ARCHITECTURE

The adenohypophysis and the neurohypophysis are the two major components of the human pituitary gland. The adenohypophysis develops from Rathke's pouch, an evagination of the primitive oral ectoderm, whereas the neurohypophysis originates from the infundibular process of the diencephalon. The pituitary can be recognized by the third month of fetal development, and the hormone-producing cells of the anterior gland can be identified as early as 5 weeks of gestation, with cell differentiation dependent on transcriptional regulators such as TPIT, PIT1, SF1, and others (Table 14.2).

The anterior pituitary constitutes approximately 70–80% of the pituitary gland and comprises the pars distalis, pars intermedia, and pars tuberalis. The pars intermedia separates the pars distalis from the posterior

Table 14.2 Cells of the Anterior Pituitary, Identification of Cell Types in Fetal Development, Cell Percentages in Adults, and Location

CELL TYPE (HORMONES)	WEEKS OF GESTATION	CELL % IN ADULTS	LOCATION
Corticotroph (ACTH)	5	10–20	Mucoid edge
Somatotroph (GH)	8	40–50	Lateral wings
Multiple lineages (α subunit)	9	Variable	Diffuse throughout
Thyrotroph (TSH)	12	5	Anterior mucoid edge
Lactotroph (PRL)	12	10–30	Lateral wings
Gonadotroph (FSH/LH)	15–20	10	Diffuse throughout

ACTH, adrenocorticotrophic hormone; FSH, follicle-stimulating hormone; GH, growth hormone; LH, luteinizing hormone; PRL, prolactin; TSH, thyroid-stimulating hormone.

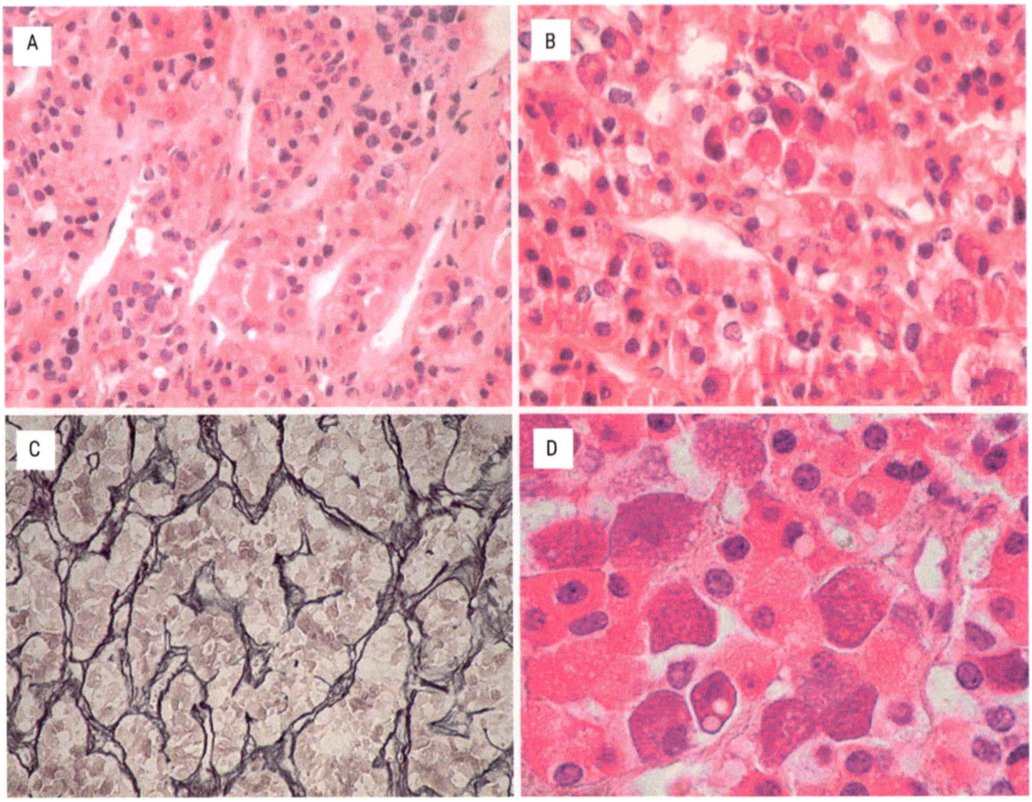

FIGURE 14.1 Normal adenohypophysis histology. (**A**) Normal acinar cells (H&E). (**B**) Acinar staining cell types: acidophils, basophils, and chromophobes (H&E). (**C**) A reticulin network defines normal acinar architecture (reticulin). (**D**) Basophils tend to be corticotroph cells, and acidophils tend to be mammosomatotrophy cells (H&E).

pituitary; in humans, it is vestigial and includes gland-like spaces and some corticotroph acini. The epithelial cells within the anterior pituitary form cords, nests, and small acini that are surrounded by an extensive network of capillaries, which can be clearly outlined using reticulin staining (Fig. 14.1). Folliculostellate sustentacular cells are distinct from the epithelial cells and surround the acini of normal pituitary hormone-producing cells; these supporting cells stain for S-100 protein and glial fibrillary acidic protein.

The epithelial cells can be subdivided into three groups based on the staining properties of their cytoplasm in hematoxylin and eosin (H&E) preparations: acidophils stain with acidic dyes (eosin), basophils stain with basic dyes (hematoxylin), and chromophobes exhibit faint staining (Figure 14.1). The variability in staining properties of normal cells within the pituitary is essential in diagnosing and distinguishing normal tissue from neoplastic tissue, given that the cells in pituitary tumors often display relatively uniform staining properties.

Notably, the distribution of the hormone-producing cell types within the pituitary gland is not uniform (Table 14.2): Acidophils (40%) are concentrated in the lateral "acidophilic" wings, basophils (10%) in the central "mucoid" wedge, and chromophobes (50%) are diffusely spread across the pituitary (Fig. 14.2A).

The posterior pituitary constitutes 20–30% of the gland and comprises the infundibulum or median eminence, the infundibular stem or pituitary stalk, and the posterior lobe. Within this region, basophils in the central "mucoid" wedge tend to infiltrate adjacent portions of the neurohypophysis, a phenomenon termed *basophilic invasion*. The axon terminals of the neurohypophysis are part of a neurosecretory unit that stores oxytocin and vasopressin hormones, along with the carrier protein neurophysin. Distinctive ovoid eosinophilic swellings called Herring bodies are a hallmark of the neurohypophysis in both the pituitary stalk and the posterior pituitary. These structures have a granular appearance

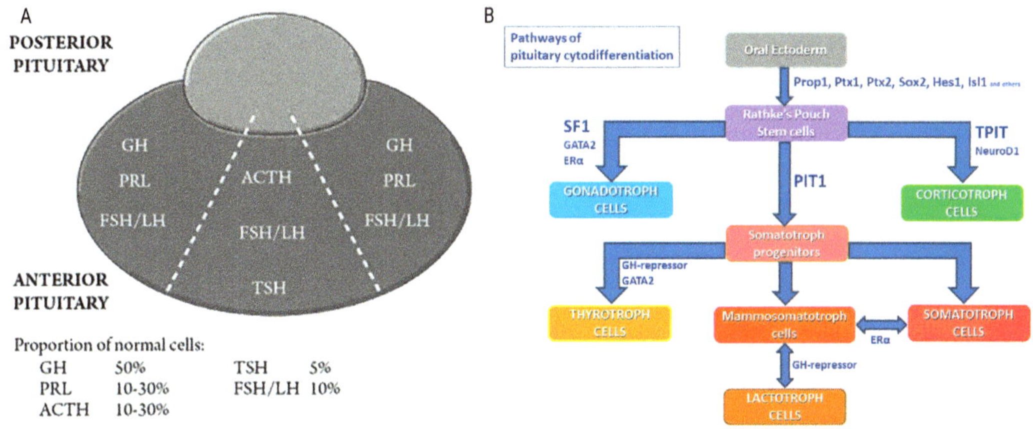

FIGURE 14.2 Anterior pituitary cell types: (**A**) cell type distribution in the anterior pituitary in horizontal plane; note the distribution and proportion of cell types (ACTH, corticotroph; FSH/LH, gonadotroph; GH, somatotroph; PRL, lactotroph; TSH, thyrotroph); (**B**) pathway of pituitary cytodifferentiation: transcription factor expression during fetal development.

and correspond to accumulations of oxytocin and vasopressin (antidiuretic hormone) secretion.

14.3. LESIONS OF THE PITUITARY GLAND

Abnormalities of the pituitary include a wide range of distinct entities (Table 14.3).

The primary cause of hormone abnormal secretion is a functional pituitary neuroendocrine tumor (PitNET)/pituitary adenoma, although less frequently, this can be caused by pituitary hyperplasia and very rarely by a metastatic PitNET/pituitary carcinoma. Seldom, hormone excess may be related to tumors arising in other sites with paraneoplastic hormone production. The clinical and endocrinological manifestations of the tumors are determined by the specific hormone that is produced in excess (Table 14.4). The most common clinical features include (1) galactorrhea and disruptions in ovulation among women, and decreased libido and erectile dysfunction in men related to excess prolactin (PRL) production; (2) Cushing disease due to the overproduction of adrenocorticotrophic hormone (ACTH); (3) gigantism/acromegaly due to the overproduction of growth hormone (GH); and (4) central hyperthyroidism related to thyroid-stimulating hormone (TSH) excess. Rarely, an overproduction of the gonadotrophic hormones follicle-stimulating hormone (FSH) and luteinizing hormone (LH) can lead to hypergonadism.

Pituitary tumors can cause the deficiency of one or more hormones due to compression of the pituitary or hypothalamus. Less commonly, hormone deficiencies may result from inflammatory diseases, intrasellar hemorrhage, infarction (known as pituitary apoplexy), or complications arising from pituitary surgery. When all hormone-secreting cells are lost, resulting in the absence of trophic hormones, it leads to a condition termed panhypopituitarism.

The primary clinical syndrome associated with neurohypophysis injury is diabetes insipidus, resulting from insufficient secretion of antidiuretic hormone. Alterations in the secretion of oxytocin, the other posterior pituitary hormone, rarely produce noticeable clinical features. Tumor growth can lead to mass effects within the sellar region, causing sellar expansion, bone erosion, and disruption of the sellar diaphragm. Given its proximity to visual pathways, an expanding pituitary mass can cause visual field deficits, including bitemporal hemianopsia due to optic chiasm compression or homonymous hemianopsia due to optic tract compression. Patients with PitNET/pituitary adenoma may also experience other neurologic syndromes, including increased intracranial pressure, headaches, seizures, obstructive hydrocephalus, and cranial nerve palsies.

14.4. PITUITARY NEUROENDOCRINE TUMORS/ PITUITARY ADENOMA

Up to 20% of "normal" pituitary glands harbor incidental lesions that can be detected by radiological

Table 14.3 Lesions of the Pituitary and Sellar Region

Benign Neoplasms	
Pituitary neuroendocrine tumor (PitNET)/pituitary adenoma	
Craniopharyngioma	Glomangioma
Meningioma	Hemangioma
Granular cell tumor	Hemangioblastoma
Pituicytoma	Myxoma
Spindle cell oncocytoma	Fibrous dysplasia of bone
Gangliocytoma	Osteoma
Ganglioglioma	Giant cell tumor of bone
Paraganglioma	
Glioma	
Inflammatory Disorders	
Xanthomatous hypophysitis	Giant cell granuloma
Lymphocytic hypophysitis	Granulomatous hypophysitis
Vascular Lesions	
Pituitary infarction	Aneurysm
Pituitary apoplexy	Vascular malformation
Cysts/Malformations	
Rathke's cleft cyst	Mucocele
Arachnoid cyst	Dermoid cyst
Epidermoid cyst	Hamartoma
Choristoma	Congenital malformations
Malignant Neoplasms	
Metastatic PitNET/pituitary carcinoma	
Chordoma	
Germ cell tumors	Leukemia
Hemangiopericytoma	Metastatic lymphoma
Postirradiation sarcoma	Plasmacytoma
Osteosarcoma	Fibrosarcoma
Hemangiosarcoma	Melanoma
Histiocytosis	Malignant peripheral nerve sheath tumor
Chondrosarcoma	Pituitary blastoma
Infectious Diseases	
Bacterial abscess	Syphilis
Tuberculosis	Cysticercosis
Fungal abscess	Hydatid cyst
Systemic Diseases	
Hemosiderosis/hemochromatosis	Amyloidosis
Mucopolysaccharidoses	Sarcoidosis
Injury	
Trauma	Radionecrosis
Empty sella syndrome	

imaging. In recent years, several studies have revealed a prevalence ranging from 78 to 116 cases per 100,000 people. According to data from the Central Brain Tumor Registry of the United States spanning from 2016 to 2020, pituitary tumors are the second most common tumor type arising in the brain (~17%), second only to meningiomas (~41%), and more common than glioblastoma (~14%). Incidence rates for tumors of the pituitary are 4.54 per 100,000 people. Pituitary adenomas are slightly more common in females (56%) than males (44%). The vast majority of PitNET/pituitary adenoma occurs in adults (>98% occur in individuals older than age 14 years; median age of diagnosis is 51 years) and are benign (99.9%). Five-year survival rates are very favorable (>99%).

The clinicopathological classification of PitNETs/pituitary adenomas relies on multiple factors, including the histological and immunohistochemical characterization using anterior pituitary hormones and lineage-restricted pituitary transcription factors (Table 14.4), evaluation of endocrine status (Table 14.5), and imaging data and operative findings.

Most PitNETs/pituitary adenomas consist of a clonal proliferation of well-differentiated neoplastic cells originating from anterior pituitary neuroendocrine cells. Generally, they remain benign, although approximately 50% of cases in surgical studies have been reported to show locally invasive behavior. Metastatic PitNET, also termed "pituitary carcinoma," is rare, accounting for only 0.1–0.4% of all PitNETs. A subset of these tumors may lack metastases but nonetheless show aggressive clinical behavior characterized by invasive and rapid growth with early and multiple relapses despite undergoing multimodal treatment (Box 14.1). The prevalence of these clinically aggressive tumors is unknown, and establishing tumor registries could assist with better defining these entities.

14.4.1. PitNET/pituitary adenoma of PIT1 lineage

The PIT1 group of PitNET/pituitary adenoma is complex and heterogeneous given the early expression of PIT1 lineage-restricted transcription factor during pituitary development (Fig. 14.2B). Thus, expression of this transcription factor is common to several types of PitNET/pituitary adenoma: lactotroph, somatotroph, thyrotroph, and bihormonal or plurihormonal PitNET/pituitary adenoma.

14.4.1.1. LACTOTROPH PITNET/PITUITARY ADENOMA

The majority of lactotroph PitNETs/pituitary adenomas, previously referred to as prolactinomas or prolactin cell adenomas, typically comprise diffuse, uniformly round cells. These cells usually appear chromophobic in the common subtype (sparsely granulated lactotroph tumor) or, less frequently, appear acidophilic in the rare subtype (densely granulated lactotroph tumor). They generally have few secretory granules and, therefore, are negative on periodic acid–Schiff (PAS) stain. The homogeneous population of small cells generally lacks pleomorphism (Fig. 14.3A) and occasionally contains microcalcifications and psammoma bodies. The PRL immunoreactivity in the sparsely granulated tumors is paranuclear, located around

Table 14.4 Pituitary Neuroendocrine Tumors and Immunohistochemical Findings

IMMUNOHISTOCHEMICAL FINDINGS OF ADENOHYPOPHYSEAL TUMORS

PITNET TYPE	PITUITARY HORMONES	TRANSCRIPTION FACTOR IMMUNOREACTIVITY
Somatotroph	GH, α subunit, ± PRL	PIT1
Lactotroph	PRL	PIT1, ER
Mammosomatotroph	GH, PRL, α subunit	PIT1, ER
Corticotroph	ACTH	T-PiT
Thyrotroph	TSH, α subunit	PIT1, GATA2/3
Mature plurihormonal PiT-1	GH, PRL, TSH, α subunit	PIT1, ER, GATA2/3
Acidophil stem cell tumor	PRL, GH focal	PIT1, ER
Immature PiT-1 lineage tumor	GH, PRL, α subunit, βTSH	PIT1, ER, GATA2/3
Gonadotropic	FSH/LH	SF-1, GATA2, ER
Null cell	Hormone negative	TF negative

ACTH, adrenocorticotrophic hormone; ER, estrogen receptor; FSH, follicle-stimulating hormone; GH, growth hormone; LH, luteinizing hormone; PRL, prolactin; TF, transcription factor; TSH, thyroid-stimulating hormone.

Table 14.5 Major Causes of Hormone Excess/Deficit Syndrome

SYNDROME	PITUITARY ORIGIN	OTHER ORIGIN (DIFFERENTIAL DIAGNOSIS)
Excess Hormone Syndromes		
Acromegaly/gigantism	Somatotroph tumor Mixed somatotroph and lactotroph tumors Mammosomatotroph tumor Mature plurihormonal PIT1 lineage tumor Immature PIT1 lineage tumor	Central excess growth hormone–releasing hormone secretion Hypothalamic hamartoma Choristoma Ganglioneuroma Peripheral excess growth hormone–releasing hormone secretion Bronchial carcinoid Pancreatic NETs Small cell lung cancer Adrenal tumor Excess growth factor activity Acromegaly
Cushing syndrome (CS)	ACTH-dependent CS Corticotroph tumor Pituitary blastoma	Ectopic ACTH/CRH dependent CS Phaeochromocytoma Pancreatic NETs Bronchial carcinoid Medullary thyroid cancer Small cell lung cancer Thymic neuroendocrine tumor Appendiceal neuroendocrine tumor ACTH-Independent CS Adrenal adenoma and carcinoma Micro- and macronodular hyperplasia Primary pigmented nodular adrenocortical disease Pseudo-CS Neuropsychiatric disorders Alcoholism Eating disorders Obesity Chronic high-dose glucocorticoid therapy (iatrogenic CS)
Hyperthyroidism	Thyrotroph tumor Mature plurihormonal PIT1 lineage tumor Immature PIT1 lineage tumor	Thyroid origin Graves disease Toxic nodular/multinodular goiter Subacute thyroiditis Resistance to thyroid hormone Amiodarone-induced Struma ovarii Metastatic differentiated thyroid cancer Factitious thyrotoxicosis

Table 14.5 Continued

SYNDROME	PITUITARY ORIGIN	OTHER ORIGIN (DIFFERENTIAL DIAGNOSIS)
Hyperprolactinemia	Lactotroph tumors Mammosomatotroph tumor Mature plurihormonal PIT1 lineage tumor Acidophil stem cell tumor Immature PIT1 lineage tumor • Sellar tumors with suprasellar extension (pituitary stalk compression)	Hypothalamic–pituitary stalk damage Granulomas Infiltrations Rathke's cyst Trauma: pituitary stalk section, suprasellar surgery Tumors: craniopharyngioma, germinoma, hypothalamic metastases, meningioma Drugs induced Hypothyroidism Chronic renal failure Polycystic ovary syndrome Physiological states Pregnancy Breastfeeding Stress Exercise
Hypergonadism (extremely rare)	Pituitary/sellar tumors Hypophysitis Pituitary infarction and apoplexy Sheehan syndrome Empty sella syndrome Genetic diseases	Iatrogenic causes Pituitary surgery and radiation Radiation for central nervous system and nasopharyngeal malignancies Glucocorticoid induced (hypoadrenalism) Trauma with fracture of skull base Hypothalamic impairment Mass effect from benign or malignant tumors of surrounding structures Infiltrative/inflammatory lesions
Deficit Hormone Syndrome		
Hypopituitarism	Pituitary/sellar tumors Hypophysitis Pituitary infarction and apoplexy Sheehan syndrome Empty sella syndrome Genetic diseases	Iatrogenic causes Pituitary surgery and radiation Radiation for central nervous system and nasopharyngeal malignancies Glucocorticoid induced (hypoadrenalism) Trauma with fracture of skull base Hypothalamic impairment Mass effect from benign or malignant tumors of surrounding structures Infiltrative/inflammatory lesions

the Golgi apparatus. By contrast, the rarer densely granulated PRL cell adenoma shows diffuse cytoplasmic PRL positivity (Fig. 14.3D). Both subtypes are immunoreactive for PIT1 and are generally positive for estrogen receptor-α (ER).

These adenomas occur most often in young adult women aged 20–40 years. In males, lactotroph PitNETs/pituitary adenomas are typically identified when they have grown to be macrotumors (>1 cm in greatest dimension). Patients with this tumor

Box 14.1 Pituitary Neuroendocrine Tumors with Aggressive Behavior

PitNET

PitNET with elevated MIB-1 index
Sparsely granulated somatotroph PitNET
Silent corticotroph PitNET
Crooke cell PitNET
Lactotroph PitNET in men
Plurihormonal PIT1-positive PitNET

are often resistant to dopamine agonist treatment and manifests aggressive clinical behavior. In females, the tumor is typically small, *a microtumor (<1 cm)*. Dopamine agonist therapy commonly results in involution/growth arrest and exhibits microcalcifications.

Lactotroph PitNET/pituitary adenoma needs to be distinguished from other lesions producing hyperprolactinemia, such as those that compress the pituitary stalk and the axons of hypothalamic nerves that release dopamine. Dopamine inhibits the production and secretion of prolactin; therefore, lesions that compress the pituitary stalk reduce the release of dopamine and result in elevated prolactin. Typically, serum PRL levels in stalk compression are less than 300 IU/μL, whereas patients with a PRL-secreting tumor usually have PRL levels greater than 1,000 IU/μL.

14.4.1.2. SOMATOTROPH PITNET/PITUITARY ADENOMA

Blood tests and tissue immunohistochemistry show evidence of GH production in approximately 30% of PitNETs/pituitary adenomas. These tumors can exclusively produce GH, a combination

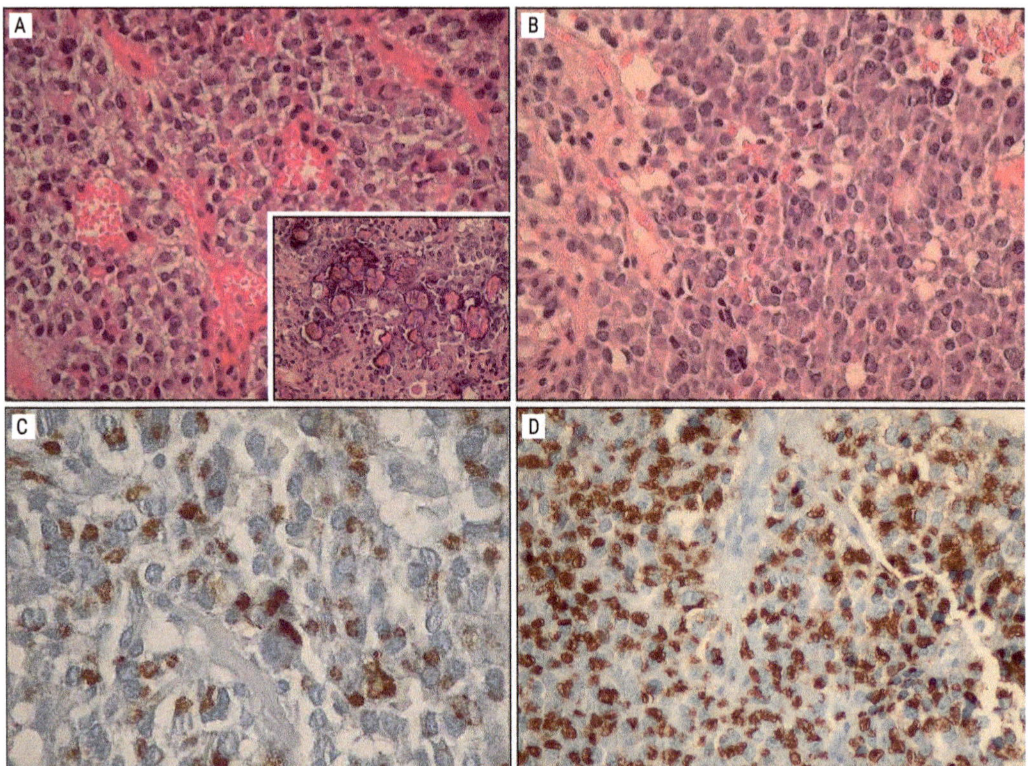

FIGURE 14.3 Lactotroph PitNET (adenoma). (**A**) Sparsely granulated lactotroph composed of chromophobic or slightly acidophilic cells with microcalcifications and psammoma bodies (inset) (H&E). (**B**) Densely granulated lactotroph composed of acidophilic cells (H&E). (**C**) PRL in sparsely granulated tumors is paranuclear/Golgi-like (PRL IHC), and (**D**) in densely granulated lactotroph it shows diffuse cytoplasmic positivity (PRL IHC).

of GH and PRL, or they can also be plurihormonal PIT1-positive. These PitNETs/pituitary adenomas are the primary cause of acromegaly/gigantism (Table 14.5).

14.4.1.2.1. GH-only PitNET/pituitary adenoma. PitNETs/pituitary adenomas producing GH only have a uniform population of round to oval cells that have eosinophilic (acidophilic) cytoplasm. The GH molecule lacks a carbohydrate component, so PAS stains are uniformly negative. Immunohistochemistry for GH shows variable expression (weak to very strong). If the tumor is densely granulated, there is strong and diffuse cytoplasmic GH staining, whereas sparsely granulated tumors have low levels of GH. These sparsely granulated tumors are often refractory to systemic treatment with somatostatin analogs, and patients are candidates for treatment with GH receptor antagonists. Sparsely and densely granulated tumors can also be distinguished using antibodies to low-molecular-weight cytokeratins such as CAM5.2. Densely granulated tumors predominantly have perinuclear cytoplasmic CAM5.2 reactivity, whereas sparsely granulated GH-producing PitNET/pituitary adenoma, CAM5.2 recognizes globular perinuclear structures termed fibrous bodies in the majority of cells with little staining in the cytoplasm outside of these bodies. These structures can also be observed in H&E-stained slides. Sparsely granulated tumors also have reduced expression of E-cadherin.

14.4.1.3. MIXED SOMATOTROPH-LACTOTROPH PITNET/PITUITARY ADENOMA

Patients with acromegaly can also have evidence of hyperprolactinemia as a result of production of both GH and PRL hormones in separate cell populations (Fig. 14.4). The mixed GH cell/PRL cell PitNET/pituitary adenoma contains two different cell types

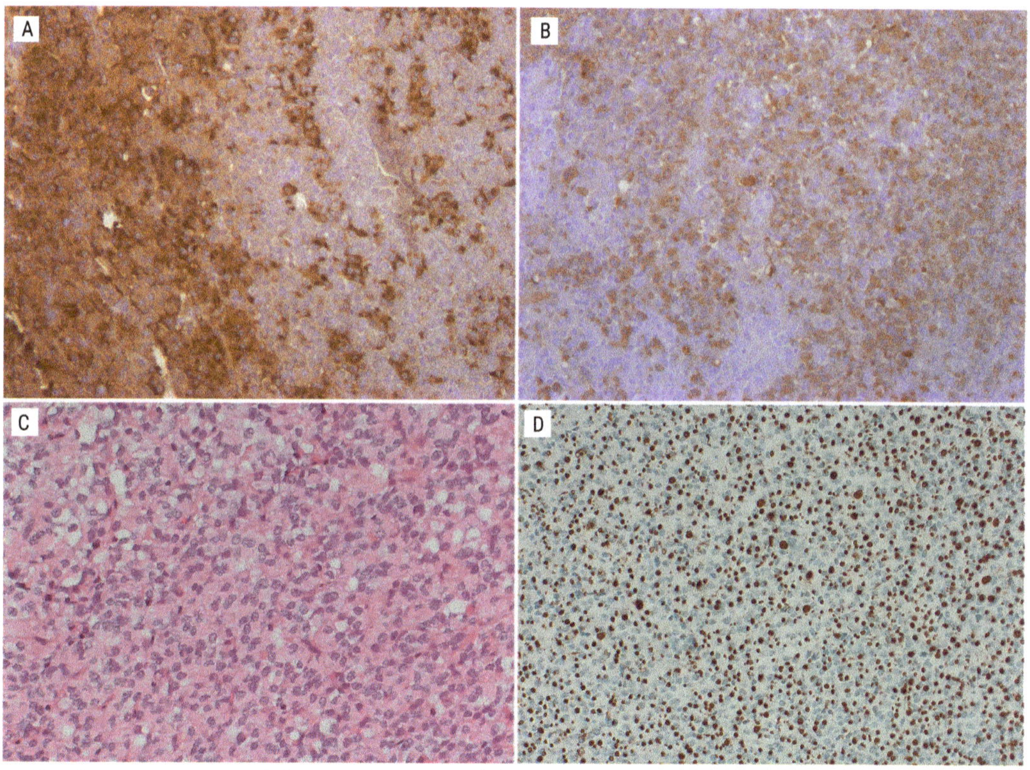

FIGURE 14.4 Somatotroph lactotroph PitNETs: (**A**) Mixed somatotroph/lactotroph expressing GH in a subset of tumor cells (GH IHC); (**B**) on adjacent section stained with anti-PRL antibody, GH-producing cells are negative for PRL and the PRL-producing cells are positive (PRL IHC); (**C**) sparsely granulated somatotroph PitNET composed of chromophobic or slightly acidophilic cells (H&E); (**D**) sparsely granulated somatotroph PitNET with perinuclear fibrous bodies (CAM 5.2 IHC).

which both express PIT1, well characterized by both their distinctive ultrastructural appearance and immunohistochemistry. These lesions are not aggressive.

14.4.1.4. MAMMOSOMATOTROPH PITNET/PITUITARY ADENOMA

The rare mammosomatotroph cell PitNET/pituitary adenoma is characterized by a monomorphous eosinophilic cell population and dual immunopositivity for PRL and GH. Unlike other mixed bicellular tumors, these cells by electron microscopy exhibit both lactotroph and somatotroph differentiation in the same cell.

14.4.1.5. ACIDOPHIL STEM CELL PITNET/PITUITARY ADENOMA

Acidophil stem cell PitNET/pituitary adenoma is a rare PIT1 lineage tumor showing characteristics of partial lactotroph differentiation and limited somatotroph differentiation. The tumor cells display oncocytic histologic features with chromophobic and acidophilic cytoplasm that contains large clear vacuoles, attributed to the accumulation of giant mitochondria. Many tumor cells show strong PRL expression, whereas GH expression tends to be weak or absent. Oncocytic features can be highlighted using anti-mitochondrial antibodies. Hyperprolactinemia may occur, and acromegaly features can also be present. Although large studies are not available, the current data suggest that these tumors display aggressive clinical behavior and are unresponsive to treatment with dopamine agonists and somatostatin analogues.

14.4.1.6. THYROTROPH PITNET/PITUITARY ADENOMA

TSH-producing tumors are a rare PitNET/pituitary adenoma subtype. These are often invasive macrotumors, and they can present with hyperthyroidism, hypothyroidism, or, rarely, euthyroidism. The thyrotroph cell PitNET/pituitary adenoma represents less than 1% of PitNETs/pituitary adenomas. Most of these tumors have polygonal and chromophobic tumor cells that are faintly PAS positive. The tumor cells are diffusely positive for PIT1 and are positive for β-TSH, the α subunit of glycoprotein hormones, and GATA3. Most of these lesions are located in the anterior mucoid wedge, where the thyrotroph cells are usually concentrated. Electron microscopy shows peripherally placed sparse secretory granules.

14.4.1.7. PLURIHORMONAL PITNET/PITUITARY ADENOMA

The plurihormonal PIT1-positive PitNETs/pituitary adenomas are rare tumors derived from PIT1 lineage characterized by the production of multiple hormones. They produce high levels of GH and have variable expression of PRL, TSH, and the α subunit of the glycoprotein hormones. The plurihormonal PitNETs/pituitary adenomas may be functioning, partially functioning, or silent. One or more cell types, as detected by electron microscopy, can form these tumors. The monomorphous type is composed of one cell type that can produce multiple hormones. The plurimorphous type comprises at least two cell types with distinct immunohistochemical and electron microscopic characteristics. Some of these latter lesions may represent a collision tumor.

14.4.2. PitNET/pituitary adenoma of TPIT lineage

Many types of lesions can cause excess production of ACTH. The most common cause is ACTH-dependent Cushing syndrome, stemming from a PitNET/pituitary adenoma that produces ACTH, which leads to adrenal cortical hyperplasia (Table 14.5). ACTH-independent Cushing disease is less frequent.

14.4.2.1. CORTICOTROPH PITNET/PITUITARY ADENOMA

Corticotroph cell PitNETs/pituitary adenomas account for approximately 20% of all PitNETs/pituitary adenomas and are more prevalent in women than in men. Typically, these tumors manifest as microtumors and arise in the central mucoid wedge of the anterior pituitary, where most normal ACTH-producing cells are located. These tumors have uniform positivity for the TPIT lineage transcription factor. ACTH-producing macrotumors are rare but tend to be invasive. These tumors consist of a uniform population of basophilic cells with PAS-positive cytoplasm, expressing ACTH or other proopiomelanocortin derivatives demonstrated by immunohistochemistry (Fig. 14.5).

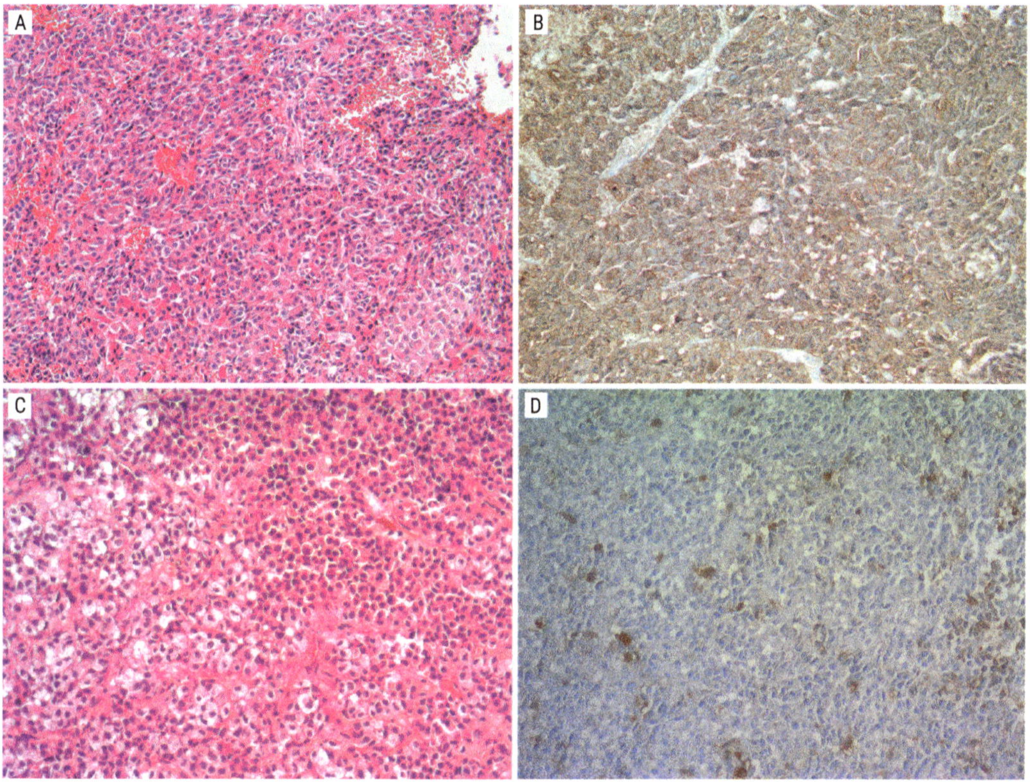

FIGURE 14.5 Corticotroph PitNET/pituitary adenoma: (**A**) Densely granulated corticotroph PitNET composed of basophilic cells (H&E); (**B**) diffuse cytoplasmic ACTH expression in densely granulated corticotroph tumor (ACTH IHC); (**C**) sparsely granulated corticotroph PitNET, composed of slightly basophilic or chromophobic cells with (**D**) low ACTH expression in a subset of tumor cells (ACTH IHC).

Corticotroph PitNETs are classified into three subtypes: densely granulated, sparsely granulated, and Crooke cell tumors. Both densely granulated and sparsely granulated corticotroph tumors have diffuse and strong cytoplasmic CAM5.2 staining, whereas Crooke cell tumors have a strong perinuclear and ring-like expression of CAM5.2 corresponding to the "hyaline" material that collects in this subtype. Whereas PAS staining and ACTH immunoreactivity are strong in densely granulated tumors, the staining is weak and variable in sparsely granulated tumors. In Crooke cell tumors, the staining is localized to the periphery of the cytoplasm. Crooke cell PitNETs should not be confused with resident Crooke cells in the surrounding adenohypophysis. In the majority of functioning corticotroph PitNETs, non-neoplastic cells surrounding the PitNET may show Crooke hyaline change, which is a marker of chronic exposure to elevated cortisol. Diffuse Crooke hyalinization of ACTH-producing PitNET/pituitary adenoma is rare and is associated with larger size neoplasms (i.e., macrotumors with invasion). ATRX mutations are present in a subset of aggressive pituitary tumors and are enriched in corticotroph tumors that exhibit aggressive behavior.

14.4.2.2. SILENT CORTICOTROPH PITNET/PITUITARY ADENOMA

Although most corticotrophs are functioning, approximately 40% of patients present with macrotumors that do not exhibit hormone activity (i.e., they are endocrinologically nonfunctioning; silent). The tumor cells, nonetheless, have immunoreactivity for ACTH. These tumors are believed to either produce abnormal biologically inactive products or fail to release the hormone. In some cases, patients present with mildly elevated serum ACTH. Silent corticotroph PitNETs/pituitary adenomas have basophilic-to-chromophobic cells with immunoreactivity to ACTH or other proopiomelanocortin derivatives, similar to the typical corticotroph cell PitNET/pituitary adenoma. Although previous studies reported that silent corticotroph PitNETs/pituitary adenomas are more invasive and have elevated rates of recurrence, recent studies have not confirmed this. Further research is needed to establish the behavior and characteristics of these tumors.

14.4.3. PitNET/pituitary adenoma of SF1 lineage

Most gonadotroph PitNETs are clinically nonfunctioning, and patients present with signs and symptoms that arise from mass effect, such a headache, hypopituitarism, and visual defects. There is marked variability of expression of FSH and LH in these tumors; however, they have uniform positivity for the SF1 lineage transcription factor. Some demonstrate diffuse positive immunoreactivity for the β subunits of human chorionic gonadotrophin, FSH, and LH, with or without immunoreactivity for the α subunit, and others fail to demonstrate immunoreactivity for these hormones (Fig. 14.6). Gonadotroph PitNETs are believed to be nonfunctional because of a failure to appropriately combine the α and β subunits of the glycoprotein hormones to make the active hormone. These macrotumors are generally not aggressive and less frequently invade surrounding structures.

14.4.4. PitNET/pituitary adenoma with neuronal metaplasia

Rare GH-producing PitNET/pituitary adenoma and, even more rarely, other types of PitNET/pituitary adenoma may contain ganglion cells and are referred to as "gangliocytoma and mixed gangliocytoma–PitNET/pituitary adenoma." The ganglion cells may be dysplastic with multiple nuclei, and they react with neuronal markers such as NeuN and neurofilament protein as well as epithelial markers; they also have the hormonal immunoprofile of PitNET/pituitary adenoma cells. These ganglion cells may be scant or may represent the great majority of tumor cells and may or may not be accompanied by neuropil. The ganglion cells are thought to represent neuronal metaplasia of PitNET cells (i.e., "transdifferentiation"), and this is supported by immunocytochemical and ultrastructural demonstration of cells with transitional features between neurons and pituitary neuroendocrine cells. Alternatively, the presence of neurons in a PitNET/pituitary adenoma might be interpreted as a developmental malformation.

14.4.5. PitNET/pituitary adenoma not associated with hormone production

The term "null cell adenoma" was used in the past to describe approximately one-third of all pituitary adenomas, which lacked clinical evidence of hormonal production. Patients with these tumors often seek medical attention when the tumors are large and they are experiencing symptoms and signs related to compression of surrounding structures. Extensive destruction of normal pituitary tissue can lead to hypopituitarism, and compression of the pituitary stalk can lead to mild hyperprolactinemia. However, although hormone expression is absent in most of these tumors, they retain the expression of lineage transcription factors. The majority of these tumors express SF1 (without FSH or LH) and are designated gonadotroph PitNET, a smaller fraction express TPIT (without ACTH) and are designated corticotroph PitNET, and a very small percentage express PIT1 (without PRL, GH, or TSH) and are designated PIT1 lineage PitNET. Thus, the vast majority of tumors that were previously recognized as "null cell adenomas" are now considered to be silent (hormone-negative) gonadotroph or corticotroph PitNETs. Less than 5% of PitNETs do not express pituitary hormones or the pituitary lineage transcription factors PIT1, TPIT, or SF1 but do express neuroendocrine markers, such as synaptophysin and chromogranin A. The diagnosis of null cell PitNET/pituitary adenoma is now used for this subset of nonfunctioning PitNETs/pituitary adenomas. When evaluating tumors in the pituitary that are negative for transcription factors and hormones, it is important to exclude other tumor entities that can arise in the pituitary or metastasize to it.

The overall algorithm for the classification of PitNETs (pituitary adenomas) begins with determination of the primary hormonal syndrome (Table 14.6) and follows the format of an integrated classification. The clinical secretion phenotype is then subclassified based on hormonal immunophenotype, low-molecular-weight keratin distribution, and, when needed, transcription factor expression.

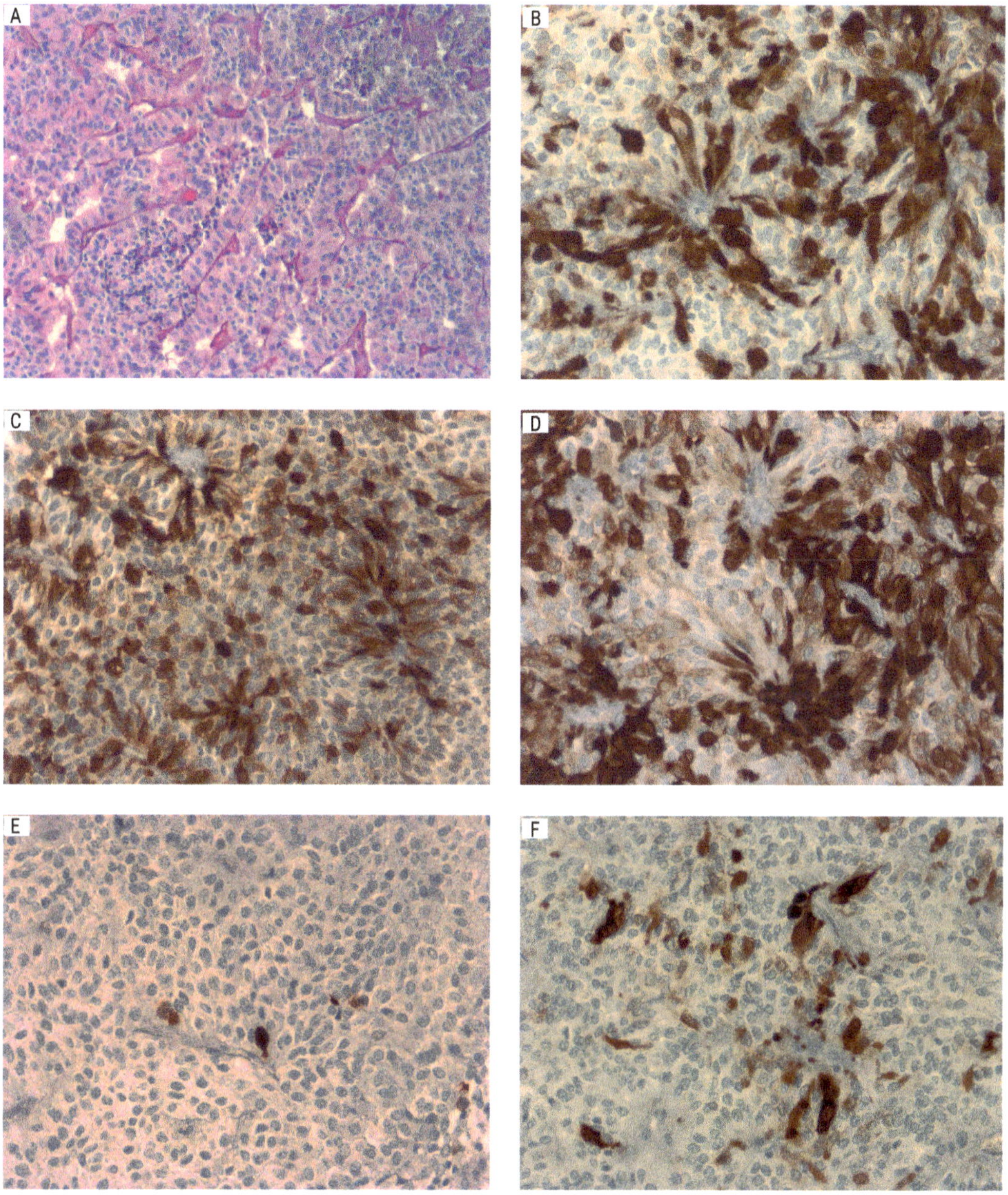

FIGURE 14.6 Gonadotrophic PitNET/pituitary adenoma. (**A**) Tumor cells are arranged in papillary and frond architecture around fine capillaries (H&E). Using immunohistochemistry, scattered tumor cells express (**B**) the α subunit of human chorionic gonadotropin, (**C**) LH, (**D**) FSH, (**E**) TSH, and (**F**) the α subunit.

14.4.6. Genetic aberrations in PitNET/pituitary adenoma

Recurrent genetic aberrations are common in GH- and ACTH-producing PitNET/pituitary adenoma. *GNAS1*, a gene encoding a guanine nucleotide–binding protein that transduces signals from G-protein–coupled receptors and regulates cAMP (cyclic adenosine monophosphate) levels, is mutated in approximately 50% of GH-only and GH-producing plurihormonal PitNETs. GNAS R201C is the most commonly observed mutation. Approximately 50% of ACTH-producing PitNETs/pituitary adenomas harbor mutations in *USP8*, a gene encoding a deubiquitinating enzyme. These mutations are present most often in densely granulated corticotroph tumors, but not in silent corticotroph tumors. The mutations enhance the catalytic activity of USP8 and lead to increased deubiquitination of targets such as the epidermal growth factor receptor (EGFR), thereby impairing the degradation of EGFR and supporting sustained EGF signaling in these tumors. Lactotroph PitNETs/pituitary adenomas do not have a consistent mutation, but a recurrent mutation has been identified in the *SF3B1* gene (R625H) in approximately 20% of these tumors.

Although most PitNETs/pituitary adenomas do not harbor specific recurrent mutations that have been identified, many PitNETs/pituitary adenomas have high levels of chromosome arm-level copy number alterations across large fractions of the genome with few accompanying focal events. Genomic disruption is enriched in functioning PitNET.

14.4.7. Ectopic PitNET/pituitary adenoma

Ectopic PitNETs/pituitary adenomas are rare. They are derived from pituitary cells in the pharynx and can occur in the cavernous sinus, sphenoid sinus, mouth, nasal cavity, or the suprasellar region. These ectopic PitNETs/pituitary adenomas can be null cell or hormonally producing tumors, often producing ACTH.

14.4.8. Invasive PitNET/pituitary adenoma

PitNETs/pituitary adenomas are classified as invasive if invasion of the dura, adjacent bone, cavernous sinus, or sinus mucosa can be demonstrated based on either imaging or operative findings. There are no light microscopic or ultrastructural features that distinguish noninvasive from invasive PitNETs/pituitary adenomas. Mitoses are more often present in invasive tumors than in noninvasive lesions.

14.4.9. Metastatic PitNET/pituitary carcinoma

Adenohypophyseal neoplasms with craniospinal spread, brain invasion, and metastases to extracranial sites are designated pituitary or adenohypophyseal carcinomas (metastatic PitNETs). They are extremely rare. Metastatic potential distinguishes pituitary carcinoma from the other adenohypophyseal tumors. The metastases are usually to lymph nodes, bone, liver, or skull. Pituitary carcinomas (Fig. 14.7) are more frequently hormonally inactive tumors; however, PRL-producing and ACTH-producing carcinomas have been described.

The diagnosis of pituitary carcinoma is not based on histologic criteria alone but, rather, on the basis of metastases. In fact, most carcinomas do not show much cellular pleomorphism or nuclear atypia. However, they have increased mitotic activity, high MIB-1 labeling index, and p53 immunoreactivity compared with typical PitNETs (Figs. 14.7 and 14.8).

14.4.10. Pituitary blastoma

Pituitary blastoma is defined in the 2022 World Health Organization (WHO) classification as an embryonal sellar neoplasm composed of primitive blastemal cells, neuroendocrine cells, and Rathke pouch epithelium. This tumor has been reported to occur in children younger than age 2 years, and Cushing disease is the most common clinical presentation. These tumors are reported to occur in the DICER1 tumor predisposition syndrome. All tumors are reported to harbor *DICER1* gene alterations. Pituitary blastomas resemble the fetal pituitary gland of 10–12 weeks and are composed of three cellular components: (1) usually large adenohypophysial neuroendocrine cells organized in lobules or diffuse sheets, (2) scattered small undifferentiated blastemal cells, and (3) cuboidal primitive Rathke pouch epithelium that has rosettes or glands and follicles. These components are immunoreactive for CAM5.2.

14.4.11. Pituitary hyperplasia

A rare cause of pituitary hyperfunction is pituitary hyperplasia. It may cause a clinical syndrome such as acromegaly, Cushing syndrome, or hypothyroidism. By definition, pituitary hyperplasia is an increase in the number of one or more specific anterior pituitary cell types; it is a nonneoplastic proliferation distinct from pituitary neuroendocrine tumors. Anterior pituitary hyperplasia can be classified as primary hyperplasia (idiopathic), secondary hyperplasia due to lack of negative-feedback stimulation and end-organ failure, or tertiary hyperplasia due to hypothalamic or ectopic hormone stimulation. Idiopathic pituitary hyperplasia is probably due to hypothalamic dysfunction with an excess of hypothalamic hormone production.

Table 14.6 Diagnostic Algorithms for PitNETs of PIT1, TPIT, and SF1 lineage, and for nonfunctioning PitNETs

SECRETION/FUNCTION	LINEAGE	ROUTINE STAINING	IMMUNOPHENOTYPE	TRANSCRIPTION FACTOR	INTEGRATED DIAGNOSIS
Hyperprolactinemia, or galactorrhea	PIT1 lineage (somato-lacto-thyrotroph PitNET)	Neuroendocrine tumor morphology (often chromophobe), may have calcifications	PRL+	PIT1+	Lactotroph PitNET, prolactin producing
Acromegaly, or gigantism, with or without hyperprolactinemia		Neuroendocrine tumor morphology (may be acidophils; PAS negative)	HGH+ (cytoplasmic, often weak staining) CAM5.2 fibrous body staining only	PIT1+	Somatotroph PitNET, sparsely granulated, growth hormone producing
		Neuroendocrine tumor, strongly PAS positive (may be acidophils; PAS negative)	HGH+++ (perinuclear, strong staining) CAM5.2 perinuclear	PIT1+	Somatotroph PitNET, densely granulated, growth hormone producing
		Neuroendocrine tumor morphology	HGH+ and PRL+ in separate cells (rare mixed tumors with dual expression in same cells)	PIT1+	Mixed somatotroph/lactotroph PitNET, growth hormone and prolactin-producing
Central hyperthyroidism		Neuroendocrine tumor morphology, chromophobe with weak PAS staining	TSH+, α subunit+, GATA3+	PIT1+	Thyrotroph PitNET, TSH producing
Acromegaly or gigantism, and central hyperthyroidism (with or without hyperprolactinemia)		Neuroendocrine tumor morphology	TSH+ and second hormone production (either GH, PRL)	PIT1+ (required for diagnosis)	Somatotroph plurihormonal PitNET, PIT1 expressing

(continued)

Table 14.6 Continued

SECRETION/FUNCTION	LINEAGE	ROUTINE STAINING	IMMUNOPHENOTYPE	TRANSCRIPTION FACTOR	INTEGRATED DIAGNOSIS
Cushing disease (reticulin or collagen IV may be required for microadenomas)	TPIT lineage (corticotroph PitNET)	Neuroendocrine tumor morphology; weak or negative PAS staining	Cam5.2+++, ACTH variable (may be negative)	TPIT+	Corticotroph PitNET, sparsely granulated, ACTH producing
		Neuroendocrine tumor morphology; strong PAS staining	Cam5.2+++, ACTH+ strongly	TPIT+	Corticotroph PitNET, densely granulated, ACTH producing
		Neuroendocrine tumor morphology; Crooke hyalin may be seen on H&E	Cam5.2+ ring-like encircling the nucleus; ACTH+	TPIT+	Corticotroph PitNET, Crooke cell type, ACTH producing
Nonfunctioning (>80% are SF1 lineage, with or without hypergonadotrophism)	SF1 lineage (gonadotroph PitNET)	Neuroendocrine tumor morphology	FSH+, LH+	SF1+	Gonadotroph PitNET, LH and/or FSH producing
Nonfunctioning (without hypergonadotrophism)	TPIT lineage	Neuroendocrine tumor morphology, basophilic-to-chromophobic	Cam5.2+, ACTH+	TPIT+	Corticotroph PitNET, clinically silent, ACTH producing
		Neuroendocrine tumor morphology, basophilic-to-chromophobic	Cam5.2+, ACTH variable (may be negative)	TPIT+ (required for diagnosis)	Corticotroph PitNET, clinically silent, weakly ACTH producing (or non-ACTH producing)
Nonfunctioning (with or without mildly elevated serum GH, PRL, or TSH)	PIT1 lineage (somato-lacto-thyrotroph PitNET)	Neuroendocrine tumor morphology	HGH+ or PRL+ or TSH+ (mixed hormone production may occur)	PIT1+ (required for diagnosis)	PitNET, clinically silent, PIT1 lineage, weakly (GH, PRL, or TSH) producing

Nonfunctioning PitNET	SF1 lineage (gonadotroph PitNET)	Neuroendocrine tumor morphology	All negative hormones negative (or only very rare cells positive)	SF1+ (required for diagnosis)	Gonadotroph PitNET, SF1 expressing
	TPIT lineage (somato-lacto-thyrotroph PitNET)	Neuroendocrine tumor morphology	All negative hormones negative (or only very rare cells positive)	TPIT+ (required for diagnosis)	Corticotroph PitNET, silent clinically, TPIT expressing
	PIT1 lineage (somato-lacto-thyrotroph PitNET)	Neuroendocrine tumor morphology	All negative hormones negative (or only very rare cells positive)	PIT1+ (required for diagnosis)	PitNET, clinically silent, PIT1 lineage, non-hormone producing
	Negative for all transcription factors	Neuroendocrine tumor morphology, synaptophysin+ or chromogranin+	All negative hormones negative (or only very rare cells positive)	All transcription factors negative	Null cell PitNET, clinically silent, non-hormone producing

+, positive for expression; +++, strongly positive for expression.
ACTH, adrenocorticotropic hormone; CAM 5.2, cytokeratin CAM5.2; FSH, follicle-stimulating hormone; GATA3, GATA-binding protein; H&E, hematoxylin and eosin; HGH, human growth hormone; LH, luteinizing hormone; PAS, periodic acid–Schiff; PRL, prolactin; TSH, thyroid-stimulating hormone; TPIT, PIT1, SF1, transcription factors.

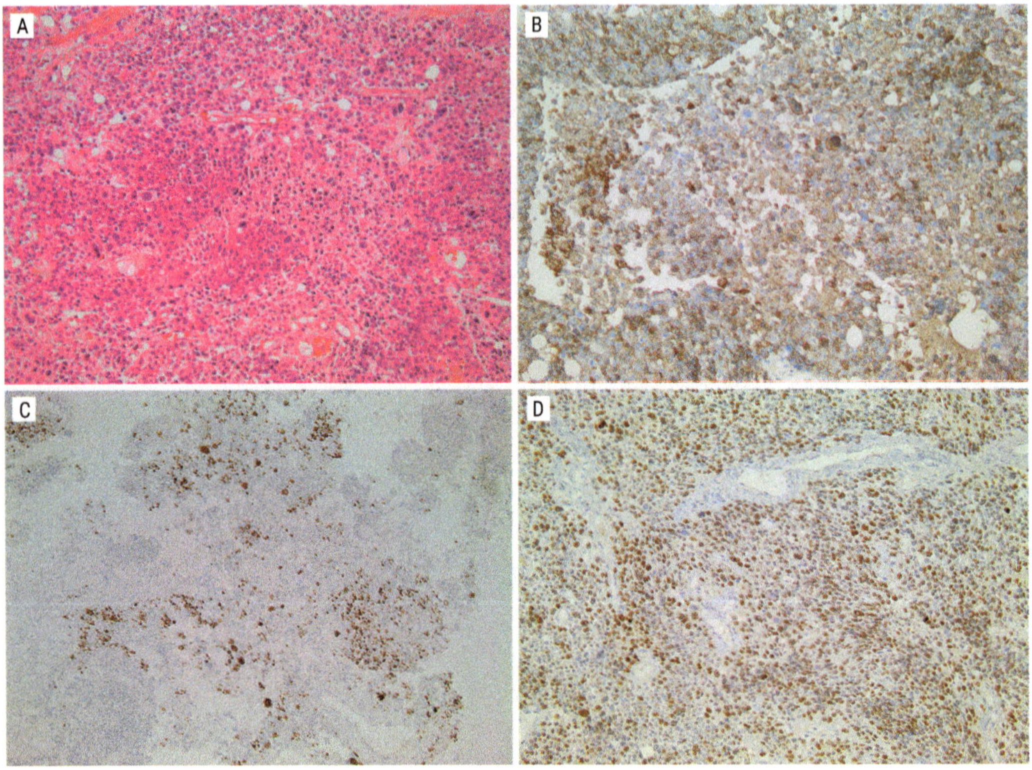

FIGURE 14.7 Metastatic PitNET/pituitary carcinoma: (**A**) histological appearance; numerous mitoses are present (H&E); (**B**) ACTH expression in this densely granulated corticotroph carcinoma (ACTH IHC); (**C**) focal areas with high proliferative activity "hot spots" (Ki-67/MIB-1 IHC); (**D**) diffuse and intense p53 expression (p53 IHC).

Hyperplastic cells are usually found in foci, but the process can be nodular or diffuse. The diagnosis is based on histological findings of expansion of the acinar architecture, seen with a reticulin stain. Immunohistochemistry can help in identifying the hyperplastic cell type. Differentiating pituitary hyperplasia from PitNET can be difficult.

14.5. HYPOPITUITARISM AND INFLAMMATORY AND VASCULAR LESIONS

Hypopituitarism is caused by deficiency of the pituitary trophic hormones due to a variety of causes.

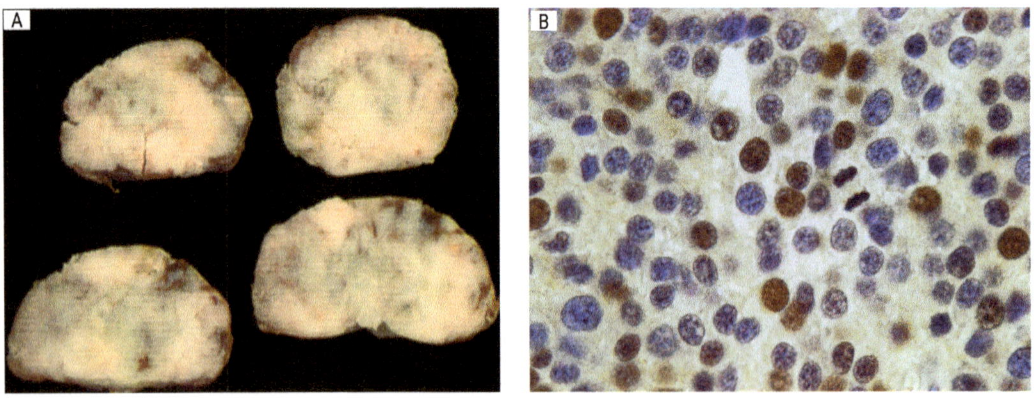

FIGURE 14.8 Metastatic PitNET/pituitary carcinoma: (**A**) gross appearance of tumor with (**B**) high proliferative index and increased mitotic activity (Ki-67/MIB-1 IHC).

> **Box 14.2 Inflammatory Lesions of the Pituitary Gland**
>
> **Primary or Idiopathic**
> Lymphocytic hypophysitis
> Granulomatous hypophysitis
> Xanthomatous hypophysitis
> Giant cell granuloma
>
> **Secondary**
> Infections: pneumocystis, toxoplasma, cytomegalovirus, meningitis, syphilis, brucellosis, fungi, mycobacteria
> - Systemic diseases: sarcoidosis, Wegener granulomatosis, Takayasu disease, Crohn disease
> - PitNET undergoing necrosis
> - Ruptured Rathke's cleft cyst

With the loss of 50% of the pituitary cells, the patient may be asymptomatic. When more than 80% of the anterior pituitary cells are destroyed, hypopituitarism becomes evident.

14.5.1. Inflammatory lesions

Inflammatory lesions of the pituitary (Box 14.2) can cause hypopituitarism, mass effect, or diabetes insipidus. Inflammatory disorders of the pituitary can be divided into those that are primary (or idiopathic) and those that are secondary to lesions elsewhere in the body.

14.5.1.1. PRIMARY OR IDIOPATHIC INFLAMMATORY LESIONS

14.5.1.1.1. Lymphocytic hypophysitis. Lymphocytic hypophysitis is a chronic autoimmune process that is particularly associated with pregnancy or the postpartum period; it is a cause of pituitary insufficiency of pregnancy. The clinical presentation is that of panhypopituitarism, often with headache. Decompressive biopsy is part of the treatment. The adenohypophyseal interstitium and the acini are infiltrated by lymphocytes and plasma cells with occasional histiocytes. Lymphoid infiltrates with well-developed germinal centers may occur (Fig. 14.9). Fibrosis may be found in chronic phases. Both humoral and cell-mediated immunity are apparently involved, with the development of anti-pituitary antibodies.

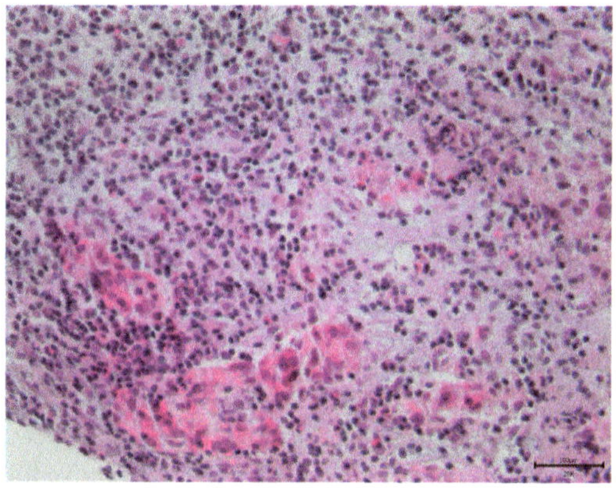

FIGURE 14.9 Lymphocytic hypophysitis. The anterior pituitary tissue is almost replaced by a dense lymphocytic infiltrate (H&E).

14.5.1.1.2. Granulomatous hypophysitis. Granulomatous hypophysitis is a rare chronic inflammatory disease of unknown pathogenesis. Unlike lymphocytic hypophysitis, granulomatous hypophysitis occurs equally in both sexes. The usual clinical presentation is a variable degree of adenohypophyseal failure, hyperprolactinemia, headache with nausea and vomiting, and diabetes insipidus.

Microscopically, granulomatous hypophysitis is characterized by large collections of histiocytes, sometimes with occasional multinucleated giant cells, and a lymphoplasmacytic infiltrate (Fig. 14.10).

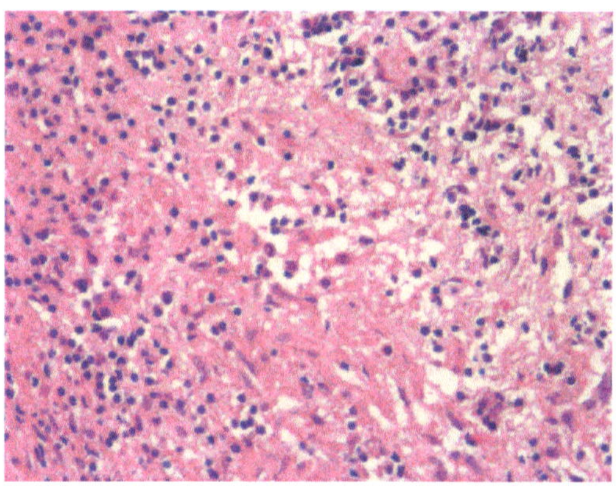

FIGURE 14.10 Granulomatous hypophysitis. There is a well-formed granuloma in the anterior pituitary with epithelioid cells and some scattered, multinucleated giant cells at the periphery (H&E).

It must be differentiated from other causes of granulomatous inflammation, such as tuberculosis, fungi, and sarcoidosis.

14.5.1.1.3. Xanthomatous hypophysitis. Xanthomatous hypophysitis is a rare idiopathic entity that may represent a reactive process. It occurs in young women who present to medical attention with a combination of menstrual irregularities, diabetes insipidus, headache, and nausea with a localized lesion in the pituitary. Histologically, the adenohypophysis is infiltrated by foamy histiocytes, immunoreactive for CD68 and immunonegative for CD1a and S-100 protein.

14.5.1.1.4. Giant cell granuloma of the pituitary. Giant cell granuloma of the pituitary is another rare cause of hypophysitis. It occurs in both sexes and is not associated with pregnancy. Histologically, the pituitary is infiltrated by noncaseating granulomas with occasional Schaumann bodies. Systemic evidence of sarcoidosis or other diseases has to be excluded.

14.5.1.2. SECONDARY HYPOPHYSITIS

A variety of systemic diseases and infections can also cause hypophysitis. Involvement of the pituitary may occur in sarcoidosis, Langerhans cell histiocytosis, vasculitis, and other immune-mediated disorders.

14.5.2. Vascular lesions of the pituitary

14.5.2.1. PITUITARY INFARCTION

Diverse diseases can cause ischemic necrosis of the pituitary gland, such as hemorrhagic shock, thrombocytopenia, other coagulopathies, head injury, massive cerebrovascular accidents, and heparin therapy. This condition is followed by hypopituitarism.

14.5.2.2. PITUITARY APOPLEXY

Pituitary apoplexy is a medical emergency presenting with acute headache and sometimes visual loss, secondary to hemorrhage or infarction of the pituitary. It is most often due to a pituitary macrotumor. It can occur in the setting of an enlarged pituitary gland during pregnancy. Often, much of a resection specimen contains necrotic tissue. Nonetheless, a reticulin stain can be used to assess whether there is effacement of the normal pituitary architecture, and immunohistochemistry (particularly on small viable areas of the tumor) can be used to guide tumor classification.

14.5.2.3. SHEEHAN SYNDROME

Sheehan syndrome is postpartum hypopituitarism in women and is due to necrosis of the pituitary gland secondary to hypotension from postpartum hemorrhage. The posterior pituitary is spared due to its independent blood supply. There is a rim of normal viable adenohypophyseal cells at the periphery of the gland, with almost total necrosis of the gland. Subsequent fibrosis follows the necrosis.

14.6. HEREDITARY AND DEVELOPMENTAL DISORDERS

14.6.1. Persistence of Rathke's pouch remnants

Rathke's pouch remnants are small nests of epithelial cells in the posterior lobe adjacent to the cleft. They can be found in 30% of normal human pituitaries at autopsy. The nests have no hormonal function and are an unlikely origin of a neoplasm, although it has been postulated that craniopharyngiomas may arise from these remnants.

14.6.2. Persistence of cleft of Rathke's pouch

The developmental abnormality of persistence of the cleft of Rathke's pouch is frequent, without significant functional or clinical consequences. It is a colloid-filled space between the anterior and posterior pituitary that can give rise to Rathke's cleft cysts. These cysts are usually small, but when large, they can be symptomatic from either pressure or hypopituitarism, including diabetes insipidus. When suprasellar extension is present, headaches and visual field defects can occur.

The Rathke's cleft cyst contains watery to mucinous fluid, and it is lined by columnar epithelium (Fig. 14.11) or ciliated cuboidal epithelium with occasional goblet cells. Squamous metaplasia, xanthomatous inflammation, and amyloid deposition can be seen.

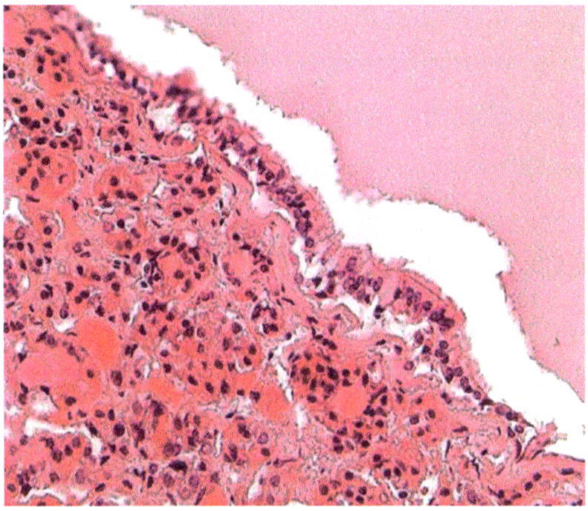

FIGURE 14.11 Rathke's pouch cyst. Note the ciliated cuboidal epithelium adjacent to pituitary parenchyma, with a colloid-filled cyst (H&E).

14.6.3. Cysts

Arachnoid cysts, congenital or acquired, and *dermoid* or, more commonly, *epidermoid cysts* originating from ectopic or implanted epithelial cells can be found in the sella or parasellar regions. The clinical presentation of patients with these cysts is due to the mass effect from suprasellar extension or hypopituitarism due to pituitary compression.

14.6.4. Pituitary aplasia and hypoplasia

Congenital absence of the pituitary is rare and is usually associated with hypoplasia of the adrenals, thyroid, and gonads. Even if the anterior pituitary is not formed, the posterior pituitary may be present. Pituitary hypoplasia is an incomplete pituitary gland development due to atrophy or a developmental defect. It may be associated with anencephaly, where the number of cells may be normal, but the ACTH-producing cells are decreased and have poorly developed organelles.

14.6.5. Empty sella syndrome

Empty sella syndrome refers to a condition in which the sella appears fluid-filled radiologically. The syndrome may be either primary or secondary. The primary empty sella syndrome is a developmental disorder due to incomplete development of the diaphragma sella. The arachnoid membrane invaginates and compresses the pituitary. This condition is usually asymptomatic; however, imaging studies may reveal an enlarged sella, mimicking a PitNET. The secondary empty sella syndrome occurs after resection, irradiation, necrosis, or infarction of a PitNET.

14.7. OTHER LESIONS

14.7.1. Familial genetic disorders associated with PitNETs

The great majority of PitNETs occur in a sporadic way. These tumors are clonal, but only a minority have documented genetic alterations. The rare cases arising in a familial setting have clarified the involved pathways.

PitNETs are integral components of type 1 multiple endocrine neoplasia syndrome (MEN1), an autosomal dominant disorder resulting from mutations in the *MEN1* gene, a tumor suppressor gene on chromosome 11q13. The menin1 protein is an important component of chromatin-remodeling complexes, and mutations lead to hyperplasia and neoplasms of the pituitary, pancreas, and parathyroid glands (Table 14.7). Both alleles of MEN1 have to be mutated to develop pituitary neoplasia: One copy harbors an inherited germline mutation, and the other copy acquires a somatic mutation. Other genes may be mutated, and some hormonal factors may be involved both in the formation of PitNET and in the hormone production of PitNET associated with MEN1. The PitNETs in the MEN1 syndrome are usually hormonally active, with a preponderance of PRL or GH production.

Carney complex is due to mutations in a component of protein kinase A (*PRKAR1A*). Affected patients develop pigmented mucosal and skin lesions; multiple myxomas; endocrine tumors, including PitNET; ovarian and testicular tumors; and Cushing syndrome due to a pigmented nodular adrenal disease.

Familial isolated somatotropinoma and familial isolated pituitary adenoma, which can result from mutations in the *AIP* gene, is a familial syndrome that predisposes patients to GH-producing PitNETs.

PitNETs may occur in the pheochromocytoma/paraganglioma syndromes associated with germline mutations in the genes for succinate dehydrogenase (SDHA-D). This syndrome predisposes the development of tumors of diverse organs, including renal cell carcinomas and gastrointestinal stromal tumor, besides paragangliomas and pheochromocytomas.

Table 14.7 Inherited Genetic Susceptibility to Pituitary Tumors

DISEASE	GENE(S)	PITUITARY LESIONS (IN ORDER OF FREQUENCY)	ASSOCIATED CLINICAL FEATURES
Isolated Pituitary Tumors			
Familial isolated pituitary adenoma	*AIP* or unknown	Somatotroph, lactotroph, mammosomatotroph, corticotroph, and other tumors Rarely, somatotroph hyperplasia	/
X-linked acrogigantism	*GPR101a*	Mammosomatotroph adenomas and/or hyperplasia	/
Syndromes Associated with Pituitary Tumors			
Multiple endocrine neoplasia type 1	*MEN1*	Lactotroph, nonfunctioning, somatotroph, and corticotroph tumors Multiple or plurihormonal tumors Somatotroph or mammosomatotroph hyperplasia	Primary hyperparathyroidism and duodenopancreatic neuroendocrine tumors Rarely cutaneous tumors, central nervous system tumors, and breast cancer
Multiple endocrine neoplasia type 4	*CDKN1B*	Somatotroph, nonfunctioning, and corticotroph tumors	Primary hyperparathyroidism and duodenopancreatic neuroendocrine tumors
Carney complex	*PRKAR1A*	Somatotroph, lactotroph, and corticotroph tumors Mammosomatotroph or somatotroph hyperplasia	Cardiac, endocrine, cutaneous, and neural tumors; variety of pigmented lesions of the skin and mucosae
McCune–Albright syndrome	*GNAS* (mosaic)	Mammosomatotroph and somatotroph tumors Mammosomatotroph or somatotroph hyperplasia	Fibrous dysplasia of bone, café-au-lait skin macules, and endocrinopathies (thyroid, gonadal, adrenal abnormalities)
Leigh syndrome	*SDHA*	Lactotroph, somatotroph, gonadotroph, and (rarely) corticotroph tumors	Phaeochromocytoma, thoracoabdominal paraganglioma, head and neck paraganglioma, clear cell renal cell carcinoma, gastrointestinal stromal tumor
Carney–Stratakis syndrome	*SDHB, SDHC, SDHD*	Lactotroph, somatotroph, gonadotroph, and (rarely) corticotroph tumors	Phaeochromocytoma, thoracoabdominal paraganglioma, clear cell renal cell carcinoma, gastrointestinal stromal tumor

Table 14.7 Continued

DISEASE	GENE(S)	PITUITARY LESIONS (IN ORDER OF FREQUENCY)	ASSOCIATED CLINICAL FEATURES
DICER1 syndrome	*DICER1*	Pituitary blastoma (majority ACTH-secreting; rarely, growth hormone-secreting and prolactin-secreting)	Pleuropulmonary blastoma, thyroid follicular nodular disease, differentiated thyroid carcinoma in children, and other neoplasms
Neurofibromatosis type 1	*NF1*	Corticotroph and somatotroph adenomas Pituitary duplication	Pigmentary lesions (café-au-lait macules, skinfold freckling, and Lisch nodules) and dermal neurofibromas
Lynch syndrome	*MSH2, MSH6, MLH1, PMS2*	Corticotroph and lactotroph tumors	Colorectal cancer and endometrial cancer Less frequent: stomach, pancreas, urinary tract, ovary, prostate cancer
USP8-related syndrome	*USP8*	Corticotroph tumors	

14.7.2. Metastatic neoplasms to the pituitary gland

Metastatic neoplasms to the pituitary gland are rare (Fig. 14.12). The metastases are usually from carcinomas in patients with widespread systemic metastases. Metastatic sarcomas are extremely rare. Metastases often present with diabetes insipidus due to involvement of the posterior lobe. The most common primary sites of origin are breast, prostate, and lung. In some cases, the anterior lobe can be the only region involved by metastatic tumor; in such cases, the differential diagnosis includes PitNETs, which can be resolved by immunohistochemistry (Table 14.8).

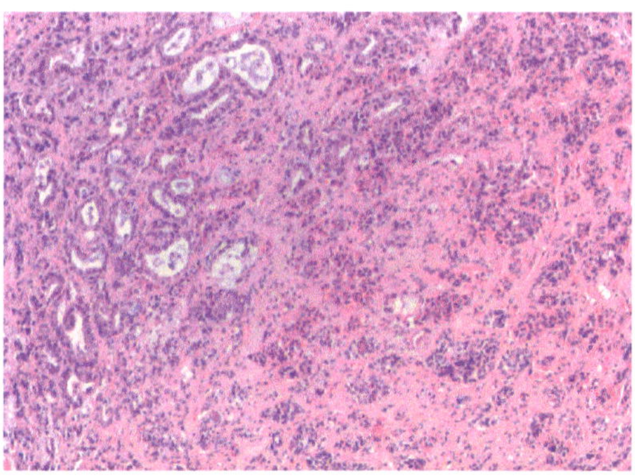

FIGURE 14.12 Metastatic carcinoma involving the pituitary gland. The malignant glandular cells (on the left) are surrounded by pituitary acinar cells (on the right). The patient had widely metastatic lung adenocarcinoma.

14.7.3. Tumors of the hypothalamus, neurohypophysis, and sellar region

The sellar region has a variety of tissues and cell types, including the central and peripheral nervous systems, endocrine, germinal, epithelial, meningeal, mesenchymal, and hematopoietic cells. In addition to the great variety of neoplasms that can occur in this region, the neoplasms can mimic each other clinically and morphologically, making the classification of tumors in this region difficult.

14.7.3.1. CRANIOPHARYNGIOMA

Although craniopharyngiomas are uncommon neoplasms overall, they are the second most common neoplasm of the sellar region, second only to PitNETs, and the most common sellar/suprasellar neoplasm in children, in whom PitNETs are rare. Usual symptoms include headache and visual changes, such as diplopia, as well as endocrine abnormalities. Two types of craniopharyngioma have been defined based on histologic and molecular features.

Table 14.8 Immunoreactivity of Tumors of the Pituitary and Sellar Region

TUMOR	PITUITARY HORMONES	EMA	CK	S100 PROTEIN	SYN	CHROMOGRANIN	CEA	PLAP	LCA	VIMENTIN
PitNET	+ (null cell –)	ACTH +	ACTH + GH ±	–	+	Null cell > LH/FSH, TSH	–	–	–	–
Metastatic carcinoma	–	+	+	±	±	±	±		–	±
Myeloma	–	±	–	–	–	–	–	–	±	–
Germinoma	–	–	10% +	–	–	–	–	+	–	15% +
Granular cell tumor	–	–	–	+	–	–	±	–	–	+
Chordoma	–	+	+	+	–	–	+10%	–	–	+

ACTH, adrenocorticotrophic hormone; CEA, carcinoembryonic antigen; CK, cytokeratin; EMA, epithelial membrane antigen; FSH, follicle-stimulating hormone; GH, growth hormone; LCA, leukocyte common antigen; LH, luteinizing hormone; PLAP, placental alkaline phosphatase; SYN, synaptophysin; TSH, thyroid-stimulating hormone.

Adamantinomatous craniopharyngiomas (ACPs) occur in both children and adults and are usually cystic, irregular nodular masses of firm tissue with yellow-brown viscid contents, often described as "crankcase oil" (Fig. 14.13A). The fluid contains cholesterol crystals. These tumors have well-differentiated neoplastic epithelium arranged in cords, lobules, and whorls with basal palisading. Some areas have loosely arranged microcystic areas called stellate reticulum. There are often nests of anucleated squamous ghost cells called *wet keratin*. A squamous cell pattern with keratinization can be intermixed with the adamantinomatous, forming a mixed pattern (Fig. 14.13B, C). The tumors frequently contain calcific debris, cholesterol clefts, and foreign body giant cells.

Most ACPs harbor mutations in the *CTNNB1* gene, which encodes the β-catenin protein, a major component of the Wnt signaling pathway. The mutations are in *CTNNB1* exon 3, disrupting phosphorylation by GSK-3b and subsequent proteasome-mediated degradation. Accumulation of β-catenin results in nuclear translocation. However, this occurs in only a subset of the neoplastic epithelial cells, which coincides with SHH, BMP, and FGF expression and is common in cells present in whorls. Currently, there are no effective system medical treatments for ACP. Radical excision is potentially curative but is seldom accomplished, and it may lead to hypothalamic dysfunction and psychological abnormalities as well as hypopituitarism. Despite their designation as WHO grade 1 tumors, ACPs commonly recur. Radiation therapy can play a role in combined management.

Papillary craniopharyngiomas (PCPs) occur almost exclusively in adults. These tumors exhibit distinctive histologic features compared to ACPs, including squamous epithelium covering fibrovascular cores, lack of wet keratin, lack of basal palisading, calcification, and cholesterol

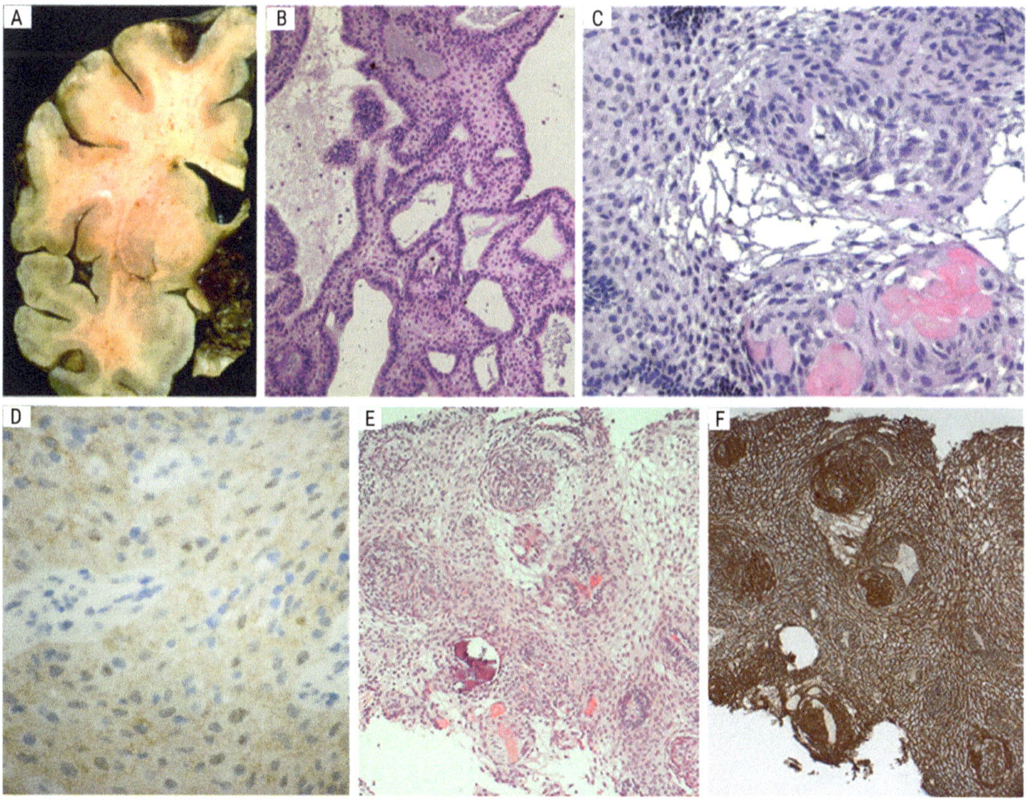

FIGURE 14.13 Craniopharyngioma: (**A**) gross appearance on coronal section showing a craniopharyngioma occupying the region of the hypothalamus; (**B**) adamantinomatous pattern with the basaloid epithelium (H&E); (**C**) lacy type of epithelial maturation with keratin nests; (**D**) BRAF mutant protein cytoplasmic positivity in a papillary craniopharyngioma (BRAF V600E IHC); (**E**) epithelium in islands with whorls and calcification in adamantinomatous craniopharyngioma (H&E); (**F**) β-catenin nuclear localization in whorls in an adamantinomatous type (β-catenin IHC).

crystals. These tumors are managed surgically with combined radiation therapy, as needed. PCPs have *BRAF* mutations and respond to *BRAF/MEK* targeted therapies (Fig. 14.13D). They do not have nuclear β-catenin localization.

14.7.3.2. GRANULAR CELL TUMORS

Granular cell tumors are benign tumors of the neurohypophysis or distal pituitary stalk with uncertain histogenesis. Most are slow-growing tumors, and affected patients are asymptomatic. When careful pituitary sectioning is performed, the tumors may be found incidentally in 1–17% of autopsies. Macroscopically, they are firm, well-demarcated, nonencapsulated tumors. The characteristic histological findings are similar to those for granular cell tumors of other locations, with clusters of plump cells with abundant eosinophilic granular cytoplasm and uniform small round nuclei.

14.7.3.3. CHORDOMA

Chordomas of the sellar region, clivus, and sphenoid bone account for approximately half of all chordomas, corresponding to the most cranial portion of the notochord. Visual field changes are the most common presentation, and bony destruction of the sella and clivus is frequent. The myxoid multilobular neoplasm has characteristic histological features. It is composed of cords of epithelioid cells, with vacuolated physaliferous cells (Fig. 14.14) containing mucin. The extracellular matrix is Alcian blue positive, and the cells express the brachyury protein, encoded by the *TBXT* gene.

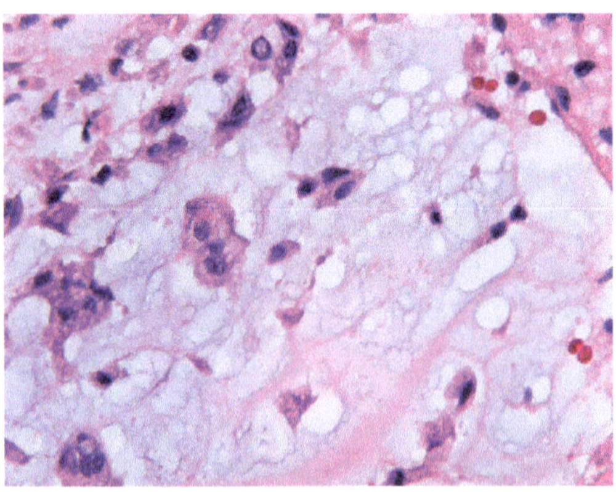

FIGURE 14.14 Chordoma. The neoplasm is derived from notochord and has a similar histological appearance (H&E).

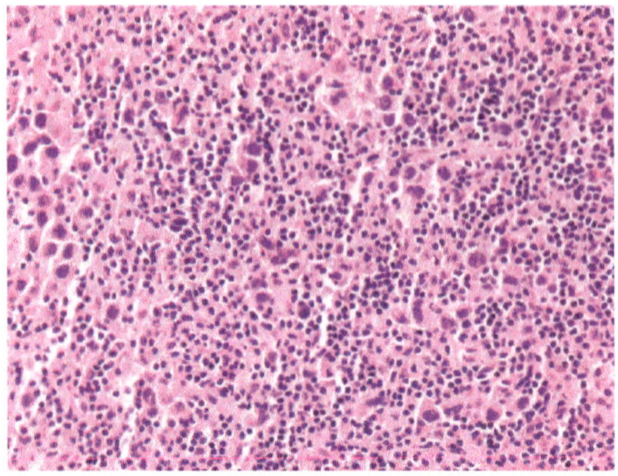

FIGURE 14.15 Germinoma. The histology shows a densely cellular tumor composed mostly of lymphocytes, with less frequent interspersed larger malignant germinoma cells with clear cytoplasm and prominent nucleoli (H&E).

14.7.3.4. GERM CELL TUMORS

Germ cell tumors (GCTs) are usually in the midline and derived from residual germ cells. The GCTs of the pituitary and suprasellar sites are rare and include germinomas (Fig. 14.15), embryonal carcinomas, endodermal sinus tumors, teratomas, and choriocarcinomas. The histological findings are identical to those for the corresponding extra-gonadal germ cell tumors found elsewhere. Suprasellar GCTs occur more often in females, whereas pineal region GCTs occur more often in males. Expression of OCT4 and NANOG, two transcription factors that are involved in stem cell pluripotency, is characteristic of these lesions.

14.7.3.5. PLASMACYTOMA

A difficult histological differential diagnosis from PitNET is a plasmacytoma of the sellar region (Fig. 14.16). The majority of the sellar plasmacytomas will evolve into systemic multiple myeloma. Immunohistochemistry is helpful in distinguishing these entities.

14.7.3.6. HAMARTOMA OR CHORISTOMA

Hamartomas or choristomas are rare and located usually in the hypothalamus. Hamartomas are lesions attached to the tuber cinereum or the mammillary bodies, located usually behind the pituitary stalk. The patient may present with visual

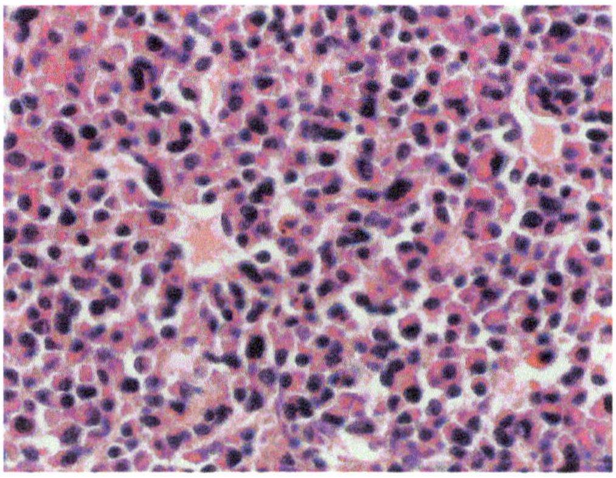

FIGURE 14.16 Plasmacytoma: a rare neoplasm of the pituitary, usually in association with systemic multiple myeloma, composed of pleomorphic plasma cells (H&E).

field defects or endocrinologic disturbances, such as precocious puberty. The association of neuronal hamartomas and GH-producing PitNET has suggested that the GH-releasing factor has a paracrine effect. Hamartomas and choristomas are firm, round masses formed by mature neurons in clusters separated by unmyelinated axons.

14.7.3.7. OTHER TUMORS

Other primary neoplasms in the region of the sella turcica are rare and include meningioma, paraganglioma, oligodendroglioma, ependymoma, glioma, esthesioneuroblastoma, Langerhans cell histiocytosis, fibromas, sarcomas, giant cell tumor of bone, osteosarcoma, melanoma, vascular tumors, and lymphomas, among others (Table 14.3).

Appendix

Brief Survey of Neuropathology Techniques

DAVID MEREDITH AND FRANCK BIELLE

The practice of neuropathology depends on several specialized techniques, some of which are derived from those used in general pathology.

A.1. METHODS OF REMOVAL

A.1.1. Autopsy

Autopsy of the nervous system cannot be regarded as an isolated procedure, and the findings should be correlated with those of the general autopsy. The procedure should be performed without delay because the central nervous system (CNS) deteriorates very rapidly, resulting in postmortem autolysis. CNS tissue is delicate, and being enclosed within bony structures (skull and spine), dissection is complex and requires special training.

A.1.1.1. REMOVAL OF THE SPINAL CORD

Removal of the spinal cord may proceed at the beginning of the autopsy or can occur after evisceration (anterior approach) or via the posterior approach when the entire length of the spinal cord and dorsal root ganglia need to be examined. The procedure includes the following steps:

A.1.1.1.1. Posterior approach

- The body is turned face down.
- The skin and underlying soft tissues are incised along the spinous processes from the external occipital protuberance to the base of the sacrum.
- The soft tissues are freed, first with the knife and then with a scraper, to expose the vertebral

lamina on either side of the spinous processes. The prosector should angle the blade of the saw to cut as far laterally as possible from the posterior spinous processes.
- The vertebral laminae are then sectioned along the entire spine.
- The spinous processes down the length of the dissection, together with their connecting tendinous aponeuroses, are lifted and pulled off.
- The rostral end of the cervical cord, as high up as possible, is severed with a scalpel.
- The spinal cord is then carefully removed by lifting the dura with a pair of forceps at each segmental level, working carefully from the top, down to the cauda equina, cutting with a scalpel or scissors each of the spinal nerve roots and sequentially dissecting out the dorsal root ganglia.

A.1.1.1.2. Anterior approach

- The bodies of the vertebrae are exposed and the peduncles of the vertebrae are cut along the length of the cord. The anterior vertebral arch is then lifted, and the spinal cord is removed following the procedure described above.

Once the cord is removed, the dural sheath is opened longitudinally with scissors along the midline, on both the dorsal and ventral surface, to identify any lesions and to permit better penetration by the fixative and thus avoid possible shrinkage and distortion of the underlying cord.

The spinal cord is then stretched out flat, secured on a cardboard or other suitable surface, and fixed by immersion in 10% formalin.

A.1.1.2. REMOVAL OF THE BRAIN

Removal of the brain entails the following steps:

- The body is laying face up.
- The scalp is incised along a coronal plane from one pinna to the other.
- The scalp is freed and reflected forward up to the supraorbital ridges and backward to the external occipital protuberance.
- The cranial cavity is opened with an electric saw.
- The skullcap thus obtained is lifted by exerting firm traction from front to back, using the wedge of the autopsy hammer inserted in the center of the cut frontal bone. The dura should remain intact up to this point.
- The dura is then incised first longitudinally, approximately 2 cm on either side of the midline from front to back, and then in a semicircular fashion, along the edge of the cut bone.
- The anterior attachment of the falx cerebri is incised down to the crista galli.
- The olfactory bulbs are lifted and gently dissected off the base of the skull.
- The frontal lobes are very gradually raised and freed from front to back, sequentially sectioning with scissors the anterior connecting structures (optic nerves, internal carotid arteries, pituitary stalk).
- The tentorium cerebelli is incised along the outer edge of its attachment to the upper border of the petrous bone.
- The posterior connecting structures (cranial nerves, vertebral arteries) are sectioned while, with one hand, the prosector supports the brain, which will otherwise tend to topple backward.
- The brain is then removed; with one hand, the prosector continues to support the brain while placing the palm of the other hand on the ventral surface of the pons, inserting the index finger to the left and the middle finger to the right of the medulla. If the spinal cord has not been removed beforehand, it will be necessary to section the upper cervical cord with a long, thin scalpel. The cut end of the medulla is then extracted, following which the prosector inserts two fingers under each cerebellar hemisphere. With the left hand, the prosector is then able to lift the entire brain, and it only remains for the dura of the posterior fossa to be incised for the brain to be completely freed.
- The brain is weighed.
- A string is tied dorsal to the basilar artery (or other method of suspending the brain), and the brain is immediately immersed in 10% formalin, base facing up, within a receptacle large enough to allow it to float and thus avoid future distortion resulting from potential postmortem compression.

In cases of suspected infection, meningeal swabs or portions of the brain itself are sent to the microbiology laboratory for culture. These specimens must be secured before immersion of the brain in formalin. Similarly, if the case is part of a research protocol, or if tissue is needed for biochemical analysis, selected samples are taken and, if necessary, frozen before fixation.

A.1.1.3. REMOVAL OF PORTIONS OF THE PERIPHERAL NERVOUS SYSTEM AND SAMPLES OF THE SKELETAL MUSCULATURE

The removal of samples of skeletal muscle and peripheral nerves is both easy and essential, although because of various artifacts, histopathological examination of autopsy material gives less valuable information than examination of biopsies. In obtaining these samples, it is important to avoid multiple skin incisions and disfigurement of the body.

A.1.1.4. SPECIAL PROCEDURES

Removal of the spinal cord, brain, samples of peripheral nervous system, and skeletal musculature is part of a complete routine autopsy. Removal of the pituitary gland is part of any routine autopsy. In some cases, these procedures may be supplemented by dissection of certain areas of the body that are not ordinarily examined as part of a routine autopsy procedure. This includes, for example, removal of the eyes and petrous portion of the temporal bone and inner ear, examination and sampling of the base and the vault of the skull, and removal en bloc of the cervical spine to include the vasculature of the neck.

Consent must be obtained if necropsy studies are to be performed. Indeed, the legal consent requirements for the autopsy have greatly changed in many areas of the world, and the prosector must adhere to the authorization as stipulated in the autopsy consent, including, for example, when determining if retention of organs is permitted or if it is required that any of these be returned to the body. In general, even if organs are to be returned for funeral arrangements, most permits allow for retention of small portions of tissue necessary for diagnosis. The physician requesting the autopsy must inform the family that a restricted autopsy will necessarily limit the extent of information expected from a postmortem examination under such circumstances. This limitation is particularly problematic regarding a nonhomogeneous organ, such as the brain. Tissue retained for research purposes may require specific consent in many countries.

A.1.2. Surgical specimens

Neurosurgical specimens must be immediately placed in fixative after their removal by the neurosurgeon. Ideally, separate portions of the specimen should also be snap frozen for molecular studies in most brain tumor biopsy, in muscle and nerve biopsy specimens, and in cases in which there is a strong clinical suspicion of prion disease or certain infectious diseases.

For purposes of intraoperative consultation with the neurosurgeon, frozen sections and smear and touch preparations are prepared; these permit a general diagnostic assessment to be rendered within a few minutes. This information can be very useful, providing the intrinsic interpretative shortcomings of the procedure are recognized by all involved.

A.1.3. Biopsy procedures

A.1.3.1. MUSCLE BIOPSY

Muscle biopsy is a minor surgical procedure, but it is important to stress the strict and meticulous technical care with which it must be performed. Muscle tissue is indeed very delicate, and if it is not removed with all necessary precautions, the microscopic evaluation of lesions may be hampered by the presence of artifacts (see Chapter 12). The operation is performed under local anesthesia, care being taken not to inject the local anesthetic beneath the level of the investing aponeurotic fascia. The incision should be generous enough to permit easy dissection of the muscle. After the deep fascia has been incised, the muscle is dissected by following the plane of cleavage of the muscle bundles in a direction parallel to that of the muscle fibers. A segment of muscle measuring approximately 2 cm in length by 1 cm in thickness (smaller in young children) is then isolated, care being taken to avoid traction, and, finally, sectioned at either end (Fig. A.1).

A.1.3.2. PERIPHERAL NERVE BIOPSY

Biopsy of a sensory peripheral nerve is most commonly performed on the sural nerve at its retromalleolar portion, midway between the lateral malleolus and the Achilles tendon. It may also be done on the musculocutaneous (superficial peroneal) nerve at the junction of the middle and inferior thirds of the lateral surface of the lower leg. This permits concomitant sampling of the peroneus brevis muscle (see Chapter 13). A skin incision is made 1 cm anterior to a line that joins the head of the fibula to the lateral malleolus, two-thirds of the way to the malleolus (Fig. A.2A, B). A 2-cm-long segment of the entire nerve (Fig. A.2A), or

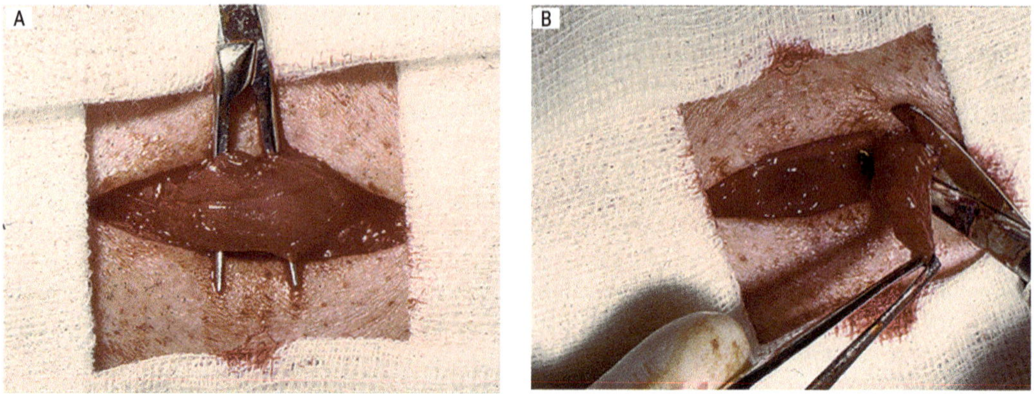

FIGURE A.1 Muscle biopsy: (**A**) dissection and isolation; (**B**) removal of muscle fragment.

a selected number of fascicles within the nerve (Fig. A.2B), may be sampled, first by sectioning the proximal end of the nerve. Care must be taken to avoid compressing the nerve. Peripheral nerve biopsy results in permanent hypesthesia of the dorsum of foot and sometimes paresthesias.

A.1.3.3. BRAIN BIOPSY

Diagnostic biopsy of the cerebral cortex or subcortical lesions is performed in selected cases in which crucial diagnostic information is unrevealing by noninvasive studies. After administration of the local anesthetic and incision of the scalp, a small disk of bone is drilled with the lobotomy trephine, the dura is incised, and a small fragment of cortex and underlying white matter is removed with the scalpel or a cutting curette. Following this procedure, the bone disk is placed back in position, and the scalp is closed. The risk of hemorrhage, infection, reactive edema, or post-traumatic epilepsy is minimal ordinarily.

A.1.3.4. STEREOTACTIC BIOPSY

Stereotactic biopsy samplings are obtained with a trocar guided by computed tomography/magnetic resonance imaging (CT/MRI). The indications for stereotactic biopsy most often involve expanding space-occupying lesions, especially tumors.

A.1.3.5. OTHER BIOPSY PROCEDURES

In some neurological disorders, particularly lipidoses, rectal biopsy is sometimes performed to examine the ganglion cells of Meissner's plexus. It is also possible to examine these structures in the intestinal appendix. Skin and conjunctival biopsies may provide additional information in some cases (e.g., capillary blood vessel walls, terminal nerve

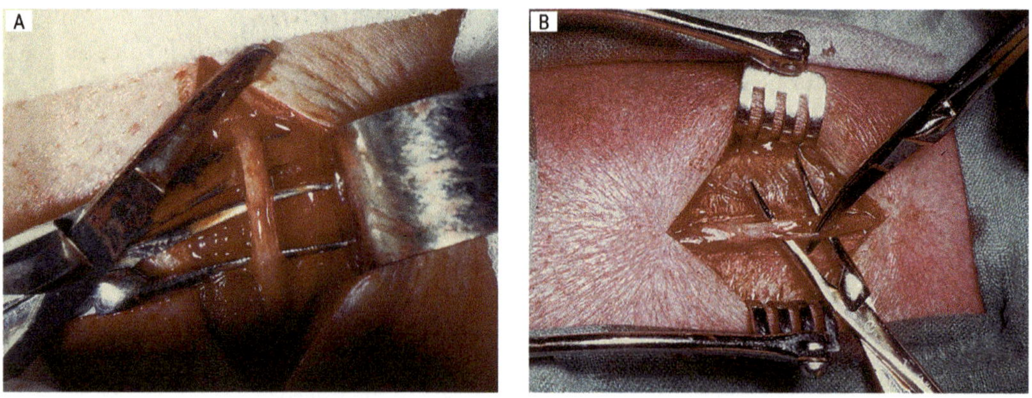

FIGURE A.2 Peripheral nerve biopsy: (**A**) dissection of a fragment of the superficial branch of the musculocutaneous nerve of the leg; (**B**) removal of nerve segment.

endings, and cellular inflammatory infiltrates). Skin biopsy can be used to obtain fibroblast cultures, allowing for genetic analysis in hereditary diseases, although with the advent of more sophisticated methods for molecular diagnosis, these procedures are now less frequent.

A.1.4. Cerebrospinal fluid cytologic examination

Cytologic study of the lumbar puncture cerebrospinal fluid (CSF) is a simple and rapid method of diagnosis. It allows for the study of neoplastic and inflammatory processes spreading through the CSF pathways. Sampling of CSF for cytologic analysis can also be obtained by the neurosurgeon during operative procedures.

A.2. FIXATION OF TISSUES

Formalin is almost always the fixative of choice used in routine surgical neuropathology. The most frequently employed formalin concentration is 10% formalin (3.7% formaldehyde), which is widely available commercially as a neutral buffered solution. This percentage formalin represents a solution prepared by mixing 10 mL of commercial formalin with 90 mL of buffered aqueous solution.

The amount of fixative to be used depends on the amount of tissue to be fixed and should be approximately 15–20 times the volume of tissue. Thus, for the brain, 5 or 6 L of a formalin solution is required for optimum results; the fixative may be renewed at regular intervals.

Good fixation requires a minimum amount of time, depending on the size of the tissue (2 or 3 weeks for a whole brain). The preservation of tissues in formalin is almost indefinite, provided the fluid, which turns yellow with age, is changed from time to time and provided the container is well sealed to avoid evaporation. Long-term fixation or decalcification will jeopardize some staining procedures and immunohistochemical techniques.

A.3. MACROSCOPIC EXAMINATION OF THE CENTRAL NERVOUS SYSTEM

Gross dissection of the CNS (brain and spinal cord) is performed traditionally after 2 or 3 weeks of formalin fixation; some have preferred to shorten this period of fixation, but in our opinion this is not the best approach. When organs are required to be returned to the body, the brain must be cut fresh and photographed. Selected blocks are then fixed in formalin for shorter time periods.

Tissue for microbiological, toxicological, or molecular studies or for brain banking must be obtained fresh at the time of autopsy.

A.3.1. Inspection of the brain and spinal cord

The brain and spinal cord are carefully examined, and any abnormal or interesting features are recorded on schematic diagrams and photographed before and after fixation.

A.3.2. Cutting of gross slices

A.3.2.1. USUAL PROTOCOL

The usual protocol includes the following steps:

- *Severing the cerebral hemispheres from the brainstem.* The arachnoid membranes, which usually obscure the structures of the interpeduncular fossa and the floor of the third ventricle, are first delicately removed with forceps or fine scissors. The blood vessels of the circle of Willis are then inspected, and the cranial nerves are identified in sequence. The posterior fossa structures are then separated from the supratentorial portion of the brain by cutting through the rostral part of the cerebral peduncles with a scalpel, along a plane parallel to the base of the brain.
- *Coronal hemispheric slices.* The brain resting on the convexity is placed sideways on a suitable cutting board. The first section is through the mammillary bodies, and all subsequent sections are cut from the base by placing the cut surface flat on the board and cutting slices parallel to the ground at approximately 1-cm thick from the frontal to the occipital poles (Figs. A.3 and A.4). The slices are then placed on an examining board in sequence from front to back.
- *Horizontal sections through the brainstem and cerebellum.* Without separating the cerebellum from the brainstem, horizontal sections approximately 1 cm thick are cut from the

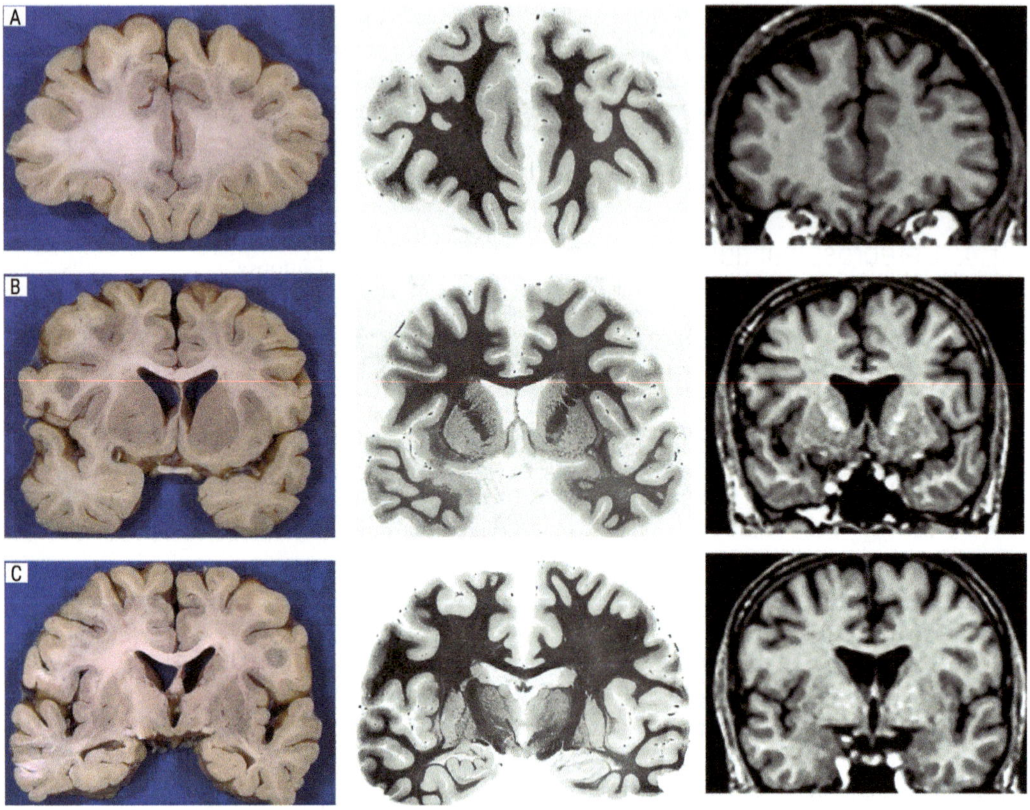

FIGURE A.3 Coronal sections through the cerebral hemispheres: gross appearance after fixation (*left*); myelin stain of corresponding slices after celloidin embedding (*middle*); corresponding T1-weighted MRI images (*right*). (**A**) Frontal poles; (**B**) section through the rostral portion of the basal ganglia; (**C**) section through the mammillary bodies. (MRI images courtesy of Dr. Liangge Hsu, Brigham and Women's Hospital, Boston, MA.)

cerebral peduncles to the medulla (Fig. A.5). An alternative method is to separate the brainstem from the cerebellum by cutting through the peduncles. In such a case, the cerebellar hemispheres are hemisected in the sagittal plane at the vermis and subsequently cut in the same plane from medial to lateral. The brainstem is then cut in serial horizontal sections. For purposes of orientation at the time of microscopic examination, either the right or the left side of the brainstem (depending on convention) is nicked superficially.

- *Transverse sections through the spinal cord.* The spinal cord is placed flat on the cutting board, and transverse sections, approximately 1 cm thick, are made using a fresh razor blade held by forceps (Fig. A.6). For precise macroscopic localization of the segmental level of the cord lesion, careful counting of dorsal roots is required, usually by identifying the T1 level, just below the cervical enlargement, as a starting point.
- *Documentation.* After the hemispheric, brainstem, and spinal cord slices have been examined with the naked eye and a magnifying glass, the lesions are recorded on standard stenciled diagrams that depict the main neuroanatomic structures, and photographs are taken.

A.3.2.2. SECTIONING IN THE AXIAL PLANE OF COMPUTERIZED TOMOGRAPHY OR MRI

In some cases, it may be preferable to compare axial CT scan or MRI images to neuropathological data; the brain is then sectioned in the appropriate plane.

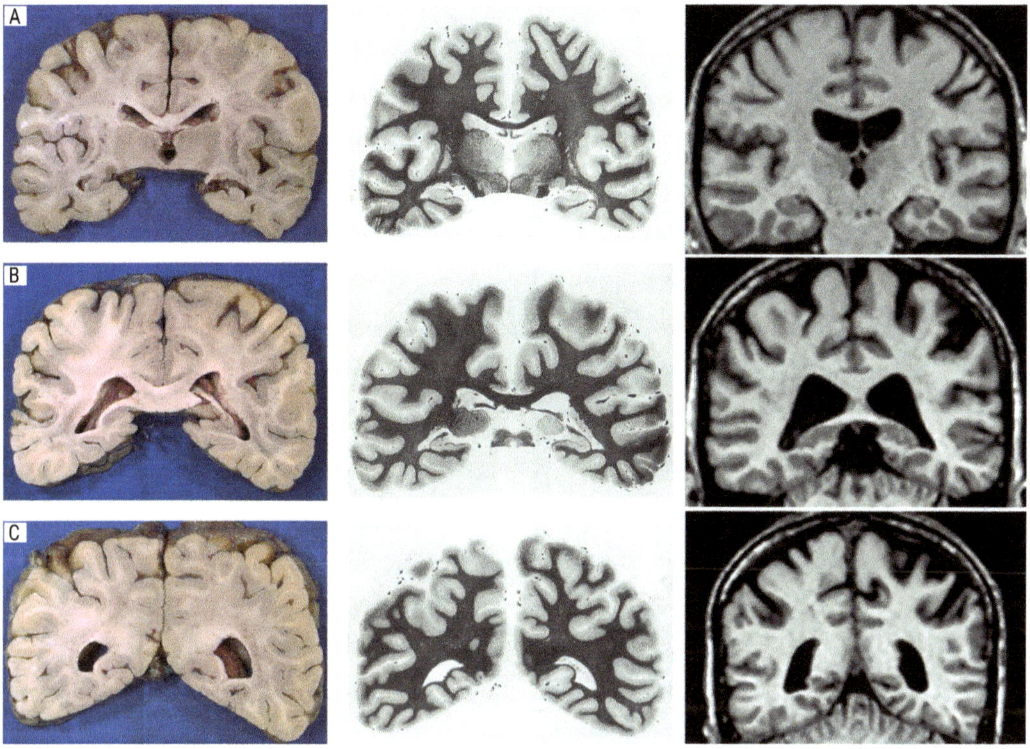

FIGURE A.4 Coronal sections through the cerebral hemispheres: gross appearance after fixation (*left*); myelin stain of corresponding slices after celloidin embedding (*middle*); corresponding T1-weighted MRI images (*right*). (**A**) Section through the thalamus and lateral geniculate bodies; (**B**) section through the splenium of the corpus callosum; (**C**) posterior section through the occipital horns. (MRI images courtesy of Dr. Liangge Hsu, Brigham and Women's Hospital, Boston, MA.)

A.3.3. Histological sampling

After the brain slices have been examined grossly, the tissue is sampled for histological study. In this selection, the neuropathologist is guided by the clinical data, the general autopsy findings, the gross study of the slices, and the type of histological technique to be applied to the tissues. The samples are then carefully identified and labeled. Many laboratories have a standardized series of blocks required, particularly for the systematic analysis of certain diseases (e.g., Alzheimer disease and other dementias).

A.4. EMBEDDING, SECTIONING, AND STAINING METHODS

The indications, advantages, and disadvantages of the various techniques are reviewed here solely in the context of neuropathological practice. For details on embedding and sectioning techniques, the reader is referred to general reference works on histological methods.

A.4.1. Paraffin embedding

- *Advantages*. In most neuropathology laboratories, paraffin embedding is the embedding method of choice for autopsy and biopsy samples. It is rapid and allows for relatively thin sections (5–7 μm) as well as serial or step sections. Many stains and immunostains can be performed on paraffin sections. Utilizing special microtomes, it is now also possible to cut large paraffin-embedded blocks of brain and even an entire slab of brain cut in the coronal or horizontal plane.
- *Disadvantages*. Paraffin embedding requires preliminary treatment with alcohol and toluene, which are lipid solvents. Part of the procedure

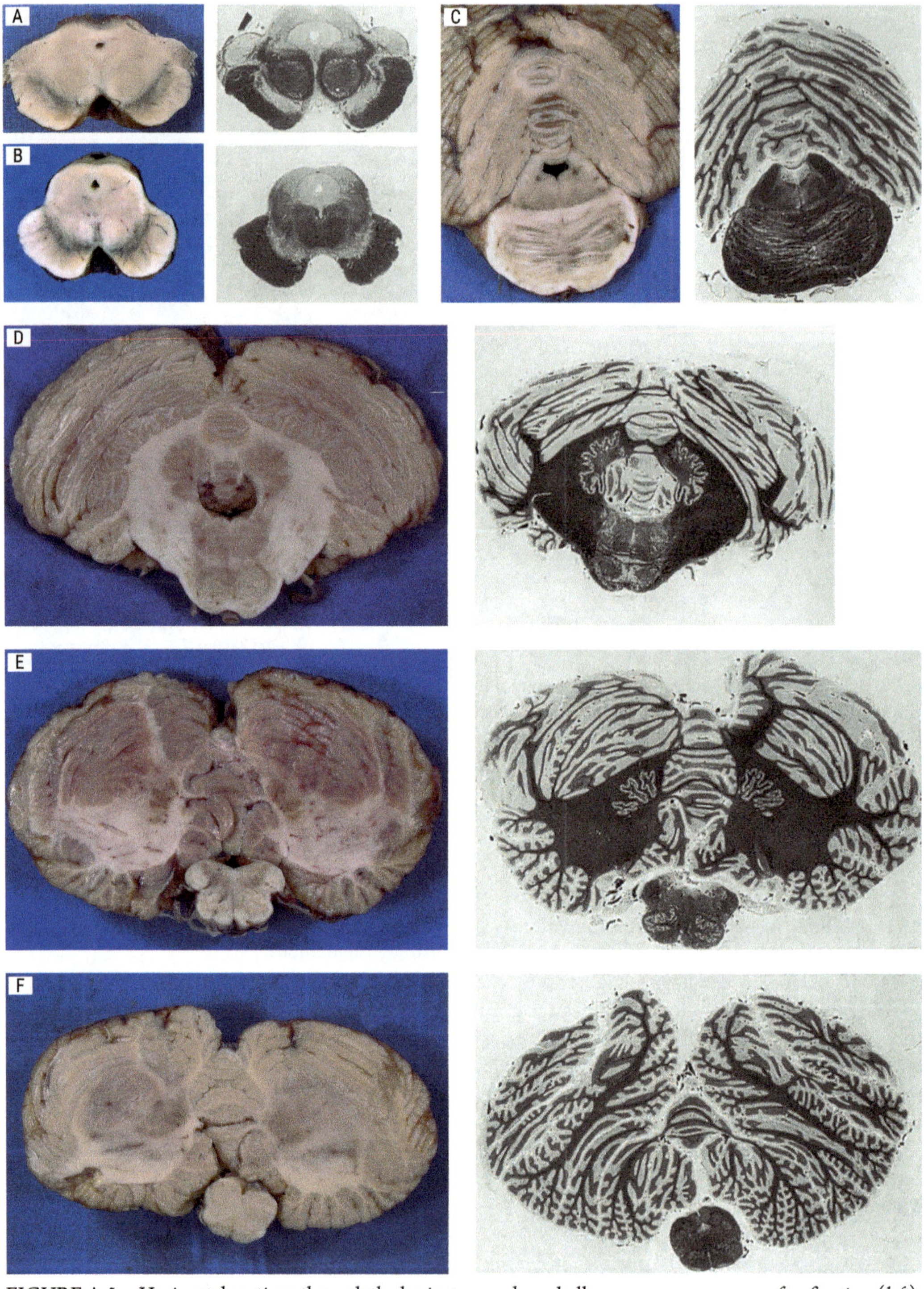

FIGURE A.5 Horizontal sections through the brainstem and cerebellum: gross appearance after fixation (*left*); myelin stain of corresponding slices after celloidin embedding (*right*). (**A**) Rostral midbrain (cerebral peduncles, red nuclei, superior colliculi); (**B**) caudal midbrain (dentatorubral decussation, inferior colliculi); (**C**) upper pons and superior cerebellar vermis; (**D**) midpons and cerebellar hemispheres with dentate nuclei; (**E**) upper medulla and cerebellar hemispheres with dentate nuclei and inferior vermis; (**F**) lower medulla and inferior portion of cerebellar hemispheres.

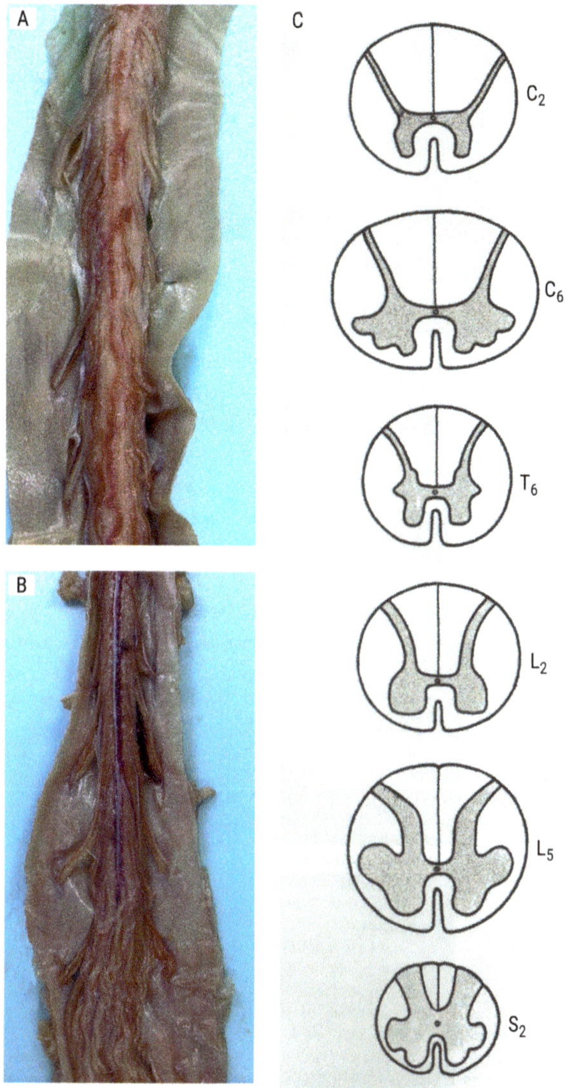

FIGURE A.6 Gross appearances of the spinal cord: (**A**) Cervicothoracic cord. Note the smaller thoracic roots compared to the cervical roots. (**B**) Lower part of spinal cord and cauda equina. Note exits of L1 roots from the dura at the level of conus medullaris. (**C**) Diagrammatic depiction of the gray and white matter of the spinal cord sectioned at various levels.

requires that the tissues be heated in an oven at a temperature of 56°C (for the paraffin to be melted). Nervous tissue tolerates this level of temperature relatively poorly, and this may result in some artifacts.

- *Stains.* See Table A.1.

A.4.2. Celloidin embedding

Celloidin embedding is no longer utilized in most laboratories throughout the world. It is mentioned here for completeness and in historical context.

- *Advantages.* The technique permitted embedding and sectioning of very large sections, such as a cerebral hemisphere or even an uncut whole brain.
- *Disadvantages.* The procedure has been abandoned because it is lengthy, time-consuming, and very expensive. Its use has been prohibited for safety reasons (mixture with explosive ether-alcohol).
- *Stains.* See Table A.1.

A.4.3. Frozen sections

- *Advantages.* The tissues are not processed through lipid solvents, thus permitting preservation of several cell constituents, which disappear after paraffin or celloidin embedding, and the application of special techniques (histochemistry, enzyme analysis, and immunocytochemistry) that are not always possible otherwise. Frozen sections can be examined under the microscope soon after removal of tissue (after a few minutes); this is of practical importance when rapid histological diagnosis is important (e.g., in intraoperative consultations of brain biopsies).
- *Disadvantages.* These sections are usually not as thin as those obtained after paraffin embedding. The technique also carries distinctive artifactual problems. The preparations are less permanent than embedded specimens.
- *Stains.* See Table A.1.

A.4.4. Special techniques

A.4.4.1. ELECTRON MICROSCOPY

For electron microscopy, immediate fixation is necessary. This is done with a buffered glutaraldehyde in solution at 0–4°C, followed by post-fixation in osmic acid.

A.4.4.2. IMMUNOHISTOCHEMISTRY

All immunohistochemistry (IHC) methods have as a common aim the visualization on histological sections of antigenic sites that have become immunoreactive with antibodies with which the sections have been incubated. These techniques may also be applied to dissociated cells, as in the CSF. There are numerous technical variants that are based on the demonstration of different antigens. These can be demonstrated by immunofluorescence or immunoperoxidase techniques. Various procedures may be used to retrieve the antigens. The specificity of monoclonal antibodies may sometimes be

Table A.1 Traditional Staining Methods

General histological stains		Hematoxylin–eosin
		Masson trichrome
		Van Gieson
Neuron stains	Nissl bodies	Thionin (Nissl variant)
		Cresyl violet
	Neurofibrils	Bielschowsky
		Gallyas
	Axons	Bodian
		Gros
Myelin stains		Luxol fast blue
		Heidenhain–Woelcke
Glial cell stains	Astrocytes	Holzer
		Mallory PTAH
	Microglia	Silver carbonate
Connective and vascular tissue stains	Collagen	Masson trichrome
	Reticulin	Van Gieson
		Perdrau
		Wilder
		Gordon–Sweets
		Gomori
		Laidlaw
		Foot
	Elastic fibers	Elastic tissue
		Van Gieson

Table A.2 Antibodies Widely Used in General Neuropathology

CELL TYPES	ANTIBODY	CHARACTERISTICS
Neuronal compartment	NF	Family of neuronal intermediate filaments: three subunits expressed separately or together (NFL, NFM, NFH)
	NeuN	"Neuron-specific nuclear protein"; expressed in several postmitotic neuronal cell types in the central and peripheral nervous systems; not expressed in Purkinje, mitral, and photoreceptor cells
	MAP2	Belongs to the microtubule-associated protein family
	Calbindin 2	Calcium-binding protein labeling interneurons; 29-kDa calbindin also known as calretinin
	Synaptophysin	Integral membrane protein of small synaptic vesicles
	Chromogranin	Secretory protein; found in secretory vesicles of neurons and endocrine cells
	APP	Amyloid-β (A4) precursor protein: a cell surface receptor and transmembrane precursor protein accumulated early in axonal lesions
Astrocytes	GFAP	Glial fibrillary acidic protein: filament of mature astrocytes
Oligodendrocytes	Olig2	Oligodendrocyte lineage transcription factor 2
Microglia	Iba-1	Calcium-binding protein, specifically expressed in macrophages/microglia
	CD68	110-kDa transmembrane glycoprotein highly expressed by human monocytes and tissue macrophages
Stem cells	Nestin	Intermediate filament protein that is expressed predominantly in stem cells of the CNS in the neural tube
Myelin	MBP	Myelin basic antibody
	PLP	Myelin proteolipid protein

superior to that of polyclonal antisera, but their sensitivity may be inferior.

Positive and negative controls are mandatory. IHC methods have replaced many staining techniques used in the past (Table A.1).

However, in some circumstances, the highly specific detection of a single target molecule may give a restricted view of a disease and may need to be combined with classical stains. Commonly used antibodies in general neuropathology are listed in Table A.2).

A.4.4.3. IN SITU HYBRIDIZATION

In situ hybridization refers to the utilization of nucleic acid probes (DNA or RNA) to demonstrate and localize within cells or tissues the nucleic acid sequences that show base pairing with the probe. The probes used are most often double-stranded DNA, less often single-stranded DNA or messenger RNA. The probes may be tagged with radioactive isotopes, such as ^{3}H, ^{32}P, or ^{35}S, or with nonradioactive compounds, such as biotin (so-called cold probes). With the former, demonstration is made by autoradiography; with the latter, it is made by different means—for example, by the avidin–biotin complex technique. Counting the silver grains in autoradiographs allows for semiquantitative analysis.

A.4.4.4. HISTOBLOT AND PARAFFIN-EMBEDDED TISSUE BLOT

The histoblot and paraffin-embedded tissue (PET) techniques are mainly used in prion protein research. Based on a combination of IHC and Western blot, they allow sensitive detection of the scrapie prion protein (PrPSc) isoforms and the analysis of their general distribution in different areas of the CNS. A nitrocellulose membrane is used instead of a glass slide as a mount for tissue sections. This porous membrane allows optimal proteolysis of the cellular isoform of the prion protein (proteinase K) and protein denaturation (guanidine thiocyanate), enhancing the immunoreactivity. Histoblot was first described using cryostat sections, but PET sections can also be processed. Both are more sensitive than IHC, which in turn has better cellular and subcellular resolution.

A.4.4.5. OTHER TECHNIQUES

Neurochemical studies must be performed on freshly unfixed material (e.g., biopsy samples or necropsy tissues that are promptly frozen).

For virological studies, particularly in tissue culture, sampling is performed in a sterile fashion on the brain in situ, after aseptic removal of the skullcap and dura.

A.5. MOLECULAR TECHNIQUES

As modern molecular tools have become increasingly more available and utilized, our understanding of the genetic basis of many CNS neoplasms has advanced tremendously. Similar advancements in IHC algorithms have permitted indirect assessment of genetics for many tumors in a quick and inexpensive fashion, especially for many laboratories that may not have access to advanced molecular testing. Several such antibodies are listed in Table A.3. A summary of the major diagnostic, prognostic, and predictive biomarkers for the most common CNS tumor types is presented next.

A.5.1. Diffuse gliomas

A.5.1.1. IDH MUTANT GLIOMAS

The IDH mutant gliomas show highly characteristic genetic signatures, which are easily separable from IDH wild-type tumors (Table A.4). Although high-grade tumors frequently exhibit multiple copy number alterations, distinct signatures for tumor progression have not yet been identified. Importantly, *MGMT* promoter methylation is

Table A.3 Immunohistochemical Markers for Common Mutation Events

MARKER	STAINING PATTERN	ABERRATION	TUMOR TYPES
p53	>10% positivity, nuclear	LOF mutations	Glioblastoma, IDH mutant astrocytoma
ATRX	Lost in tumor cells	LOF mutations	IDH mutant astrocytoma, diffuse midline/hemispheric glioma, small subset giant cell glioblastoma
IDH1 R132H	Positive, cytoplasmic and nuclear	GOF mutations	IDH mutant astrocytoma, oligodendroglioma
H3 K27M	Positive, nuclear	LOF mutation	Diffuse midline glioma
H3 K27me3	Lost in tumor cells	Surrogate marker for H3.3 K27M	Diffuse midline glioma
INI-1	Lost in tumor cells	Deletion, mutation	AT/RT, cribriform neuroepithelial tumor
SMARCA4	Lost in tumor cells	Deletion, mutation	AT/RT, small subset group 3/4 medulloblastomas
MYB	Positive, nuclear	MYB rearrangements	Angiocentric glioma
BRAF V600E	Positive, cytoplasmic	GOF mutation	Ganglioglioma, PXA, PA, DNET, pediatric DA, eGBM
LIN28A	Positive, nuclear	Marker of *C19MC* activation	EMTR
L1CAM	Positive, cytoplasmic	Marker of nuclear factor κB activation	ZFTA rearranged ependymomas, other gliomas
β-Catenin	Positive, nuclear	GOF mutation, WNT pathway activation	WNT-activated medulloblastoma

DA, diffuse astrocytoma; DNET, dysembryoplastic neuroepithelial tumor; eGBM, epithelioid glioblastoma; EMTR, embryonal tumor with multilayer rosettes; GOF, gain of function; LOF, loss of function; PA, pilocytic astrocytoma; PXA, pleomorphic xanthoastrocytoma.

Table A.4 Summary of Genomic Aberrations in Adult Gliomas

MARKER	ABERRATION	CLINICAL SIGNIFICANCE	IDH WILD TYPE	IDH MUTANT	METHOD OF DETECTION
MGMT	Promoter methylation	Prognostic, predictor of temozolomide response	50% methylated	>75% methylated	Bisulfite sequencing, MS-PCR, pyrosequencing
TERT	Promoter mutation	Diagnostic, prognostic	+	Oligo only	Sequencing
EGFR	Amplification, internal deletions (EGFRvIII), SNVs	Diagnostic, therapeutic target	40%	Rare	FISH, CMA, IHC, PCR, sequencing
PTEN	Deletion, LOF mutations	Diagnostic	Up to 95%	Rare	FISH, CMA, IHC, sequencing
PDGFRA	Amplification, mutations	Diagnostic, therapeutic target	13%	–	FISH, CMA, sequencing
TP53	LOF mutations, deletions	Prognostic	42%	Astro only	IHC, sequencing
CDKN2A/B	Homozygous deletions, LOF mutations	Diagnostic, prognostic	Up to 50%	May be present in high-grade tumors	FISH, CMA, sequencing
Polysomy 7	Whole-chromosome gain	Diagnostic	Up to 95%	Rare	FISH, CMA, sequencing
Monosomy 10	Whole-chromosome loss	Diagnostic	Up to 95%	Rare	FISH, CMA, sequencing
1p/19q	Whole arm codeletion	Diagnostic, prognostic	–	Oligo only	FISH, CMA, sequencing
ATRX	LOF mutations	Diagnostic	Subset of giant cell GBM	Astro only	IHC, sequencing
IDH1/2	GOF mutation	Diagnostic, prognostic, therapeutic target	–	+ (IDH2 mostly in oligos)	IHC (IDH1 R132H only), sequencing
CIC	LOF mutations	Diagnostic	–	Oligo only	Sequencing
FUBP1	LOF mutations	Diagnostic	–	Oligo only	Sequencing

CMA, chromosomal microarray; FISH, fluorescence in situ hybridization; GOF, gain of function; IHC, immunohistochemistry; LOF, loss of function; MS-PCR, methylation-specific polymerase chain reaction.

usually present in the vast majority (>75%) of IDH mutant tumors of all grades and classes.

A.5.1.2. IDH WILD-TYPE GLIOMAS

The IDH wild-type gliomas are driven primarily by copy number changes and often include amplification events that activate RTK/RAS/PI3K signaling. Their characteristic signature includes polysomy 7, monosomy 10, and homozygous deletion of CDKN2A/B. *TERT* promoter mutations are commonly seen, as are *TP53* mutations, although at a lower frequency than in IDH mutant astrocytomas. Amplifications of *EGFR* are present in roughly 40% of tumors, while amplifications of *PDGFRA, CDK4, CDK6, MDM2, MDM4,* and *MET* may also occur less frequently. Importantly, glioblastomas may show amplifications of multiple receptor tyrosine kinases, each present in a separate tumor subclone. This phenomenon of tumor heterogeneity can be easily demonstrated by fluorescence in situ hybridization (FISH), but array comparative genomic hybridization or sequencing assays may instead show low-level gains of these genes as each subclone's genetic material is diluted by the others' in the whole specimen. Methylation of the *MGMT* promoter is less frequent than in IDH mutant gliomas, comprising as much as 50% of all tumors.

A.5.2. Pediatric gliomas

Many pediatric gliomas are characterized by defining point mutations or gene fusion driver events, usually with otherwise stable genomes. The most common events are summarized in Table A.5.

A.5.2.1. PILOCYTIC ASTROCYTOMA

The *KIAA1549–BRAF* fusion gene is the most common genetic aberration in pilocytic astrocytomas and is diagnostic of this entity. Supratentorial tumors also frequently contain *KIAA1549–BRAF* but have a higher proportion of other nonspecific driver events, including mutations in *BRAF, KRAS, FGFR1, NF1* (germline), or other fusions involving *BRAF, NTRK* genes, or *FGFR1*. In addition, tumors in older children or adults may show one or more polysomies by copy number analysis.

Table A.5 Summary of Genomic Aberrations in Pediatric Gliomas

MARKER	ABERRATION	CLINICAL SIGNIFICANCE	DIAGNOSIS	METHOD OF DETECTION
H3F3A K27M	LOF mutations	Diagnostic, prognostic	Diffuse midline glioma	IHC, sequencing
H3F3A G34R/V	LOF mutations	Diagnostic, prognostic	Diffuse hemispheric glioma	Sequencing
BRAF V600E	GOF mutation	Diagnostic, predictor of targeted therapy	Ganglioglioma (50%), PXA (50%), PA (rare), DNET (20%–30%), DLGG, PLNTY. DIG/DIA	IHC, sequencing
KIAA1549-BRAF	BRAF rearrangements	Diagnostic, predictor of targeted therapy	PA, DLGNT	FISH, CMA, sequencing
FGFR1	Duplication, mutations	Diagnostic, predictor of targeted therapy	DLGG, DNET, RGNT	Sequencing
FGFR2	Rearrangements	Diagnostic	PLNTY	
MYB	Rearrangements, usually MYB-QKI fusion	Diagnostic	Angiocentric glioma (100%), DA-MYB/MYBL1 (25%)	FISH, CMA, sequencing
NF1	Deletions, LOF mutations	Diagnostic	PA (optic pathway)	FISH, CMA, sequencing
KRAS	GOF mutation	Diagnostic, predictor of targeted therapy	PA (supratentorial/adult)	Sequencing
MYBL1	Rearrangements	Diagnostic	DA-MYB/MYBL1	FISH, CMA, sequencing
PDGFRA K385I/L	GOF mutation	Diagnostic	Myxoid glioneuronal tumor	Sequencing
PRKCA	Rearrangements	Diagnostic	Papillary glioneuronal tumor	Sequencing

CMA, chromosomal microarray; DA-MYB/MYBL1, diffuse astrocytoma, MYB/MYBL1-altered; DIG/DIA, desmoplastic infantile ganglioglioma/astrocytoma; DLGG, diffuse low-grade glioma, MAPK pathway-altered; DLGNT, diffuse leptomeningeal glioneuronal tumor; DNET, dysembryoplastic neuroepithelial tumor; FISH, fluorescence in situ hybridization; GOF, gain of function; IHC, immunohistochemistry; LOF, loss of function; PA, pilocytic astrocytoma; PLNTY, polymorphous neuroepithelial tumor of the young; PXA, pleomorphic xanthoastrocytoma; RGNT, rosette-forming glioneuronal tumor.

A.5.2.2. ANGIOCENTRIC GLIOMA

Angiocentric gliomas universally contain rearrangements of the *MYB* locus, with *QKI* the most recurrent fusion partner. As a result, many of these tumors show overexpression of *MYB*, which may be detectable with IHC.

A.5.2.3. PEDIATRIC DIFFUSE GLIOMAS

A.5.2.3.1. Low-grade diffuse gliomas. Low-grade diffuse gliomas frequently show alterations in the MAPK signaling pathway, including *BRAF* V600E mutations, rearrangements of *MYBL1*, or alterations of *FGFR1*. High-grade tumors, by contrast, usually demonstrate different genetic events.

A.5.2.3.2. Pediatric high-grade gliomas. Pediatric high-grade gliomas may contain mutations in the H3.1/3 histone encoding genes (e.g., *H3-3A/B*). The K27M mutant in either of these genes is defining for diffuse midline gliomas, whereas H3 G34R/V occurs in diffuse hemispheric gliomas. Because mutations in *TP53* and *ATRX* often occur, care must be taken to exclude mutations in *IDH1* or *IDH2*. Similarly, amplifications of various RTKs or mutations in RTK/RAS/PI3K pathway components may be present, mimicking the profile of IDH wild-type adult glioblastoma in diffuse pediatric-type high-grade glioma, H3-wildtype and IDH-wildtype.

A.5.2.4. GLIONEURONAL TUMORS

Most glioneuronal tumors share overlapping driver mutation events, making molecular classification especially challenging. By far the most prevalent genetic alteration is the *BRAF* V600E mutation, which may accompany variably complex cytogenetic changes in pleomorphic xanthoastrocytoma and ganglioglioma. Duplication or activating mutations of *FGFR1* are also highly common and can be found in dysembryoplastic neuroepithelial tumor and rosette-forming glioneuronal tumor. Certain entities, such as myxoid glioneuronal tumor (PDGFRA K385I/L mutations) and papillary glioneuronal tumor (*SLC44A1–PRKCA* fusion), have characteristic alterations not yet described in other tumors.

A.5.3. Embryonal tumors

A.5.3.1. MEDULLOBLASTOMA

The current molecular classification scheme for medulloblastoma is summarized in Table A.6, with histologic patterns included for reference.

A.5.3.1.1. WNT-activated subgroup. The WNT-activated subgroup of tumors characteristically possess mutations in exon 3 of *CTNNB1*, and monosomy 6 is often the only detectable cytogenetic aberration. Furthermore, activation of the WNT pathway can be assessed indirectly by IHC against β-catenin, which should exhibit nuclear

Table A.6 Medulloblastoma Molecular Subgroups

	WNT ACTIVATED	SHH ACTIVATED		NON-WNT/NON-SHH	
		TP53-WT	TP53-MUT	GROUP 3	GROUP 4
Histologic pattern	Classic	Desmoplastic/ nodular	Large cell/ anaplastic	Classic, large cell/anaplastic	Classic, large cell/ anaplastic
Characteristic CNAs	Monosomy 6	PTCH1 deletion, 10q deletion	Amplification of MYCN, GLI2; 17p deletion	Isodicentric 17q, MYC amplification	Isodicentric 17q, MYCN amplification
Characteristic mutations and structural variants	CTNNB1, DDX3X, TP53	PTCH1, SMO, SUFU, TERT promoter	TP53	PVT1-MYC fusion, GFI1/ GFI1B structural variants	KDM6A mutations, GFI1/ GFI1B structural variants, SNCAIP duplication

CNAs, copy number alterations.

positivity, occasionally very focally. Unlike SHH-activated tumors, mutations in *TP53* carry no prognostic significance in this subgroup.

A.5.3.1.2. SHH-activated subgroup. The SHH-activated subgroup is defined by activation of the SHH pathway, usually in the form of loss-of-function mutations in *PTCH1*, although mutations in other pathway components such as *SMO* and *SUFU* may also be seen. Tumors with *TP53* mutations are more likely to possess amplifications of *MYCN* and *GLI2* rather than *PTCH1* mutations.

A.5.3.1.3. Non-WNT/non-SHH. Tumors not conforming to the WNT and SHH subgroups may be categorized into either group 3 or group 4 and usually show isodicentric 17q by copy number analysis.

Group 3 medulloblastomas are characterized by amplification of *MYC* on chromosome 8 when present, although this feature is mainly present in infants and represents fewer than 25% of group 3 tumors overall. *MYC–PVT1* fusion is another common finding in group 3 tumors, as are *GFI1* enhancer activation; *OTX2* amplifications; and mutations in *SMARCA4*, *CTDNEP1*, *LRP1B*, and *KMT2D*.

Group 4 medulloblastomas, by contrast, may show amplification of *MYCN* on chromosome 2, albeit in a minority of cases. More specific to the group is a tandem duplication of *SNCAIP* (synuclein, α-interacting protein), occurring in only approximately 10% of tumors. Relatively few other recurrent events are characteristic of group 4 medulloblastomas, except for mutations in *KDM6A*, which occur in approximately 13% of cases.

A.5.3.2. EMBRYONAL TUMOR WITH MULTILAYERED ROSETTES

The embryonal tumor with multilayer rosettes contains a defining amplification or rearrangement of the *C19MC* microRNA cluster on chromosome 19, which can be evaluated indirectly by IHC for LIN28A.

A.5.3.3. ATYPICAL TERATOID/RHABDOID TUMOR

Deficiency of *SMARCB1* (INI1) must be demonstrated to make the diagnosis of atypical teratoid/rhabdoid tumor (AT/RT). *SMARCB1* status can be easily assessed by IHC, which will show complete loss of staining in tumor cells. Inactivation of *SMARCA4* has been reported in very rare cases of AT/RT and can be similarly assessed by IHC (if available) or more advanced molecular techniques.

A.5.3.4. OTHER EMBRYONAL TUMORS

Embryonal neoplasms not fitting into the categories mentioned comprise a small subset of tumors often showing characteristic gene rearrangement events, such as CNS neuroblastoma, *FOXR2*-activated, and CNS tumor with *BCOR* internal tandem duplication. Clinically available sequencing panels frequently lack coverage of these key gene regions, necessitating methylation analysis for accurate classification.

A.5.4. Meningioma

Although meningiomas usually pose little diagnostic difficulty, their well-characterized genetic features make ancillary molecular testing especially helpful in certain settings. Many copy number alterations correlate strongly with tumor grade, and several morphologic subtypes of meningioma possess unique mutational signatures (Table A.7).

A.5.5. Ependymoma

Ependymomas may be subclassified molecularly, largely based on their anatomic site of origin (Table A.8). Within the supratentorial compartment, ependymomas usually demonstrate the highly recurrent fusion events involving *ZFTA* (70%) or *YAP1* (10%). *ZFTA*-fused ependymomas are usually associated with chromothripsis of chromosome 11, which may be used as a surrogate marker if FISH probes or sequencing assays are not available. Multiple other copy number changes are usually also present, although outside of 9p losses, none is significantly recurrent. IHC for L1CAM is typically positive in these tumors; however, this marker may be positive in other glial neoplasms. *YAP1*-fused ependymomas rarely show additional cytogenetic aberrations.

Posterior fossa ependymomas have traditionally been split into group A and group B tumors. Group A typically exhibits few, if any, cytogenetic changes, whereas group B usually possesses numerous whole-chromosome gains and losses, with monosomy 6 the most common.

Table A.7 Summary of Genomic Aberrations in Meningiomas

MARKER	ABERRATION	CLINICAL SIGNIFICANCE	DIAGNOSIS	METHOD OF DETECTION
NF2	Deletions, LOF mutation	Diagnostic	Transitional or fibrous meningioma	FISH, CMA, sequencing
AKT1	E17K mutation	Diagnostic, therapeutic target	Anterior skull base, meningothelial meningioma	Sequencing
SMO	Mutations	Diagnostic, therapeutic target	Anterior skull base, meningothelial meningioma	Sequencing
KLF4	K409Q mutation	Diagnostic	Secretory meningioma	Sequencing
TRAF7	Mutations	Diagnostic	Secretory meningioma	Sequencing
1p, 6q, 10, 14q, or 18q loss; 1q gain	Deletions, gains	Prognostic	Atypical meningioma	FISH, CMA
Multiple polysomies	Single-copy gains	Diagnostic	Angiomatous meningioma	FISH, CMA, sequencing
CDKN2A	Deletions, LOF mutation	Prognostic	Anaplastic meningioma	FISH, CMA, sequencing
BAP1	Deletions, LOF mutation	Prognostic	Rhabdoid meningioma	IHC, FISH, CMA, sequencing
SMARCE1	Deletions, LOF mutation	Diagnostic	Clear cell meningioma	IHC, FISH, CMA, sequencing
TERT	Promoter mutations	Prognostic	Grade 2–3 meningiomas	Sequencing

CMA, chromosomal microarray; FISH, fluorescence in situ hybridization; IHC, immunohistochemistry; LOF, loss of function.

Similar to group B ependymomas of the posterior fossa, spinal ependymomas are characterized by extensive aneuploidy. Myxopapillary ependymomas usually show only whole-chromosome gains, whereas classic ependymomas exhibit a mixture of chromosome gains and losses, with the most common being 22q. An aggressive subset of spinal ependymomas show amplification of *MYCN*.

The subependymoma generally shows stable genomes regardless of location but may occasionally demonstrate partial or complete loss of chromosome 6.

A.5.6. Methylation profiling

Epigenetic analysis has proven highly powerful when used in concert with machine learning algorithms to classify a wide array of tumors with great accuracy. The fifth edition of the World Health Organization Classification of Tumors of the Central Nervous System (2021) permits inclusion of DNA methylation classifier results as desirable or essential criteria for many tumor types, especially in instances when centers lack access to DNA/RNA-based assays necessary to demonstrate diagnostic alterations.

A.6. BRAIN BANK

Tissue samples from biopsies and autopsies are collected in tissue banks for research purposes. Brain tissue may be collected specifically in brain banks. Some samples (e.g., from tumors) are also kept for diagnostic purposes because new molecular tools are developing at an accelerating pace.

The samples must be neuropathologically documented and clinically and, as far as possible, genetically annotated. Neuroimaging and biomarkers (blood and CSF) data must be integrated. To allow the collection of many samples necessary for scientific investigation, collaboration with multiple centers is required. The diagnostic criteria must

Table A.8 Ependymoma Molecular Subgroups by Anatomic Location

	SE	SUPRATENTORIAL		INFRATENTORIAL		SPINAL		
		ZFTA FUSED	YAP1 FUSED	GROUP A	GROUP B	MPE	CLASSIC EPENDYMOMA	MYCN AMPLIFIED
WHO grade	1	2/3	2/3	2/3	2/3	2	2/3	2/3
Characteristic CNAs	6q loss	Chromothripsis 11	–	1q (poor prognosis)	Multiple polysomies and monosomies	Multiple polysomies	Multiple polysomies and monosomies	MYCN amplification
Characteristic structural variants	–	ZFTA–RELA fusion	YAP1–MAMLD1 fusion	–	–		–	–

CNA, copy number alteration; MPE, myxopapillary ependymoma; SE, subependymoma.

therefore be reliable with high interrater agreement. The quality control of the samples, biopsies, and postmortem tissues must be ensured. The collection of control cases often appears difficult, and the definition of normal and pathological material may raise problems.

Legal and ethical restrictions vary from country to country, but informed consent from the patient or next of kin is generally required before any investigational use of the samples begins.

The ideal utilization of large collections of neuropathological data and of clinical and molecular records requires powerful computer databases. Most tissue banks have adopted a thematic approach, bringing together experts in a specific field of research, sometimes with the help of patient advocacy associations.

A.7. ARTIFACTS

Neural tissue is subject to a wide range of artifacts. These may be the result of agonal changes (i.e., terminal circulatory and hypoxic disturbances); the conditions of removal and fixation; or problems related to embedding, sectioning, and staining procedures.

A.7.1. Macroscopic artifacts

Large bullous cavities with sharp edges ("Swiss-cheese artifact"), visible to the naked eye, are the result of postmortem putrefaction in the setting of overgrowth of gas-forming organisms consequent to inadequate or delayed fixation.

Inadequate fixation is likewise responsible for the pinkish appearance (pink spots) and soft consistency of the white matter (formalin solution of insufficient concentration). Conversely, fixation that is either excessive (because of a formalin solution of excessive concentration) or unduly prolonged may be responsible for a yellowish, parchment-like appearance of the cortex. Under these circumstances, the application of most histological techniques is difficult or impossible.

Congestion with vascular dilation is most frequently the result of terminal asphyxial disturbances. The so-called respiratory brain is a swollen and soft organ that cannot be fixed properly or studied histologically in a meaningful manner.

A.7.2. Microscopic artifacts

Many of the artifacts encountered in histologic preparation of any organ may also be seen in microscopic neuropathology. Some, however, are specific to brain tissue.

Multiple microscopic, elongated cavities, often predominating in the cortex, are sometimes seen as the result of improper freezing of tissue.

Nerve cell retraction, with clear pericellular spaces, is very frequently seen in PETs and is related to the temperature to which the paraffin has been heated. The same applies to the apparent dilation of the perivascular spaces, which needs to be differentiated from possible edema.

Dark neurons result from neuronal retraction with nuclear shrinkage and basophilia. These abnormal neurons are frequently found in material removed by cerebral biopsy and related to poking at the tissue at the time of removal or to immersion fixation.

Pale, ballooned *neurons* may be caused by excessive washing of the nervous tissue fragments with water before fixation. An artifact consisting of cellular pallor with blurring of the nuclear outlines of the neurons in the cerebellar granular layer ("état glacé" or "conglutination artifact") is the result of a postmortem autolytic change, particularly when the body has not been refrigerated properly. It is seen more often in lateral lobes.

Index

For the benefit of digital users, indexed terms that span two pages (e.g., 52–53) may, on occasion, appear on only one of those pages.

Note: Index terms are listed in their full form, followed by acronyms in parentheses, except for antigens, genes, proteins, and markers.

Tables, figures, and boxes are indicated by an italic *t*, *f*, and *b* following the page number.